Drugs and Human Lactation

Second Edition

Drugs and Human Lactation

Second Edition

A comprehensive guide to the content and consequences of drugs, micronutrients, radiopharmaceuticals and environmental and occupational chemicals in human milk

Editor:

Peter N. Bennett

Co-authors:

Allan Astrup-Jensen
Christopher J. Bates
Evan J. Begg
Susan Edwards
Colin R. Lazarus
Ingrid Matheson
Peter J. Mountford
Margaret C. Neville
Lidia J. Notarianni
Ann Prentice
Anders Rane
Dietrich Reinhardt
Carol T. Walsh

1996
ELSEVIER
Amsterdam – Lausanne – New York – Oxford – Shannon – Tokyo

ISBN 0 444 81981-9

Library of Congress Cataloging-in-Publication Data

Drugs and human lactation : a comprehensive guide to the content and
consequences of drugs, micronutrients, radiopharmaceuticals, and
environmental and occupational chemicals in human milk / editor,
Peter N. Bennett ; co-authors, Allan Astrup-Jensen ... [et al.]. --
2nd ed.
p. cm.
Includes bibliographical references and index.
ISBN 0-444-81981-9 (alk. paper)
1. Breast feeding--Health aspects. 2. Breast milk--Contamination.
3. Infants (Newborn)--Effect of drugs on. I. Bennett, P. N.
[DNLM: 1. Lactation--drug effects. 2. Milk, Human--drug effects.
WP 825 D7936 1996]
RJ216.D69 1996
613.2'69--dc21
DNLM/DLC 96-38943
for Library of Congress CIP

Printed in The Netherlands on acid-free paper

List of contributors

PETER N. BENNETT, M.D., F.R.C.P.
School of Postgraduate Medicine
University of Bath
Wolfson Centre
Royal United Hospital
Combe Park
Bath BA1 3NG
United Kingdom

ALLAN ASTRUP-JENSEN, Ph.D.
DK-Teknik Energy & Environment
15 Gladsaxe Møllevej
DK-2860 Søborg
Denmark

CHRISTOPHER J. BATES, M.A., D.Phil.
MRC Dunn Nutrition Unit
Downham's Lane
Milton Road
Cambridge
CB4 1KJ
United Kingdom

EVAN J. BEGG, M.B.Ch.B,F.R.A.C.P.
Clinical Pharmacology
Christchurch Hospital
Private Bag 4710
Christchurch
New Zealand

SUSAN EDWARDS, B.Sc.
Women, Children and Families
Directorate
Essex County Hospital
Lexden Road
Colchester CO3 3NB
United Kingdom

COLIN LAZARUS, Ph.D.
Department of Nuclear Medicine
Guy's Hospital
St. Thomas Street
London SE1 9RT
United Kingdom

INGRID MATHESON, Ph.D.
Department of Pharmacotherapeutics
University of Oslo
Postboks 1065 Blindern
0316 Oslo
Norway

PETER J. MOUNTFORD, Ph.D.
Department of Biomedical
Engineering and Medical Physics
North Staffordshire Hospital
Princes Road
Hartshill
Stoke on Trent ST4 7LN
United Kingdom

MARGARET C. NEVILLE, Ph.D.
Department of Physiology
University of Colorado Health
Sciences Center
Denver, CO 80262
USA

LIDIA J. NOTARIANNI, M.Sc.,Ph.D.
School of Pharmacy and
Pharmacology
University of Bath
Claverton Down
Bath BA2 7AY
United Kingdom

ANN PRENTICE, D.Phil.
MRC Dunn Nutrition Unit
Downham's Lane
Milton Road
Cambridge CB4 1KJ
United Kingdom

DIETRICH REINHARDT, M.D.
Kinderpoliklinik
Universität München
Pettenkoferstrasse 8a
80336 München 2
Germany

ANDERS RANE, M.D., Ph.D.
Department of Clinical Pharmacology
University Hospital
S-751 85 Uppsala
Sweden

CAROL WALSH, Ph.D.
Department of Pharmacology
Boston University School of Medicine
80 E. Concord Street
Boston, MA 02118-2394
USA

Preface

In 1985 the European Office of the World Health Organization called together a group of experts with the remit of evaluating and rationalising the rather confused literature on the dangers, real and perceived, of substances in human milk. Over the next two years the WHO Group met in Copenhagen, Bath, Oslo and, memorably, amid the pine and birch trees of a more remote part of Norway, and developed principles for assessing reports and allocating levels of risk for breast-feeding mothers. These principles and their application to the current literature on drugs, radiopharmaceuticals, micronutrients and pollutants comprised the first edition of this book, which appeared in 1988.

It is a pleasure to record the contribution of the European Office of WHO and in particular Graham Dukes in overseeing the original project. In addition, the first edition owed a great deal to the input of Chris van Boxtel, Elisabet Helsing, Per-Knut Lunde, Michael Orme, John Philip, Hans Seyberth, Paivi Soderman and John Wilson; although they are not participating in the new edition, their part in the development of the methodology for the book and its application to individual substances is gratefully acknowledged.

This second edition welcomes the contributions of Evan Begg, Peter Mountford, Margaret Neville and Carol Walsh. New material has been analysed according to the methods established for the first edition, bringing the various subject-areas up to date. The book remains what its sub-title claims: a comprehensive guide to the content and consequences of substances in milk. We hope it will continue to provide a rational basis for making therapeutic decisions in women who seek to breast-feed.

Peter N. Bennett

Contents

Drugs and Human Lactation
P.N. Bennett, editor

1. Is breast best? Milk and formula feeds

Lidia J Notarianni

SUMMARY

Breast-feeding has important clinical, economic and sociological consequences. Nursing mothers benefit from drug therapy, as we all do. But when bottle-feeding supplants breast-feeding purely from lack of knowledge of whether a drug will reach the infant in sufficient quantities to cause harm, a mother may unnecessarily deny her child important benefits; these are outlined in this chapter.

INTRODUCTION

Preparation for breast-feeding begins soon after conception. Changes in breast size and the colour of the areola are often the first physical indications of pregnancy noticed by the expectant mother. During gestation some of the energy that will be required for milk production in the first few weeks is stored in the form of fat, typically 2–4 kg. Milk production usually commences within 48 h of birth, although it may precede parturition. Lactating women have been shown to have an increased metabolic efficiency which reduces the overall increase in energy required in milk production (1). Food intake required to maintain milk production is considered to be less than the minimum 500 kcal (2100 kJ) that has previously been recommended (2).

Breast milk is the only nourishment an infant needs for the first 4 months of life, with the possible exceptions of vitamins D and K. Its composition changes from the initial high protein, low fat content of colostrum to that of mature milk in a matter of 2–3 weeks to suit the requirements of the infant. Milk flow is essentially a demand and supply system controlled by the amount of infant suckling; the greater the suckling the more milk is produced. As well as adapting to the needs of the growing child this system allows the successful nursing of twins. Breast-feeding can continue well into the second year of life although supplementation with other foods is necessary from 4–6 months.

USE OF FORMULA FEEDS

Although breast-feeding is associated with a wide range of sociological and health benefits, formula milks have been used throughout this century. The use of diluted cows' milk, and from 1904 'roller-dried' cow milk powder, became popular for reasons of convenience or, as women entered the work force, of necessity. Following the Second World War aggressive marketing techniques associated their use with modern affluent societies and large healthy babies. Formula milks were promoted world-wide and propagated through local health care systems, particularly maternity and baby clinics giving them respectability and the status of medicines. New mothers were frequently given free samples. Early use of these formulae, possibly on a trial basis with the sample packs, could lead to incomplete establishment of lactation and hence 'no turning back' for the mother.

From the 1950s through to the late 1970s, formula milks became widely used not only in the Western world but also in less developed countries where contaminated water supplies, lack of storage facilities and poor hygiene made their use inappropriate. Poverty and high levels of illiteracy meant that the feeds were often not made up correctly. The net result was that in the developing countries, infant mortality, directly related to the use of breast milk substitutes, increased significantly (4, 5).

The issue of the use of these milk formulae in the poorer countries began to receive international attention in the mid-1970s and led in 1981 to the adoption of a resolution by the World Health Assembly recommending member states to implement a World Health Organization (WHO) code of practice for marketing breast milk substitutes (3). The substance of this code was to (a) restrict advertising of

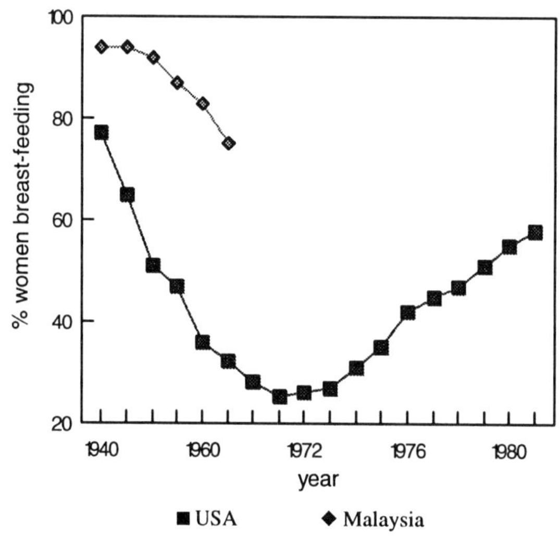

FIG. 1 *Breast-feeding trends in the USA (1936–1980) (68–72) and Malaysia (1936–1965) (63).*

breast milk substitutes directly to the public; (b) prevent personnel paid by manufacturers or distributors of these products from 'educating' mothers via the health care system; (c) stop the distribution of samples to new mothers; (d) eliminate financial inducements to health professionals to promote commercial products; (e) require formula products to contain the necessary information about the appropriate use of the product and the superiority of breast milk; and (f) promote breast-feeding through adequate information and education.

In developing countries a decrease in neonatal mortality and morbidity in breast-fed as opposed to formula-fed infants was demonstrated following the adoption of the WHO code of practice (4, 5). In many Western cultures in the 1970s, breast-feeding rates were slowly increasing for other reasons. Groups were formed to promote and advise on lactational problems as breast-feeding was perceived to be healthier for the child and important in the establishment of the mother–infant bond. The incidence of breast-feeding has subsequently increased in all parts of the globe (Fig. 1, Table 1).

TABLE 1 *Breast-feeding statistics in relation to infant age*

Country	Year	Duration of feeding	% Breast-feeding	Source[a]
Austria	1980	1 week	83.7	a
Austria	1980	3 months	41.2	a
Austria	1980	6 months	17.0	a
Denmark	1988	1 week	99.5	a
Denmark	1988	6 months	71.0	a
Denmark	1988	9 months	33.0	a
Gambia	1989	6 months	99.5	a
Gambia	1989	7–12 months	98.4	a
Gambia	1989	18–27 months	63.9	a
Iceland	1983	2 months	53.0	a
Iceland	1983	4 months	46.0	a
Iceland	1983	6 months	18.0	a
Mexico	1979	1 months	76.8	b
Mexico	1979	6 months	52.4	b
Mexico	1979	15 months	29.0	b
Norway	1993	3 months	84.0	a
Norway	1993	6 months	65.0	a
Norway	1993	9 months	40.0	a
Sweden	1992	1 week	97.0	a
Sweden	1992	3 months	78.0	a
Sweden	1992	9 months	58.0	a
Thailand	1978	1 month	69.0	b
Thailand	1978	2 months	16.0	b
Thailand	1978	6 months	2.0	b
USSR	1984	3 months	76.0	a

[a]Includes mixed infant feeding.
[b]Source a, personal communication from appropriate Ministry of Health or similar authority or data submitted to WHO by member states (67). Source b, from reference (66).

INCIDENCE OF BREAST-FEEDING

Almost all mothers have the capacity to breast-feed (6). Even in times of drought, famine and stress such as captivity or ritual fasting such as Ramadan (although nursing mothers are exempt they often participate), this capacity remains (7). Norwegian statistics show that from 1860 until about 1950 some 75% of mothers breast-fed their infants at 3 months; there was then a sharp decline to 25% participation, followed by a return to the previous level by the 1980s (73). Records on the percentage of mothers suckling their infants from the late 1930s reported 77% of mothers in the USA choosing this method to feed their infants. From the 1940s until the beginning of the 1970s there was a significant downward trend in breast-feeding as the promotion and variety of available formula feeds gathered momentum. In 1972 it was estimated that less than 25% mothers in the USA breast-fed their infants (Fig. 1), not necessary for health or social reasons but rather because the practice was seen as old fashioned. Knowledge that the developed world had apparently abandoned breast-feeding, combined with the promotion of formulae, led to women in less developed nations following their example.

The downward trend in breast-feeding did no harm to infants born to mothers of high socio-economic groups so far as could be established from infant mortality figures, although the incidence of some conditions (allergies, gastrointestinal, respiratory) did appear to be greater in bottle-fed children. The effect of the use of formula feeds in lower socio-economic groups and poorer nations, however, was extremely serious. Rates of infant mortality and serious disease increased with the decline in breast-feeding as did the incidence of post-partum conception due to the loss of the contraceptive effect of lactation. Part of the neonatal mortality was attributed directly to the use of contaminated water or incorrect preparation of the feed leading to dehydration or malnutrition.

As well as the decline in the numbers of infants that were breast-fed, those who were nursed were often suckled for a significantly shorter period and/or mixed feeding (breast and bottle) was practised. These infants may not have derived the full benefit of breast-feeding. Because of these trends, statistics on the number of breast-fed infants are frequently difficult to interpret. Should an infant count as being breast-fed only if s/he were fed exclusively for a minimum period (e.g. 3 months) or did a shorter period qualify? Did mixed feeding qualify as breast-feeding? Any statistics on the percentage of women breast-feeding should clearly define duration and exclusivity. Variation in the criteria applied may yield very different conclusions.

The decline in the number of breast-fed infants rapidly became a cause for concern for various influential groups including health professionals, child psychologists and government agencies. In less developed nations and lower socio-economic groups in richer nations, the return to breast-feeding became appreciated as the safest, most economical way to promote infant health. Consequently, from the early 1970s there was a conscious attempt to educate, encourage and promote breast-feeding. Surveys were performed to discover why and when women stopped feeding their children and the WHO code of practice was introduced to many countries. The success of this campaign can be judged by the steady increase in the numbers of breast-fed infants in Europe and America while the decline in the developing nations was halted.

Currently the incidence of breast-feeding varies greatly between countries; motivation, necessity, and the socio-economic group of the mother all contribute. In less developed countries, the percentage of women breast-feeding at 3 months is generally over 75% (Table 1). In developed countries, Scandinavia has the highest number of breast-fed infants and also the longest duration of breast-feeding; in 1980 only 2.5% of Norwegian mothers did not breast-feed on discharge from hospital in contrast to 67% in Belfast (8, 9). The numbers of Scottish mothers breast-feeding at 7 days in 1990–1991 varied between 21.1% and 59.1% in different parts of the country (10). In the United Kingdom as a whole in 1985–86, 65% of mothers breast-fed at birth and 22% at 6 months; these figures represented no alteration from the position 5 years before and may herald another decline (11). In the United States the number of women who breast-feed is estimated at 61.4% although marked racial differences exist; 64% of white infants are breast-fed but only 32% of black infants (12). Variation between and within countries of similar social structure may be influenced by the degree of promotion of breast-feeding and support available, and the length and flexibility of maternity leave for working mothers. Additionally, the proportion appears to relate to social group, being 87% for social class 1 (professional) against 43% for class 5 (unskilled) (11). These figures should be taken into account when comparing the merits of different forms of feeding. It is now believed that to increase the number of women nursing their infants in areas and groups where the numbers are low and experience limited, a 'warm chain of breast-feeding' is required, i.e. an investment in education and practical help from experienced health professionals on a one-to-one basis (13).

BENEFITS OF BREAST-FEEDING

The benefits of breast-feeding are varied and range from sociological benefits through to improved health for the young infant and eventually the grown person. Some are pertinent to all socio-economic groups whilst others relate largely to less developed nations. A summary of reported advantages of this form of infant feeding appears below:

Clinical benefits

Breast-feeding exclusively for a minimum period of time is now believed to give protection from various conditions, some of which may not appear until middle age.

Allergies

The incidence in children of IgE-associated disorders such as eczema, asthma and allergic rhinitis is increasing (14, 15). Childhood eczema often precedes the onset of asthma which may persist into adulthood. As far back as 1936 Grulee and Sanford (16) reported a sevenfold increase in the incidence of eczema in babies fed cow's milk. Avoiding early exposure to cow's milk as well as to egg, wheat and beef in the diet could reduce the incidence of eczema and asthma in childhood (17, 18) although other studies have found no difference (19, 20) or a delayed onset of eczema in breast-fed infants (21). Other environmental factors such as exposure to cigarette smoke and chemicals, house-dust mite, housing and social conditions are considered to be more potent than food components in promoting allergies (22, 23). It is now generally believed that breast-feeding diminishes the incidence of diet-related hypersensitivity disorders because of its relatively low allergen nature, although breast milk may for some infants still contain sufficient maternally ingested dietary (dairy based) antigens to promote hypersensitivity reactions. Goat's milk and soya-based preparations however, are generally believed to have a low allergenic nature and may be used in the absence of breast-feeding where infants cannot tolerate cow's milk.

Insulin-dependent diabetes mellitus (IDDM)

Both genetic and environmental components contribute to the aetiology of IDDM. Susceptibility to IDDM is highly correlated with specific genes (24) but its development may be precipitated by some factor in the infant diet. Various studies have indicated that infants breast-fed for >3 months have a lower risk of IDDM than those breast-fed for shorter periods (25, 26) although this view is challenged (27, 28); other environmental factors may also precipitate the condition. Bovine milk proteins have been reported as being the trigger initiating antibody production and the initiating of an autoimmune response resulting in IDDM (29, 30). Early cow's milk exposure has been reported to increase the risk of Type I diabetes by approximately 1.5 in susceptible individuals (31).

Cardiovascular disease

Prolonged breast-feeding (>1 year) has been associated with increased low density lipoprotein cholesterol and higher death rates from ischaemic heart disease in adult life (32), although other studies have been inconclusive (33). Breast-feeding elevates plasma cholesterol which is maintained until weaning (34), throughout childhood (35) or even throughout adult life (32). Additionally the HDL/LDL cholesterol ratio is higher in formula-fed than in breast-fed infants at 2 and 6 months of age (36). A possible explanation for this observation is that the infant absorbs thyroid hormones from breast milk and, through hormonal imprinting, the point of thyroid homeostasis is permanently set at a higher level (37).

Neurological status
Children who were breast-fed for a minimum of 3 weeks after birth appeared to have a small but significantly improved neurological status 9 years later compared to children who had been formula-fed (38). Breast milk contains longer-chain polyunsaturated fatty acids which are absent from formula milk and it has been proposed that these are essential for brain development. Other studies suggest that the method of feeding has a long-term effect on cognitive development (39,40)

Weight
Breast-fed infants are reported to weigh less at 3 and 12 months compared to weaned infants although body length is not different. Statistical data on weight and body length suggest that bottle-fed infants are overweight rather than that breast-fed infants are underweight (34). The difference in weight rapidly disappears after weaning.

Immunity
Maternal antibodies, immunoglobulins and other protective agents are transferred to the infant in milk. Agents such as secretory IgA, lactoferrin, interleukin-6, memory T-cells, PAF-acetylhydrolase, lysozyme and antibodies are not produced until some months after birth (41), and their passage to the infant in breast milk complements the agents transferred while in utero.

Sudden infant death syndrome(SIDS)
Over the past 25 years 11 studies have reported an increased incidence of SIDS in bottle-fed infants while another 7 found no effect. A recent study (42) found full bottle-feeding not to be a significant independent risk factor for SIDS but that bottle-fed babies are more likely to have mothers who smoke, to be born preterm and to come from poorer families. The issue of risk from bottle-feeding appears to remain unresolved.

Sociological benefits

These may be summarised as follows: (a) rapid establishment of infant-mother bond is believed to be invoked whilst breast-feeding; (b) demand feeding is more practical and successful when breast-feeding; (c) the infant obtains the right nutritional balance since milk composition changes both with time and on a circadian rhythm; (d) intelligence quotient at 8 years of age is reported to be increased by eight points in children who breast-fed as infants, particularly premature infants (43), although this finding is in contention with results attributed to other social factors (44, 45). An increased rate in learning disorders has been reported among formula fed infants which may relate to minor neurological dysfunction in these children (46).

Additional benefits pertinent to less developed nations and poorer communities

(a) Breast-feeding is convenient and low cost, and avoids problems of contamination of feed with polluted water and inadequate sterilisation facilities. Additionally, breast-feeding negates problems that may be associated with the making up of a feed to the correct strength. (b) Onset of ovulation is delayed thereby allowing children to be 'spaced' when other forms of contraception are not available, particularly when demand feeding is practised. (c) Breast-feeding protects against environmental infections especially in the gastrointestinal and respiratory tracts. Mortality and morbidity rates are higher among bottle-fed infants living in unfavourable and/or disadvantaged conditions. Specific reports, for example, have shown protective effects of breast milk against *Campylobacter jejuni* diarrhoea (milk contains IgA antibodies which neutralise bacterial surface antigens) (47) and *Escherichia coli* and salmonella infections (48). In countries with a moderate or high infant mortality rate, babies fed on formula milk are at least 14 times more likely to die from diarrhoea than are breast-fed children, and 4 times more likely to die of pneumonia. Even in countries where infant mortality is low, formula fed infants require hospital treatment up to 5 times more often than those who are fully or partly breast-fed (49).

WHEN BREAST-FEEDING MAY NOT NECESSARILY BE BEST

The composition of formula milk has changed greatly over the years. Prior to the second world war the commonest infant 'formula' was diluted cows' milk to which sugar was added. Available dried formulae were also derived from cows' milk by the addition of fat and carbohydrate, the product being diluted to resemble breast milk in its major components. Dietary supplements such as vitamin D and iron were introduced into formulae although the amount of vitamin D was reduced after 1957 (50). In 1972 attention was drawn to the high incidence of babies with gastro-enteritis and dehydration caused by over-concentrated feeds and the high concentrations of protein and electrolytes in the formulae (51). The UK Department of Health and Social Security (DHSS) consequently commissioned a study to examine all aspects of infant nutrition (52). This found that all the fat in formula milks was butterfat, and manufacturers were directed to change within 2 years the fat content to short chain fatty acids. Further research into the composition of human milk prompted a radical alteration of formula milks after 1977. The lipid component became 90–100% vegetable fat, mainly short chain fatty acids, and the content of protein, electrolytes, water-soluble and trace elements was reduced (53). These alterations in the composition of formula milks after 1974 may diminish perceived risks of disorders such as atherosclerosis associated with the use of the earlier formulations (32). Thus the new generation formula feeds do not necessarily disadvantage infants when circumstances dictate that breast-feeding may not confer advantage or may actually be is inadvisable. Some of these are considered below.

Premature infants

The milk of women delivering prematurely differs from that of mature milk in its energy, protein and sodium content (all greater) and its carbohydrate content (lower). Feeding donated human milk to a very low birth-weight infant may lead to insufficient intakes of protein and energy, since available human milk is likely to be mature rather than colostrum. Premature infants fed milk from mothers delivering prematurely grow significantly better than those fed mature breast milk (55). In such circumstances mature milk may be supplemented with protein, fat and carbohydrate derived from human or cow's milk to improve its nutritional content (56, 57). Mature milk may also contain insufficient vitamin D for such infants (58).

Infectious disease

Human immunodeficiency virus (HIV) can be transmitted in breast milk (59, 60) but the risk of transmission has been difficult to separate from other risk factors such as prior transmission of the virus to the infant in utero. Evidence suggests a 14% additional risk of transmission of HIV by breast-feeding (60, 61).

Contamination of milk

Breast milk may suffer contamination with insecticides, pesticides and other environmental chemicals including heavy metals (see Chapter 00). As exposure to these substances also occurs in utero, there is difficult in establishing the extent to which contamination occurs prenatally or during lactation. Advice issued in Canada encourages women to breast-feed despite the presence of pollutants in milk (54).

Drug utilisation during lactation

Women use a variety of drugs, both prescribed and over-the-counter, in the early stages of lactation. In surveys 90% (9), 99% (8), and 95% (62) of women were taking at least one form of medication in the week after delivery. The number of agents taken in this period reached a maximum of 7 (mean 2.1). Reports from Canada (62), Norway (9), England (63) and Northern Ireland (8, 64) find that the drugs most commonly prescribed are analgesics, laxatives, vitamins, antimicrobials, anti-emetics, sedatives and hypnotics. Table 2 indicates the percentages of hospitalised women using some of these agents in the immediate post-partum period. After discharge from hospital drug utilisation declines although some 17% of mothers

TABLE 2 *Drug utilisation by mothers in maternity wards in Norway (9) and Northern Ireland (8)*

	Norway[a] (n = 970)	N. Ireland[b] (n = 2004)
Drug class		
Analgesic	82	78
Hypnotic	85	36
Antimicrobial (systemic)	4	14
Specific drug		
Codeine	54	41
Dextropropoxyphene	25	1
Nitrazepam	60	17
Ergometrine	15	1
Diazepam	4	2
Mean number of drugs	2.1	3.6

[a]98% mothers breast-feeding.
[b]33% mothers breast-feeding.

breast-feeding at 4 months take at least one drug per day. Some 5% of mothers who continued to breast-feed were receiving regular medication for asthma, allergy, hypertension, arthritis, diabetes, epilepsy or migraine (65).

For many years the drugs commonly administered during lactation were either assumed to be safe or to present hazard to the suckling infant without being subjected to a rational process of analysis. Table 3 shows that warnings are given more often about drugs use during pregnancy and childhood than during lactation. Consciousness of possible unwanted effects of drugs transmitted in milk appears to be increasing as caveats or proscriptions on drugs for nursing women listed in the UK Monthly Index of Medical Specialities (MIMS) rose from 22% in January 1985 to 32% in 1994.

It is common practice carefully to assess the case for any drug that is administered to a pregnant woman. Since most drugs will find their way into milk to some extent there is an equal case to make a rational assessment of risk to the infant before prescribing medication to a nursing mother. While the quantities of drug transferred may be small in absolute terms, new-born infants have a low capacity to metabolise and excrete these foreign substances. Now that breast-feeding is again

TABLE 3 *Warnings on the use of medicines*

Users	Contraindicated (%)	Special precautions (%)
Children	35.3 (39)	–
Pregnant women	18.0 (15)	27.6 (22)
Nursing mothers	14.8 (4)	17.3 (18)

Data from MIMS, July 1994. Figures in parentheses refer to MIMS, January 1985.

popular, it is especially important to attempt a rational evaluation of the medicines that may be taken with safety during lactation both to avoid harm to the child and permit the mother to breast-feed with confidence.

REFERENCES

1. Illingworth PJ, Jung RT, Howie PW, Leslie P, Isles TE (1986) Diminution in energy expenditure during lactation. *Br. Med. J., 292*, 437–441.
2. National Research Council (1980) *Recommended Dietary Allowances, 9th edn.* National Academy of Sciences, Washington DC.
3. WHO (1981) *International Code of Marketing of Breast Milk Substitutes.* WHO, Geneva.
4. Lepage P, Munyakazi C, Hennart P (1981) Breastfeeding and hospital mortality in children in Rwanda. *Lancet, 2*, 409–411.
5. Clavano NR (1982) Mode of feeding and its effect on infant mortality and morbidity. *J. Trop. Pediatr., 28*, 287–293.
6. Applebaum RM (1975) The obstetrician's approach to the breasts and breast-feeding. *J. Reprod. Med., 14*, 98.
7. Prentice AM, Lamb WH, Prentice A, Coward WA (1984) The effect of water abstention on milk synthesis in lactating women. *Clin. Sci., 66*, 291–298.
8. Passmore CM, McElnay J, D'Arcy P (1984) Drugs taken by mothers in the puerperium: inpatient survey in Northern Ireland. *Br. Med. J., 289*, 1593–1596.
9. Matheson I (1985) Drugs taken by mothers in the puerperium. *Br. Med. J.*, 290, 1588–1589.
10. Ferusin AE, Tappin DM, Girdwood RW, Kennedy R, Cockburn F (1994) Breast feeding in Scotland. *Br. Med. J., 308*, 824–825.
11. Department of Health and Social Security (1988) *Present Day Practice in Infant Feeding: Third Report.* HMSO, London.
12. Office of Disease Prevention and Health Promotion (1988) Disease Prevention/Health Promotion – *The Facts.* US Dept. Health and Human Services, Bethesda, MD.
13. Editorial (1994) A warm chain for breastfeeding. *Lancet, 344*, 1239–1241.
14. Burr ML, Butland BH, Kings S, Vaughan-Williams E (1989). Changes in asthma prevalence: two studies (fifteen years apart). *Arch Dis Child, 64*, 1452–1456.
15. Mitchell EA (1986). Increasing prevalence of asthma in children. *N.Z. Med. J., 96*, 463–464.
16. Grulee CG, Stanford HN (1936) The influence of breast and artificial feeding on infantile eczema. *J. Pediatr., 9*, 223–225.
17. Hill DJ, Hosking CS (1993) Preventing childhood allergy. *Med. J. Aust., 158*, 367–369.
18. Matthew D, Taylor B, Norman A, Turner M, Soothill J (1977) Prevention of eczema. *Lancet, i*, 321–324.
19. Hide DW, Guyer BM. (1981) Clinical manifestations of allergy related to breast and cows' milk feeding. *Arch. Dis. Child., 56*, 172–175.
20. Kramer MS, Moroz B (1981) Do breast feeding and delayed introduction of solid foods protect against subsequent atopic eczema. *J. Pediatr., 98*, 546–550.
21. Halpern SR, Sellars WA, Johnson RB, Anderson DW, Saperstein S, Reisch JS (1973) Development of childhood allergy in infants fed breast milk, soy or cow's milk. *J. Allergy Clin. Immunol., 51*, 139–151.
22. Arshad SH, Hide DW (1992) Effect of environmental factors on the development of allergic disorders in infancy. *J. Allergy Clin. Immunol., 90*, 235–241.
23. Kershaw CR (1987) Passive smoking, potential atopy and asthma in the first five years. *J. R. Soc. Med., 80*, 683–688.

24. Dosch H-M (1993). The possible link between insulin dependent (juvenile) diabetes mellitus and dietary cow milk. *Clin. Biochem., 26*, 307–308.
25. Kostraba JN, Cruickshanks J, Lawler-Heavner J, Jobim LF, Rewers MJ, Gay EC, Chase P, Klingensmith G, Hamman RF (1993) Early exposure to cow's milk and solid foods in infancy, genetic predisposition and risk of IDDM. *Diabetes, 42*, 288–295.
26. Mayer EJ, Hamman RF, Gay EC, Lezotte DC, Savitz DA, Klingensmith GJ (1988). Reduced risk of IDDM among breast-fed children. *Diabetes, 37*, 1625–1632.
27. Fort P, Lanes R, Dahlem S (1986) Breast feeding and insulin-dependent diabetes mellitus in children. *J. Am. Coll. Nutr., 5*, 439–441.
28. Scott FW (1990). Cow milk and insulin-dependent diabetes mellitus: is there a relationship? *Am. J. Clin. Nutr., 51*, 489–491.
29. Martin JM, Daneman D, Dorsch H-M, Robinson B. (1991) Milk proteins in the etiology of insulin-dependent diabetes mellitus. *Ann. Med., 23*, 447–452.
30. Savilahti E, Saukkonen TT, Virtala ET (1993) Increased levels of cow's milk and β-lactoglobulin antibodies in young children with newly diagnosed IDDM. *Diabetes Care, 16*, 984–989.
31. Gerstein HC (1994) Cow's milk exposure and type I diabetes Mellitus. *Diabetes Care, 17*, 13–19.
32. Fall CHD, Barker DJP, Osmond C, Winter PD, Clark PMS, Hales CN (1992) Relation of infant feeding to adult serum cholesterol concentration and death from ischaemic heart disease. *Br. Med. J., 304*, 801–805.
33. Huttenen JK, Saarinen UM, Kostiainen E, Sümes MA (1983) Fat composition of the infant diet does not influence subsequent serum lipid levels in man. *Atherosclerosis, 46*, 87–94.
34. Jooste PL, Rossouw LJ, Steenkamp HJ, Rossouw JE, Swanepoel ASP, Charlton DO (1991) Effect of breast feeding on the plasma cholesterol and growth of infants. *J. Pediatr. Gastroenterol. Nutr., 13*, 139–142.
35. Sporik R, Johnstone JH, Cogswell JJ (1991) Longitudinal study of cholesterol values in 68 children from birth to 11 years of age. *Arch. Dis. Child., 66*, 134–137.
36. Kallio MJT, Salmenperä L, Siimes MA, Perheentupa J, Miettinen TA (1992) Exclusive breast-feeding and weaning: effect on serum cholesterol and lipoprotein concentrations in infants during the first year of life. *Pediatr., 89*, 663–666.
37. Phillips DIW, Barker DJP, Osmond C (1993) Infant feeding, fetal growth and adult thyroid function. *Acta Endocrinol., 129*, 134–138.
38. Lanting CI, Fidler V, Huisman M, Touwen BCL, Boersma ER (1994) Neurological differences between 9-year-old children fed breast milk or formula-milk as babies. *Lancet, 344*, 1319–1322.
39. Fergusson DM, Beautrais AL, Silva PA (1982) Breast feeding and cognitive development in the first seven years of life. *Soc. Sci. Med., 16*, 1705–1708.
40. Morrow-Tlucak M, Haude RH, Ernhart CB (1988). Breastfeeding and cognitive development in the first 2 years of life. *Soc. Sci. Med., 23*, 635–639.
41. Goldman AS (1993) The immune system of human milk: antimicrobial, antiinflammatory and immunomodulating properties. *Pediatr. Infect. Dis. J., 12*, 664–671.
42. Gilbert RE, Wigfield RE, Fleming PJ, Berry PJ, Rudd PT (1995) Bottle feeding and the sudden infant death syndrome. *Br. Med. J., 310*, 88–90.
43. Lucas A, Morley R, Cole TJ, Lister G, Leeson-Payne C (1992) Breast milk and subsequent intelligence quotient in children born preterm. *Lancet, 339*, 261–264.
44. Wright P, Deary IJ (1992) Breastfeeding and intelligence. *Lancet, 339*, 612–613.
45. MacArthur C, Knox EG, Simins KJ (1992) Letter. *Lancet, 339*, 612–613
46. Menkes JH (1977) Early feeding history of children with learning disorders. *Dev. Med. Child Neurol., 19*, 169–171.

47. Torres O, Cruz JR (1993) Protection against *Campylobacter* diarrhea: role of milk IgA antibodies against bacterial surfact antigens. *Acta Paediatr.*, *82*, 838–838.
48. Blake PA, Ramos S, MacDonald KL, Rassi V, Gomes TAT, Ivey C, Bean NH, Trabulsi LR (1993) Pathogen-specific risk factors and protective factors for acute diarrheal disease in urban Brazilian infants. *J. Infect. Dis.*, *167*, 627–632.
49. De Zoysa I, Rea M, Martines J (1991) Why promote breastfeeding in diarrhoeal disease control programmes? *Health Policy Planning, 6*, 371–379.
50. Walker A and Rolls B (Eds) (1994) *Infant Nutrition, Issues in Nutrition and Toxicology 2.* Chapman and Hall, London.
51. Taitz LS, Byers HD (1972) High calorie osmolar feeding and hypertonic dehydration. *Arch. Dis. Child.*, *47*, 257–260.
52. Department of Health and Social Security (UK) (1974) Present day practice in infant feeding. *Reports on Health and Social Subjects, No. 9.* HMSO, London.
53. Department of Health and Social Security (UK) (1977) The composition of mature human milk. *Reports on Health and Social Subjects. No. 12.* HMSO, London.
54. Frank JW, Newman J (1993) Breast-feeding in a polluted world: uncertain risks, clear benefits. *Can. Med. Assoc.*, *149*, 33–37.
55. Gross SJ (1983) Growth and biochemical response of preterm infants fed human milk or modified infant formula. *N. Engl. J. Med.*, *308*, 237–241.
56. Ronnholm KAR, Perheentupa J, Siimes MA (1986) Supplementation with human milk protein improves growth of small premature infants fed human milk. *Pediatrics, 77*, 649–653.
57. Bustamante SA, Fiello A, Pollack PF (1987) Growth of premature infants fed formulas with 10%, 30%, or 50% medium chain triglycerides. *Am. J. Dis. Child.*, *141*, 516–519.
58. Senterre J, Putet G, Salle B, Rigo J (1983) Effect of vitamin D and phosphorus supplementation on calcium retention in preterm infants fed banked human milk. *J. Pediatr.*, *103*, 305–307.
59. Van de Perre P, Lepage P, Homsy J, Dabis F (1992) Mother to infant transmission of human immnunodeficiency virus by breast milk: presumed innocent or presumed guilty? *Clin. Infect. Dis.*, *15*, 502–507.
60. De Martino, M, Tovo P-A, Tozzi AE (1992) HIV-1 transmission through breast-milk: appraisal of risk according to duration of feeding. *AIDS*, *6*, 991–997.
61. Dunn DT, Newell M-L, Ades AE, Peckham CS (1992). Risk of human immunodeficiency virus type 1 transmission through breast feeding. *Lancet, 340*, 585–588.
62. Shore MF (1970) Drugs can be dangerous during pregnancy and lactation. *Can. Pharm. J.*, *103*, 358–367.
63. Lewis PJ, Boylan P, Bulpitt CJ (1980) An audit of prescribing in an obstetric service. *Br. J. Obstet. Gynaecol.*, *87*, 1043–1046.
64. Treacy V, McDonald D (1981) Drug utilization in antenatal and postnatal wards. *Ir. Med. J.*, *74*, 159–160.
65. Matheson I, Kristensen K, Lunde PKM (1986) Drug utilization during breast feeding. A comparison of questionnaire and interview data on mother and child, Oslo 1985. *Report World Health Organisation Drug Utilization Research Group, ICP/BSE/103/M04*, pp 69–70. WHO Regional Office for Europe, Copenhagen.
66. Notzon F (1984) Trends in infant feeding in developing countries. *Pediatrics*, *74 (Suppl. 2)*, 648–666.
67. WHO Regional Office for Europe (1985) *Infant and Young Child Nutrition in Europe*. WHO, Copenhagen.
68. Henderson GE (1980) *Trends in Breast Feeding*. US Dept of Health and Human Services Publication No. 80–1250. National center for Health Statistics, Washington, DC.

69. Hendershot GE (1981) *Trends in Breast-Feeding in the United States, 1970–1975*. Working Paper Series, No. 5. National Center for Health Statistics, Washington, DC.
70. Bain K (1947) The incidence of breast-feeding in the US. *Pediatrics, 2*, 313–320.
71. Martinez GA (1979) The recent trend in breast feeding. *Pediatrics, 64*, 686–692.
72. Martinez GA, Nalezienski JP (1981). 1980 update: the recent trend in breast feeding. *Pediatrics, 67*, 260–263.
73. Rosenberg M (1989) Breast-feeding and infant mortality in Norway 1860–1930. *J. Biosocial Sci., 21*, 335–348.

Drugs and Human Lactation
P.N. Bennett, editor

2. Effects of drugs on milk secretion and composition

Margaret C. Neville and Carol T. Walsh

SUMMARY

The rate of milk secretion or milk composition potentially can be altered by agents that act in a number of ways: they may act directly on the mammary epithelium affecting its growth or its function; they may affect the hormonal milieu that regulates milk secretion or ejection or they may alter the delivery of nutrients to the lactating mammary cell. After a brief review of mammary development and the mechanisms of milk secretion we discuss the potential effects of drugs on mammary development, focussing on anti-estrogens. During lactation a large number of drugs act through the dopamine receptor on the lactotroph to increase or decrease prolactin secretion. Alcohol and opioids, on the other hand inhibit oxytocin release, interfering with the let-down reflex. A great deal of information is available about the effects of sex steroids on milk secretion from studies of oral contraceptive agents. In general estrogens, particularly at high doses, inhibit milk secretion whereas progesterone appears to have little effect. Other points where drugs might be expected to act are the secretory architecture of the mammary secretory cell and the enzymes of lipid synthesis. More research is indicated to determine whether therapeutic agents, as opposed to environmental chemicals, alter milk secretion by affecting these pathways.

INTRODUCTION

Although the greatest concern about drugs and lactation is rightfully directed toward the secretion of drugs in breast milk and their effects on the newborn, there are also potential effects of drugs on lactation itself, without which no treatise on this subject would be complete. Drugs have the potential of intervening at all stages in the development and function of the mammary gland. In particular drugs may interfere with the following processes:

a. normal mammary gland development;
b. milk secretion;
c. the hormonal milieu of the lactating mammary gland;
d. nutrient delivery to the lactating mammary cell.

The effects of drugs on some of these process have been well-defined. For example, a great deal of information is available on the role of dopaminergic compounds on secretion of prolactin, a major lactogenic hormone. In these instances we will present a concise summary of the available information. In other areas, for example, mammary development, the effects of pharmacological agents can only be suspected as definitive research is lacking. In this realm we can only make suggestions about fruitful areas for further investigation. To set the stage for both types of discussion the first part of this chapter summarises normal mammary development and function.

NORMAL MAMMARY DEVELOPMENT AND FUNCTION

Mammary gland development takes place in several stages known as *mammogenesis*, *lactogenesis* or the onset of copious milk secretion, *galactopoiesis* or sustained milk production and *involution* or dedifferentiation of the mammary gland at the cessation of lactation.

Mammogenesis takes place in several stages. In embryonic life the fat pad into which the alveolar elements must grow is laid down subcutaneously and rudimentary ducts composed of epithelial cells develop below the nipple (1). Little further development occurs until puberty when estrogen stimulates ductile growth (2, 3) into the fat pad in a highly regulated manner that probably involves the local secretion of a number of growth factors. With the onset of the menses progesterone secretion by the corpus luteum stimulates limited development of lobulo-alveolar complexes. By the end of puberty the normal gland is composed of ducts that course throughout the mammary stroma and terminate in small alveolar clusters as shown by the beautiful camera lucida drawing of Dabelow (Fig. 1) (4). Again development pauses until the complex hormonal milieu of pregnancy brings about additional growth and differentiation of the mammary epithelium. Although the specific roles of the hormones of pregnancy are not completely understood, it is clear that the lactogenic hormones prolactin and placental lactogen (also known as chorionic somatomammotrophin) play a role in this process as does progesterone (5). The role of estrogens is more problematic since levels are low throughout most of pregnancy in many species, although not humans. Progesterone probably enhances alveolar development while inhibiting milk secretion. In humans increasing levels of estrogens may also play a role in the inhibition of milk secretion, particularly if the woman is lactating at the onset of pregnancy.

The process of lactogenesis is set in motion with the birth of the young and depends on the presence of a differentiated mammary epithelium, the withdrawal of

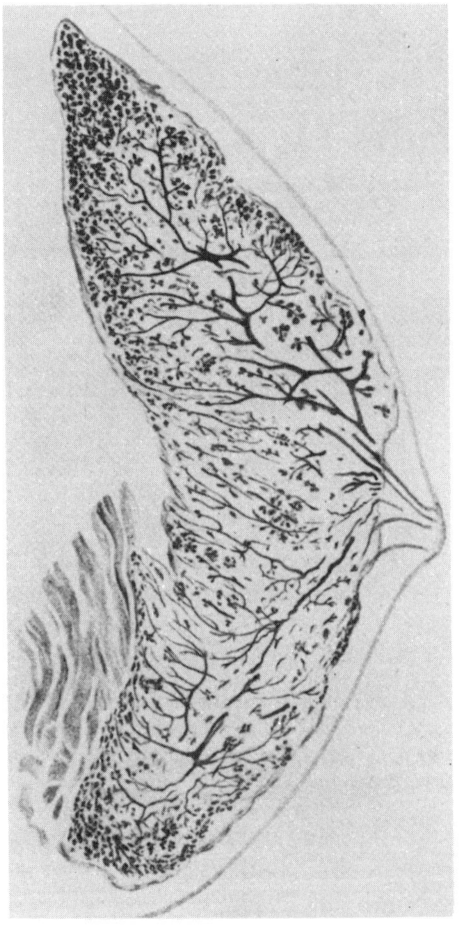

FIG. 1 *Camera lucida drawing of a cross section through the breast of a 19-year-old woman who had never been pregnant. Several ducts coursing from the alveolar complexes at the periphery of the gland are shown terminating on the nipple. From Ref. (4).*

high levels of sex steroids and the maintenance of prolactin secretion. The timing of lactogenesis is thought to depend most directly on the withdrawal of progesterone (6), since the process can be inhibited if progesterone levels are maintained from exogenous sources after parturition. In addition, the timing of lactogenesis across species is temporally related to the fall in progesterone. In humans, unlike most other mammals in which lactogenesis occurs around the time of birth, the onset of lactation is delayed until about 40 h after birth (7, 8). The decline in estrogen and the abrupt fall in placental lactogen are also likely to contribute to lactogenesis, but these effects are as yet poorly defined. Evidence that prolactin must

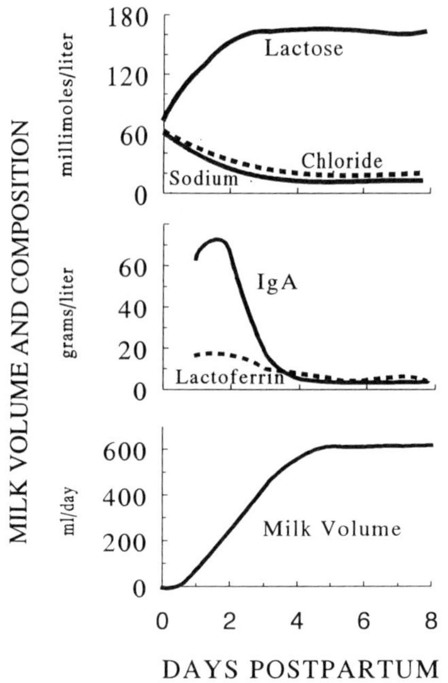

FIG. 2 *Changes in milk volume and composition during lactogenesis. Milk volume increases most rapidly between days 2 and 4 postpartum, thereafter leveling off. Sodium, chloride and lactose concentrations change most rapidly during the first 2 days postpartum as a result of closure of the tight junctions. The total protein concentration of the mammary secretion also decreases rapidly during this period, largely as a result of changes in secretory IgA and lactoferrin concentrations.*

be maintained at high levels for lactogenesis to occur is clear from the repression of lactogenesis by dopaminergic agonists that inhibit prolactin secretion (vide infra).

The composition of the mammary secretion undergoes profound changes during lactogenesis (Fig. 2). Although the product of the mammary gland is commonly termed colostrum during the first 5 days post-partum, its composition is far from constant with profound changes in sodium, chloride and lactose occurring during the first 48 h post-partum and changes in other constituents and milk volume being completed closer to 120 h. The early changes are the result of closure of the tight junctions between mammary epithelial cells that prevent plasma constituents such as sodium and chloride from passing directly from the interstitial space into the milk (8). The process of lactogenesis is normally complete by day 5 in women, although it may be delayed in diabetics for reasons that are incompletely understood (9, 10). Milk removal by the infant becomes necessary by day 2 or 3 postpartum if lactogenesis is to be completed (11). The average amount of milk transferred to the infant per day is about 500 ml by day 5 and continues to increase reaching ap-

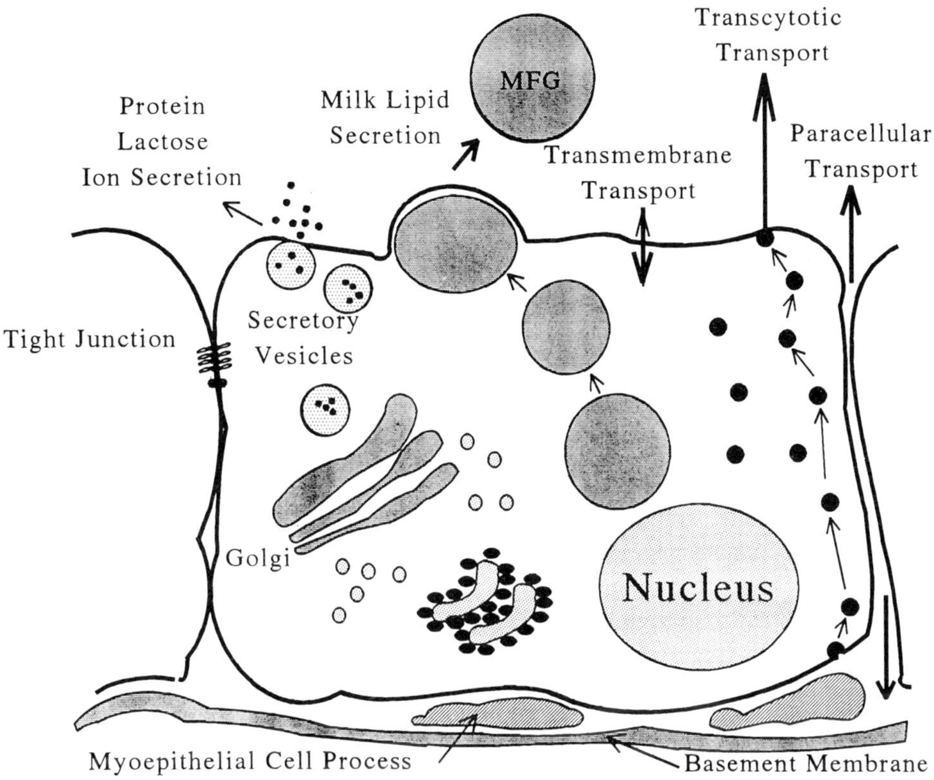

FIG. 3 *Pathways for the secretion of milk constituents. See text for explanation.*

proximately 700 ml at 1 month postpartum and about 800 ml at 6 months (7). The rate of milk secretion declines rapidly if suckling is discontinued for more than about 24 h once lactogenesis is complete.

The secretion of milk is accomplished by the mammary alveolar cell utilizing several pathways and a number of processes unique to the mammary gland (Fig. 3) (12). Most components of the aqueous fraction of milk are secreted via the exocytotic pathway responsible for the secretion of casein and other milk proteins as well as citrate and phosphate. Lactose is synthesized within Golgi vesicles of this pathway and secreted by the same pathway along with sufficient water to maintain an isotonic secretion. Milk lipids, largely triglycerides, are synthesized in the mammary gland and secreted as milk fat globules (MFG) surrounded by plasma membrane. A transmembrane pathway confined largely to monovalent ions and glucose probably keeps these substances equilibrated with the cellular cytoplasm. Finally, a transcytotic pathway is responsible for the secretion of secretory IgA into milk and is probably the route by which most plasma and interstitial proteins including protein hormones find their way into milk. During pregnancy, involution and mastitis an open paracellular pathway allows direct exchange between the interstitial fluid and milk. This pathway is closed in lactation when milk formation is carried out in its entirety by activities of mammary cells.

The hormones prolactin and oxytocin are critical for the maintenance of lactation (5). The secretion of both is stimulated by suckling. Prolactin, however, is secreted by lactotrophs in the anterior pituitary and acts on mammary epithelial cells to stimulate the secretion of milk components. Some level of prolactin is necessary for continuation of milk secretion, at least in women; it does not, however, seem to be responsible for day to day regulation of milk volume. Oxytocin, on the other hand, is secreted by the posterior pituitary and is responsible for the let-down reflex. Milk is secreted into the alveolar lumen where it remains until the network of myoepithelial cells that surrounds the mammary ducts and alveoli contracts, forcing milk into the mammary ducts and sinuses and making it available for the suckling infant. Letdown is normally the result of a neuroendocrine reflex whose afferent arm is the sensory stimulation provided by suckling and whose efferent arm is provided by oxytocin secretion. It can, however, be conditioned; in many women it is stimulated by the cry or even the thought of the infant. Strong emotional states are also thought to inhibit the reflex (13). Without this reflex milk cannot be removed from the alveoli.

It is becoming increasingly clear that regulation of the rate of milk secretion has a very large local component, mediated by removal of milk itself from the mammary alveoli. Thus if larger amounts of milk are required by the nursing infant, increased removal of residual milk from the alveoli stimulates milk secretion. Conversely, if the infant removes less milk because of illness or increased supplementation with other foods, removal of milk from the gland is less complete and milk secretion is down-regulated. A feedback inhibitor of lactation (FIL) (14,15), present in milk, is thought to be responsible for the effects of residual milk in the gland mediating the effects of infant demand on the amount of milk secreted. An understanding of this concept is crucial to the design and interpretation of experiments on the effects of drugs on milk secretion. If, for example, an agent like a combined oral contraceptive partially inhibits milk secretion, its effects can be overcome by increased removal of residual milk by the infant. If this occurs, neither a change in the daily transfer of milk to the infant nor in infant growth may be observed. However, the volume of residual milk will be decreased. For this reason procedures that measure residual milk volume are likely to provide important information about the effects of drugs on milk secretion.

Involution occurs when milk secretion is inhibited either by withdrawal of prolactin or cessation of regular milk removal (5). Although it has not been thoroughly studied, partial loss of the mammary epithelium appears to occur after weaning of the infant with further loss of both epithelium and stroma on withdrawal of sex steroids at menopause.

EFFECT OF DRUGS ON MAMMARY DEVELOPMENT

Estrogens and antiestrogens

Estrogens play an essential role in the pubertal development of the mammary gland, bringing about extension of the mammary ducts throughout the preexisting fat pad. Extensive evidence that estrogen replacement in ovariectomized prepubertal animals brings about ductule development (2) has recently been reinforced by the studies of Silberstein et al. (3) in which a specific estrogen antagonist, ICI 163,438, implanted into the mammary glands of pubertal mice, was shown to inhibit local ductule growth. This experiment constitutes proof that any agent that disrupts the action of estrogen has the potential to inhibit mammary growth. Such observations provide the experimental justification for the administration of antiestrogens such as tamoxifen in patients at high risk for breast cancer (16). Because a wide variety of estrogens and antiestrogens appear to be present in the environment (17, 18), the risk of exposure may not be restricted to the small number of women for whom such agents are prescribed as anticancer agents.

Anti-estrogens can act in a number of ways. The classic mechanism is interaction with the estrogen receptor directly inhibiting the effects of estrogen on estrogen-responsive cells (19). Some compounds, however, like the triphenylene antiestrogens may also bind to membrane-associated antiestrogen binding sites (20). Compounds such as 2,3,7,8-tetrachlorodibenzo-*p*-dioxin (TCDD) may enhance estrogen degradation (21) by upregulating estrogen metabolising enzymes. Others such as 6-hydroximinoandrostenedione may inhibit aromatases and thereby suppress estrogen synthesis (22, 23). There is an extensive literature in this area that can be reviewed only briefly here.

Antagonists like tamoxifen and ICI 163,438 bind directly to the estrogen receptor, competitively inhibiting the actions of estrogen as a transcription regulator. Biswas and Vonderhaar (20, 24) showed that tamoxifen and related triphenylene anti-estrogens also bind to the prolactin receptor, inhibiting prolactin binding. This interaction appears to be the basis of the inhibition of prolactin-stimulated casein synthesis in mammary explants by tamoxifen. The effects of tamoxifen and estradiol on mammary growth in prepubertal pigs were compared by Lin and Buttle (25). Tamoxifen, which is a partial estrogen agonist, stimulated mammary growth when given alone but partially inhibited the effect of estradiol when both agents were given together. When the treatment was repeated in pregnant pigs (26), neither mammary development nor the ability to lactate at parturition was affected although mammary progesterone receptor content was lower than the controls at day 90 of pregnancy. The currently available data make it difficult to predict the effects of tamoxifen and its congeners on mammary development and ultimately on milk secretion.

Epidemiological evidence that polychlorinated hydrocarbons exemplified by TCDD decrease growth of mammary epithelial cells was provided by an investigation of the effects of an industrial accident in Seveso, Italy (27). Although high levels of exposure to TCDD were associated with an increase in breast cancer, in this study a significant decrease in breast cancer incidence in a population exposed to chronic low levels of TCDD was found. In vitro TCDD and its congeners have been shown to reduce growth of estrogen-dependent mammary tumors (28, 29) and suppress estrogen-induced growth of MCF-7 breast cancer cells (21) as well as their secretion of tissue plasminogen activator (30). These agents are thought to act at least in part by combining with the Ah (aryl-hydrocarbon) receptor (31), up-regulating such estrogen metabolising enzymes as CYP1A2 (cytochrome P-4501A2). CYP1A2, in turn, catalyses the formation of 2-OH-estradiol and 16-OH-estradiol from estradiol-17β, thereby decreasing the half-life of the active hormone. Although CYP1A2 is thought to be confined to the liver there is experimental evidence (21) that TCDD increases the rate of estrogen metabolism in mammary cells as well. There is also evidence that TCDD decreases the level of estrogen receptor in the mammary gland (31). Chronic exposure of rats to TCDD in vivo has been observed to decrease the incidence of mammary tumours (32).

Another category of compounds may inhibit estrogen synthesis by interfering with the aromatase that converts androgenic precursors into active estrogens. For example, Gervais and Tan (22) have identified a male steroid hormone analogue, 6-hydroximinoandrostenedione, that acts as both an aromatase and growth inhibitor in cultured human T47D breast cancer cells. Kadohama and colleagues (23) found that tobacco constituents, acyl derivatives of nornicotine and anabasine, suppressed estrogen production by breast cancer cell lines.

The possibility does not seem to have been investigated that a crucial time window exists during pubertal formation of the mammary ducts when reductions in estrogen activity might effect a permanent decrease in mammary alveolar tissue. The accumulating evidence that estrogenic and anti-estrogenic compounds are widespread in the environment including cigarette smoke (23, 33), and that activities such as smoking have a deleterious effect on milk production, suggests that much more research is needed to relate the growing field of environmental estrogens and antiestrogens to their effects on mammary development and function.

DRUGS THAT ALTER THE HORMONAL MILIEU THAT SUPPORTS LACTATION

Prolactin

Prolactin is necessary for milk secretion in humans and may also play a role in mammary development. The secretion of prolactin from the anterior pituitary is regulated primarily by dopaminergic neurons of the tuberoinfundibular pathway with cell bodies in the periventricular and more caudal regions of the arcuate nucleus and terminals in the external layer of the median eminence of the hypothalamus (34). Dopamine released from these neurons diffuses into capillary loops of the hypophysial portal system and is transported to the anterior pituitary. The activity of these neurons is not regulated by dopaminergic feedback loops or autoreceptors; their activity, however, is inhibited by suckling and during lactation these neurons become less responsive to feedback inhibition by prolactin (34). In the anterior pituitary, dopamine interacts with the D_2 subtype of membrane receptor on prolactin-secreting cells or lactotrophs. Activation of these receptors by dopaminergic agonists inhibits prolactin release, in part through G-protein-dependent inhibition of cAMP (35). Signal transduction may be mediated through activation of potassium channels and cell hyperpolarisation, but not by direct inhibition of voltage-gated calcium channels (36).

Pharmacologic agents alter prolactin release by modifying the activity of dopaminergic neurons, by competing with dopamine for its receptor, or by directly activating dopaminergic receptors on prolactin-secreting cells (37). Drugs of therapeutic importance for their ability to decrease prolactin secretion selectively activate the D_2 receptor subtype. Many of these agents are ergot alkaloid derivatives. The prototype, approved in the United States for treatment of hyperprolactinemia, is bromocriptine. This drug has been documented in numerous clinical studies to inhibit postpartum lactation by bringing about a significant reduction in plasma prolactin (38). Bromocriptine is currently the drug of first choice in treating hyperprolactinemia associated with pituitary tumors (39). The drug is typically administered orally twice a day, but is also efficacious by the intravaginal route in women who cannot tolerate oral administration (40). The drug has a markedly longer duration of action when injected in a microsphere formulation by the intramuscular route (41–44). Analogues of bromocriptine which have also been shown clinically to inhibit lactation include dihydroergocristine (45), lisuride (46), terguride (47), pergolide (48), and cabergoline. Cabergoline is unique with respect to its long duration of action after oral administration (49–53). These other agents are not approved for use in the United States, except for pergolide which has other indications. Approval for the use of bromocriptine to inhibit post-partum lactation has recently been withdrawn in the United States because of cardiovascular complications (54, 55).

Other dopaminergic agonists have also been demonstrated clinically to decrease prolactin secretion. Examples include ibopamine, a structural analogue of dopamine, and the aminoquinolone quinagolide (CV205-502) both of which have been shown to inhibit puerperal lactation (56, 57). L-Dopa, metabolised to dopamine in the brain, has been shown to inhibit abnormal lactation (58). Indirect-acting agonists such as amphetamine (59) and nomifensine (60) decrease prolactin but have not been used clinically to suppress lactation.

In contrast to dopaminergic agonists, drugs with affinity for the D_2 receptor but no intrinsic activity can inhibit the effect of endogenous dopamine and typically produce hyperprolactinemia in both female and male subjects (37, 61). The effect may be manifested in some patients as galactorrhea or gynecomastia (62). D_2 receptor antagonists, used clinically for their neuroleptic effects, encompass a variety of chemical classes, including phenothiazines such as chlorpromazine, butyrophenones such as haloperidol, benzisoxazoles such as risperidone, and benzamides such as remoxipride and sulpiride (63). There is generally a correlation between their potency in modifying behaviour and in producing hyperprolactinemia (37). There has been concern about the relation between long-term use of neuroleptics and increased risk of breast cancer (64), but this issue is not resolved. The atypical neuroleptic agents such as clozapine are relatively weak D_2 antagonists, do not antagonise dopamine-induced inhibition of prolactin release from pituitary cells in vitro (65) and at most produce a transient rise in prolactin with usual clinical regimens (66).

D_2 receptor antagonists used as anti-emetic or prokinetic agents also can be expected to produce hyperprolactinemia. The benzamide metoclopramide, in a regimen for treating gastric stasis, has been shown to elevate serum prolactin levels (67) primarily the non-glycosylated form of the hormone (68). Use of metoclopramide post-partum has been reported to increase the volume of milk produced by lactating women without changing the concentration in milk of prolactin or sodium (69). Domperidone, another dopaminergic antagonist used in gastrointestinal motility disorders, increases serum prolactin as well (70).

Prolactin secretion is also enhanced by agonists which activate cholinergic, opioidergic, and tryptaminergic receptors in the central nervous system. There is evidence to suggest that these effects are mediated by actions within the dorsal arcuate nucleus that reduce dopaminergic neurotransmission in the tuberoinfundibular pathway (71). The increase in prolactin secretion from cholinergic activation has been demonstrated in unrestrained male rats with nicotine as agonists, this effect undergoes rapid desensitisation (72). Opioid agonists, both alkaloids and peptides, also increase prolactin secretion in part by decreasing dopamine release (35). The opioid-induced increase in prolactin is attenuated during lactation, possibly because of increased secretion of adrenal cortical hormones (73). The role of endogenous opioid peptides in prolactin secretion is unclear, since administration of the antagonist naloxone generally does not alter basal serum levels or hyperprolactinemia from a variety of causes (74). Some studies in animal models, including the cynomolgus monkey (75) and rat (76), suggest that opioids contribute to the rise in prolactin that occurs in response to suckling. It has been hypothesised that endogenous opioids may play a role in amenorrhea in athletes, but studies with the non-selective opioid antagonist naloxone have been inconclusive (77).

Tryptaminergic agonists shown to increase serum prolactin include serotonin (5-HT) (78), tryptophan (the 5-HT precursor) (79), fenfluramine (a 5-HT releasing agent) (80), fluoxetine (a 5-HT reuptake inhibitor) (81), moclobenmide (an MAO-A inhibitor) (82), the non-selective agonist m-chlorophenylpiperazine (83), and the 5-HT1$_A$ receptor selective agents, buspirone (84) and 8-hydroxy-2-(di-n-propyl-amino)tetralin (71). Serotonin-releasing neurons are believed to contribute to the increase in prolactin which occurs in response to suckling (35).

The release of prolactin is also induced by thyrotropin-releasing hormone (TRH) which acts directly on the pituitary lactotroph (85, 86). The physiological significance of TRH-mediated secretion is not clear (35). A synthetic form of this tripeptide, protirelin, is available for clinical use and has been used diagnostically to evaluate prolactin secretion (68, 87, 88).

Oxytocin

Oxytocin is released in response to suckling as well as certain psychological stimuli such as the cry of an infant. It causes contraction of myoepithelial cells around the mammary alveoli and ducts and brings about milk ejection. The compound is available as a nasal solution containing 40 USP units per ml. The compound is readily absorbed across the nasal epithelium and is prescribed during the first week after parturition to aid the let-down reflex. It has also been used in experimental protocols to produce hourly milk samples that represent complete emptying of the breast (7). As stated above, let-down is essential to milk removal from the breast. In the presence of inadequate let-down milk accumulates in the mammary alveoli, resulting in inhibition of milk secretion.

Ethyl alcohol is a potent inhibitor of oxytocin release. Chronic ethanol ingestion by lactating rats led to both a decrease in milk production and a change in milk composition, with decreased lactose and increased lipid content (89). An elegant, early study in which intramammary pressure was measured in response to suckling by the infant demonstrated that ethanol inhibited milk ejection in a dose-dependent manner (Fig. 4) (90). In this study Cobo found that doses of alcohol up to 0.45 g/kg, doses that produce a blood level less than 0.1%, had no effect on intramammary pressure although they did abolish uterine contractures, suggesting that the myoepithelial cells in the breast are more sensitive to the hormone than is the myometrium or that the effect of alcohol on oxytocin release is attenuated in lactating compared to parturient women. More recently Coiro and colleagues (91) measured the plasma oxytocin concentrations in response to breast-stimulation in non-lactating women and found that 50 ml of ethyl alcohol completely abolished the oxytocin rise. Minor effects of chronic maternal alcohol consumption were observed on motor development of breast-fed infants in a well-controlled study in humans (92). These effects were attributed to alcohol transfer to the infant rather than suppression of milk secretion.

A potent effect of opioids on oxytocin release is suggested by the observation in rats that morphine inhibits the let-down reflex (93, 94) and the mechanism of this response has been extensively studied in this species. In one carefully done study evidence for involvement of kappa receptors on magnocellular neurons was obtained, whereas morphine, a mu-receptor agonist appeared to depress the mammary response to oxytocin (95) with no effect on oxytocin-secreting neurons. The effects of opioids have not been extensively studied in lactating women. In a single report (91), naloxone, an opioid antagonist, had no effect on oxytocin release but partially abrogated the inhibition produced by alcohol, suggesting both that ethanol acts through an opioid pathway and that oxytocin is not subject to chronic inhibition by opioids during lactation.

Prostaglandins

The effects of prostaglandins on milk let-down were studied in a number of laboratories in the early 1970s with conflicting results (summarised in Ref. 96). Cobo and colleagues (97) found that milk ejection was stimulated in women by $PGF_{2\alpha}$ and McNeilly and Fox (98) found that PGE_1, E_2, $F_{1\alpha}$, and $F_{2\alpha}$ all possessed inherent milk-ejecting ability in the guinea pig. Consistent with a direct effect on prostaglandins on the mammary gland, Batta et al. (99) found that $PGF_{2\alpha}$ caused milk ejection from isolated fragments of lactating mammary gland. In rats, however, $PGF_{2\alpha}$ appeared to interfere with oxytocin release and thus inhibit the letdown reflex (96). In a more recent study prostaglandin E_2 was found to be as effective as bromocriptine in suppressing post-partum lactation in women (100) adding to the general confusion about the effects of prostaglandins on lactation.

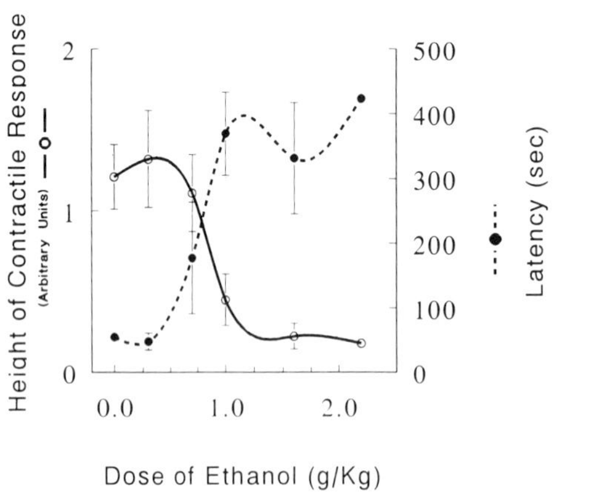

FIG. 4 *Effect of alcohol on the let-down reflex. Intramammary pressure was measured in one breast with a catheter while the infant suckled the other. Control measurements were obtained from each subject prior to ethanol ingestion. All women responded to exogenous oxytocin with increased mammary pressure after ingestion of ethanol, indicating that the inhibition is centrally mediated. Plotted from data in Ref. (90).*

Other hormones

Glucocorticoids have been shown both in vivo and in vitro to be necessary for milk secretion in animal and tissue culture models (101, 102). There are, however, no studies of the effects of chronic glucocorticoid treatment on milk secretion, possibly because breast-feeding is not recommended in women on high doses of glucocorticoids which have the potential to accumulate in milk. Adequate levels of *thyroid hormone* have long been known to be essential for lactation in goats and rats (103–105) and thyroid hormone has been shown to increase milk output in cows with some effects on milk composition (106). Its effects, however, have not been studied in women. Anecdotally, women who are clinically hypothyroid may have difficulty initiating lactation (N. Powers, pers. commun.) but this effect has not received systematic study.

EFFECTS OF SEX STEROIDS AND THEIR CONGENERS ON MILK SECRETION

Much information is available on the effects of sex steroids on milk secretion in women because of the world-wide importance of hormonal contraception. In addition, before the serious side effects of many of these hormones and their congeners were appreciated, very high doses of sex steroids were used to suppress puerperal lactation. While such high doses of drugs have not been used in lactating women for two decades, the effects that were observed in the 1960s and early 1970s provide us with important information about the consequences of high dose steroids on lactation. In this section we review the most important work on the use of steroid hormones to suppress puerpural lactation and discuss the use of combined oral contraceptive agents containing a combination of compounds with estrogen- and progestin-like actions. Finally, the use of progestin-only agents in the lactating woman is discussed.

All extant studies on the effects of sex steroids suffer from inadequate measurements of the rate of milk secretion. Nontheless, some general conclusions can be drawn. In many studies on steroid contraceptive agents a major parameter was the amount of milk that could be extracted from the breast under controlled conditions. This parameter is likely to be sensitive to subtle effects of inhibitory agents because, as discussed above, it includes the residual milk volume. In general changes in duration of lactation tended to parallel changes in extractable milk volume. Infant growth appeared to be much less sensitive to oral contraceptive agents, probably because increased suckling by the infant is able to compensate for partial inhibition of milk secretion. For studies of puerperal lactation suppression, where it was necessary to depend heavily on personal evaluations by the subjects themselves, reliable quantitative data on the inhibition of milk secretion are not available.

Lactation suppression with sex steroids

In several studies doses of steroid hormones, unacceptably high by today's standards, were given to puerperal women under reasonably controlled circumstances for the suppression of puerperal lactation. The parameters investigated included the ability to express milk from the breast and the apparent degree of engorgement and pain. A large, placebo-controlled experiment by Markin and Wolst (107), published in 1960, used five different agents, four of which had their own placebo controls, in about 500 postpartum women. As can be seen from Table 1 all agents, including both a potent estrogen alone (diethylstilbesterol) as well as a number of combinations of an androgen with an estrogen, significantly reduced the signs and symptoms of milk secretion compared to the placebo. Four of the agents were associated with significant rebound milk secretion after termination of daily dosing and for that reason, the clinical impression was that they were no more efficacious than controls. The fifth agent, a high dose of testosterone and estrogen given intramuscularly was not associated with any rebound in this group of patients, possibly because of prolonged absorption of this very large dose from the muscle. Results similar to the effects of diethylstilbesterol were found with the estrogenic agents quinestrel (108) and chlorotriansene (109).

The question of whether estrogens inhibit lactation by suppressing prolactin secretion was answered by a 1975 study (108) in which quinestrol (4 mg immediately after delivery) followed by placebo was compared with placebo alone or with bromocriptine (Fig. 5). It is quite clear that the estrogenic compound increased plasma prolactin levels. Numerous more recent studies confirm a potent stimulation of prolactin secretion by estrogens. From such indirect evidence we surmise that estrogen suppresses lactation by acting locally on the mammary gland. The mechanism is unknown and the finding is, in fact, rather puzzling since studies on the mammary glands of rodents suggest that estrogen neither stimulates formation of progesterone receptors nor binds to chromatin isolated from the lactating gland of mice (110).

It is important to emphasize that sex steroids are now absolutely contraindicated in the post-partum period because they promote blood clotting (111) and thromboembolism, and have been associated with cervical cancer.

Combined oral contraceptive agents and lactation

Tables 2 and 3 summarize data from a large number of studies of the effects of steroid contraceptives on various parameters related to milk secretion. These studies were selected for citation here because they included reasonable control groups. Those parameters that were most often measured were:

a. *Duration of breast-feeding* (112–122). This parameter is best measured by the mean duration of breast-feeding in a population of women who are observed

TABLE 1 *Effect of sex steroids on the initiation of lactation*

Agent	Regimen[a] Day postpartum 1	2	3	4	5	N Drug	Placebo	Effects on lactation: Milk secretion	Engorgement	Pain	Rebound secretion	Ref.	Year
Diethylstilbesterol	15	15	15	15	15	52	40	↓↓	↓↓	↓↓↓	+	(107)	1960
Dienestrol +	2.3	2.3	1.5	1.5	0.8	49	65	↓	↓	↓	+	(107)	1960
methyl testosterone	45	45	30	30	15								
Conjugated estrogen, equine +	7.5	5.3	2.5	1.3	1.3	49	65	↓↓	↓	↓↓	+	(107)	1960
methyl testosterone	60	40	20	10	10								
Testosterone proprionate +	50 i.m.	50 i.m.				67	0	↓↓↓	↓↓↓	↓↓↓	+	(107)	1960
diethyl stilbesterol			15	15	15								
Testosterone enanthate +	360[b]					42	41	↓↓↓	↓↓↓	↓↓↓	None	(107)	1960
estradiol valerate	16												
Quinestrol	4[c]					28	27	↓	↓↓	↓↓	None	(108)	1975
Chlorotriansene (progestagen)	125	100	75			94	96	↓	↓	↓	↓	(109)	1975
Testosterone enanthate	360[b]					96	96	↓	↓	↓	↓	(109)	1975
Estradiol valerate	16[b]												

[a]All doses in mg per day given orally unless intramuscular (i.m.) is specified.
[b]i.m., day of birth only.
[c]Oral, day of birth only.

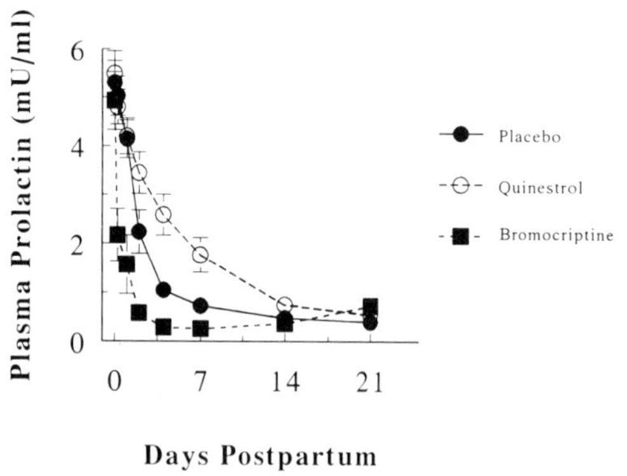

FIG. 5 *The effect of an estrogenic agent, quinestrel, and bromocriptine on prolactin secretion in the puerperium. Quinestrel (4 mg)was given as a single dose on the day of birth followed by placebo (N = 32). Bromocriptine was given orally 2.5 mg twice a day for 14 days (N = 28). Placebo identical in appearance was given on the same schedule (N = 27). Redrawn from Ref. (108).*

throughout the entire period of lactation. In shorter studies it can also be estimated by the number of women who are still lactating at a given time postpartum. In a few studies the use of supplemental feeds has been reported. Supplemental feeds are, however, difficult to quantitate without very intensive observation and, in general, the results in oral contraceptive trials have not been reported reliably.

b. *Milk volume*, as represented by the amount of milk that can be extracted from one or both breasts by breast pump, usually at a defined interval after a feed (112, 113, 118, 123–126). The milk extracted includes residual milk, i.e. milk in excess of that taken by the infant. If studies implicating a local inhibitor of milk secretion are correct (see above), the extracted milk volume may be a better measure of the secretory capacity of the breast than the actual amount taken by the infant.

c. *Milk composition* has been measured in relatively few studies, and then on relatively few parameters (123, 124, 127–129). The mechanism of the few observations of changes in composition is unknown.

d. *Infant growth and development* have been measured either acutely (112, 113, 115–118, 120, 125, 129–131) while the mother is taking the contraceptive agent or much later, after lactation has ceased (119, 121, 132). Changes in growth during contraceptive use are probably more reflective of effects on lactation since 'catch-up' growth may compensate for early growth retardation, at least in well-nourished children.

e. *Other parameters* that have been measured include maternal and infant metabolic state (120, 121, 130, 133), infant morbidity (estimated from clinic visits or school records) (119) and intellectual development (from school records) (119).

Early studies, in the 1970s for the most part, utilised the large dose combined oral contraceptive agents available at the time (112–114, 123, 125, 126) (e.g. those compounds whose labels begin with HD in Table 2). In some cases the estrogenic compound was combined with a progestagen like quingestanol that has some estrogenic or androgenic activity as well. In most of these studies convincing reductions were seen in the duration of breast-feeding, the volume of milk that could be expressed from the breast, and infant growth. Although the effects of these agents on milk production are attributed to the estrogens they contain, in one study where the estrogenic compounds were studied alone (126) in mothers who were expressing all their milk with a breast pump, no effects were observed compared with placebo. With none of the combined agents was a change in composition noted.

In the late 1970s low dose combined preparations containing levonorgestrel 150 μg, a progestagen, and ethinylestradiol 30 μg became available and were shown to have very high contraceptive efficacy with few side effects. The effects of these agents on lactation were most carefully studied by the World Health Organization in Hungary and Thailand (118). They were consistently found in this and other studies (115–119, 124, 131) to decrease the duration of breast-feeding and milk volume with little effect on infant growth (Table 2). In one long-term follow-up study in Sweden (119) that was carefully case-controlled, no effects on growth, morbidity, or intellectual achievement could be discerned from school or clinic records.

Progestagen only agents

Progestagens are often used in a long-term injectable form such as depot medroxyprogesterone acetate (DMPA), and were found in some studies to increase the duration of lactation compared to no contraceptive use or use of IUDs, barrier methods or sterilization (114, 121, 122) (Table 3). In one fairly careful study (114), however, there was little difference between the effects of progestagen injections and the use of an IUD on duration of lactation. No consistent effects on milk volume, infant growth or morbidity, or biochemical parameters in mothers and infants have been observed (118, 120, 123, 124, 129, 130, 133), with no effect found in long-term follow-up studies (121, 132). Inconsistent effects on milk composition were observed in early studies (124, 129) but were not reproduced in a more recent investigation (128). In one inquiry (121) where decreased growth, measured as infant weight at 3–4 years old, was observed in infants whose mothers had received DMPA by injection, an apparent decrease in weight disappeared when the statistical analysis was adjusted for breast-feeding duration. Progesterone-containing contraceptives are, therefore, usually recommended as the best means of steroidal contraception in the lactating woman.

The physiologic basis for the lack of responsiveness of the lactating mammary gland to progestins has been shown to reside in a lack of progesterone receptors, at

TABLE 2 *Effects of combined oral contraceptives on lactation*

Variable	Start OC time postpartum	End study	Country	*N*	Drug[a]	Control	Outcome[b]	Ref.	Year
Duration of breast-feeding	2–6 weeks	3 months	US	47	HD1	No OC, placebo	Dec	(112)	1970
	6 weeks	16 weeks	Thailand	20	HD2	No OC	Dec	(113)	1972
	1 months	Weaning	Chile	40	HD4	IUD	Dec 30%	(114)	1974
				81	E3		Dec 40%		
				194	HD5		Dec 67%		
				81	HD6		Dec 67%		
				50	HD3		Dec 52%		
	1 months	3 months pp	Chile	103	LD1	Placebo	Dec	(115)	1983
	2 months	12 months	Chile	103	LD1	No OC	Dec	(116)	1983
	3 months	12 months	Chile	59	LD1	IUD or barrier	NC	(117)	1983
	6 weeks	24 weeks	Hungary, Thailand	86	LD1	IUD, barrier, sterilization, none	Dec	(118)	1984
	2 months	8 years	Sweden	48	LD2	Case control	Dec 20%	(119)	1984
Milk volume[c]	4–24 weeks	8 weeks later	India	62	HD2	No steroid	Dec 25%	(125)	1970
	2 weeks	5 weeks	US	21	HD1	Placebo	NC	(112)	1970
	Not stated;	3 weeks later	Sweden	8	HD7	Placebo	Dec 60%	(126)	1971
	pumping			8	E1	(Mothers of hospitalized	NC		
				8	E2	infants)	NC		
	6 weeks	16 weeks	Thailand	20	HD2	No OC	Dec 75%	(113)	1972
				20	HD3		Dec 32%		
	6 weeks	18 weeks	India	34	HD8	Sterilization, barrier	Dec 56%	(123)	1974
				30	HD4		Dec 63%		
	2 months	6 months	India	6	LD3	No OC	NC	(124)	1977
	6 weeks	24 weeks	Hungary, Thailand	86	LD1	IUD, barrier, sterilization, none	Dec 32%	(118)	1984

Milk composition: protein, lactose, lipid, calcium	2 months	6 months	India	6	LD3	No OC	NC	(124)	1977
	6 weeks	24 weeks	Hungary, Thailand	86	LD1	IUD, barrier, sterilization, none	Small changes	(127)	1988
			Brazil	12	LD1	IUD	NC	(128)	1992
				13	LD4		NC		
Infant growth	6 weeks	24 weeks	Bombay	62	HD2	No steroid	Dec 20%	(125)	1969
			US	24	HD1	Placebo	Dec 25%	(112)	1970
	6 weeks	16 weeks	Thailand	20	HD2	No contraceptive	Dec 25%	(113)	1972
			Thailand	20	HD3		NC		
	25–20 days	120 days	Chile	60	LD1	No contraceptive or IUD	Dec 10%	(115)	1978
	1 months	3 months	Chile	103	LD1	Placebo; weight gain	NC	(116)	1983
	2 months	12 months	Chile	103	LD1	IUD; weight	NC	(117)	1983
	3 months	12 months	Chile	59	LD1	IUD, barrier; weight	NC	(131)	1983
	6 weeks	24 weeks	Hungary, Thailand	86	LD1	IUD, barrier, sterilization, none	NC	(118)	1984
	Any	8 years	Sweden	48	LD2	Case control; weight, height	NC	(119	1986
Infant development	Any	8 years	Sweden	48	LD2	Case control; from school and hospital records	NC	(119)	1986

[a]Key to drugs used: *High dose combined agents:* HD1, norethisterone, 1 mg, mestranol, 80 μg; daily; HD2, ethynodiol diacetate 1 mg; mestranol, 100 μg, sequential; HD3, chlormadinone acetate, 2 mg; mestanol, 80 μg, daily; HD4, norethisterone, 1 mg; ethinylestradiol, 50 μg, daily; HD5, quinestrol, 2 mg; quingestanol acetate, 5 mg monthly; HD6, quinestrol, 2 mg; quingestanol acetate, 2.5 mg monthly; HD7, levonorgestrel, 2.5 mg; mestanol, 75 μg; daily; HD8, levonorgestrel, 500 μg; ethinylestradiol, 50 μg; daily. *Estrogens alone:* E1, ethinylestradiol , 50 μg; daily; E2, mestanol, 75 μg; daily; E3, quingestanol acetate, 300 μg; daily. *Low dose combined agents:* LD1, levonorgestrel, 150 μg; ethinylestradiol, 30 μg, daily; LD2, progestin; ethinylestradiol, 50 μg, daily; LD3, norethisterone, 350 μg; ethinylestradiol, 10 μg; daily; LD4, levonorgestrel, 250 μg; ethinylestradiol, 50 μg; daily.
[b]Abbreviations: OC, oral contraceptive; Dec, decrease; NC, no change; IUD, intrauterine device; N.S., not significant.
[c]Methods: (125), 1 feed test weigh; (126), pumping by mothers of hospitalized infants; remainder, defined pumping regimen 2–4 h after previous feed.

TABLE 3 *Effects of progestin only oral contraceptives on lactation*

Effect	Start OC time postpartum	End study	Country	*N*	Drug[a]	Control	Outcome[b]	Ref.	Year pub
Duration of breast-feeding	1–2 days	Wean	Chile	80	IP3	Previous lactation; IUD	Inc. NC	(114)	1974
	1 months	Wean		33	IP3		Inc 20%		
	1 months	Wean		54	IP5		Inc. NC		
	6 weeks	12 months	Finland	29	IUD1	Copper IUD	NC	(120)	1982
				34	IUD2	Copper IUD	NC		
	2 months	3–6 years	Chile	128	IP1	IUD, barrier, sterilization, none	Inc 60%	(121)	1984
	6 weeks	24 weeks	Hungary	85	OP1	IUD, barrier, sterilization, none	NC	(118)	1984
			Thailand	58	IP1		NC		
	2–4 months	Wean	Chile	228	IP1	No contraception, IUD	Inc	(122)	1986
				185	OP2		Inc		
Milk volume	6 weeks	18 weeks	India	30	OP3	Sterilization, barrier	NC	(123)	1979
	2–6 weeks	12 weeks	India	6	IP1	No OC	Inc	(124)	1977
				6	IP2		Dec		
				7	IP7		NC		
	6 weeks	24 weeks	Hungary,	85	OP1	IUD, barrier, sterilization, none	NC	(118)	1984
			Thailand	58	IP1		NC		
Milk composition	6 weeks	18 weeks	India	30	OP3	Barrier, sterilization	NC	(123)	1974
	2–6 weeks	12 weeks	India	6	IP1	IUD, barrier, sterilization, none	Inc (prot)[c]	(124)	1977
				6	IP2		Dec (prot, lip, Ca)		
				7	IP7		Dec (lip, Ca)		
		9 weeks	Brazil		OP4	No OC; Pretreatment values	NC	(128)	1992
		5 weeks			IP1		NC		

Infant growth	6 weeks	12 months	Finland	29	UD1	Copper IUD	NC	(120)	1982
				34	IUD2		NC		
	6 weeks	24 weeks	Hungary,	85	OP1	IUD, barrier, sterilization, none	NC	(118)	1984
			Thailand	58	IP1		NC		
	2 months	3–6 years	Chile	128	IP1	IUD, barrier, sterilization, none	Dec[d]	(121)	1984
	4–6 weeks	6 months	Indonesia	60	IP6	Copper IUD	NC	(130)	1986
	1–3 months	4–6 years	Thailand	857	IP1	No DMPA	NC	(132)	1992
Other									
Infant biochemistry and morbidity	6 weeks	12 months	Finland	29	IUD1	Copper IUD	NC	(120)	1982
			Finland	34	IUD2		NC		
Infant morbidity	2 months	3–6 years	Chile	128	IP1	IUD, barrier, sterilization, none	NC	(121)	1984
	4–6 weeks	6 months	Indonesia	60	IP6	Cu-71 IUD	NC	(130)	1986
Maternal biochemistry	3 months	8 months	India Thailand	844	IP1	Non-lactating women	NC	(133)	1986

[a]Key to progestin-only drugs: *Oral agents:* CP1, *dl*-norgestrel, 75 μg daily; OP2, clogestone acetate, 600 μg/daily, oral; OP3, norgestrel, 50 μg daily; OP4, norethindrol 350 μg daily. *Injections (intramuscular):* IP1, DMPA, 150 mg/6 months; IP2, DMPA, 300 mg/ 6 months; IP3, DMPA, 250 mg/6 months; IP4, norethisterone enanthate, 20 mg monthly; IP5, chlormadione, 250 mg/3 months; IP6, levonorgestrel, 30–50 pg/day (Norplant); IP7, norethisterone, 350 mg; IP8, algestone acetofenide, 150 mg. *IUD:* IUD1, levonorgestrel, 10 μg; IUD2, levonorgestrel, 30 μg.

[b]Abbreviations: OC, oral contraceptive; Dec, decrease; NC, no change; Inc, increase; IUD, intrauterine device; DMPA, medroxyprogesterone (depot provera).

[c]In this study protein (prot), lipid (lip), lactose(lact), calcium (Ca) and phosphorus (P) were measured; only changes are noted.

[d]Attributed to increased duration of breast-feeding in the group receiving depot medroxyprogesterone injections.

least in rodents (134). One may speculate on the reasons for the apparent improvement in lactation performance in some studies where DMPA was used for contraception. This agent usually prevents the onset of the menses during the period of lactation; the attendant reduction in endogenous estrogens may remove the potentially inhibitory influence of these agents on milk secretion.

Steroid contraception during lactation

Many factors need to be taken into account in the choice of contraceptive agent in the lactating woman, including not only effects on lactation but also the duration of the planned lactation, the efficacy of the agent in preventing pregnancy, the sexual habits of the mother and the degree of side effects such as spotting or uncontrolled bleeding. While this is not the place for a thorough discussion of these issues, some points should be made from the data in Tables 1 and 2. As stated above most authorities recommend progestin-only contraceptives as the method of choice in the lactating woman. This recommendation is probably valid for women in less developed countries where prolonged lactation is desirable, DMPA or Norplant are widely available and used, and women are highly motivated to breast-feed and willing to tolerate the increased side effects of progestagens. However, combined oral contraceptive agents containing 30–50 μg of estradiol are in wide use in developed countries where breast-feeding duration is usually less than 1 year and where supplemental foods are of high quality. The data in the most careful studies of the effects of combined agents on infant growth (115–117) indicate that growth suppression is temporary, particularly if the agent is started after 2 months postpartum, and amounts to no more than 300 g over the first year of life. In an otherwise well-nourished, healthy infant this effect must be balanced against the efficacy of the agent in preventing pregnancy.

DRUGS THAT ALTER NUTRIENT TRANSPORT TO THE MAMMARY GLAND

Growth hormone

Under the appellation bovine somatotropin (bST) growth hormone is seeing increasingly widespread use to enhance milk yield in cows in the last two-thirds of the lactation cycle. Because of the commercial importance of this effect, it has received a great deal of scientific attention the details of which can be found in an excellent review by Bauman and Vernon (135). Because it is unlikely that the hormone will be widely used in the same manner in humans (but see Ref. 136), only the high points of the current knowledge in the field are summarised here. The hormone has no effect on gross milk composition or the concentration of vitamins or nutritionally important minerals. The biological effects of the hormone appear to be due to partitioning of nutrients to lactation and away from endogenous nutrient stores in the animal, resulting in an increase in milk production per unit of feed. With appropriate nutrition, however, animals can be maintained in positive energy balance because of an increase in food intake. The detailed mechanisms involved are incompletely understood but it is well-established that the major targets of bST are adipose tissue and the liver; effects on the mammary gland are thought to be indirect, most likely mediated by insulin-like growth factor I (IGF I) (135). The changes involved include increased hepatic gluconeogenesis and decreased peripheral glucose utilisation resulting in increased glucose flux to the mammary gland. Changes in whole-body lipid metabolism depend on the animal's energy balance but involve a decrease in lipid synthesis and a possible increase in lipolysis likely acting through a decrease in insulin sensitivity through a post-receptor mechanism that is not yet understood. An increase in mammary blood flow is proportional to the increase in milk secretion. Human growth hormone has received one clinical trial in lactating women where it was found to produce a marginal increase in milk volume (136).

Potential effects of drugs on mammary blood flow

Mammary blood flow has been found to be proportional to milk secretion in several studies (reviewed in Ref. 137) but the mechanisms for its regulation are not understood. Inhibitors of blood flow potentially could diminish milk output because of diminished nutrient or hormone availability. There are, however, few studies that have reported a decrease in milk volume or change in composition after administration of a drug with vasoactive properties. Polymyxin B, a relatively toxic antibiotic that finds general use only topically, was reported to decrease mammary blood flow in starved-refed lactating rats as well as to decrease lipogenesis (138). Whether its effects are due to a direct action on blood flow or an indirect action due to metabolic effects on the mammary gland was not determined.

DRUGS THAT ACT DIRECTLY ON MILK SECRETION

There are many points at which drugs have the potential to interfere directly with milk secretion. Aside from the oral contraceptive agents reviewed above, however, there is very little information available from direct studies of milk secretion. In this section of the chapter we review briefly agents that potentially disrupt either the secretory architecture of the gland or the secretion of milk lipid. The little data that are available suggest further directions for research into the effects of drugs on secretion of other milk components such as lactose, proteins, trace elements and vitamins.

A number of agents have the potential to alter the cytoarchitecture of the secretory cell and interfere with actual secretory mechanisms (137). For example the microtubule-disrupting agent colchicine inhibited milk secretion when given intraluminally into the udder of the lactating goat (139, 140) and decreased milk secretion by rabbit mammary explants. Tumour promoters such as the phorbol esters have been known for a long time to alter epithelial morphology (141) and their effects on the mammary gland have been studied both in vivo and in vitro. In primary cultures of the mouse mammary gland the phorbol ester, 12-*O*-tetradecanolphorbol-13-acetate (TPA) inhibited milk protein synthesis at concentrations as low as 0.1 ng/ml (142, 143). TPA altered the expression of neutral metalloproteinases in cultured mammary cells (144). Injection of TPA 4 mg into lactating mice twice daily for 2.5 days completely inhibited pup growth (145). Although a direct effect on the pups through TPA in milk was not ruled out by these experiments, the authors suggest a direct action on milk secretion. Because phorbol esters are now known to exert their actions through the protein kinase C pathway (146), any agent that acts through this pathway, for example, epidermal growth factor or diacylglycerol, has the potential for disrupting milk secretion. A multitude of additional agents including heavy metals, cytochalasin D, 9,10-dimethyl-1,2-benzanthracene (DMBA), retinoic acid, phalloidin and TCDD all have been shown to alter cytoskeletal morphology in tissues other than the mammary gland at very low concentrations indicating a potential for effects on milk secretion as well (reviewed in Ref. 137).

Mammary lipid synthesis involves both utilisation of lipids transported in the plasma to the mammary gland and endogenous lipid synthesis. Two key enzymes involved in these processes, lipoprotein lipase (LPL) and fatty acid synthetase are highly sensitive to metabolic regulation, suggesting that they might represent points of action of drugs. LPL has been shown to be regulated by insulin, β-adrenergic agents, cytokines such as tumour necrosis factor as well as environmental agents such as dioxins suggesting that its role in milk fat synthesis may be a potential target of a wide variety of drugs (137). High doses of the plasticiser, di(2-ethylhexyl) phthalate, were administered to laboratory rats and shown increase milk fat and decrease pup growth (147). When the pups were directly dosed with similar doses of phthalate there was no effect on growth, suggesting that this chemical, which is widespread in the environment (148), may have deleterious effects either on milk lipid synthesis or milk synthesis in general.

CONCLUSIONS

The major classes of agents that have been thoroughly investigated for their effects on milk secretion have largely been studied because of their effects on systems other than lactation. For example, dopaminergic agonists have received attention because they have a potential to decrease hyperprolactinemia of anterior pituitary origin. Sex steroids have received a great deal of attention because of their usage as oral contraceptive agents. Our understanding of the effects of these drugs on lactation has often been achieved almost as a byproduct of research targeted at other processes. Whether this is because lactation is a relatively robust process on which therapeutic agents generally have little effect or because breast-feeding is terminated when serious therapeutic regimens are undertaken is not entirely clear. There are some areas, such as the effect of antiestrogens on normal mammary development, where significant research efforts that include studies of the amount of parenchyma are clearly warranted. Other drugs, particularly those that are found in high concentrations in milk, or that have a potential to be use on a long-term basis during breast-feeding, e.g., psychotropic agents, should be more thoroughly investigated for their effects both on milk volume and composition. Until information about effects on milk secretion is available for such agents, clinicians will be forced to proceed with great caution or to advise termination of breast-feeding when these drugs must be used in the lactating woman.

ACKNOWLEDGEMENT

The writing of this review article was supported in part by grant no. HD15437 to MCN.

REFERENCES

1. Anderson RR (1978) Embryonic and fetal development of the mammary apparatus. In: Larson BL (Ed) *Lactation IV: The Mammary Gland/Human Lactation/Milk Synthesis*, pp 3–41. Academic Press, New York.
2. Daniel CW, Silberstein GB (1987) Postnatal development of the rodent mammary gland. In: Neville MC, Daniel CW (Eds) *The Mammary Gland: Development, Regulation and Function*, pp 3–36. Plenum Press, New York.
3. Silberstein GB, Van Horn K, Shyamala G, Daniel CW (1994) Essential role of endogenous estrogen in directly stimulating mammary growth demonstrated by implants containing pure antiestrogens. *Endocrinology, 134,* 84–90.
4. Dabelow A (1941) Die postnatale Entwicklung der menschlichen Milchdruse und ihre Korrelationen. *Morphol. J., 85,* 361–416.
5. Neville MC (1983) Regulation of mammary development and lactation. In: Neville MC, Neifert MR (Eds) *Lactation: Physiology, Nutrition and Breast-feeding*, pp 103–140. Plenum Press, New York.
6. Kuhn NJ (1983) The biochemistry of lactogenesis. In: Mepham TB (Ed) *Biochemistry of Lactation*, pp 351–380. Elsevier, Amsterdam.
7. Neville MC, Keller RP, Seacat J, Lutes V, Neifert M, Casey CE, Allen JC, Archer P (1988) Studies in human lactation: milk volumes in lactating women during the onset of lactation and full lactation. *Am. J. Clin. Nutr., 48,* 1375–1386.
8. Neville MC, Allen JC, Archer PC, Dasey DE, Seacat J, Keller RP, Lutes V, Rasbach J, Neifert M (1991) Studies in human lactation: milk volume and nutrient composition during weaning and lactogenesis. *Am. J. Clin. Nutr., 54,* 81–92.
9. Arthur PG, Smith M, Hartmann P (1989) Milk lactose, citrate and glucose as markers of lactogenesis in normal and diabetic women. *J. Ped. Gastroenterol. Nutr., 90,* 488–496.

10. Neubauer SH, Ferris AM, Chase CG, Fanelli J, Thompson CA, Lammi-Keefe CJ, Clark RM, Bendel RB, Green KW (1993) Delayed lactogenesis in women with insulin-dependent diabetes mellitus. *Am. J. Clin. Nutr., 58,* 54–60.
11. Kulski JK, Hartmann PE (1981) Changes in human milk composition during the initiation of lactation. *Aust. J. Exp. Biol. Med. Sci., 59,* 101–114.
12. Neville MC, Allen JC, Watters C (1983) The mechanisms of milk secretion. In: Neville MC, Neifert MR (Eds) *Lactation: Physiology, Nutrition and Breast-feeding*, pp 49–104 Plenum Press, New York.
13. Newton N, Newton M (1967) Psychologic aspects of lactation. *N. Engl. J. Med., 277,* 1179–1183.
14. Prentice A, Addey CP, Wilde CJ (1989) Evidence for local feedback control of human milk secretion. *Biochem. Soc. Trans., 16,* 122.
15. Wilde CJ, Addey CVP, Boddy LM, Peaker M (1995) Autocrine regulation of milk secretion by a protein in milk. *Biochem. J., 305,* 51–58.
16. Lerner L, Jordan VC (1990) Development of antiestrogens and their use in breast cancer: Eighth Cain memorial award lecture. *Cancer Res., 50,* 4177–4189.
17. McLachlan JA (1993) Functional Toxicology: A new approach to detect biologically active xenobiotics. *Environ. Health Perspect., 101,* 386–387.
18. McLachlan JA, Newbold RR, Korach KS, Hogan M (1987) Risk assessment considerations for reproductive and developmental toxicity of oestrogenic xenobiotics. In: Roloff MV, Wilson AW (Eds) *Human Risk Assessment: the Roles of Animal Selection and Extrapolation*, pp 187–193. Taylor and Francis, London.
19. Coezy E, Borgna JL, Rochefort H (1982) Tamoxifen and metabolites in MCF-7 cells. Correlation between binding to estrogen receptor and inhibition of cell growth. *Cancer Res., 42,* 317–323.
20. Biswas R, Vonderhaar BK (1991) Tamoxifen inhibition of prolactin action in the mouse mammary gland. *Endocrinology, 128,* 532–538.
21. Gierthy JF, Lincoln DW (1988) Inhibition of postconfluent focus production in cultures of MCF-7 breast cancer cells by 2,3,7,8-tetrachlorodibenzo-p-dioxin. *Breast Cancer Res. Treat., 12,* 227–233.
22. Gervais M, Tan L (1993) 6-Hydroximinoandrostenedione, a new specific inhibitor of estrogen biosynthesis and its effect on T47D human breast cancer cells. *Anticancer Res., 13,* 383–388.
23. Kadohama N, Shintani K, Osawa Y (1993) Tobacco alkaloid derivatives as inhibitors of breast cancer aromatase. *Cancer Lett., 75,* 175–182.
24. Das RB, Biswas R, Vonderhaar BK (1993) Characteristics of a membrane associated antilactogen binding site for tamoxifen. *Mol. Cell Endocrinol., 98,* 1–8.
25. Lin CL, Buttle HL (1991) Effect of oestradiol benzoate and tamoxifen on the growth of and induction of progesterone receptors in the uterus and mammary gland of immature pigs. *J. Endocrinol., 130,* 259–265.
26. Lin CL, Buttle HL (1994) Progesterone receptor in the mammary tissue of pregnant and lactating gilts and the effect of tamoxifen treatment during late gestation. *J. Endocrinol., 130,* 251–257.
27. Bertazzi PA, Zocchetti C, Pesatori AC, Guerciliena S, Sanarico M, Radice L (1989) Ten-year mortality study of the population involvedin the Seveso indicent in 1976. *Am. J. Epidemiol., 129,* 1187–1200.
28. Safe S, Astroff B, Harris M, Zacharewski T, Dickerson R, Romkes M, Biegel L (1991) 2,3,7,8-tetrchlorodibenzo-p-dioxin (TCDD) and related compounds as antioestrogens: characterization and mechanisms of action. *Pharmacol. Toxicol., 69,* 400–409.
29. Safe S, Krishnan V (1995) Chlorinated hydrocarbons: estrogens and antiestrogens. *Toxicol. Lett., 82–83,* 731–736.

30. Gierthy JF, Lincoln DW, Gillespie MB, Seeger JI, Martinez HL, Dickerman HW, Kuman SA (1987) Suppression of estrogen-regulated extracellular plasminogen activator activity of MCF-7 cells by 2,3,7,8-tetrachlorodibenzo-p-dioxin. *Cancer Res., 47,* 6198–6203.
31. Huff J, Lucier G, Tritscher A (1994) Carcinogenicity of TCDD: experimental, mechanistic, and epidemiologic evidence. *Annu. Rev. Pharmacol. Toxicol., 34,* 343–372.
32. Kociba RJ, Keyes DG, Beyer JE, Carreon RM, Wade CE et al. (1978) Results of a two-year chronic toxicity study and oncogenicity study of 2,3,7,8-tetrachlorodibenzo-p-dioxin in rats. *Toxicol. Appl. Pharmacol., 46,* 279–304.
33. Baron JA, La Vecchia C, Levi F (1990) The antiestrogenic effect of cigarette smoking in women. *Am. J. Obstet. Gynecol., 162,* 502–514.
34. Moore KE (1987) Interactions between prolactin and dopaminergic neurons. *Biol. Reprod., 36,* 47–58.
35. Ben-Jonathan N (1985) Dopamine: a prolactin-inhibiting hormone. *Endocr. Rev., 6,* 564–589.
36. Rendt J, Oxford GS (1994) Absence of coupling between D2 dopamine receptors and calcium channels in lactotrophs from cycling female rats. *Endocrinology, 135,* 501–508.
37. Muller EE, Locatelli V, Cella S, Penalva A, Novelli A, Cocchi D (1983) Prolactin-lowering and -releasing drugs. Mechanisms of action and therapeutic applications. *Drugs, 25,* 399–432.
38. Nyboe Andersen A, Damm P, Tabor A, Pedersen IM, Harring M (1990) Prevention of breast pain and milk secretion with bromocriptine after second-trimester abortion. *Acta Obstet. Gynecol. Scand., 69,* 235–238.
39. Sarapura V, Schlaff WD (1993) Recent advances in the understanding of the pathophysiology and treatment of hyperprolactinemia. *Curr. Opin. Obstet. Gynecol., 5,* 360–367.
40. Jasonni VM, Raffelli R, de March A, Frank G, Flamigni C (1991) Vaginal bromocriptine in hyperprolactinemic patients and puerperal women. *Acta Obstet. Gynecol. Scand., 70,* 493–495.
41. Defoort P, Thiery M, Baele G, Clement D, Dhont M (1987) Bromocriptine in an injectable retard form for puerperal lactation suppression: comparison with Estandron prolongatum. *Obstet. Gynecol., 70,* 866–869.
42. Kremer JA, Rolland R, van der Heijden PF, Schellekens LA, Vosmar MB, Lancranjan I (1990) Lactation inhibition by a single injection of a new depot-bromocriptine. *Br. J. Obstet. Gynaecol., 97,* 527–532.
43. Svanberg L, Lancranjan I, Arvidsson T, Andersch B (1987) Single dose bromocriptine microcapsules in postpartum lactation inhibition. *Acta Obstet. Gynecol. Scand., 66,* 61–62.
44. Valsamis J, Chavez H, Westelinck K, Haemers M, Francis G, L'Hermite M (1987) Inhibition of puerperal lactation by means of a single injection of bromocriptine retard. *Eur. J. Obstet. Gynecol. Reprod. Biol., 25,* 43–51.
45. de Aloysio D, Pamparana F, Zanotti A, Fabiani AG, Bottiglioni F (1988) Dihydroergocristine in stopping lactation: double-blind study vs bromocriptine. *Gynecol. Endocrinol., 2,* 67–71.
46. Zanagnolo VL, Pollini F, Falsetti L, Gastaldi A (1987) Endocrine and clinical results in administering lisuride for inhibiting lactation. *Acta Eur. Fertil., 18,* 21–24.
47. Venturini PL, Horowski R, Fasce V, Valenzano M, Ferreri C, Badino G, Rainer E, Scholz A, De Cecco L (1988) Suppression of puerperal lactation by terguride. A double-blind study. *Gynecol. Obste.t Invest., 26,* 33–38.
48. Franks S, Horrocks PM, Lynch SS, Butt WR, London DR (1981) Treatment of hyperprolactinaemia with pergolide mesylate: acute effects and preliminary evaluation of long-term treatment. *Lancet, 2,* 659–661.
49. Caballero-Gordo A, Lopez-Nazareno N, Calderay M, Caballero JL, Mancheno E, Sghedoni D (1991) Oral cabergoline. Single-dose inhibition of puerperal lactation. *J. Reprod. Med., 36,* 717–721.

50. Giorda G, de Vincentiis S, Motta T, Casazza S, Fadin M, D'Alberton A (1991) Cabergoline versus bromocriptine in suppression of lactation after cesarean delivery. *Gynecol. Obstet. Invest., 31,* 93–96.
51. European Multicentre Study Group for Cabergoline in Lactation Inhibition (1991) Single dose cabergoline versus bromocriptine in inhibition of puerperal lactation: randomised, double blind, multicentre study. *Br. Med. J., 302,* 1367–1371.
52. Melis GB, Gambacciani M, Paoletti AM, Beneventi F, Mais V, Baroldi P, Fioretti P (1987) Dose-related prolactin inhibitory effect of the new long-acting dopamine receptor agonist cabergoline in normal cycling, puerperal, and hyperprolactinemic women. *J. Clin. Endocrinol. Metabol., 65,* 541–545.
53. Melis GB, Mais V, Paoletti AM, Beneventi F, Gambacciani M, Fioretti P (1988) Prevention of puerperal lactation by a single oral administration of the new prolactin-inhibiting drug, cabergoline. *Obstet. Gynecol., 71,* 311–314.
54. Katz M, Kroll D, Pak I, Osimoni A, Hirsch M (1985) Puerperal hypertension, stroke, and seizures after suppression of lactation with bromocriptine. *Obstet. Gynecol., 66,* 822–824.
55. Watson DL, Bhatia RK, Norman GS, Brindley BA, Sokol RJ (1989) Bromocriptine mesylate for lactation suppression: a risk for postpartum hypertension? *Obstet. Gynecol., 74,* 573–576.
56. Nappi C, Colace G, Affinito P, Taglialatela M, Di Renzo GF, Montemagno U, Annunziato L (1990) Ibopamine-induced reduction of serum prolactin level and milk secretion in puerperal women. *Eur. J. Clin. Pharmacol., 39,* 133–135.
57. van der Heijden PF, Kremer JA, Brownell J, Rolland R (1991) Lactation inhibition by the dopamine agonist CV 205–502. *Br. J. Obstet. Gynaecol., 98,* 270–276.
58. Turkington RW (1972) Inhibition of prolactin secretion and successful therapy of the Forbes-Albright syndrome with L-dopa. *J. Clin. Endocrinol. Metabol., 34,* 306–311.
59. DeLeo V, Cella SG, Camanni F, Genazzani AR, Muller EE (1983) Prolactin lowering effect of amphetamine in normoprolactinemic subjects and in physiological and pathological hyperprolactinemia. *Horm. Metabol. Res., 15,* 439–443.
60. Scanlon MF, Gomez-Pan A, Mora B, Cook DB, Dewar JH, Hildyard A, Weightman DR, Evered DC, Hall R (1977) Effects of nomifensine, an inhibitor of endogenous catecholamine re-uptake, in acromegaly, in hyperprolactinaemia, and against stimulated prolactin release in man. *Br. J. Clin. Pharmacol., 4 (Suppl 2),* 191S–197S.
61. Kuruvilla A, Peedicayil J, Srikrishna G, Kuruvilla K, Kanagasabapathy AS (1992) A study of serum prolactin levels in schizophrenia: comparison of males and females. *Clin. Exp. Pharmacol. Physiol., 19,* 603–606.
62. Meltzer HY (1985) Long-term effects of neuroleptic drugs on the neuroendocrine system. *Adv. Biochem. Psychopharmacol., 40,* 59–68.
63. von Bahr C, Wiesel FA, Movin G, Eneroth P, Jansson P, Nilsson L, Ogenstad S (1991) Neuroendocrine responses to single oral doses of remoxipride and sulpiride in healthy female and male volunteers. *Psychopharmacology (Berlin), 103,* 443–448.
64. Tsubura A, Hatano T, Murata A, Shoji T, Shikata N, Morii S (1992) Breast carcinoma in patients receiving neuroleptic therapy. Morphologic and clinicopathologic features of thirteen cases. *Acta. Pathol. Jpn., 42,* 494–499.
65. Lamberts SW, van Koetsveld PM, Hofland LJ (1990) The effect of clozapine on prolactin secretion at the level of the lactotroph. *Life Sci., 46,* 1013–1019.
66. Meltzer HY, Goode DJ, Schyve PM, Young M, Fang VS (1979) Effect of clozapine on human serum prolactin levels. *Am. J. Psychiatry, 136,* 1550–1555.
67. McCallum RW, Valenzuela G, Polepalle S, Spyker D (1991) Subcutaneous metoclopramide in the treatment of symptomatic gastroparesis: clinical efficacy and pharmacokinetics. *J. Pharmacol. Exp. Ther., 258,* 136–142.

68. Liu JH, Lee DW, Markoff E (1990) Differential release of prolactin variants in postpartum and early follicular phase women. *J. Clin. Endocrinol. Metabol., 71,* 605–610.
69. Ertl T, Sulyok E, Ezer E, Sarkany I, Thurzo V, Csaba IF (1991) The influence of metoclopramide on the composition of human breast milk. *Acta Paediatr. Hung., 31,* 415–422.
70. Hofmeyr G, Van Iddekinge B, Blott J (1985) Domperidone: secretion in breast milk and effect on puerperal prolactin levels. *Br. J. Obstet. Gynecol., 92,* 141–144.
71. Flores CM, Hulihan-Giblin BA, Hornby PJ, Lumpkin MD, Kellar KJ (1992) Partial characterization of a neurotransmitter pathway regulating the in vivo release of prolactin. *Neuroendocrinology, 55,* 519–528.
72. Hulihan-Giblin BA, Lumpkin MD, Kellar KJ (1990) Acute effects of nicotine on prolactin release in the rat: agonist and antagonist effects of a single injection of nicotine. *J. Pharmacol. Exp. Ther., 252,* 15–20.
73. Kiem DT, Fekete MI, Bartha L, Nagy G, Makara GB (1991) Prolactin response to morphine in intact and adrenalectomized lactating rats. *Brain Res., 563,* 171–174.
74. Grossman A (1988) Opioids and stress in man. *J. Endocrinol., 119,* 377–381.
75. Gordon K, Hodgen GD, Richardson DW (1992) Postpartum lactational anovulation in a nonhuman primate (Macaca fascicularis): endogenous opiate mediation of suckling-induced hyperprolactinemia. *J. Clin. Endocrinol. Metabol., 75,* 59–67.
76. Baumann MH, Rabii J (1991) Inhibition of suckling-induced prolactin release by mu- and kappa-opioid antagonists. *Brain Res., 567,* 224–230.
77. Samuels MH, Sanborn CF, Hofeldt F, Robbins R (1991) The role of endogenous opiates in athletic amenorrhea. *Fertil. Steril., 55,* 507–512.
78. Jorgensen H, Knigge U, Warberg J (1992) Involvement of 5-HT1, 5-HT2, and 5-HT3 receptors in the mediation of the prolactin response to serotonin and 5-hydroxytryptophan. *Neuroendocrinology, 55,* 336–343.
79. Price LH, Charney DS, Delgado PL, Goodman WK, Krystal JH, Woods SW, Heninger GR (1990) Clinical data on the role of serotonin in the mechanism(s) of action of antidepressant drugs. *J. Clin. Psychiatry, 51 (Suppl),* 44–50; discussion 51–2.
80. Mitchell PB, Smythe GA (1991) Endocrine and amine responses to D,L-fenfluramine in normal subjects. *Psychiatry Res., 39,* 141–153.
81. Urban RJ, Veldhuis JD (1991) A selective serotonin reuptake inhibitor, fluoxetine hydrochloride, modulates the pulsatile release of prolactin in postmenopausal women. *Am. J. Obstet. Gynecol., 164,* 147–152.
82. Scheinin M, Koulu M, Karhuvaara S, Zimmer RH (1990) Evidence that the reversible MAO-A inhibitor moclobemide increases prolactin secretion by a serotonergic mechanism in healthy male volunteers. *Life Sci., 47,* 1491–1499.
83. Kahn RS, Wetzler S (1991) m-Chlorophenylpiperazine as a probe of serotonin function. *Biol. Psychiatry, 30,* 1139–1166.
84. Dinan TG, Yatham LN, Barry S, Chua A, Keeling PW (1990) Serotonin supersensitivity: the pathophysiologic basis of non-ulcer dyspepsia? A preliminary report of buspirone/prolactin responses. *Scand. J. Gastroenterol., 25,* 541–544.
85. Bjoro T, Sand O, Ostberg BC, Gordeladze JO, Torjesen P, Gautvik KM, Haug E (1990) The mechanisms by which vasoactive intestinal peptide (VIP) and thyrotropin releasing hormone (TRH) stimulate prolactin release from pituitary cells. *Biosci. Rep., 10,* 189–199.
86. Martinez de la Escalera G, Weiner RI (1992) Dissociation of dopamine from its receptor as a signal in the pleiotropic hypothalamic regulation of prolactin secretion. *Endocr. Rev., 13,* 241–255.
87. Asukai K, Uemura T, Minaguchi H (1993) Occult hyperprolactinemia in infertile women. *Fertil. Steril., 60,* 423–427.

88. Kira J, Harada M, Yamaguchi Y, Shida N, Goto I (1991) Hyperprolactinemia in multiple sclerosis. *J. Neurol. Sci., 102,* 61–66.
89. Vilaro S, Vinas O, Remesar X, Herrera E (1987) Effects of chronic ethanol consumption on lactational performance in rat: mammary gland and milk composition and pups' growth and metabolism. *Pharmacol. Biochem. Behav., 27,* 333–339.
90. Cobo E (1973) Effect of different doses of ethanol on the milk ejection reflex in lactating women. *Am. J. Obstet. Gynecol., 115,* 817–821.
91. Coiro V, Alboni A, Gramellini D, Cigarini C, Bianconi L, Pignatti D, Volpi R, Chiodera P (1992) Inhibition by ethanol of the oxytocin response to breast stimulation in normal women and the role of endogenous opioids. *Acta Endocrinol., 126,* 213–216.
92. Little RE, Anderson EW, Ervin CH, Worthington-Roberts B, Clarret SK (1989) Maternal alcohol use during breast-feeding and infant mental and motor development at one year. *N. Engl. J. Med., 321,* 425–430.
93. Haldar J, Sawyer WH (1978) Inhibition of oxytocin release by morphine and its analogs. *Proc. Soc. Exp. Biol. Med., 157,* 476–480.
94. Rayner VC, Robinson IC, Russell JA (1988) Chronic intracerebroventricular morphine and lactation in rats: dependence and tolerance in relation to oxytocin neurones. *J. Physiol., 396,* 319–347.
95. Russell JA, Coombes JE, Leng G, Bicknell RJ (1993) Morphine tolerance and inhibition of oxytocin secretion by kappa-opioids acting on the rat neurohypophysis. *J. Physiol., 469,* 365–386.
96. Prilusky J, Deis RP (1976) Inhibitory effect of prostaglandin F2 alpha (PGF2alpha) on oxytocin rlease and on milk ejection in lactating rats. *J. Endocrinol., 69,* 395–399.
97. Cobo E, Rodriguez A, De Villamizar M (1974) Milk-ejecting activity induced by prostaglandin F2 alpha. *Am. J. Obstet. Gynecol., 118,* 831–836.
98. McNeilly AS, Fox CA (1971) The effect of prostaglandins on the guinea-pig mammary gland. *J. Endocrinol., 51,* 603–604.
99. Batta SK, Gagliano PG, Martini L (1974) Effect of prostaglandins E_1 and F_{2a} on the isolated mammary gland of nursing rats. *Proc. Soc. Exp. Biol. Med., 146,* 912–917.
100. England MJ, Tjallinks A, Hofmeyr J, Harber J (1988) Suppression of lactation. A comparison of bromocriptine and prostaglandin E2. *J. Reprod. Med., 33,* 630–632.
101. Neville MC, Berga SE (1983) Cellular and molecular aspects of the hormonal control of mammary function. In: Neville MC, Neifert MR (Eds) *Lactation: Physiology, Nutrition and Breast-feeding*, pp 141–177. Plenum Press, New York.
102. Bissell MJ, Hall HG (1987) Form and function in the mammary gland: the role of extracellular matrix. In: Neville MC, Daniel CW (Eds) *The Mammary Gland: Development, Regulation and Function.* Plenum Press, New York.
103. Cowie AT, Lyons WR (1959) Mammogenesis and lactogenesis in hypophysectomized, ovariectomized, adrenalectomized rats. *J. Endocrinol., 19,* 29–32.
104. Cowie AT (1969) General hormonal factors involved in lactogenesis. In: Reynolds M, Folley SJ (Eds) *Lactogenesis, the Initiation of Milk Secretion at Parturition*, pp 157–169. University of Pennsylvania Press, Philadelphia, PA.
105. Bhattacharjee M, Vonderhaar BK (1984) Thyroid hormones enhance the synthesis and secretion of alpha-lactalbumin by mouse mammary tissue in vitro. *Endocrinology, 115,* 1070–1077.
106. Davis SR, Gluckman PD, Hart IC, Henderson HV (1987) Effects of injecting growth hormone or thyroxine on milk production and blood plasma concentrations of insulin-like growth factors I and II in dairy cows. *J. Endocrinol., 114,* 17–24.
107. Markin KE, Wolst MD (1960) A comparative controlled study of hormones used in the prevention of postpartum breast engorgement and lactation. *Am. J. Obstet. Gynecol., 80,* 128–137.
108. Walker S, Hibbard BM, Groom G, Griffiths K, Harvard-Davis R (1975) Controlled trial of bro-

mocriptine, quinoestrol, and placebo in suppression of puerperal lactation. *Lancet, 2,* 842–845.
109. Morris JA, Creasy RK, Hohe PT (1970) Inhibition of puerperal lactation: double blind comparison of chlorotrianisene, testosterone ethanate with estradiol valerate and placebo. *Obstet. Gynecol., 36,* 107–114.
110. Shyamala G, Singh RK, Ruh MF, Ruh TS (1986) Relationships between mammary estrogen receptor and estrogenic sensitivity. II. Binding of cytoplasmic receptor to chromatin. *Endocrinology, 119,* 819–826.
111. Nilson PA, Meling AB, Abildgaard U (1976) Study of the suppression of lactation and influence on blood clotting with bromocriptine (CB 154) (Parlodel): a double blind comparison with diethylstilbestrol. *Acta Obstet. Gynecol., 55,* 39–44.
112. Miller GH, Hughes LR (1970) Lactation and genital involution effects of a new low-dose oral contraceptive on breastfeeding mothers and their infants. *Obstet. Gynecol., 35,* 44–50.
113. Koetsawang S, Bhiraleus P, Chiemprajert T (1972) Effects of oral contraceptives on lactation. *Fertil. Steril., 23,* 24–28.
114. Guiloff E, Ibarra-olo A, Zanartu J, Toscanini C, Mischler TW, Gomez-Rogers C (1974) Effect of contraception on lactation. *Am. J. Obstet. Gynecol., 118,* 42–45.
115. Diaz S, Peralta O, Juez F, Herreros C, Casado ME, Salvatierra AM, Miranda P, Durán E, Croxatto HB (1983) Fertility regulation in nursing women. III. Short term influence of a low dose combined oral contraceptive upon lactation and infant growth. *Contraception, 27,* 1–11.
116. Croxatto HB, Diaz S, Peralta O, Juez G, Casado ME, Salvatierra AM, Miranda P, Durán E (1983) Fertility regulation in nursing women. IV. Long term influence of a low dose combined oral contraceptive initiated at day 30 postpartum upon lactation and infant growth. *Contraception, 27,* 13–25.
117. Peralta O, Diaz S, Juez G, Herreros C, Casado ME, Salvatierra AM, Miranda P, Durán E, Croxatto HB (1983) Fertility regulation in nursing women. V. Long term effect of a low dose combined oral contraceptive initiated at day 90 postpartum upon lactation and infant growth. *Contraception, 27,* 27–38.
118. Tankeyoon M, Dusitsin N, Chalapati S, Koetsawang S, Saibiang S, Sas M, Gellen JJ, Ayeni O, Gray R, Pinol A (1984) Effects of hormonal contraceptives on milk volume and infant growth. WHO special programme of research, development and research training in human reproduction task force on oral contraceptives. *Contraception, 30,* 505–522.
119. Nilsson S, Mellibin T, Hofvander Y, Sundelin C, Valentin J, Nygren KG (1984) Long term follow-up of children breastfed by mothers using oral contraceptives. *Contraception, 34,* 443–457.
120. Heikkilå M, Luukkainen T (1982) Duration of beastfeeding and development of children after insertion of a levonorgestrel-releasing intrauterine contraceptive device. *Contraception, 25,* 279–292.
121. Jimenez J, Ochoa M, Soler MP, Portales P (1984) Long-term follow-up of children breast-fed by mothers receiving depot-medroxyprogesterone acetate. *Contraception, 30,* 523–533.
122. Zacharias S, Aguilera E, Assenzo JR, Zanartu J (1986) Effects of hormonal and nonhormonal contraceptives on lactation and incidence of pregnancy. *Contraception, 33,* 203–213.
123. Gupta AM, Mathur VS, Garg SK (1974) Effect of oral contraceptives on quantity and quality of mlk secretion in human beings. *Indian J. Med. Res., 62,* 964–970.
124. Toddywalla VS, Joshi L, Virkar K (1977) Effect of contraceptive steroids on human lactation. *Am. J. Obstet. Gynecol., 127,* 245–249.
125. Kora SJ (1969) Effect of oral contraceptives on lactation. *Fertil. Steril., 20,* 419–423.
126. Borglin NE, Sandholm L-E (1971) Effect of oral contraceptives on lactation. *Fertil. Steril., 22,* 48–51.
127. World Health Organization (WHO) Task Force on Oral Contraceptives (1988) Effects of hormo-

nal contraceptives on breast milk composition and infant growth. *Studies Fam. Planning, 19,* 361–369.
128. Costa TH, Dorea JG (1992) Concentration of fat, protein, lactose and energy in milk of mothers using hormonal contraceptives. *Ann. Trop. Paediatr., 12,* 203–209.
129. Abdel Kader MM (1975) Effect of two long acting injectable progestogens on lactation in the human. *Acta Biol. Med. Germ., 34,* 1199–1204.
130. Affandi B, Karmadibrata S, Prihartono J, Lubis F, Samil RS (1986) Effect of Norplant on mothers and infants in the postpartum period. *Adv. Contracept., 2,* 371–380.
131. Campodonico I, Guerro B, Landa LI (1978) Effectof a low-dose oral contraceptive (150 micrograms levonorgestrel and 30 micrograms ethinylestradiol) on lactation. *Clin. Therap., 1,* 454–459.
132. Pardthaisong T, Yenchit C, Gray R (1992) The long-term growth and development of children exposed to Depo-Provera during pregnancy or lactation. *Contraception, 45,* 313–324.
133. Who Task Force on Long-Acting Agents for Fertility Regulation (1986) Metabolic side-effects of injectable depot-medroxyprogesterone acetate, 150 mg three-monthly, in undernourished lactating women. *Bull. WHO, 64,* 587–594.
134. Shyamala G, Schneider W, Schott D (1990) Developmental regulation of murine mammary progesterone receptor gene expression. *Endocrinology, 126,* 2882–2889.
135. Bauman DE, Vernon RG (1993) Effects of exogenous bovine somatotropin on lactation. *Annu. Rev. Nutr., 13,* 437–461.
136. Milsom SR, Breier BH, Gallaher BW, Cox VA, Gluckman PD (1992) Growth hormone stimulates galactopoiesis in healthy lactating women. *Acta Endocrinol., 127,* 337–343.
137. Walsh C, Neville MC (1994) Effect of xenobiotics on milk secretion and composition. *J. Nutr. Biochem., 5,* 418–441.
138. Tedstone AE, Tedoldi B, Ilic V, Williamson DH (1989) Polymyxcin B diminshes blood flow to brown adipose tissue and lactating mammary gland in the rat. Possible mechanism of its action to decrease the stimulation of lipogenesis on refeeding. *Biochem. J., 261,* 445–450.
139. Patton S (1974) Reversible supppression of lactation by colchicine. *FEBS Lett., 48,* 85–87.
140. Henderson AJ, Peaker M (1980) The effects of colchicine on milk secretion, mammary metabolism and blood flow in the goat. *Q. J. Exp. Physiol., 65,* 367–378.
141. Ben-Ze'ev A (1987) The role of changes in cell shape and contacts in the regulation of cytoskeleton expression during differentiation. *J. Cell Sci., 8(Suppl),* 293–312.
142. Taketani Y, Oka T (1983) Tumor promoter 12-O-tetradecanoylphorbol 13-acetate, like epidermal growth factor, stimulates cell proliferation and inhibits differentiation of mouse mammary epithelial cells in culture. *Proc. Natl. Acad. Sci. USA, 80,* 1646–1649.
143. Martel P, Houdebine LM, Teyssot B, Djiane J (1983) Effects of phorbol esters on multiplication and differentiation of mammary cells. *Biol. Cell, 49,* 119–126.
144. Werb A, Clark EJ (1989) Phorbol diesters regulate expression of the membrane neutral metalloendopeptidase (EC 3.4.24.11) in rabbit synovial fibroblasts and mammary epithelial cells. *J. Biol. Chem., 264,* 9111–9113.
145. Nagasawa H, Yanai R, Nakajima Y (1980) Suppression of lactation by tumor promoters in mice. *Proc. Soc. Exp. Biol. Med., 165,* 394–397.
146. Carpenter G (1990) PLC and PKC: A tale of two messengers. *New Biologist, 2,* 965–969.
147. Dostal LA, Weaver RP, Schwetz BA (1987) Transfer of di(2-ethyl) phthalate through rat milk and effects on milk composition and the mammary gland. *Toxicol. App. Pharmacol., 91,* 315–325.
148. Menzer RE (1991) Water and soil pollutants. In: Amdur MO, Doull J, Klaassen C (Eds) *Casarett and Doull's Toxicology*, pp 872–902. Pergamon, New York.

Drugs and Human Lactation
P.N. Bennett, editor

3. Determinants of drug transfer into human milk

Evan J Begg

There are three major components affecting drug transfer into human milk and thence into the suckling infant (Table 1). These are maternal pharmacokinetics, mammary pharmacokinetics and neonatal pharmacology. The first two components are discussed here. The third component is reviewed in Chapter 4.

The interdependent nature of these components is illustrated in Fig. 1. The cascade of events begins with ingestion of drug by the mother. The dose regimen and the pharmacokinetics of the drug determine the concentration in maternal plasma. The milk concentration is in turn related to the maternal plasma concentration.

The amount of drug ingested by the infant (the infant dose) depends on the milk concentration and the volume of milk consumed over time. The final concentration of the drug in the infant's plasma depends on the dose ingested via milk and the infant's pharmacokinetics.

THE MILK TO PLASMA CONCENTRATION RATIO (M/P)

The milk to plasma concentration ratio (M/P) captures the net effect of maternal and mammary pharmacokinetics. The M/P ratio is crucial to the estimation of the 'dose' ingested by the infant (Table 2).

It follows that the M/P ratio must be known accurately if doses of drugs ingested by the infant via milk are to be calculated. Unfortunately the M/P ratio may vary according to a wide variety of factors including the time of sampling after maternal

TABLE 1 *Components of drug transfer from mother to suckling infant*

1. Maternal pharmacokinetics	Drug disposition in the mother as it relates to presentation of drug to the breast for secretion in milk
2. Mammary pharmacokinetics	Transfer and sojourn of drugs in milk in relation to the formation and excretion of milk
3. Neonatal pharmacology	Absorption and disposition (distribution and elimination) of drugs delivered in milk to the child, and the effects on the child

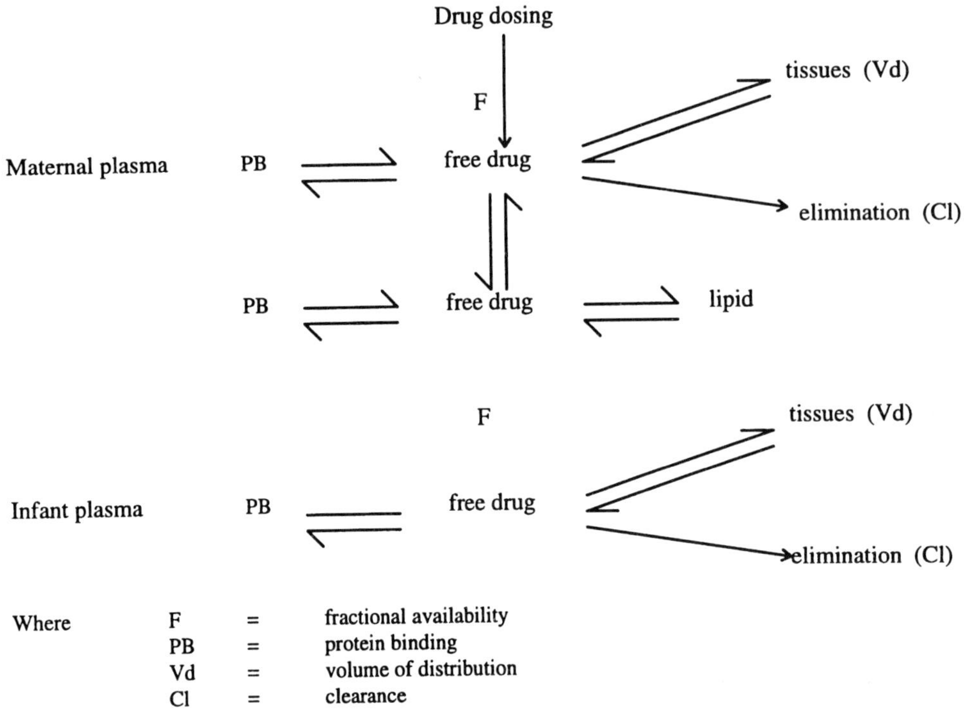

FIG. 1 *Passage of drug from maternal ingestion to the infant.*

ingestion, the route of administration, single dosing versus steady-state dosing, immature versus mature milk, and fore- versus hind-milk samples (1).

A pitfall in the understanding of the M/P ratio is the assumption that the milk and plasma concentrations parallel each other throughout the maternal dosing interval. This is often true, but equally it is sometimes not true. Fig. 2(a) illustrates the simplest case (one-compartment model) where milk and plasma concentrations do parallel each other throughout the dosing interval. Fig. 2(b) illustrates the more complex case where milk and plasma concentrations do not parallel each other. In this case the milk 'compartment' is behaving as a peripheral pharmacokinetic com-

TABLE 2 *Drug dose received by the infant via breast milk*

General calculation	Dose (mg/kg/day)	=	C_{avg} × M/P × milk volume (ml/kg/day)
Worst case analysis	Dose (mg/kg/day)	=	C_{max} × M/P × milk volume (ml/kg/day)

where C_{avg} and C_{max} are respective average and maximum drug concentrations in maternal plasma at the time of feeding; M/P is the milk to plasma ratio; milk volume is 150 ml/kg per day on average

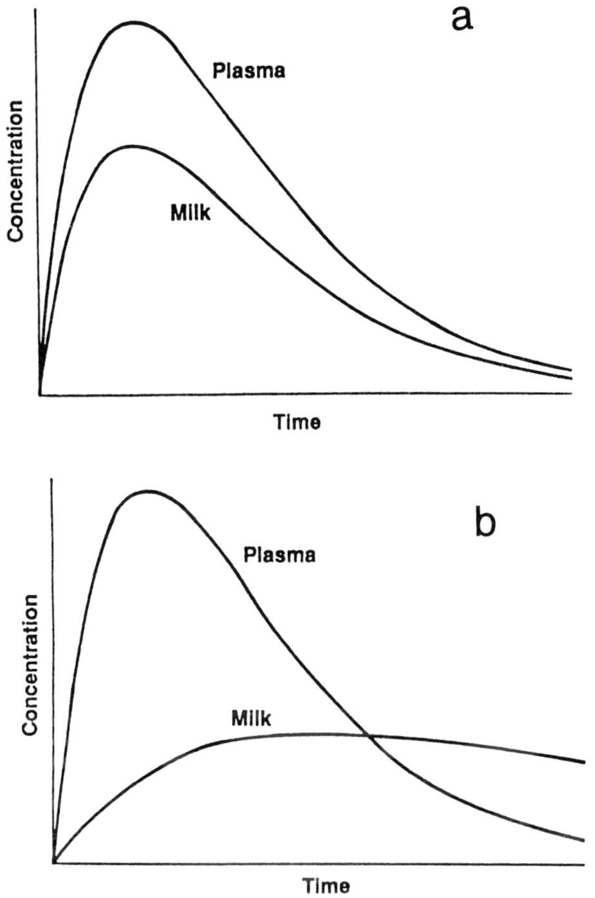

FIG. 2 *Concentration–time profile of drug in milk and plasma. (a) M/P ratio constant at all times. (b) M/P ratio varies with time.*

partment. Drugs which distribute slowly into milk will show peripheral compartment characteristics. Such drugs will accumulate in milk over time with multiple dosing, and the M/P ratio will rise slowly. The folly of single time-point estimations of M/P ratio is self-evident.

Inaccuracy in the estimation of the M/P ratio can be avoided by the use of the M/P_{AUC} ratio. The M/P_{AUC} ratio is based on the areas under the respective milk and plasma concentration–time curves.

The AUC in plasma and milk can be calculated using the trapezoidal rule. After single doses, the AUC from zero to infinity ($AUC_{0-\infty}$) is calculated. The trapezoidal rule enables the area up until the time of the last concentration measured (C_{last}) to be calculated, after which an extrapolation to infinity is necessary.

The extrapolated area is calculated by dividing the last concentration by the slope of the terminal part of the log-linear concentration-time curve. The larger the extrapolated area compared with the measured area, the less accurate is the overall assessment of the AUC. Generally the extrapolated area should be <10% of the total area.

After multiple samples the AUC is calculated in plasma and milk over a dose interval ($AUC_{0-\delta}$). Because no extrapolation is needed such AUCs are likely to be more accurate than those after single doses. The $AUC_{0-\infty}$ after single doses in fact equals the $AUC_{0-\delta}$ at steady-state after multiple administration of the same dose, providing the pharmacokinetics are not concentration dependent.

MATERNAL PHARMACOKINETICS

The dose regimen and maternal pharmacokinetics determine the maternal plasma concentration–time profile. The shape of this profile is determined by the rate of absorption (if the route is not i.v.), the volume of distribution (Vd), the clearance (Cl), and plasma protein binding (PB) (see Fig. 1). The net effect of all these parameters determines the unbound drug concentration in plasma. Unbound drug in plasma equilibrates with that in milk in mammary tissue according to the physicochemical properties of the drug and the physiological properties of the plasma and milk. The M/P ratio reflects this equilibrium.

Unfortunately the maternal pharmacokinetics are by no means constant in the lactation period. The early postpartum period is a time of physiological turmoil for the mother as her body adjusts from the pregnant to the postpartum state. The M/P ratio is therefore likely to vary according to the physiological state existing at the time of drug administration.

MATERNAL PHARMACOKINETICS DURING LACTATION

It is important to understand the maternal pharmacokinetics during lactation for two reasons. Firstly, it allows the mother to be dosed appropriately for her medical condition. Secondly, it enables the maternal plasma concentrations to be estimated, which in turn allows the estimation of the dose received by the infant through suckling (see Table 2).

Little is known about the kinetics of drugs during lactation. More is known about drug disposition during late pregnancy, which is therefore a useful starting point for discussion (Fig. 3).

Pharmacokinetics in the early postpartum period can be viewed as having characteristics similar to those of late pregnancy before settling down to the true lactational state as the effects of pregnancy wear off. This is discussed under three headings: clearance, volume of distribution, and protein binding.

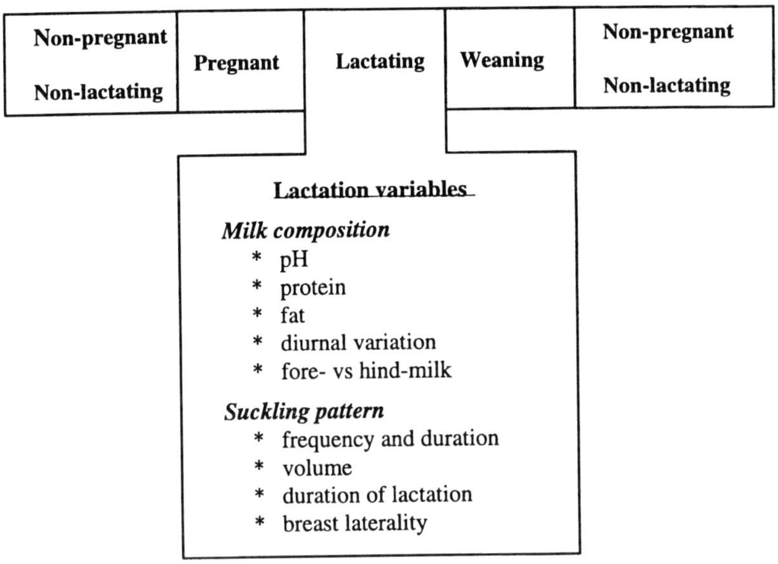

FIG. 3 *Sequence of cyclic events in the life of a woman, and variables in relation to lactation.*

Clearance

Clearance (Cl) determines the average steady-state concentrations (Cp_{ss}) of drug in the plasma during maintenance dosing (MD), i.e. MD = Cl $\times$ Cp_{ss}.

The state of pregnancy is associated with increased clearance of many drugs. Pregnancy is a hyperdynamic state in which the primary processes of drug elimination are enhanced. Clearance is related to both the rate of presentation of the drug to the eliminating organ (mainly liver and kidney) and to the intrinsic capacity of the organ to eliminate the drug. Drugs which are eliminated unchanged through the kidney have increased clearance in pregnancy because of increased renal plasma flow and glomerular filtration rate. Drugs which undergo hepatic metabolism may have increased clearance because at least some important enzymes of the cytochrome P450 mixed function oxidase system seem to be induced (2, 3). Just how many drugs are affected and how long these changes persist after parturition is not known. A review of this area was provided by Nation (1980) (4).

The state of lactation provides a potential additional route for drug elimination, via the milk itself; i.e. $Cl_{total} = Cl_{renal} + Cl_{metabolic} + Cl_{milk} + Cl_{...}$

Drug clearance in milk can occur simply by elimination of unchanged drug contained in the milk, or by metabolism within the milk. Such metabolism has been shown for sulphonilamide which undergoes N-acetylation (5). Although there will always be some clearance of drug via the milk through these processes, it is unlikely that the contribution of this to total drug clearance is very important. Calculations based on M/P ratios and milk volumes indicate that for most drugs the contribution of Cl_{milk} to Cl_{total} is inconsequential (6).

Maternal clearance is relevant to discussion about drug transfer into milk only because it determines the unbound concentration of drug in maternal plasma and therefore the amount of drug that can equilibrate with milk (see Fig. 1). The unbound concentration of drug in plasma is also considered to be the most important component for determining drug action in the mother. The steady-state unbound drug concentrations are likely to be the same in the non-pregnant/non-lactating state, even though doses to achieve these concentrations might be different. Therefore, provided dosing in the mother is appropriate to achieve a given unbound plasma concentration, the clearance can be effectively ignored and only the unbound concentration needs to be considered in relation to drug transfer into milk.

Volume of distribution (Vd)

During pregnancy, body water and fat are both increased and there is the extra 'compartment' of the fetus/placenta to consider. The Vd of most drugs, both water soluble and lipid soluble, will therefore be increased, although the degree is not great. The Vd determines the loading dose (LD) of drug to achieve a desired peak concentration (i.e. $LD = Vd \times Cp_{desired}$). It is important for drugs in which the action relates to the peak plasma concentration, e.g. paracetamol, frusemide, or for drugs which require loading doses for early drug effect, e.g. phenytoin.

In lactation the Vd is also potentially larger than in the non-pregnant, non-lactating state because of the additional milk 'compartment'. The volume of distribution of the milk compartment (Vd_{milk}) can be calculated using the M/P ratio and the volume of milk (6). For most drugs the milk compartment is very small and contributes little to the total volume of distribution (<1%) (6). It is therefore unlikely that the milk compartment has a significant influence on maternal drug concentrations. The absolute value of the Vd of a drug is important, however, in calculating the peak plasma concentration which will result after a loading dose, or during the dose interval. This concentration will influence the amount of drug in milk, via the M/P ratio.

Protein binding (PB)

Plasma protein binding is a much abused and misunderstood pharmacokinetic parameter (7). Its importance lies only in the fact that drug concentrations, as usually measured in body fluids, reflect both protein bound and unbound drug; i.e. plasma concentration = unbound drug + protein bound drug (Fig. 4).

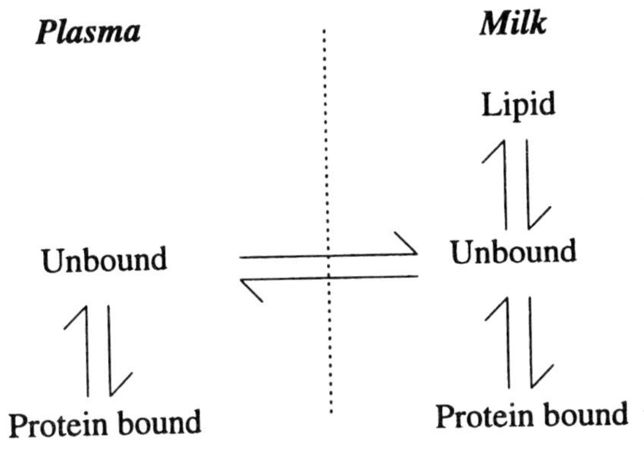

FIG. 4 *Milk:plasma partitioning of drug.*

If it were practical routinely to measure unbound concentrations of drug, then no discussion about protein binding would be necessary, because only unbound drug is able to cross into breast milk (Fig. 1). Protein bound drug in plasma could then be thought of as part of the volume of distribution of unbound drug.

Because the total drug, i.e. both protein bound and unbound is measured in conventional assays, the M/P ratio is based on the total drug concentration. Protein binding is therefore important in our understanding of the M/P ratio.

Protein binding of many drugs is altered in pregnancy and in the early postpartum period. Acidic drugs, such as phenytoin (8), diazepam (9, 10) and salicylate (10), which are largely bound to albumin, show the greatest change in protein binding. This is a result of a decrease in the albumin concentration, a change in binding affinity, and the presence of endogenous compounds which displace drugs from protein binding sites (10). Plasma protein binding returns to normal about 5–7 weeks after parturition.

The importance of altered protein binding, from the maternal perspective, is that the total drug concentration necessary for a given effect will be different. Unbound concentrations, if measured, would not be different because these arc determined solely by unbound drug clearance.

For practical purposes, the assessment of drugs whose concentrations are measured in therapeutic drug monitoring, e.g. phenytoin, needs to take into account altered protein binding so that a realistic assessment of the unbound drug concentration can be made and dosing is appropriate, i.e. the 'normal therapeutic range' for total phenytoin does not apply (7).

As far as the drug concentration in milk is concerned, altered protein binding will affect the measured M/P ratio based on total plasma drug concentrations. The M/P ratio thus measured would be expected to be different in the early, versus the later, postpartum period.

MAMMARY PHARMACOKINETICS

Breast physiology (see also Chapter 2)

Mammary tissue has the gross appearance of a multilobular structure composed of alveoli and ducts (11). Macroscopic anatomy reveals multiple acini which empty into small milk ducts (both surrounded by myoepithelial cells) from which milk is then discharged into lactiferous ducts (11). These ducts terminate in a lactiferous sinus which ends in the nipple for milk delivery. A licking and sucking manoeuvre by the infant allows milk to be expressed by compression of these sinuses. Morphological changes in breast structure and alveolar organelles occur during pregnancy, lactation and following cessation of feeding.

In the resting state the alveolus is free of secretary material and the lumen is small. The alveolar cells are also small and contain few organelles. The lactating alveolus has secretary material in the lumen and the cell contains abundant endoplasmic reticulum and Golgi apparatus. The cytoplasm is markedly increased relative to the nucleus at the time of parturition (12). There is increased intracellular storage of protein and fat, and enlargement of intercellular spaces. Both synthetic and glycolytic enzyme changes occur with lactation (13) which could impact on milk transport or metabolism.

Hormonal regulation

Milk production is dependent on hormones. Prolactin is required for lactose formation, and oestrogens and progesterone promote duct, lobular and alveolar development. Supportive hormones for milk production include growth hormone, parathormone, thyroid hormone, insulin and cortisol (14). Insulin, hydrocortisone and prolactin are important in cellular differentiation. Oxytocin contracts myoepithelial cells to express milk into ducts. Oxytocin and prolactin production corresponds to the amount of milk consumed by the infant, and the suckling vigour.

Milk composition

Milk is a suspension of fat droplets in an aqueous phase containing protein, lactose and electrolytes. The three main constituents of breast milk which are important for drug distribution are the aqueous itself, protein and fat (Table 3). Variations in the concentrations of these components will be accompanied by altered M/P ratios.

Drug in the aqueous phase

Milk and plasma are separated from each other by a biological barrier through which unbound drug passes in accordance with the principles of passive diffusion and pH partitioning theory.

TABLE 3 *Drug distribution in breast milk*

Fat		**Aqueous**		**Protein**
Drug dissolved in or on milk lipid	$\rightleftharpoons$	Free drug	$\rightleftharpoons$	Drug bound to: – albumin – lactoferrin – α-lactalbumin – other

The mean pH of milk is lower than that of plasma, and steady-state distribution of unbound drug between milk and plasma (Mu/Pu ratio) may be predicted by a rearrangement of the Henderson–Hasselbalch equation (13).
For acidic drugs:

$$\text{Mu} / \text{Pu} = \frac{1 + 10^{(\text{pHm}-\text{pKa})}}{1 + 10^{(\text{pKa}-\text{pHp})}}$$

For basic drugs:

$$\text{Mu} / \text{Pu} = \frac{1 + 10^{(\text{pKa}-\text{pHm})}}{1 + 10^{(\text{pKa}-\text{pHp})}}$$

where pHm and pHp are the pH of milk and plasma, respectively.

These equations predict that the Mu/Pu ratio will be <1 for acidic drugs, >1 for basic drugs, and 1 for neutral drugs. Variations in pH during breast feeding may, in theory, alter the Mu/Pu ratio (14). Just how important this is in clinical practice is not known.

Drugs in lipid

Lipid is present in milk as triglycerides, cholesterol and free fatty acids, coalescing into fat droplets. Drugs partition into milk lipid in accordance with their lipophilic characteristics. There is a high degree of correlation ($r^2 = 0.94$) between the log milk lipid/ultrafiltrate partition coefficient and the log of the octanol/water partition coefficient (15). The octanol/water partition coefficient can be used to predict the milk lipid/ultrafiltrate partition coefficient.

Drugs bound to milk protein

The total protein concentration in milk (10.3 g/l) (16) is lower than in plasma (74.6 g/l) (17). Whey proteins account for 70–80% of milk proteins and comprise, in order of decreasing concentrations, α-lactalbumin, lactoferrin, IgA, albumin and lysozyme. Casein accounts for the remainder. Alpha 1 acid glycoprotein is not a

TABLE 4 *General guidelines regarding drug transfer into milk*

1.	Highly ionised drugs tend not to concentrate in milk
2.	Basic drugs have higher milk concentrations than acidic drugs
3.	Drugs with high lipid solubility (high octanol/water partition coefficients) will tend to concentrate in milk
4.	Highly protein bound drugs are less likely to achieve high concentrations in milk

significant component of milk. The protein binding of drugs in milk is less than in plasma, and can be predicted with reasonable accuracy from the protein binding in plasma (16). Virtually all the binding of drugs in milk is to albumin and lactoferrin (17).

The influences outlined above are summarised in Fig. 4. It is possible to predict M/P ratios based on the pKa of the drug, the octanol/water coefficient and the protein binding of the drug in plasma (6, 18, 19).

Total drug concentrations in milk

The sum of the amounts of drug in each of the aqueous, lipid and protein phases of milk makes up the total amount of drug in milk.

Variations in the M/P ratio

Milk is by no means a constant medium. There is marked inter-individual variation in milk yield, and fat and protein content (20). There is also marked intra-individual variation in the characteristics and content of the aqueous, fat and protein phases. Milk pH varies (6.8–7.7) substantially more than that of plasma, owing to limited buffering capacity (21, 22). Fore-milk is more acidic than hind-milk.

Milk lipid content increases during the time-course of lactation from around 2.9% in early milk (colostrum) to 5.4% in mature milk (>15 days postpartum) (23). Lipid composition also changes during a feed, with hind-milk containing 4–5 times as much lipid as fore-milk (24). Lipid content is also subject to diurnal variation, being higher in the morning and reaching a nadir between 1800 h and 2200 h (25, 26). An effect of breast laterality has also been demonstrated (27) but not confirmed (26).

The milk protein concentration is highest in colostrum, declines over 15 days postpartum, and is relatively constant thereafter. The main changes are in the concentrations of immunoglobulins, lactoferrin and α-lactalbumin, while the albumin concentration is relatively constant (28). Protein content also varies within a feed, with hind milk containing around 1.5 times more protein than fore-milk.

The potential variability of M/P ratios, based on changes in pH, fat, and protein, appears to be substantial. In practice, however, the extent of variation seems to be minimal (29). More studies are needed on the effect of suckling patterns before firm conclusions are reached.

INTEGRATED MATERNAL AND MAMMARY PHARMACOKINETICS

Maternal and mammary pharmacokinetics come together in the M/P ratio

Maternal dosing and pharmacokinetics determine the unbound plasma concentration of drug, which equilibrates with unbound drug in the aqueous phase of milk. In turn, the unbound drug in milk equilibrates with milk lipids and proteins. The dose of drug ingested by the infant depends on the total concentration of the drug in the milk and the volume of milk ingested (Table 2).

REFERENCES

1. Anderson P (1991) Drug use during breast-feeding. *Clin. Pharmacol., 10,* 594–624.
2. Högstedt S, Lindberg B, Rane A (1983) Increased oral clearance of metoprolol in pregnancy. *Eur. J. Clin. Pharmacol., 24,* 217–220.
3. Högstedt S, Rane A (1993) Plasma concentration - effect relationship of metoprolol during and after pregnancy. *Eur. J. Clin. Pharmacol., 44,* 243–264.
4. Nation RL (1980) Drug kinetics in childbirth. *Clin. Pharmacokinet., 5,* 340–364.
5. Rasmussen F, Linzell JL (1967) The acetylation of sulphanilamide by mammary tissue of lactating goats. *Biochem. Pharmacol., 16,* 918–919.
6. Begg EJ, Atkinson HC (1993) Modelling of the passage of drugs into milk. *Pharmacol. Therapeut., 59,* 301–310.
7. Du Souich P, Verges J, Erill S (1993) Plasma protein binding and pharmacological response. *Clin. Pharmacokinet., 24,* 435–440.
8. Chen SS, Perucca E, Lee JN, Richens A (1982) Serum protein binding and free concentration of phenytoin and phenobarbitone in pregnancy. *Br. J. Clin. Pharmacol., 13,* 547–552.
9. Lee JN, Chen SS, Richens A, Menabawey M, Chard T (1982) Serum protein binding of diazepam in maternal and fetal serum during pregnancy. *Br. J. Clin. Pharmacol., 14,* 551–554.
10. Yoshikowa T, Sugiyama Y, Sawada Y, Iga T, Hanano M, Kawasaki S, Yanagida M (1984) Effect of late pregnancy on salicylate, diazepam, warfarin and propranolol binding: use of fluorescent probes. *Clin. Pharmacol. Ther., 36,* 201–208.
11. Vorherr H (1974) In: Vorherr H (Ed) *The Breast: Morphology, Physiology, and Lactation*, pp 1–62. Academic Press, New York.
12. Hollman K (1974) Cytology and fine structure of the mammary gland. In: Larson BL, Smith VR (Eds) *Lactation*, pp 3–95. Academic Press, New York.
13. Baldwin R, Yang T (1974) Enzymatic and metabolic changes in the development of lactation. In: Larson BL, Smith VR (Eds) *Lactation*, pp 349–411. Academic Press, New York.
14. Wilson JT (1981) Production and characteristics of breast milk. In: Wilson JT (Ed) *Drugs in Breast Milk*, pp 4–14. ADIS Press, New York.
15. Atkinson HC, Begg EJ (1988). Relationship between human milk lipid-ultrafiltrate and octanol-water partition coefficient. *J. Pharm. Sci., 77,* 796–798.
16. Atkinson HC, Begg EJ (1988) Prediction of drug concentrations in human skim milk from plasma protein binding and acid-base characteristics. *Br. J. Clin. Pharmacol., 25,* 495–503.
17. Atkinson HC, Begg EJ (1988) The binding of drugs to major human milk whey proteins. *Br. J. Clin. Pharmacol., 26,* 107–109.
18. Atkinson HC, Begg EJ (1990) Prediction of drug distribution into human milk from physicochemical characteristics. *Clin. Pharmacokinet., 18,* 151–167.

19. Begg EJ, Atkinson HC, Duffull SB (1992) Prospective evaluation of a model for the prediction of milk:plasma drug concentrations from physicochemical characteristics. *Br. J. Clin. Pharmacol., 33,* 501–505.
20. Gross SJ, Getler MS, Tomarelli RM (1981) Composition of breast milk from mothers of preterm infants. *Pediatrics, 68,* 490–493.
21. Ansell C, Moore A, Barrie H (1977) Electrolyte and pH changes in human milk. *Pediatr. Res., 11,* 1177–1179.
22. Harrison VC, Peat G (1972) Significance of milk pH in new born infants. *Br. Med. J., 4,* 515–518.
23. Ferris AM, Jensen RG (1984) Lipids in human milk: a review. 1: Sampling, determination and content. *J. Pediatr. Gastroenterol. Nutr., 3,* 103–122.
24. Hall B (1975) Changing composition of human milk and early development of appetite control. *Lancet, 1,* 779–781.
25. Hytten FE (1954) Clinical and chemical studies of human lactation. *Br. Med. J., 1,* 175–182.
26. Prentice A, Prentice AM, Whitehead RG (1981) Breast-milk fat concentrations of rural African women. I. Short-term variations within individuals. *Br. J. Nutr., 45,* 483–494.
27. Neville MC, Keller RP, Secat J, Casey CE, Allen JC, Archer P (1984) Studies on human lactation. I. Within feed and between breast variation in selected components of human milk. *Am. J. Clin. Nutr., 40,* 635–646.
28. Lonnerdahl B, Forsum E, Hambraeus L (1976) A longitudinal study of the protein, nitrogen and lactose contents of human milk in Swedish well-nourished mothers. *Am. J. Clin. Nutr., 29,* 1127–1133.
29. Fleishaker JC, Desai N, McNamara PJ (1989). Possible effect of lactational period on the milk-to-plasma drug concentration ratio in lactating women: results of an in vitro evaluation. *J. Pharm. Sci., 28,* 137–141.

Drugs and Human Lactation
P.N. Bennett, editor

4. Determinants of drug disposition in infants

Anders Rane

Drug exposure of infants by transmission from breast milk is a common clinical reality. The infant's response depends not only on the pharmacodynamic properties of the drug but also on the disposition of the drug in the infant. Adverse reactions to a drug may be due to its slow elimination from the body as much as to tissue sensitivity. When excretion is retarded a drug may accumulate to toxic amounts despite ingestion of a small quantity in milk.

With the development of sensitive analytical methods a body of data about infant drug kinetics has become available. Such data are indispensable in the assessment of the risk to an infant that is nursed by a drug-treated mother.

THE PHARMACOKINETIC BASIS

The effects of drug exposure depend not only on the dose ingested in milk, but also on its distribution and elimination in the infant. The issue may be approached by considering the individual factors that determine the steady state concentration of a drug in plasma (C_{ss}), namely: bioavailability (F), a measure of the fraction of oral dose that reaches the systemic circulation, the dose (D), the rate constant for elimination (k), the apparent volume of distribution (V_d) and the dosing interval. These are related as follows:

$$C_{ss} = \frac{F \times \text{Dose}}{k \times V_d \times T} \quad \text{(i)}$$

The oral bioavailability (F) gives an indication of the amount of drug that reaches the presumed site of drug action in the systemic circulation. A low value of F may be due to incomplete absorption from the gastrointestinal tract and/or extensive metabolism in the gut and/or liver. Little is known about the developmental influence on drug absorption from the alimentary tract, but physiological changes are likely to have some effect. The pH partition hypothesis provides a basis for the theory that the acidic environment of the stomach favours absorption of acidic drugs. In fact, the gastric pH is 6–8 at birth, remains high during the first few weeks of life (1) and attains adult values only after the age of 3 years. Gastrointestinal motility is irregular in the neonate and slow gastric emptying may affect the time-course but not the degree of drug absorption. The gastrointestinal tract of the new-born is rapidly colonised by microorganisms, some of which are capable of decon-jugating drug metabolites that are secreted in the bile to release active drug.

The rate constant k is the fraction of the amount of drug in the body that is eliminated in unit time. It reflects the sum of the contributions to elimination from hepatic metabolism, renal excretion and biliary excretion. In subprimate mammals, drug oxidising capacity generally presents postnatally, whereas the human fetus can oxidise drugs and other xenobiotics already in the first trimester (2). The capacity to inactivate foreign compounds by metabolism may generally be considered an advantage although the same processes may transform some xenobiotics into active or even toxic metabolites (3). The rate constant k may also be thought of as the fraction of the total distribution volume (V_d) from which drug is completely cleared in unit time and this provides a pharmacokinetic expression for clearance (Cl)

$$\mathrm{Cl} = k \times V_d \qquad \text{(ii)}$$

Cl is a useful measure of elimination capacity and is expressed as the volume of blood or plasma cleared in unit time. From equation (i) its relation to steady state drug concentration is:

$$C_{ss} = \frac{F \times D}{\mathrm{Cl} \times T} \qquad \text{(iii)}$$

The *half-life* ($t_{1/2}$) of a drug in plasma is a poor, yet often used, estimate of elimination capacity. Clearance is a better indicator. The relation between them is:

$$t_{1/2} = \frac{0.693 \times V_d}{\mathrm{Cl}} \qquad \text{(iv)}$$

This equation shows that $t_{1/2}$ is a function of the drug's distribution as well as of clearance. The $t_{1/2}$ reflects the elimination capacity only if V_d remains constant. V_d may change rapidly in the neonatal period with alteration in body composition (4) and with changes in binding to plasma proteins. Therefore, clearance is the preferred method of comparing elimination capacity between children of different ages. Nevertheless, drug half-lives are quoted in this chapter, as most information in the literature is presented in this form.

HEPATIC CLEARANCE

The metabolic activity of the hepatocyte, the hepatic blood flow and the binding to plasma proteins are the major determinants of drug clearance in the liver (5, 6). Drugs cleared by liver metabolism are often classified into: (a) those that have a low extraction in a single pass through the liver, i.e. the rate of metabolism by hepatocytes determines their inactivation, and (b) those that are extensively extracted, i.e. the rate at which they are presented to the liver in the blood, namely hepatic blood flow, is the important determinant of the clearance. Examples of group (a) include phenytoin (7), tolbutamide, warfarin (8) and carbamazepine (9). Drugs of group (b) include acetylsalicylic acid, morphine (7), pethidine (10), some tricyclic antidepressants (11, 12), and lignocaine (lidocaine) (13). In general, drug metabolic reactions initially involve molecular modification through oxidation, reduction or hydrolysis; the drug metabolite may then be conjugated with various endogenous water-soluble molecules and the resulting polar compound is then excreted by the kidney. Drug disposition data relevant to infants in respect of these metabolic reactions appear in Tables 1 and 2.

Low extraction drugs

Drugs such as amobarbital and tolbutamide have a longer $t_{1/2}$ in newborn infants than in adults due to a lower rate of oxidation in the newborn (Table 1). If the drug has been used by the mother throughout pregnancy, transplacental induction of the fetal drug-metabolising enzymes may have taken place so that the $t_{1/2}$ in the newborn approaches the same value as in the adult (cf. phenytoin and carbamazepine in Table 1). It has long been known that children under 30 kg body weight (29) and newborn infants (30) require higher weight-related doses of phenytoin than adults to achieve similar plasma concentrations. The V_d of phenytoin is similar in newborn infants and adults (31).

Intermediate-to-high extraction drugs

The disposition of these drugs is poorly studied in infants. Plasma concentrations of propoxyphene and propranolol exhibit interindividual variation in children (32) and the $t_{1/2}$ of propoxyphene is similar in children and adults (15).

Drugs that are conjugated

The capacity to conjugate is often deficient in the newborn; the $t_{1/2}$ values of oxazepam and bilirubin, which are glucuronidated, are respectively 3–4 times and 3–6 times longer in neonates than in adults (33, 34). Bromosulfophthalein is conjugated with glutathione and cysteine and has a $t_{1/2}$ in the neonate that is twice that in older

TABLE 1 *Plasma half-lives in newborns and adults of drugs that are metabolised by oxidation*

Drug name	Newborns (N) (h)	Adults(A) (h)	N/A	Reference
Aminopyrine	30–40	3–4	>1	(16)
Amobarbital	17–60	12–27	>1	(17)
Bupivicaine	25	1.3	>1	(18)
Caffeine	95	4	>1	(19)
Carbamazepine	8–28	21–36	1	(20)
Diazepam	25–100	15–25	>1	(21)
Indometacin	14–20	2–11	>1	(22)
Mepivacaine	8.7	3.2	>1	(14)
Nortriptyline	56	18–22	>1	(23)
Pethidine	22	3–4	>1	(24)
Phenytoin	21	11–19	1	(26)
Theophylline	24–36	3–9	>1	(27)
Tolbutamide	10–40	4.4–9	>1	(28)

infants (35, 36). Conjugation with glycine and sulphate also occurs, e.g. with salicylic acid and paracetamol (acetaminophen). The developmental pattern of these pathways is illustrated in Table 2.

Binding to plasma proteins

Several drugs are less bound to proteins in infant or umbilical cord plasma than in adult plasma (Table 3). Displacement of drugs from protein-binding sites may be caused by endogenous substances such as bilirubin (46) or free fatty acids (52), and possibly by qualitative differences in albumin. The possible consequences of reduced binding are mostly related to drugs with low hepatic extraction; as more of the unbound fraction is available for metabolism a lower total plasma concentration can be expected. This may partly explain the low steady state plasma concentrations of phenytoin (low drug extraction) in young infants. In contrast, alterations in binding do not limit the clearance of drugs that are extensively extracted by the liver.

TABLE 2 *Age-dependent metabolism and kinetics of salicylic acid and paracetamol*

Drug	Conjugated with	Urinary excretion (%)			Plasma $t_{1/2}$ (h)		
		Newborns	Older infants	Adults	Newborns	Older infants	Adults
Salicylic acid	Glycine	75	–	40–50	4.0–11.5	–	
	Glucuronic acid	10	–	35			
Paracetamol	Glucuronic acid	13–18	32–47	50–72	3.5	1–3.5	
	Sulphate	48–50	30–43	15–30			

TABLE 3 *Drugs with lower plasma protein binding in cord (or infant) serum than in adult serum*

Drug group	
Antibiotics	Ampicillin, benzypenicillin (38), nafcillin (39)
Antimicrobials	Sulfamethoxypyrazine (40), sulfaphenazole (41), sulfadimethoxine, sulfamethoxydiazin (42)
Cardiac glycosides	Digoxin (43)
Anxiolytics	Diazepam (44)
Tricyclic antidepressants	Imipramine (45), desmethylimipramine (46)
Analgesics	Salicylates (47), phenylbutazone (25)
Local anaesthetics	Bupivicaine, lidocaine (48)
Sedatives	Pentobarbitone (50), phenobarbital (49)
Antiepileptics	Phenytoin (26), clonazepam (51)

Reprinted from Rane (37), by courtesy of the Publishers.

RENAL CLEARANCE

Glomerular filtration and tubular secretary processes are functionally immature at birth (53, 54) and during the first year of life. Calculations show that a drug distributed in the extracellular water and eliminated only by glomerular filtration would have a $t_{1/2}$ of 100 min in a 1.5-month-old infant but only 67 min in an adult; if the drug were eliminated only by tubular secretion the $t_{1/2}$ would be 40 min in this infant and 13 min in an adult (55). Due caution must thus be exercised in the use of drugs that are excreted in the kidneys, e.g. aminoglycoside antibiotics and digoxin.

CONCLUSION

Physiological maturation with increasing age has a significant influence on drug bioavailability and distribution, and on hepatic and renal clearance, which are important determinants of steady state drug concentrations in plasma. These changes are particularly pronounced in early infancy when a child is likely to be breastfed. In addition, the type of drug, e.g. whether it is metabolised or excreted directly in the kidneys, must be taken into account in the assessment of the consequences of drug intake via the breast milk.

REFERENCES

1. Weber WW, Cohen SN (1975) Aging effects and drugs in man. In: Gillette JR, Mitchell JR, (Eds) *Concepts in Biochemical Pharmacology,* pp 213–233. Springer Verlag, New York.
2. Yaffe SJ, Rane A, Sjöqvist F, Boréus LO, Orrenius S (1970) The presence of a mono-oxygenase system in human fetal liver microsomes. *Life Sci., 9,* 1189–1200.
3. Drayer DE (1982) Pharmacologically active metabolites of drugs and other foreign compounds. Clinical, pharmacological, therapeutic and toxicological considerations. *Drugs, 24,* 519–542.

4. Friis-Hansen B (1961) Body water compartments in children: changes during growth and related changes in body composition. *Pediatrics, 8,* 169–181.
5. Wilkinson GR (1975) Pharmacokinetics of drugs disposition: hemodynamic considerations. *Ann. Rev. Pharmacol., 15,* 11–27.
6. Wilkinson GR, Shand DG (1975) A physiological approach to hepatic drug clearance. *Clin. Pharmacol. Ther., 18,* 377–390.
7. Rowland M, Blaschke TF, Meffin PJ (1976) Pharmacokinetics in disease states modifying hepatic and metabolic function. In: Benet LZ (Ed) *Effect of Disease States on Drug Pharmacokinetics*, pp 53–76. American Pharmaceutical Association, Washington DC.
8. Andreassen PB, Vesell ES (1974) Comparison of plasma levels of antipyrine, tolbutamide and warfarin after oral and intravenous administration. *Clin. Pharmacol. Ther., 16,* 1059–1065.
9. Rane A, Shand DG, Wilkinson GR (1977) Disposition of carbamazepine and its 10,11-epoxide metabolite in the isolated perfused rat liver. *Drug Metab. Dispos., 5,* 179–184.
10. Nies AS, Shand DG, Wilkinson GR (1976) Altered hepatic blood flow and drug disposition. *Clin. Pharmacokinet., 1,* 135–155.
11. Gram LF, Christiansen J (1975) First–pass metabolism of imipramine in man. *Clin. Pharmacol. Ther., 17,* 555–563.
12. Gram LF, Fredricson, Overø K (1975) First–pass metabolism of nortriptyline in man. *Clin. Pharmacol. Ther., 18,* 305–314.
13. Boyes RN, Scott DB, Jebson PH, Godman MJ, Julian DG (1971) Pharmacokinetics of lidocaine in man. *Clin. Pharmacol. Ther., 12,* 105–116.
14. Moore RG, Thomas J, Triggs EJ, Thomas DB, Burnard ED, Shanks CA (1978) The pharmacokinetics and metabolism of the anilide local anaesthetics in neonates. III. Mepivacaine. *Eur. J. Clin. Pharmacol., 14,* 203–212.
15. Wolen RL, Gruber Jr CM, Kiplinger GF, Scholz NE (1971) Concentration of propoxyphene in human plasma following oral, intramuscular, and intravenous administration. *Toxicol. Appl. Pharmacol., 19,* 480–492.
16. Reinicke C, Rogner G, Franzel J (1970) Die Wirkung von Phenylbutazon und Phenobarbital auf die Amidopyrin-Elimination, die Bilirubin-Gesamt-konzentration im Serum und einige blutgerinnungsfaktoren bei neugeborenen Kindern. *Pharmacol. Clin., 2,* 167–172.
17. Krauer B, Draffan GH, Williams FM, Clare RA, Dollery CT, Hawkins DF (1973) Elimination kinetics of amobarbital in mothers and their newborn infants. *Clin. Pharmacol. Ther., 14,* 442–447.
18. Caldwell J, Mofatt JR, Smith RL (1976) Pharmacokinetics of bupivacaine administered epidurally during childbirth. *Br. J. Clin. Pharmacol., 3,* 956–957.
19. Aranda JV, Gorman W, Outerbridge EW (1977) Pharmacokinetic disposition of caffeine in premature neonates with apnea. *Pediatr. Res., 11,* 414.
20. Rane A, Bertilsson L, Palmér L (1975) Disposition of placentally transferred carbamazepine (Tegretol) in the newborn. *Eur. J. Clin. Pharmacol., 8,* 283–284.
21. Morselli PL, Principi N, Togoni G, Reali E, Belvedere G, Standen SM, Sereni F (1973) Diazepam elimination in premature and full–term infants and children. *J. Perinat. Med., 1,* 133–141.
22. Traeger A, Nöschel H, Zaumseil J (1973) Zur Pharmakokintic von Indomethazin bei Schwangeren, Kreissenden und deren Neugeborenen. *Zentralbl. Gynäkol., 95,* 635–641.
23. Sjöqvist F, Bergfors PG, Borgå O, Lind M, Ygge H (1972) Plasma disappearance of nortriptyline in a newborn following placental transfer from an intoxicated mother: evidence for drug metabolism. *J. Pediatr., 80,* 496–500.
24. Caldwell J, Wakile LA, Notarianni LJ (1978) Transplacental passage and neonatal elimination of pethidine given to mothers in childbirth. *Br. J. Pharmacol. (Abstr. Proc. B.P.S., Sept. 1977),* 716P.

25. Gladtke E (1968) Pharmacokinetic studies on phenylbutazone in children. *Farmaco Ed. Sci., 23,* 897–906.
26. Rane A, Garle M, Borgå O, Sjöqvist F (1974) Plasma disappearance of transplacentally transferred phenytoin in the newborn studied with mass fragmentography. *Clin. Pharmacol. Ther., 15,* 39–45.
27. Aranda JV, Sitar DS, Parsons DW (1976) Pharmacokinetic aspects of theophylline in premature newborns. *N. Engl. J. Med., 295,* 413–416.
28. Nitowsky HM, Matz L, Berzofsky JA (1966) Studies on oxidative drug metabolism in the full-term newborn infant. *Pediatr. Pharmacol. Ther., 69,* 1139–1149.
29. Svensmark O, Buchtal E (1964) Diphenylhydantoin and phenobarbital. Serum levels in children. *Am. J. Dis. Child., 108,* 82–87.
30. Jalling B, Boréus LO, Rane A, Sjöqvist F (1970) Plasma concentrations of diphenylhydantoin in young infants. *Pharmacol. Clin., 2,* 200–202.
31. Loughnan PM, Waters G, Aranda JV, Neims AH (1976) Age-related changes in pharmacokinetics of diphenylhydantoin (DPH) in the newborn and young infant: implications regarding treatment of neonatal convulsions. *Austr. Paediatr. J., 12,* 204–205.
32. Wilson JT, Atwood GF, Shand DG (1976) Disposition of propoxyphene and propranolol in children. *Clin. Pharmacol. Ther., 19,* 264–270.
33. Tomson G, Sundwall A, Lunell NO, Rane A (1979) Transplacental passage and kinetics in the mother and newborn of oxazepam given during labour. *Clin. Pharmacol. Ther., 25,* 74–81.
34. Gladtke E, Rind H (1967) Bilirubinstoffwechsel beim Neugeborenen. *Monatsschr. Kinderheilkd., 115,* 231–233.
35. Vest MF, Rossier R (1963) Detoxification in the newborn. The ability of the newborn infant to form conjugates with glucuronic acid, glycine, acetate and glutathione. *Ann. N. Y. Acad. Sci., 111,* 183–197.
36. Wichmann HM, Rind H, Gladtke E (1968) Die Elimination von Bromsulphalein beim Kind. Z. *Kinderheilkd., 103,* 262–276.
37. Rane A (1992) Drug disposition and action in infants and children. In: Yaffe SJ, Aranda JV (Eds) *Pediatric Pharmacology. Therapeutic Principles in Practice*, pp 10–21. WB Saunders, Philadelphia, PA.
38. Ehrnebo M, Agurell S, Jalling B (1971) Age differences in drug binding by plasma proteins: studies on human fetuses, neonates and adults. *Eur. J. Clin. Pharmacol., 3,* 189–193.
40. Krasner J, Yaffe SJ (1975) Drug protein binding in the neonate. In: Morselli P, Garattini S, Sereni F (Eds) *Basic and Therapeutic Aspects of Perinatal Pharmacology,* pp 357–366. Raven Press, New York.
40. Sereni F, Perletti L, Marubini E, Mars G (1968) Pharmacokinetic studies with a long-acting sul fonamide in subjects of different ages. *Pediatr. Res., 2,* 29–37.
41. Chignell CF, Vesell ES, Starkweather DK et al (1971) The binding of sulfaphenazole to fetal–neonatal and adult human plasma albumin. *Clin. Pharmacol. Ther., 12,* 897–901.
42. Ganshorn A, Kurz H (1968) Unterschiede zwischen der Proteinbindung Neugeborener und Erwachsener und ihre Bedeuting für die parmakologische Wirkung. *Arch. Pharm. Exp. Pathol., 260,* 117.
43. Kim PW, Krasula RW, Soyka LF, Hastreiter AR (1975) Postmortem tissue digoxin concentrations in infants and children. *Circulation, 52,* 1128–1131.
44. Kanto J, Errkola R, Sellman R (1974) Perinatal metabolism of diazepam. *Br. Med. J., 1,* 641–642.
45. Pruitt AW, Dayton PG (1972) A comparison of the binding of drugs to adult and cord plasma. *Eur. J. Clin. Pharmacol., 4,* 59–62.

46. Rane A, Lunde PKM, Jalling B, Yaffe SJ, Sjöqvist F (1971) Plasma protein binding of diphenylhydantoin in normal and hyperbilirubinemic infants. *J. Pediatr., 78,* 877–882.
47. Krasner J, Giaccoia GP, Yaffe SJ (1973) Drug protein binding in the newborn infant. *Ann. N. Y. Acad. Sci., 226,* 101–114.
48. Tucker GT, Boyes RN, Bridenbaugh PO (1970) Binding of anilide-type local anesthetics in human plasma. II. Implications in vivo, with special reference to transplacental distribution. *Anesthesiology, 33,* 304–314.
49. Boréus LO, Jalling B, Kållberg N (1975) Clinical pharmacology of phenobarbital in the neonatal period. In: Morselli P, Garattini S, Sereni F, (Eds) *Basic and Therapeutic Aspects of the Perinatal Pharmacology*, pp 331–340. Raven Press, New York.
50. Short CR, Sexton RL, McFarland I (1975) Binding of ^{14}C-salicylic acid and ^{14}C-phenobarbital to plasma proteins of several species during the perinatal period. *Biol. Neonate, 26,* 58–66.
51. Pacifici GM, Taddeucci-Brunelli G, Rane A (1984) Clonazepam serum protein binding during development. *Clin. Pharmacol. Ther., 35,* 354–359.
52. Fredholm BB, Rane A, Persson B (1975) Diphenylhydantoin binding to proteins in plasma and its dependence on free fatty acid and bilirubin concentration in dogs and newborn infants. *Pediatr. Res., 9,* 26–30.
53. West JR, Smith HW, Chasis H (1948) Glomerular filtration rate, effective renal blood flow and maximal tubular excretory capacity in infants. *J. Pediatr., 32,* 10–18.
54. Barnett HL, McNamara H, Schultz S, Tompsett R (1949) Renal clearances of sodium penicillin G, procaine penicillin G and insulin in infants and children. *Pediatrics, 3,* 418–422.
55. Rane A, Wilson JT (1976) Clinical pharmacokinetics in infants and children. *Clin. Pharmacokinet., 1,* 2–24.

Drugs and Human Lactation
P.N. Bennett, editor

5. Use of the monographs on drugs

PRESENTATION OF DATA

Drugs in this text are named according to their entries in the Cumulative List No. 8 of the International Nonproprietary Names (INN) for Pharmaceutical Substances published by the World Health Organization, Geneva, 1992. Other commonly-used names are included in the general description of a drug; these are referenced in the index to help the reader who is not familiar with the INN usage.

Clearly there is variation in the drugs contained in the pharmacopoeias of different countries and readers may be unfamiliar with, or even surprised to see, certain drugs in this book. The INN also lists the names of drugs from various national pharmacopoeias. Such listing has been taken to mean that a drug is currently in use, and thus it has been included in this book.

The text provided on each drug opens with a general section, considering briefly the clinical use of the drug, and its simple pharmacokinetics. The quoted pharmacokinetic values are taken from various standard sources and are not referenced individually. In the second section a table usually follows in which the essential data are presented. The table looks like this:

Treatment conditions	Concentration (mg/l)		Milk/ plasma ratio	Maximum observed milk conc. (mg/l)	Absolute dose to infant (mg/kg day)		Ref.
Dose × Frequency × Duration; Route; No. of patients; Lactation stage	Milk	Plasma			Ave	Max	

Treatment conditions

The treatment conditions can include a number of regimens and are represented as:

Dose × Frequency × Duration (e.g. 100 mg × 3/d × 14 d);
Route; Number of patients; Lactation stage.

The dose is usually specified in milligrams (mg); in this case 100 mg. The frequency in this example is shown by, e.g. × 3/d, which indicates 3 doses daily. The duration is shown by, e.g. × 14 d, which indicates 14 days. (A single dose is shown as × 1/d × 1 d.). The route is shown as p.o., i.v., i.m. etc. The number of subjects is shown as, e.g. $n = 6$ or $n = 10$, indicating that 6 or 10 subjects were studied. The lactation stage is often shown by a question mark which implies that the stage of lactation is unknown (many studies examined). It is presumed that this indicates established lactation. In some cases colostrum or transitional milk was examined.

Concentrations

The concentration of drug in milk or plasma is shown as mg/l in most cases (occasionally μg/l or ng/l). A figure of <50 μg/l indicates that the drug was not detectable at the sensitivity level of the assay (in this case 50 μg/l). If the assay sensitivity is not known the abbreviation n.d. (for not detected) is used. A figure in parentheses indicates a concentration of metabolite.

Milk to plasma ratio

The milk to plasma ratio (M/P) is calculated for paired samples or from the areas under the respective concentration–time curves; in some cases a range is given which reflects intersubject variation.

Dose

The assumption is made that the infant ingests milk at the rate of 150 ml/kg day. The average dose is then calculated from the data shown in column 2 and expressed as mg or mg/kg per day. The maximum dose is calculated from the maximum milk concentration. The relative dose to the infant is then given both in terms of the maternal dose and of the paediatric therapeutic dose where this is available (see assumptions on page 70).

There follow comments on any observed effects or drug measurements in the infants. The section on each drug finishes with an assessment and recommendations, and with references. The criteria used for the general recommendations are shown in the discussion on assumptions on pages 69–74.

SELECTION AND REJECTION OF EVIDENCE

Readers may notice that certain references are missing from this book, and indeed information on some drugs has been excluded altogether. In some cases no data were available, and in other cases the data were inconclusive. Many of the early studies in this field used spectrophotometric or colorimetric methods, or measured total radioactivity in breast milk after a radiolabelled dose of the drug. It is very likely that many of these studies measured not only drug, but also metabolites. In many cases very few subjects were studied: in some only one mother was examined. Unless the data were of particular interest, these studies have not been included.

Many studies examined only the situation after a single dose of the drug. It should be realised that drug concentration in breast milk may be different in a multiple-dose regimen (the usual situation) to that seen after single dosing. In particular the milk to plasma ratio, often quoted as an accurate assessment for any situation, may vary not only from the single-dose to a multiple-dose regimen, but also during a dosing interval (see Chapter 3). Even when the multiple-dose situation was studied, on some occasions the mothers were clearly not at steady state. Data are often insufficient to evaluate unexpected accumulation in milk. In general comments on these aspects of the quoted studies are included below the main table.

ASSUMPTIONS FOR CALCULATIONS AND INTERPRETATION OF DATA

a. A drug can accumulate in plasma (and in milk) during repeated dosing. This is not considered when the daily 'dose to infant' calculations are made from single-dose data. *In general, no assumptions are made about conditions of chronic dosing when only single-dose data are available.*

b. *Inter-individual variation* occurs in both the maternal plasma drug concentrations and the milk concentrations. The data are often not sufficient to assess this variation, and so the dose in the milk is calculated without this assessment.

c. *Breast-feeding practices vary* in different parts of the world. In some countries the only alternative to breast milk may be an artificial feed which may harbour bacteria. Thus the risk of a drug-contaminated milk must be weighed against that of possibly infected milk. In most cases the recommendations assume a suitable alternative source of milk.

d. Due to local circumstances or personal wishes, some women may wish to breastfeed *contrary to the recommendations of this book.* It is advisable then: (i) to use the lowest dose of drug necessary to achieve the therapeutic effect in the mother, (ii) to monitor the drug plasma concentration in the infant, and (iii) to observe the infant for drug effects.

e. The effect of the *stage of lactation* on the dose delivered to the infant is not considered, i.e. for the purposes of dose calculation it is assumed that maximum drug concentration in milk does not change as a function of stage (duration) of lactation, unless stated otherwise.

f. The calculations for the doses of drug received by infants are based on the milk concentrations and on maternal doses used in the studies quoted. Caution should be exercised when advice is given to mothers who receive *doses in excess of those studied.*

g. Whenever possible advice is given on the basis of the information available, but as a general principle, if recommendations are based on data from less than 6 women at only one stage of lactation, then it is considered that further studies are needed to validate or to refute the recommendations. In such a situation the mother should be appropriately *monitored* until more data are available.

h. *Milk to plasma (M/P) ratio estimates.* The M/P ratio is expressed in two ways.

(i) The area under the concentration-time curve in milk relative to that in plasma; when a range is quoted, this refers to the variation within or between mothers and does not indicate the variation between doses and during repeated dosing.

(ii) The concentration in milk relative to that in plasma; when a range is quoted, this may indicate the variation for all paired data points in all cases or it may indicate the variation between average M/P ratios for all cases in the study.

No assumption is made that the time-course profile of drug concentration in milk is concurrent with that in plasma. Accordingly, the M/P ratio is usually calculated when the data are sufficient to show the extent of its variation within a dose interval.

The M/P ratio derived from a single dose may not necessarily be that observed after multiple doses if a drug accumulates in milk more than in plasma. Calculations of the M/P ratio are based on the conditions of each study.

j. Pharmacokinetic parameters are quoted for adults (often healthy males) and the assumption has been made these parameters also apply to lactating females unless otherwise specified.

k. *Relative dose in milk.* The chemical form in which a drug is administered, e.g. salt or ester, may differ from the form measured in plasma or milk, e.g. free base. Where the chemical form of a drug is not specified the total maternal dose is assumed to reflect the parent drug for the purpose of calculating infant dose as a percentage of maternal dose. When an active metabolite(s) of a drug was measured in milk, the values for drug and metabolite(s) were added together (i.e. the metabolite(s) were assumed to have equal biological activity to the parent drug).

The dose of drug that an infant received in breast milk has been expressed as a dose in mg/kg rather than as dose per square metre of body surface area as follows:

Relationship to maternal dose

The dose in breast milk is expressed relative to the maternal dose and a linear relationship between age and weight-adjusted dose requirements is assumed. The maternal dose is weight-adjusted using a reference female weight of 60 kg. An infant milk consumption of 150 ml/kg per day is assumed. The average and maximum concentrations in the following calculations are quoted in mg/l.

Single dose administration

Many studies report results of single doses of drugs to mothers. For these the maximum milk concentration (either mean or single maximum concentrations as is judged appropriate in the individual study) is taken, and it is assumed that the child will suckle once at this maximum milk concentration (C_{max}). It is further assumed that the infant will suckle 5 times per day and thus will ingest a milk volume of 30 ml/kg (0.03 l/kg) in that feed. The data can then be expressed (in percent) as the dose received in a feed relative to the weight-adjusted maternal single dose. The calculation is:

$$\frac{C_{max} \times 0.03 \times 60}{\text{Maternal single dose}} \times 100 = \frac{C_{max} \times 180}{\text{Maternal single dose}} = \%$$

Multiple-dose administration

In some studies breast-milk concentrations were measured during multiple dosing. Here, the achievement of steady state is assumed unless the conditions of the study suggest otherwise. The infant daily dose is expressed as a percentage of the weight-adjusted maternal daily dose. The dose is expressed both as an *average* figure using the average milk concentration (C_{ave}) and/or as a *maximum* figure using the maximum milk concentration C_{max}, (mean or single value as is judged appropriate in the individual study). The calculations are, for average doses:

$$\frac{C_{ave} \times 0.15 \times 60}{\text{Maternal daily dose}} \times 100 = \frac{C_{ave} \times 900}{\text{Maternal daily dose}} = \%$$

and for maximum doses:

$$\frac{C_{max} \times 0.15 \times 60}{\text{Maternal daily dose}} \times 100 = \frac{C_{max} \times 900}{\text{Maternal daily dose}} = \%$$

where 0.15 is the daily milk intake of the infant in l/kg and 60 is the reference maternal weight in kg. The daily maternal dose is the dose used in the particular study.

Relationship to paediatric dose

The dose received by the infant from breast milk is also expressed as a percentage of the relevant infant therapeutic dose. Where the drug is not given to infants (e.g. sex steroids) or the paediatric dose applies to older children (e.g. antidepressants) no such relative dose is given.

Single-dose administration

When the mother is given a single dose, the maximum milk concentration is taken (C_{max} in mg/l) and it is assumed that the child suckles once at this maximum milk concentration. It is further assumed that the infant ingests a milk volume of 30 ml/kg (0.03 l/kg) in that feed. The infant single dose is normally quoted as a weight-adjusted dose (mg/kg). The calculation is:

$$\frac{C_{max} \times 0.03}{\begin{array}{c}\text{Infant single dose}\\ \text{(weight - adjusted)}\end{array}} \times 100 = \frac{C_{max} \times 3}{\begin{array}{c}\text{Infant single dose}\\ \text{(weight - adjusted)}\end{array}} = \%$$

Multiple-dose administration

The dose received by the infant in the breast milk is calculated using both average and/or maximum concentrations (in mg/l) in milk (mean or single maximum values as is judged appropriate in the individual study). The dose referred to is the lowest daily therapeutic dose (in mg/kg) as currently recommended. The amount of milk ingested is taken as 0.15 l/kg/day. The calculation for average daily intake of drug from breast milk, expressed as a percentage of daily therapeutic dose, is:

$$\frac{C_{ave} \times 0.15}{\begin{array}{c}\text{Infant single dose}\\ \text{(weight - adjusted)}\end{array}} \times 100 = \frac{C_{ave} \times 15}{\begin{array}{c}\text{Infant single dose}\\ \text{(weight - adjusted)}\end{array}} = \%$$

The calculation for maximum daily intake of drug from breast milk, expressed as a percentage of daily infant therapeutic dose, is:

$$\frac{C_{max} \times 0.15}{\begin{array}{c}\text{Infant daily dose}\\ \text{(weight - adjusted)}\end{array}} \times 100 = \frac{C_{max} \times 15}{\begin{array}{c}\text{Infant daily dose}\\ \text{(weight - adjusted)}\end{array}} = \%$$

k. In order to assign a level of risk to the infant for drugs received in breast milk, the following *criteria* are used:

- If the *inherent pharmacological action* of the drug suggests that a toxic effect may occur in the immediate or longer term, regardless of the amount of drug in milk, then the conclusion about the drug is appropriately qualified. Usually breast-feeding is not advisable, e.g. for most cytotoxic drugs.
- If there are *observed effects* in breast-fed infants which suggest that the drug may not be safe during breast-feeding, then the appropriate recommendation is made if the study results are supported by the calculated

amount of the drug in the milk or observed concentrations in the infant's plasma. Usually breast-feeding is not advisable.

- If the *relative dose* in milk calculation reveals that either: (i) during multiple dosing to the mother there is an average or maximum daily dose in milk greater than 10% of the weight-adjusted maternal or paediatric daily dose, or (ii) after a single dose to the mother there is a maximum dose in each milk feed that is greater than 10% of the weight-adjusted maternal or paediatric dose, then the drug will usually be unacceptable for breast-feeding mothers on the basis of the *dose* of drug in milk alone. In some cases qualifying statements are made, and knowledge about infant pharmacokinetic parameters may modify the recommendation. Thus it is assumed that a dose that is less than 10% of the lowest paediatric dose, or less than 10% of the weight-adjusted maternal dose, is most unlikely to create a risk of adverse effects that exceeds the risk which an infant would run by receiving the drug for therapeutic purposes.
- Under expected steady state conditions in the infant, if the plasma concentration of a drug in the suckling infant is greater than 25% of the lower end of the therapeutic concentration range, then the drug is taken to be *unacceptable* for breast-feeding women, on the basis of the *dose* of drug in milk.

Adverse effects to the infant are considered as: (i) *toxicity related to the dose* of a drug or chemical taken in milk, i.e. when a dose-response relationship appears to exist and the consequence is either an exaggerated therapeutic effect or an adverse effect (such events tend to be recognised and reported) and (ii) *toxicity unrelated to the dose,* i.e. when an idiosyncratic response occurs (much of this data is dependent on case reports).

The rationale underlying assignment of risks to the infant includes ethical and practical considerations. From an ethical point of view, the child's inability to give informed consent might require that drugs be given to children only for therapeutic indications. If this principle were to be accepted for drug exposure through breast milk, then even drugs with undetectable concentrations in milk would be unacceptable for breast-feeding women as idiosyncratic adverse response may be provoked by minute amounts of drug. This approach is obviously impractical. Therefore, a pragmatic approach is adopted whereby some exposure to drug in milk is accepted but the risk is minimised by using the guidelines (above) for the percent of dose or plasma concentration to which an infant may be exposed. While these guidelines do not guarantee safety in all infants (hypersensitivity may occur at very low doses), they are set to offer a practical margin of safety without unduly compromising drug therapy in women who wish their infants to receive the benefits of breast-feeding.

I. It is generally assumed that *no conditions coexist* with the state of lactation or the state of infancy *to alter either drug disposition,* in mother or infant, *or the pharmacological effect* in the infant. Examples of such conditions include renal or hepatic disease, or combination drug therapy. Unless stated otherwise, the interpretation of data, assessment and recommendations assumes absence of such coexisting conditions.

m. In general, *animal data have been excluded* from an assessment of the risk.

Drugs and Human Lactation
P.N. Bennett, editor

6. Monographs on individual drugs

P. Bennett, I. Matheson, L.J. Notarianni, A. Rane and D. Reinhardt

ACICLOVIR

GENERAL

Aciclovir (acyclovir) is a synthetic analogue of guanine used in the treatment and prophylaxis of infections due to herpes simplex or varicella-zoster viruses. Some 15–30% of an oral dose is absorbed from the gastrointestinal tract, 15% is bound to plasma proteins and the 80% is cleared unchanged by the kidney. The plasma half-life is 2 h.

EVALUATION OF DATA

Passage of aciclovir into human milk has been reported as follows:

Treatment conditions: Dose × Frequency × Duration; Route; No. of patients; Lactation stage	Concentration (mg/l): Milk	Concentration (mg/l): Plasma	Milk/plasma ratio	Maximum observed milk conc. (mg/l)	Absolute dose to infant (mg/kg/day): Ave	Absolute dose to infant (mg/kg/day): Max	Ref.
200 mg × 5/d × 5 d; p.o.; 1, 12 months	0.78–1.26	0.16–0.92	3.24	1.45	0.16	0.22	(1)
900 mg/d × 5 d; i.v.; 1; 6 weeks	7.3 (max.) 4.88 (ave.)	6.5	1.12	7.3	0.73	1.10	(2)

Five paired samples of milk and plasma were taken once daily during the 5-day course of aciclovir (1). The figures in (2) refer to collections taken every 6 h starting after the final aciclovir infusion on the 5th day of treatment. Steady-state conditions of dosing are assumed to apply.

RELATIVE DOSE IN MILK

The amount of aciclovir that a suckling infant would ingest in a day is on average

1.0% (1.06 × 900/1000)* and a maximum of 1.3% (1.45 × 900/1000)* of the weight-adjusted maternal daily oral dose (1). Alternatively, a suckling infant would ingest in a feed at maximum 1.5% (7.3 × 180/900)* and on average 4.9% (4.88 × 900/900)* of the weight-adjusted maternal daily i.v. dose (2).

DATA ON THE INFANT

No data are available.

ASSESSMENT AND RECOMMENDATIONS

Data from two mothers suggests that the risk to the suckling infant of administering aciclovir to its mother is low on the basis that the quantity of drug that passes into milk is small. Breast feeding can probably be regarded as safe.

REFERENCES

1. Myer LJ, de Miranda P, Sheth N, Spruance S (1988) Acyclovir in human breast milk. *Am. J. Obstet. Gynecol., 158,* 586–588.
2. Bork K, Benes (1995) Concentration and kinetic studies of intravenous acyclovir in serum and breast milk of a patient with eczema herpeticum. *J. Am. Acad. Derm., 32,* 1053–1055.

* An explanation of the calculation (s) appears on pp. 71–72.

AMIKACIN

GENERAL

Amikacin is an aminoglycoside antibiotic. It is poorly absorbed from the adult gastrointestinal tract and is given by i.m or i.v. injection or by i.v. infusion. It is negligibly bound to plasma proteins. Amikacin is eliminated unchanged in the urine and the plasma half-life is 2 h. Renal excretion of aminoglycosides is generally slower in neonates.

EVALUATION OF DATA

Passage of amikacin into human milk has been reported as follows:

Treatment conditions — Dose × Frequency × Duration; Route; No. of patients; Lactation stage	Concentration (mg/l) Milk	Concentration (mg/l) Plasma	Milk/ plasma ratio	Maximum observed milk conc. (mg/l)	Absolute dose to infant (mg/kg/day) Ave	Absolute dose to infant (mg/kg/day) Max	Ref.
100 mg × 1/d × 1 d; i.m.; 2–3; 5–7 d	Trace	1.93	–	–	–	–	(1)

The table gives average plasma concentration based in the area under the concentration-time curve, the peak concentration being 4.2 mg/l. Only trace amounts were found in milk but the lower limit of sensitivity of the assay is not stated.

RELATIVE DOSE IN MILK

As the amount in milk was not quantified, a relative dose cannot be calculated.

DATA ON THE INFANT

No data are available.

ASSESSMENT AND RECOMMENDATIONS

The quantity of amikacin in milk after a single dose to the mother was too small to quantify. There are no data on which to base an estimate of the amount ingested by the infant under steady-state conditions at an appropriate maternal dose. In common with other aminoglycosides, amikacin may be eliminated more slowly by the infant, especially the neonate, in which it may thus accumulate. Use of amikacin is best avoided when breast-feeding a neonate but is probably safe when the infant is older.

REFERENCE

1. Matsuda T (1984) Transfer of antibiotics into maternal milk. *Biol. Res. Preg., 5,* 57–60.

AMOXICILLIN

GENERAL

Amoxicillin (amoxycillin) is a penicillin antibiotic closely related to ampicillin (see p. 81) in its antibacterial spectrum, but more lipid soluble. After oral administration peak concentrations are attained in 1–2 h in the adult and absorption is little affected by food. Plasma protein binding is 20% and it is eliminated by the kidney. The plasma half-life is 1 h.

EVALUATION OF DATA

Passage of amoxicillin into human milk has been reported as follows:

Treatment conditions Dose × Frequency × Duration; Route; No. of patients; Lactation stage	Concentration (mg/l) Milk	 Plasma	Milk/ plasma ratio	Maximum observed milk conc. (mg/l)	Absolute dose to infant (mg/kg/day) Ave	 Max	Ref.
1000 mg × 1/d × 0.43; p.o.; 6; 3 d	0.43	8.75	0.05	1.3	0.45	1.29	(1)

Concentration-time profiles were defined for 3 h (serum) and 6 h (milk) after dosing. The peak concentration was observed at 2 h in serum and after 4–5 h in milk. The quoted milk and serum concentrations are average values over these times based on area measurements; the maximum concentration is the highest value recorded in an individual.

RELATIVE DOSE IN MILK

The amount of amoxicillin which a suckling infant would ingest in a feed is at maximum 0.2% (1.3 × 180/1000)* of the weight-adjusted maternal single dose (1).

DATA ON THE INFANT

No adverse effects were recorded in infants nursed by mothers taking amoxicillin in the quoted study.

ASSESSMENT AND RECOMMENDATIONS

Only single dose data are available, but the risk to the suckling infant of administering amoxicillin to its mother would appear to be low on the basis that the

* An explanation of the calculation (s) appears on pp. 71–72.

quantity of drug that passes into milk is small. Breast feeding may be regarded as safe.

REFERENCE

1. Kafetzis DA, Siafas CA, Georgakopoulos PA, Papadatos CJ (1981) Passage of cephalosporins and amoxycillin into the breast milk. *Acta Paediatr. Scand., 70*, 285–288.

AMPICILLIN

GENERAL

Ampicillin is a aminopenicillin antibiotic. It is rapidly absorbed from the adult gastrointestinal tract, is 20% bound to plasma proteins and is eliminated largely unchanged in the urine. The plasma elimination half-life is 1 h.

EVALUATION OF DATA

Passage of ampicillin into human milk has been reported as follows:

Treatment conditions	Concentration (mg/l)		Milk/ plasma ratio	Maxi-mum observed milk conc. (mg/l)	Absolute dose to infant (mg/kg/day)		Ref.
Dose × Frequency × Duration; Route; No. of patients; Lactation stage	Milk	Plasma			Ave	Max	
500 mg × 1/d × 1 d; p.o.; 2–3; 5–7 d	0.11	2.21	0.05	0.02	0.03	1	(1)
4 g/d × 5 d; p.o.; 13; ?	0.91 (ave.)	8.60 (ave.)	0.03–0.11	2.74	0.66	–	(2)
350 mg × 3/d × ?; p.o.; 12; 0–22 d	0.034–0.082	006–8.2	0.01–0.58	0.082	0.01	–	(3)
700 mg × 3/d × ?; p.o.; 2; 0–22 d	0.25–1.02	0.74–13.83	0.027–0.52	1.02	0.15	–	(3)

Average values based on the areas under the milk amd plasma concentration-time curves for 6 h are given for (1). The maximum milk concentration is the highest value recorded in an individual. In reference (3) pivampicillin was administered to mothers with puerperal infections and ampicillin was assayed. Steady-state dosing conditions are assumed to apply. A further study (4) reported milk to plasma ratios consistent with those in the table.

RELATIVE DOSE IN MILK

A suckling infant would ingest in a feed at maximum 0.1% (0.2 × 180/500)* of the maternal single dose (1) and at maximum 0.6 % (2.74 × 900/4000) of the weight-adjusted maternal daily dose (2).

DATA ON THE INFANT

Six infants whose mothers took pivampicillin for puerperal infection were estimated to have received in milk 0.06–0.37% of the maternal daily dose (5).

* An explanation of the calculation (s) appears on pp. 71–72.

ASSESSMENT AND RECOMMENDATIONS

The risk to the suckling infant of administering ampicillin to its mother is low on the basis that the quantity of drug that passes into milk is small. Breastfeeding should be regarded as safe.

REFERENCES

1. Matsuda T (1984) Transfer of antibiotics into maternal milk. *Biol. Res. Pregnancy Perinatol., 5,* 57–60.
2. Peiker G, Schröder S (1986) Investigations concerning concentrations of oxacillin and ampicillin Penstabil® in the serum and milk of mothers suffering from mastitis puerperalis. *Pharmazie, 41,* 793–795.
3. Branebjerg PE, Heisterberg L (1987) Blood and milk concentrations of ampicillin in mothers treated with pivampicillin and in their infants. *J. Perinatol. Med., 15,* 555–558.
4. Amiraslanova LA, Emelyanova AI, Fursova SA, Rukhadze TG (1985). Some aspects of ampicillin, kanamycin and cerufoxim pharmacokinetics in puerperant patients with endometritis. *Akush. Ginekol. (Mosk.), 10*, 14–17.
5. Matheson I, Samseth M, Sande HA (1988) Ampicillin in breast milk during puerperal infections. *Eur. J. Clin. Pharmacol., 34*, 657–659.

AZTREONAM

GENERAL

Aztreonam is a β-lactam antibiotic. It is poorly absorbed from the gastrointestinal tract and is administered by i.m. injection or i.v. infusion. Aztreonam is 56% bound to plasma proteins and 65% of the dose appears in the urine unchanged. The plasma half-life is 2 h in adults.

EVALUATION OF DATA

Passage of aztreonam into human milk has been reported as follows:

Treatment conditions Dose × Frequency × Duration; Route; No. of patients; Lactation stage	Concentration (mg/l)		Milk/ plasma ratio	Maximum observed milk conc. (mg/l)	Absolute dose to infant (mg/kg/day)		Ref.
	Milk	Plasma			Ave	Max	
1000 mg × 1 × 1/d; i.v.; 10; colostrum	<0.4–1.0 (3 h)	2.5–32.4 (1.5–2 h)		1.0	–	0.15	(1)

The milk and serum values while not concurrent indicate a low milk/serum ratio. Negligible transfer of aztreonam into milk is also suggested by other data (2).

RELATIVE DOSE IN MILK

The amount of aztreonam which a suckling infant would ingest in a feed is at maximum 0.2% (1 × 180/1000)* of the weight-adjusted maternal single dose. The dose to the infant would be less than this estimate if aztreonam is incompletely absorbed from its gastrointestinal tract.

DATA ON THE INFANT

No data are recorded.

ASSESSMENT AND RECOMMENDATIONS

The risk to the suckling infant of administering aztreonam to its mother is low on the basis that the quantity of drug that passes into milk is small. Breast feeding may be regarded as safe.

* An explanation of the calculation(s) appears on pp 71–72.

REFERENCES

1. Ito K, Hirose R, Tamaya T, Yamada Y, Izumi K (1990) Pharmacokinetic and clinical studies on aztreonam in the perinatal period. *Jpn. J. Antibiot.*, *43,* 719–726.
2. Matsuda S, Oh K, Hirayama H, Shimizu T, Sengoku K, Haga H, Inoue H et al. (1990) Pharmacokinetics and clinical evaluations on aztreonam in perinatal infections in obstetrics and gynecology. *Jpn. J. Antibiot.*, *43*, 736–753.

BENZYLPENICILLIN

GENERAL

Benzylpenicillin is an antibiotic that is acid labile and is not suitable for administration by mouth. Following i.m. injection in the adult, it penetrates effectively into most tissues. About 50% is bound to plasma proteins and it is rapidly excreted in the urine. The plasma half-life is 0.5 h.

EVALUATION OF DATA

Passage of penicillin into human milk has been reported as follows:

Treatment conditions	Concentration (mg/l)		Milk/ plasma ratio	Maximum observed milk conc. (mg/l)	Absolute dose to infant (mg/kg/day)		Ref.
Dose × Frequency × Duration; Route; No. of patients; Lactation stage	Milk	Plasma			Ave	Max	
360 mg × 1/d × 1 d; i.m.; 2–3; 5–7 d	0.21	0.37	0.57	0.37	0.03	0.06	(1)
120–360 mg × 1/d × 1 d; i.m.; 13; 2–8 d	0.12	0.34	0.35	0.58	0.02	0.09	(2)
60 mg × 1/d × 1 d; i.m.; 7; 2–5 d	<0.01–0.02	0.23–1.15	–	–	–	–	(3)
60 mg × 2/h × 6 h; i.m.; 3; 2–5 d	0.03	0.48	0.06	–	–	–	(3)

The milk and serum concentration-time profiles were defined over 6 h after dosing in reference (1) and were concurrent. In references (1) and (2) the quoted milk and serum concentrations were average values and the maximum concentration was the highest value recorded in an individual. In reference (3) only a single pair of milk and serum samples was taken from each mother 1–2 h after the last dose. Both references (2) and (3) give doses and concentrations in units and units/ml and a conversion of 1 unit = 0.6 μg has been used. Passage of certain derivatives of benzylpenicillin into breast milk has also been studied; these include dimethoxyphenylpenicillin, methylphenylisoxazoylylpenicillin, methylchlorophenylisoxazolylpenicillin and methyldichlorophenylisoxazolylpenicillin (1). The milk concentrations of these substances after a single dose are in general similar to those of benzylpenicillin.

RELATIVE DOSE IN MILK

The amount of benzylpenicillin that a suckling infant would ingest in a feed is at maximum 0.2% (0.37 × 180/360)* of the weight-adjusted maternal single dose (1).

* An explanation of the calculation (s) appears on pp. 71–72.

DATA ON THE INFANT

No adverse effects were reported in the infants studied.

ASSESSMENT AND RECOMMENDATIONS

Only single dose data are available, but the risk to the suckling infant of administering benzylpenicillin to its mother is low on the basis that the quantity of drug that passes into milk is small. Breast feeding may be regarded as safe.

REFERENCES

1. Matsuda S (1984) Transfer of antibiotics into maternal milk. *Biol. Res. Pregnancy Perinatol., 5,* 57–60.
2. Rozansky R, Brzezinsky A (1949) The excretion of penicillin in human milk. *J. Lab. Clin. Med., 34*, 497–500.
3. Greene HJ, Burkhart B, Hobby GL (1946) Excretion of penicillin in human milk following parturition. *Am. J. Obstet. Gynecol., 51*, 732–733.

CEFACLOR

GENERAL

Cefaclor is a cephalosporin antibiotic. It is absorbed from the adult gastrointestinal tract, is 25% bound to plasma proteins and 88% is excreted in the urine. The plasma half-life is 40 min.

EVALUATION OF DATA

Passage of cefaclor into human milk has been reported as follows:

Treatment conditions — Dose × Frequency × Duration; Route; No. of patients; Lactation stage	Concentration (mg/l)		Milk/ plasma ratio	Maximum observed milk conc. (mg/l)	Absolute dose to infant (mg/kg/day)		Ref.
	Milk	Plasma			Ave	Max	
250 mg × 1/d × 1 d; p.o.; 2; ?	0.1	–	–	0.19	0.02	0.03	(1)
500 mg × 1/d × 1 d; p.o.; 5; ?	0.16	–	–	0.35	0.02	0.05	(1)

The concentration-time profile was defined in milk over 6 h after dosing. The Table gives average values for this period based on area measurements. The maximum milk concentrations were the highest values recorded in individuals. The maximum serum concentration in mothers who received cefaclor 500 mg p.o. in another part of the same study was estimated from a graph to be 9 mg/l.

RELATIVE DOSE IN MILK

The amount of cefaclor which a suckling infant would ingest in a feed is at maximum 0.1% (0.19 × 180/250)* of the weight-adjusted single maternal dose (1).

DATA ON THE INFANT

No data are reported in the study quoted.

ASSESSMENT AND RECOMMENDATIONS

Only single dose data are available, but the risk to the suckling infant of administering cefaclor to its mother appears to be low on the basis that the quantity of drug that passes into milk is small. Breast feeding may be regarded as safe.

* An explanation of the calculation (s) appears on pp. 71–72.

REFERENCES

1. Takase Z (1979) Clinical and laboratory studies of cefaclor in the field of obstetrics and gynecology. *Chemotherapy (Tokyo), 27, (Suppl).*, 666–671.

CEFADROXIL

GENERAL

Cefadroxil is a cephalosporin antibiotic. It is well absorbed from the adult gastro-intestinal tract, 20% is bound to plasma proteins and 88% is excreted unchanged in the urine. The plasma half-life is 1.5 h.

EVALUATION OF DATA

Passage of cefadoxil into human milk has been reported as follows:

Treatment conditions Dose × Frequency × Duration; Route; No. of patients; Lactation stage	Concentration (mg/l)		Milk/ plasma ratio	Maxi- mum observed milk conc. (mg/l)	Absolute dose to infant (mg/kg/day)		Ref.
	Milk	Plasma			Ave	Max	
500 mg × 1/d × 1 d; p.o.; 2–3; 5–7 d	0 (1 h); 0.3 (6 h); 0.28 (ave.)	9.5 (1 h) 1.4 (6 h) 5.91 (ave.)	0.05	0.5	0.04	0.08	(1)
1000 mg × 1/d × 1 d; p.o.; 6; 3 d	0.1 (1 h) 0.43 (3 h) 0.81 (ave.)	11.6 (1 h); 21.6 (3 h); 13.63 (ave.)	0.06	2.4	0.12	0.36	(2)
500 mg × 1/d × 1 d; p.o.; 5; ?	0.44	–	–	0.90	0.07	0.14	(3)

The milk concentration-time profiles were defined in references (1–3) for 6–8 h after dosing and in serum for 3 h (1, 2). Maximum milk concentrations occurred 4–6 h after dosing. The variation in the average serum concentrations and the relative stability of the average milk concentrations are emphasised by the values quoted at times after dosing (1, 2). The table also gives the average concentrations based on area calculations over the periods of measurement. The maximum milk concentrations are the highest values recorded in individuals.

RELATIVE DOSE IN MILK

The amount of cefadoxil which a suckling infant would ingest in a feed is at maximum 0.4% (2.4 × 180/1000)* of the weight-adjusted maternal single dose (2).

DATA ON THE INFANT

No data are reported in the studies quoted.

* An explanation of the calculation (s) appears on pp. 71–72.

ASSESSMENT AND RECOMMENDATIONS

Only single dose data are available but the risk to the suckling infant of administering cefadroxil to its mother appears to be low on the basis that the quantity of drug that passes into milk is small. Breast feeding may be regarded as safe.

REFERENCES

1. Matsuda S. Transfer of antibiotics into maternal milk (1984) *Biol. Res. Pregnancy Perinatol., 5*, 57–60.
2. Kafetzis D, Siafas C, Georgakopoulos PA, Papadatos C (1981) Passage of cephalosporins and amoxicillin into the breast milk. *Acta Paediatr. Scand., 70*, 285–288.
3. Takase Z, Shirafuji H, Uchida M (1980) Experimental and clinical studies of cefadroxil in the treatment of infections in the field of obstetrics and gynecology. *Chemotherapy (Tokyo), 28, Suppl. 2*, 424–431.

CEFALEXIN

GENERAL

Cephalexin (cephalexin) is a cephalosporin antibiotic. It is rapidly and almost completely absorbed from the adult gastrointestinal tract, is 10–15% bound to plasma proteins and is excreted by the kidneys. The plasma half-life is 1–2 h.

EVALUATION OF DATA

Passage of cefalexin into human milk has been reported as follows:

Treatment conditions Dose × Frequency × Duration; Route; No. of patients; Lactation stage	Concentration (mg/l) Milk	 Plasma	Milk/ plasma ratio	Maximum observed milk conc. (mg/l)	Absolute dose to infant (mg/kg/day) Ave	 Max	Ref.
1000 mg × 1/d × 1 d; p.o.; 6; 3 d	0.2 (1 h) 0.39 (3 h) 0.33 (ave.)	22.9 (1 h) 0.14 (3 h) 12.6 (ave.)	0.009 (1 h) 0.14 (3 h) 0.03 (ave.)	0.85	0.05	0.13	(1)
500 mg × 1/d × 1 d; p.o.; 2–3; 5–7 d	Trace (1 h) 0.7 (4 h) 0.39 (ave.)	5.8 (1 h) 2.8 (4 h) 2.98 (ave.)	0.13 (ave.)	0.8	0.06	0.12	(2)

Reference (1) defines the concentration-time profiles for milk over 6 h and for serum over 3 h. Reference (2) defines the profiles for both milk and serum over 6 h. The table emphasises the decline in average serum concentration and the relative stability of the average milk concentration at the stated times after dosing. The table also gives the average concentrations based on area calculations over the periods of measurement. The maximum milk concentrations for both references are the highest values recorded in individuals.

RELATIVE DOSE IN MILK

The amount of cephalexin that a suckling infant would ingest in a feed is at maximum 0.3% (0.8 × 180/500)* of the weight-adjusted maternal single dose (2).

DATA ON THE INFANT

None are reported in the study quoted.

* An explanation of the calculation (s) appears on pp. 71–72.

ASSESSMENT AND RECOMMENDATIONS

Only single dose data are available, but the risk to the suckling infant of administering cephalexin to its mother would appear to be low on the basis that the quantity of drug that passes into milk is small. Breast feeding may be regarded as safe.

REFERENCES

1. Kafetzis D, Siafas C, Georgakopoulos P, Papadatos CJ (1981) Passage of cephalosporins and amoxicillin into the breast milk. *Acta Paediatr. Scand., 70,* 285–288.
2. Matsuda S (1984) Transfer of antibiotics into maternal milk. *Biol. Res. Pregnancy Perinatol., 5,* 57–60.

CEFALORIDINE

GENERAL

Cefaloridine (cephaloridine) is a cephalosporin antibiotic that is poorly absorbed from the gastrointestinal tract and must be given i.m or i.v.. In the adult it is widely distributed in body tissues and fluids and 20% is bound to plasma proteins. Over 80% of cefaloridine is eliminated in the urine unchanged and the plasma half-life is 1.5 h.

EVALUATION OF DATA

Passage of cefaloridine into human milk has been reported as follows:

Treatment conditions: Dose × Frequency × Duration; Route; No. of patients; Lactation stage	Concentration (mg/l): Milk	Concentration (mg/l): Plasma	Milk/plasma ratio	Maximum observed milk conc. (mg/l)	Absolute dose to infant (mg/kg/day): Ave	Absolute dose to infant (mg/kg/day): Max	Ref.
1000 mg × 1/d × 1 d; i.m.; 2–3; 5–7 d	0.0 (1 h)	19.0 (1 h)	–	–	–	–	(1)
	0.15 (6 h)	2.0 (6 h)	–	–		–	
	0.09 (ave.)	8.32 (ave.)	0.01	0.3	0.01	0.05	
500 mg × 1/d × 1 d; i.m.; 6; colostrum	Trace	–	–	Trace	–	–	(2)

Reference (1) defines the concentration-time profiles over 6 h after dosing. Cefaloridine could not be measured in milk at 1 and 2 h and the highest average concentration was at 6 h; the peak concentration in serum was at 1 h. The table also gives the average concentrations based on area measurements over 6 h. The maximum milk concentration was the highest value recorded in an individual. In reference (2) only 'trace' amounts of cefaloridine were recorded in milk over 12 h after dosing. The limit of sensitivity of the assay was not quoted.

RELATIVE DOSE IN MILK

The amount of cefaloridine that a suckling infant would ingest in a feed is at maximum 0.1% (0.3 × 180/1000)* of the weight-adjusted maternal single dose (1). The dose to the infant would be less than this estimate if cefaloridine is incompletely absorbed from its gastrointestinal tract.

DATA ON THE INFANT

When cefaloridine 10 or 25 mg was administered i.m. to neonates, peak plasma

* An explanation of the calculation (s) appears on pp. 71–72.

concentrations were reported 1–2 h after dosing and excretion was significantly slower than in adults (2). No adverse effects were observed.

ASSESSMENT AND RECOMMENDATION

The risk to the suckling infant of administering cefaloridine to its mother is low on the basis that the quantity of drug that passes into milk is small. Breastfeeding may be regarded as safe.

REFERENCES

1. Matsuda S (1984) Transfer of antibiotics to maternal milk. *Biol. Res. Pregnancy Perinatol., 5,* 57–60.
2. Fukada M (1973) Studies on chemotherapy during the perinatal period with special reference to such derivatives of cephalosporin C as cefazolin, cephaloridine and cephalothin. *Jpn. J. Antibiot., 26,* 197–212.

CEFALOTIN

GENERAL

Cefalotin (cefalothin) is a cephalosporin antibiotic that is poorly absorbed from the gastrointestinal tract and is consequently given by i.v. injection or infusion. In the adult it is 50% bound to plasma proteins. Cefalotin undergoes deacetylation in the liver to yield an inactive metabolite which accounts for 20–30% of the excreted dose; the remainder is eliminated unchanged in the urine. The plasma half-life is 0.5 h.

EVALUATION OF DATA

Passage of cefalotin into human milk has been reported as follows:

Treatment conditions: Dose × Frequency × Duration; Route; No. of patients; Lactation stage	Concentration (mg/l): Milk	Concentration (mg/l): Plasma	Milk/ plasma ratio	Maximum observed milk conc. (mg/l)	Absolute dose to infant (mg/kg/day): Ave	Absolute dose to infant (mg/kg/day): Max	Ref.
1000 mg × 1/d × 1 d; i.m.; 6; colostrum	Trace	–	–	–	–	–	(1)
1000 mg × 1/d × 1 d; i.v.; 6; 2–3 d	0.41 (1 h)	5.9 (1 h)	0.07 (1 h)	–	–	–	(2)
	0.36 (3 h)	0.7 (3 h)	0.5 (3 h)				
	0.31 (ave)	2.71 (ave)	0.31	0.62	0.05	0.09	

The concentration-time profiles for milk over 6 h and for serum over 3 h were defined in reference (2); the Table gives the average values at the times stated to emphasise the fluctuation in serum concentration relative to that in milk. The average concentration in milk over 6 h and in serum over 3 h based on area measurements are also given (2). The maximum milk concentration is the highest value recorded in an individual.

RELATIVE DOSE IN MILK

The amount of cefalotin that a suckling infant would ingest in a feed is at maximum 0.1% (0.62 × 180/1000)* of the weight-adjusted maternal single dose (2). The dose to the infant would be less than this estimate if cephalothin is incompletely absorbed from its gastrointestinal tract.

* An explanation of the calculation (s) appears on pp. 71–72.

DATA ON THE INFANT

Infants who received 10 or 25 mg/kg of cefalotin as a single i.m. dose produced peak plasma concentrations within 30 min and there was no trace of the drug in plasma 12 h after dosing (1). No adverse effects were observed.

ASSESSMENT AND RECOMMENDATIONS

Only single dose data are available, but the risk to the suckling infant of administering cefalotin to its mother would appear to be low on the basis that the quantity of drug that passes into milk is small. Breast feeding may be regarded as safe.

REFERENCES

1. Fukada M (1973) Studies on chemotherapy during the perinatal period with special reference to such derivatives of cephalosporin C as cefazolin, cephaloridine and cephalothin. *Jpn. J. Antibiot.*, *26*, 197–212.
2. Kafetzis DA, Siafas CA, Georgakopoulos PA, Papadatos CJ (1981) Passage of cephalosporins and amoxicillin into the breast milk. *Acta Paediatr. Scand.*, *70*, 285–288.

CEFAPIRIN

GENERAL

Cefapirin (cefapirin) is a cephalosporin antibiotic that is poorly absorbed from the gastrointestinal tract and is therefore given by i.m. or i.v. injection. In the adult cefapirin is 35–50% bound to plasma proteins and is eliminated primarily by the kidneys. The plasma half-life is 30 min.

EVALUATION OF DATA

Passage of cefapirin into human milk has been reported as follows:

Treatment conditions	Concentration (mg/l)		Milk/plasma ratio	Maximum observed milk conc. (mg/l)	Absolute dose to infant (mg/kg/day)		Ref.
Dose × Frequency × Duration; Route; No. of patients; Lactation stage	Milk	Plasma			Ave	Max	
1000 mg × 1/d × 1 d; i.v.; 6; 3 d	0.41 (1 h)	6.1 (1 h)	0.07	–	–	–	(1)
	0.33 (3 h)	0.7(3 h)	0.47	–	–	–	
	0.33 (ave)	2.75(ave)	0.12	0.64	0.05	0.1	

Concentration-time profiles were defined in milk over 6 h and in serum over 3 h after dosing in reference (1). The average values for the group at 1 and 3 h after cefapirin emphasise the decline in serum concentration and the relative stability of the milk concentration. The Table also gives the average concentrations based on area calculations over the periods of measurement. The maximum milk concentration is the highest value recorded in an individual. The half-life in milk was 2.5–3.5 h.

RELATIVE DOSE IN MILK

The amount of cefapirin which a sucking infant would ingest in a feed is at maximum 0.1% (0.64 × 180/1000)* of the weight-adjusted maternal single dose (1). The dose to the infant would be less than this estimate if cefapirin is incompletely absorbed from its gastrointestinal tract.

DATA ON THE INFANT

No adverse reactions were observed in the infants who were nursed in the quoted study.

* An explanation of the calculation (s) appears on pp. 71–72.

ASSESSMENT AND RECOMMENDATIONS

Only single dose data are available, but the risk to the suckling infant of administering cefapirin to its mother appears to be low on the basis that the quantity of drug that passes into milk is small. Breast feeding may be regarded as safe.

REFERENCES

1. Kafetzis DA, Siafas CA, Georgakopoulos PA, Papadatos CJ (1981) Passage of cephalosporins and amoxicillin into the breast milk. *Acta Paediatr. Scand., 70,* 285–288.

CEFAZEDONE

GENERAL

Cefazedone is a cephalosporin antibiotic. It is moderately lipid soluble and, being poorly absorbed from the adult gastrointestinal tract, it is administered parenterally. The half-life is 1.4 h in maternal serum and 4.2 h in neonates, based on urine data (1).

EVALUATION OF DATA

Passage of cefazedone into human milk has been reported as follows:

Treatment conditions — Dose × Frequency × Duration; Route; No. of patients; Lactation stage	Concentration (mg/l) — Milk	Concentration (mg/l) — Plasma	Milk/ plasma ratio	Maximum observed milk conc. (mg/l)	Absolute dose to infant (mg/kg/day) — Ave	Absolute dose to infant (mg/kg/day) — Max	Ref.
1000 mg × 3/d × 1–11 d; i.v.; 4; ?	0.57	47.5	0.01	1.0	0.09	0.15	(1)

Milk and serum samples were taken at intervals from mothers who received courses of cefazedone. Average values appear in the Table but the maximum milk concentration is the highest value recorded in an individual. The elimination half-life from milk was 7 h. Steady-state dosing conditions were probably achieved in 3 of the mothers.

RELATIVE DOSE IN MILK

The amount of cefazedone which a suckling infant would ingest in a day is on average 0.2% (0.57 × 900/3000)* and at maximum 0.3% (1.0 × 900/3000)* of the weight-adjusted maternal daily dose (1). The dose to the infant would be less than these estimates if cefazedone is incompletely absorbed from its gastrointestinal tract.

ASSESSMENT AND RECOMMENDATIONS

The risk to the suckling infant of administering cefazedone to its mother is low on the basis that the quantity of drug that passes into milk is small. Breast feeding may be regarded as safe.

REFERENCES

1. von Kobyletzki D, Sas M, Wahlig DH, Wiemann H (1979) Pharmacokinetic investigations of cefazedone in gynaecology and obstetrics. *Arzneim-Forsch/Drug Res., 29,* 1763–1768.

* An explanation of the calculation (s) appears on pp. 71–72.

CEFAZOLIN

GENERAL

Cefazolin (cephazolin) a cephalosporin antibiotic. It is poorly absorbed from the gastrointestinal tract and is given i.m. or by i.v. injection or infusion. In the adult 90% of the drug is weakly bound to plasma proteins. Cephazolin is excreted unchanged in the urine. The plasma half-life is 2 h.

EVALUATION OF DATA

Passage of cefazolin into human breast milk has been reported as follows:

Treatment conditions	Concentration (mg/l)		Milk/ plasma ratio	Maximum observed milk conc. (mg/l)	Absolute dose to infant (mg/kg/day)		Ref.
Dose × Frequency × Duration; Route; No. of patients; Lactation stage	Milk	Plasma			Ave	Max	
500 mg × 1/d × 1 d; i.m.; 4; colostrum	Trace	–	–	Trace	–	–	(1)
2000 mg × 1/d × 1 d; i.v.; 20; ?	0.99 (ave)	54.3 (2 h)	0.02 (2 h)	1.51	0.2	0.23	(2)
500 mg × 3/d × 2 d; i.m.; 12; ?	<0.09	–	–	<0.09	–	–	(3)

In reference (1) milk samples were taken on 4 occasions over 12 h after cefazolin. The limit of sensitivity of the assay is not given. In reference (2) cefazolin was infused over 10 min. The Table gives the average value based on the area under the plasma concentration-time curve over 4 h. Reference (3) gives data on mothers from whom milk samples were taken 11–25 h after their last dose of cefazolin. In the same study cefazolin could not be detected in any sample of milk from 10 mothers 1–14 h after a single 500 mg i.m. dose.

RELATIVE DOSE IN MILK

The amount of cefazolin which a suckling infant would ingest in a feed is at maximum 0.3% (1.51 × 180/1000)* of the weight-adjusted maternal single dose (2). The lowest recommended paediatric single dose of cefazolin is 25 mg/kg and the maximum amount a suckling infant would ingest in a feed is 0.2% (1.51 × 3/25)* of this (2). The dose to the infant would be less than these estimates if cefazolin is incompletely absorbed from its gastrointestinal tract.

* An explanation of the calculation (s) appears on pp. 71–72.

DATA ON THE INFANT

When cefazolin was administered to neonates at a single dose of 25 or 50 mg/kg, peak plasma concentrations were observed within 1–2 h and the plasma elimination half-life was 4–12 h. No adverse effects were observed in these infants (1).

ASSESSMENT AND RECOMMENDATIONS

The risk to the suckling infant of administering cefazolin to the mother is low on the basis that the quantity of drug that passes into milk is small. Breast-feeding may be regarded as safe.

REFERENCES

1. Fukada M (1973) Studies on chemotherapy during the perinatal period with special reference to such derivatives of cephalosporin C as cefazolin, cephaloridine and cephalothin. *Jpn. J. Antibiot., 26,* 197–212.
2. Yoshioka H, Cho K, Takimoto M, Maruyama S, Shimizu T (1979) Transfer of cefazolin into human milk. *J. Pediatr., 94,* 151–152.
3. Von Kobyletzki D, Reither K, Gellen J, Kanyo A, Glocke M (1974) Pharmacokinetische Utersuvhungen mit Cefazolin in Geburtshilfe und Gynäkologie. *Infection, 2, Suppl. 1,* 60–67.

CEFMENOXIME

GENERAL

Cefmenoxime is a cephalosporin antibiotic. It is poorly absorbed from the adult gastrointestinal tract and is administered by intravenous injection. Cefmenoxime is 52% bound to plasma proteins and 70% is excreted unchanged in the urine. The plasma half-life is 1 h.

EVALUATION OF DATA

Passage of cefmenoxime into human milk has been reported as follows:

Treatment conditions Dose × Frequency × Duration; Route; No. of patients; Lactation stage	Concentration (mg/l)		Milk/ plasma ratio	Maximum observed milk conc. (mg/l)	Absolute dose to infant (mg/kg/day)		Ref.
	Milk	Plasma			Ave	Max	
1000 mg × 2/d × 7 d; i.v.; 5; colostrum	1.38	1.06	1.30	1.75	0.21	0.26	(1)
1000 mg × 1/d × 1 d; i.v.; 6, colostrum	0.17	–	–	0.34	–	0.05	(2)

Mothers received cefmenoxime for obstetric infections. In (1) milk and serum were collected on 5 occasions during 72 h of treatment and average values are quoted. An average value for milk is quoted in reference (2), based on area measurements.

RELATIVE DOSE IN MILK

The amount of cefmenoxime which a suckling infant would ingest in a day is on average 0.6% (1.38 × 900/2000)* and at maximum 0.8% (1.75 × 900/2000)* of the weight-adjusted maternal daily dose (1). The dose to the infant may be less than these estimates if cefmenoxime is incompletely absorbed from its gastrointestinal tract.

DATA ON THE INFANT

No data are available.

ASSESSMENT AND RECOMMENDATIONS

The risk to the suckling infant of administering cefmenoxime to its mother is low

* An explanation of the calculation (s) appears on pp. 71–72.

on the basis that the quantity of drug that passes into milk is small. Breast feeding may be regarded as safe.

REFERENCES

1. Weissenbacher ER, Adams D, Gutschow K, Peters-Welte C, Luehr HG (1984) Clinical results and concentrations of cefmenoxime in serum, amniotic fluid, mother's milk and umbilical cord. *Am. J. Med., 77, Suppl 6A,* 11–12.
2. Cho N, Fukunaga K, Kunii K (1989) Fundamental and clinical studies on cefmenoxime in perinatal period. *Jpn. J. Antibiot., XLII,* 2692–2708.

CEFODIZIME

GENERAL

Cefodizime is a cephalosporin antibiotic with actions and uses similar to cefotaxime. It is excreted by the kidneys largely in the unchanged form and the serum half-life is 2 h.

EVALUATION OF DATA

Passage of cefodizime into human breast milk has been reported as follows:

Treatment conditions Dose × Frequency × Duration; Route; No. of patients; Lactation stage	Concentration (mg/l) Milk	Serum	Milk/plasma ratio	Maximum observed milk conc. (mg/l)	Absolute dose to infant (mg/kg/day) Ave	Max	Ref.
1 g × 1/d × 1 d; i.v.; 13; 1–2 d	0.57 (3 h) 0.25 (8 h)	–	–	0.57	–	0.09	(1)
2 g × 1/d × 1 d; i.v.; 13; 1–2 d	1.22 (2 h) 0.45 (8 h)	–	–	1.22	–	0.18	(1)
1 g × 1/d × 1 d; i.v.; 4; 1 d	0.24 (3 h) 0.16 (6 h)	–	–	0.24	–	0.04	(2)

The milk concentrations are average values for the groups at the times stated (1, 2). Concurrence of the milk and serum concentration-time profiles cannot be assessed but average values of 0.21 mg/l in milk and 77.6 mg/l in serum at 1 h after cefodizime 1.0 g i.v. suggest a very low milk to serum ratio (1).

RELATIVE DOSE IN MILK

The amount of cefodizime that a suckling infant would ingest in a feed is at maximum 0.2% (1.22 × 180/1000)* of the weight adjusted maternal single dose. The dose to the infant would be less than this estimate if cefodizime is incompletely absorbed from its gastrointestinal tract.

DATA ON THE INFANT

No data are available on breast-fed infants.

ASSESSMENT AND RECOMMENDATIONS

The risk to the suckling infant of administering cefodizime to the mother is low on the basis that the quantity of drug that passes into milk is small. Breast feeding may be regarded as safe.

* An explanation of the calculation (s) appears on pp. 71–72.

REFERENCES

1. Mikamo H, Izumi K, Ito K, TamayaT (1993). Investigation on the transfer of cefodizime to breast milk. *Chemotherapy (Japan), 41,* 1268–1271.
2. Ito K, Nakagawa M, Mabuchi M, Tamaya T, Hayasaki M, Yamada Y, Ito N (1989). Fundamental and clinical evaluation of cefodizime in obstetrics and gynecology. *Jpn. J. Antibiot., XLII*, 2107–2109.

CEFONICID

GENERAL

Cefonicid is a cephalosporin antibiotic; it is administered parentally. Cefonicid is 80% bound to plasma proteins and has a plasma half-life of 2 h in adults.

EVALUATION OF DATA

Passage of cefonicid into human milk has been reported as follows:

Treatment conditions Dose × Frequency × Duration; Route; No. of patients; Lactation stage	Concentration (mg/l)		Milk/ plasma ratio	Maximum observed milk conc. (mg/l)	Absolute dose to infant (mg/kg/day)		Ref.
	Milk	Plasma			Ave	Max	
1000 mg × 1/d × 1 d; i.m.; 10, 5 d	0.16 (trace–0.3)	67.4 (35.6–91.4)	0.002	0.3	0.02	0.05	(1)

The mothers did not breast-feed their infants. A single pair of milk and blood samples was taken 1 h after cefonicid and the table gives average values and the range of concentrations. The concentration-time profiles and peak concentrations were not defined.

RELATIVE DOSE IN MILK

The amount of cefonicid which a suckling infant would ingest in a feed is at maximum 0.1% (0.3 × 180/1000)* of the weight-adjusted maternal single dose (1). The dose to the infant would be less than this estimate if cefonicid is incompletely absorbed from its gastrointestinal tract.

DATA ON THE INFANT

No data are available.

ASSESSMENT AND RECOMMENDATIONS

Only single dose data are available, but the risk to the suckling infant of administering cefonicid to the mother would appear to be low on the basis that the quantity of drug that passes into milk is small. Breast-feeding may be regarded as safe.

* An explanation of the calculation (s) appears on pp. 71–72.

REFERENCE

1. Lou MA, Wu YH, Jacob LS, Pitkin DH (1984) Penetration of cefonicid into human breast milk and various body fluids and tissues. *Rev. Infect. Dis., 6, Suppl. 4,* S816–820.

CEFOTAXIME

GENERAL

Cefotaxime is a cephalosporin antibiotic which is poorly absorbed from the gastrointestinal tract and is administered i.m. or by i.v. injection or infusion. In the adult it is 40% bound to plasma proteins and is excreted 75% by the renal and 25% by the biliary route; the plasma half-life is 1 h. Its principal hepatic metabolite is desacetyl-cefotaxime which is 15% as active as the parent drug and is found in significant quantities in both blood and urine.

EVALUATION OF DATA

Passage of cefotaxime into human milk has been reported as follows:

Treatment conditions Dose × Frequency × Duration; Route; No. of patients; Lactation stage	Concentration (mg/l)		Milk/ plasma ratio	Maximum observed milk conc. (mg/l)	Absolute dose to infant (mg/kg/day)		Ref.
	Milk	Serum			Ave	Max	
1000 mg × 1/d × 1 d; i.v.; 12; 3 d	0.26 (1 h) 0.3 (3 h) 0.20 (ave)	9.4 (1 h) 1.9 (3 h) 4.68 (ave)	0.04	0.52	0.03	0.08	(1)
100 mg × 1/d × 1 d; i.v.; 2–3; 5–7 d	Trace (1 h) 0 (4 h)	15.5 (1 h) 1.0 (4 h)	–	–	–	–	(2)

Reference (1) defines the concentration-time profiles for milk over 6 h and for serum over 3 h after dosing. The average concentrations at the stated times emphasises the decline in serum concentration and the relative stability of the milk concentration. The table also gives the average concentration based on area measurements in milk over 6 and serum over 3 h. The maximum concentration is the highest value recorded in an individual. The milk half-life was 2.9 h compared to 0.9 h in serum and suggests that during chronic dosing the milk concentrations may be higher than those quoted above.

RELATIVE DOSE IN MILK

The amount of cefotaxime which a suckling infant would ingest in a feed is at maximum 0.1% (0.52 × 180/1000)* of the weight-adjusted maternal single dose (1). The dose to the infant would be less than this estimate if cefotaxime is incompletely absorbed from its gastrointestinal tract.

DATA ON THE INFANT

No data are available.

* An explanation of the calculation (s) appears on pp. 71–72.

ASSESSMENT AND RECOMMENDATIONS

Only single dose data are available, but the risk to the suckling infant of administering cefotaxime to its mother appears to be low on the basis that the quantity of drug that passes into milk is small. Breast-feeding may be regarded as safe.

REFERENCE

1. Kafetzis DA, Lazarides CV, Siafas CA, Georgakopoulos PA, Papadatos CJ (1980) Transfer of cefotaxime in human milk and from mother to foetus. *J. Antimicrob. Chemother., 6, Suppl. A*, 135–141.
2. Matsuda S (1984) Transfer of antibiotics into maternal milk. *Biol. Res. Pregnancy Perinatol., 5*, 57–60.

CEFOTIAM

GENERAL

Cefotiam is a cephem antibiotic. It is administered by i.m. or i.v. injection. The half-life of elimination from plasma is 3 h.

EVALUATION OF DATA

The passage of cefotiam into human milk has been reported as follows:

Treatment conditions	Concentration (mg/l)		Milk/ plasma ratio	Maximum observed milk conc. (mg/l)	Absolute dose to infant (mg/kg/day)		Ref.
Dose × Frequency × Duration; Route; No. of patients; Lactation stage	Milk	Plasma			Ave	Max	
1000 mg × 1/d × 1 d; i.v.; 6; colostrum	0.2–0.4	–	–	0.4	–	0.06	(1)
1000 mg × 1/d × 1 d; i.v.; 4; colostrum	n.d.–0.51	–	–	0.51	–	0.08	(2)

n.d. = not detected

RELATIVE DOSE IN MILK

The concentration of cefotiam that a suckling infant would ingest would be at maximum 0.1% (0.51 × 180/1000)* of the weight-adjusted maternal dose. The dose to the infant would be less than this estimate if cefotiam is incompletely absorbed from its gastrointestinal tract.

DATA ON THE INFANT

No data are available on breast-fed infants.

ASSESSMENT AND RECOMMENDATIONS

The risk to the suckling infant of administering cefotiam to its mother is low on the basis of the amount of drug that passes into milk is small. Breast-feeding may be regarded as safe.

* An explanation of the calculation (s) appears on pp. 71–72.

REFERENCES

1. Cho N, Fukunaga K, Kunii K (1986) Pharmacokinetic and clinical studies of cefotiam in perinatal period. *Jpn. J. Antibiot.*, *39*, 2488–2496.
2. Takase Z, Miyoshi T, Fujiwara M, Nakayama M, Komoto Y, Shirafuji H (1986) Study on cefotiam in the perinatal period. *Jpn. J. Antibiot.*, *39*, 2534–2542.

CEFOXITIN

GENERAL

Cefoxitin is a cephalosporin antibiotic. It is poorly absorbed from the adult gastrointestinal tract and is administered i.m. or by i.v. injection or infusion. Cefoxitin is 70% bound to plasma proteins and is excreted mainly in the urine although biliary elimination also occurs. The plasma half-life is 40 min.

EVALUATION OF DATA

Passage of cefoxitin into human milk has been reported as follows:

Treatment conditions: Dose × Frequency × Duration; Route; No. of patients; Lactation stage	Concentration (mg/l): Milk	Concentration (mg/l): Serum	Milk/plasma ratio	Maximum observed milk conc. (mg/l)	Absolute dose to infant (mg/kg/day): Ave	Absolute dose to infant (mg/kg/day): Max	Ref.
1000 mg × 1/d × 1 d; i.m.; 15; 6–10 d	<0.5	6–25	–	<0.5	–	–	(1)
2000 mg × 1/d × 1 d; i.m.; 5; 6–10 d	<0.25–0.65	22.7–77.6	–	0.65	–	0.10	(2)
1000 mg × 1/d × 1 d; i.v.; 3; 5–7 d	Trace	0.8–15.4	–	–	–	–	(3)

Mothers reported in reference (1) interrupted breast-feeding for 24 h following the injection of cefoxitin and a single pair of milk and blood samples was taken usually within 2 h of the dose. Further samples of milk were taken from 5 mothers for up to 24 h but cefoxitin was not detected in any. In reference (2) a more sensitive assay was used. Milk samples were taken 1 h and thereafter every 3 h after cefoxitin for 25 h and blood was taken after 1 h. Cefoxitin was measurable for 25 h in 2 of the 5 mothers. In both studies the range of concentrations is presented. In reference (3) the Table gives the serum concentrations 1 h and 4 h after dosing; only trace amounts of cefoxitin were noted in milk. Another study also reported negligible passage of cefoxitin into milk with 24 of 25 samples from 18 women recorded as <0.5 mg/l after 2–4 g of the drug were given (4). These samples, however, were collected on average 25 h after the last dose.

RELATIVE DOSE IN MILK

The amount of cefoxitin which a suckling infant would ingest in a feed is at maximum 0.1% (0.65 × 180/1000)* of the weight-adjusted maternal single dose (2). The lowest recommended single dose for an infant is 25 mg/kg and a suckling infant would receive in a feed at maximum 0.1% (0.65 × 3/25)* of this (2). The dose to the infant would be less than these estimates if cefoxitin is incompletely absorbed from its gastrointestinal tract.

* An explanation of the calculation (s) appears on pp. 71–72.

DATA ON THE INFANT

No adverse effects were noted in an infant whose mother's milk contained cefoxitin (4).

ASSESSMENT AND RECOMMENDATIONS

The risk to the suckling infant of administering cefoxitin to its mother would appear to be low on the basis that the quantity of drug that passes into milk is small. Breast-feeding may be regarded as safe.

REFERENCES

1. Dubois M, Delapierre D, Chanteux L, Demonty J, Lambotte R, Kramp R, Dresse A (1981) A study of the transplacental transfer and the mammary excretion of cefoxitin in humans. *J. Clin. Pharmacol., 21*, 477–483.
2. Dresse A, Lambotte R, Dubois M, Delapierre D, Kramp R (1983) Transmammary passage of cefoxitin: additional results. *J. Clin. Pharmacol., 23*, 438–440.
3. Matsuda S (1984) Transfer of antibiotics into maternal milk. *Biol. Res. Pregnancy Perinatol., 5*, 57–60.
4. Roex AJM, Loenen AC, Puyenbroek JI, Arts NFT (1987) Secretion of cefoxitin in breast milk following short-term prophylactic administration in caesarian section. *Eur. J .Obstet. Gynecol. Reprod. Biol., 25*, 299–302.

CEFPROZIL

GENERAL

Cefprozil is a cephalosporin antibiotic that is suitable for oral use. It is 40% bound to plasma proteins and is excreted in the urine mainly in the unchanged form. The half-life of elimination from plasma is 1.5 h. Cefprozil consists of *cis* and *trans* isomers in an approximately 9:1 ratio.

EVALUATION OF DATA

Passage of cefprozil into human milk has been reported as follows:

Treatment conditions — Dose × Frequency × Duration; Route; No. of patients; Lactation stage	Concentration (mg/l) Milk	Plasma	Milk/plasma ratio	Maximum observed milk conc. (mg/l)	Absolute dose to infant (mg/kg/day) Ave	Max	Ref.
1000 mg × 1/d × 1 d; p.o.; 9; 6–12 months	1.52	–	0.05 (2 h); 5.67 (12 h)	3.4	–	0.51	(1)

The quoted values relate to the *cis* isomer. The plasma and milk concentration-time curves were defined and were not concurrent, and this is reflected in the variation in the milk:plasma ratio. The quoted milk value is an average concentration based on area measurements and the maximum value is the average for the group. Milk concentrations of the *trans* isomer were <0.26 mg/l.

RELATIVE DOSE IN MILK

The amount of *cis* cefprozil which a suckling infant would ingest in a feed is at maximum 0.6% (3.4 × 180/1000)* of the weight-adjusted maternal single dose. Contribution from the *trans* isomer is negligible.

DATA ON THE INFANT

No data are available.

ASSESSMENT AND RECOMMENDATIONS

Only single dose data are available, but the risk to the suckling infant of administering cefprozil to its mother is low on the basis that the quantity of drug that passes into milk is small. Breast-feeding may be regarded as safe.

* An explanation of the calculation (s) appears on pp. 71–72.

REFERENCE

1. Shyu WC, Shah VR, Campbell DA, Venitz J, Jaganathan V, Pittman KA, Wilber RB, Barbhaiya RH (1992) Excretion of cefprozil into human breast milk. *Antimicrob. Agents Chemother.*, 36, 938–941.

CEFRADINE

GENERAL

Cefradrine (cephradine) is a cephalosporin antibiotic. It is rapidly absorbed from the adult gastrointestinal tract and is 6–20% bound to plasma proteins. Cefradine is eliminated mainly by the kidneys and the plasma half-life is 30 min.

EVALUATION OF DATA

Passage of cephradrine into human milk has been reported as follows:

Treatment conditions: Dose × Frequency × Duration; Route; No. of patients; Lactation stage	Concentration (mg/l)		Milk/ plasma ratio	Maximum observed milk conc. (mg/l)	Absolute dose to infant (mg/kg/day)		Ref.
	Milk	Serum			Ave	Max	
500 mg × 4/d × 2 d; p.o.; 6; 1–63 d	0.63 (0.61–0.68)	3.01 (0.49–5.40)	0.21	0.68	0.10	0.10	(1)

The milk and serum concentration-time profiles were defined in a dose interval. The Table gives average values for the group based on area measurements, and the range. The latter indicates that whilst the serum concentrations showed the expected rise and fall with dosing, the milk concentrations remained relatively constant. Steady-state dosing conditions were attained as judged by the serum half-life but it is not known if these conditions apply to the drug in milk.

RELATIVE DOSE IN MILK

The amount of cefradine which a suckling infant would ingest in a day is at maximum 0.3% (0.68 × 900/2000)* of the weight-adjusted maternal daily dose (1). The recommended infant daily dose is 50 mg/kg and a suckling infant would ingest in a day at maximum 0.2% (0.68 × 15/50)* of this.

DATA ON THE INFANT

No data are available.

ASSESSMENT AND RECOMMENDATIONS

The risk to the suckling infant of administering cefradine to its mother is low on the basis that the quantity of drug that passes into milk is small. Breast-feeding may be regarded as safe.

* An explanation of the calculation (s) appears on pp. 71–72.

REFERENCE

1. Mischler TW, Corson SL, Larranaga A, Bolognese RJ, Neiss ES, Vukovich RA (1978) Cephradine and epicillin in body fluids of lactating and pregnant women. *J. Reprod. Med., 21,* 130–136.

CEFSULODIN

GENERAL

Cefsulodin is a cephalosporin antibiotic that is given by the i.m or i.v. routes as its absorption from the gastrointestinal tract is negligible. In the adult cefsulodin is 30% is bound to plasma proteins and is eliminated unchanged in the urine. The plasma half-life is 1.5 h.

EVALUATION OF DATA

Passage of cefsulodin into human milk has been reported as follows:

Treatment conditions Dose × Frequency × Duration; Route; No. of patients; Lactation stage	Concentration (mg/l)		Milk/plasma ratio	Maximum observed milk conc. (mg/l)	Absolute dose to infant (mg/kg/day)		Ref.
	Milk	Plasma			Ave	Max	
1000 mg × 1/d × 1 d; i.v.; 4; ?	0.84	–	–	1.2	–	0.18	(1)

The concentration in milk is an average value based on area measurements over 6 h after administration of the drug. The maximum concentration in milk is the average for the group.

RELATIVE DOSE IN MILK

The amount of cefsulodin that a suckling infant would ingest in a day is at maximum 0.2% (1.2 × 180/1000)* of the weight adjusted maternal single dose.

DATA ON THE INFANT

No data are available in breast-fed infants.

ASSESSMENT AND RECOMMENDATIONS

The risk to the suckling infant of administering cefsulodin to its mother is low on the basis that the quantity of drug that passes into milk is small. Breast-feeding may be regarded as safe.

REFERENCE

1. Cho N, Fukunaga K, Kunii K (1989) Pharmacokinetic studies on cefsulodin in the perinatal period. *Jpn. J. Antibiot., XL11*, 2735–2742.

* An explanation of the calculation (s) appears on pp. 71–72.

CEFTAZIDIME

GENERAL

Ceftazidime is a cephalosporin antibiotic that is poorly absorbed from the gastrointestinal tract and is therefore administered i.m. or i.v. injection or infusion.. In the adult ceftazidime is 10% bound to plasma proteins and it is eliminated mainly unchanged by the kidneys. The plasma half-life is 2 h.

EVALUATION OF DATA

Passage of ceftazidime into human milk has been reported as follows:

Treatment conditions: Dose × Frequency × Duration; Route; No. of patients; Lactation stage	Concentration (mg/l): Milk	Concentration (mg/l): Plasma	Milk/ plasma ratio	Maximum observed milk conc. (mg/l)	Absolute dose to infant (mg/kg/day): Ave	Absolute dose to infant (mg/kg/day): Max	Ref.
2000 mg × 3/d × 5 d; i.v.;11; colostrum/ transitional	3.8 (pre-dose)	7.6 (pre-dose)	0.5	–	–	–	(1)
	5.2 (1 h)	71.8 (1 h)	–0.07	–	–	–	
	4.5 (3 h)	–	–	–	–	–	
	4.5 (ave)	–	–	5.2	0.68	0.78	

Ceftazidime was given to the mothers for postpartum endometritis. Milk and serum samples were taken on days 2–4 of therapy before, and at 1 and 3 h after a dose of ceftazidime. The concentrations quoted are average values for the group at these times. The Table also gives the average milk concentration over the time of the study. The serum concentration showed the expected rise after i.v. injection but the milk concentration exhibited much less fluctuation. This difference is reflected in the variation in the milk to plasma ratio.

RELATIVE DOSE IN MILK

The amount of ceftazidime that a suckling infant would ingest in a day is on average 0.7% (4.5 × 900/6000)* and at maximum 2.3% (5.2 × 900/2000)* of the weight-adjusted maternal daily dose (1). The dose to the infant would be less than these estimates if ceftazidime is incompletely absorbed from its gastrointestinal tract.

DATA ON THE INFANT

No data are reported.

* An explanation of the calculation (s) appears on pp. 71–72.

ASSESSMENT AND RECOMMENDATIONS

The risk to the suckling infant of administering ceftazidime to its mother is low on the basis that the quantity of drug that passes into milk is small. Breast-feeding may be regarded as safe.

REFERENCES

1. Blanco JD, Jorgensen JH, Castaneda YS, Crawford SA (1983) Ceftazidime levels in human breast milk. *Antimicrob. Agents Chemother., 23,* 479–480.

CEFTIBUTEN

GENERAL

Ceftibuten is a cephalosporin antibiotic. It is well absorbed from the gastrointestinal tract in adults and children, is 30% bound to plasma protein and is eliminated by the kidneys largely as the parent compound. The half-life in plasma is 3 h.

EVALUATION OF DATA

Passage of ceftibuten into human milk has been reported as follows:

Treatment conditions — Dose × Frequency × Duration; Route; No. of patients; Lactation stage	Concentration (mg/l)		Milk/ plasma ratio	Maximum observed milk conc. (mg/l)	Absolute dose to infant (mg/kg/day)		Ref.
	Milk	Plasma			Ave	Max	
200 mg × 1 × 1 d; p.o.; 6, ?	n.d.	1–10.84	–	n.d.	–	–	(1)

n.d., not detected; assay limit 1 mg/l.

RELATIVE DOSE IN MILK

The concentration in milk was below 1 mg/l. At the assay limit an infant would ingest a maximum of 0.9% (1 × 180/200)* of the weight-adjusted maternal single dose.

DATA ON THE INFANT

No data are available.

ASSESSMENT AND RECOMMENDATIONS

Only single-dose data are available but the risk to the suckling infant of administering ceftibuten to the mother is low on the basis that the quantity of drug that passes into milk is small. Breast-feeding may be regarded as safe.

REFERENCE

1. Barr WH, Lin CC, Radwanski E, Lim J, Symchowicz S, Affrime M (1991) The pharmacokinetics of ceftibuten. *Diagn. Microbiol. Infect. Dis.*, *14*, 93–100.

* An explanation of the calculation (s) appears on pp. 71–72.

CEFTIZOXIME

GENERAL

Ceftizoxime is a cephalosporin antibiotic. It is poorly absorbed from the gastrointestinal tract and is administered by i.m. or i.v. injection or by i.v. infusion. Ceftizoxime is 30% bound to plasma protein and is eliminated largely unchanged by the kidneys. The plasma half life is 2 h.

EVALUATION OF DATA

Passage of ceftizoxime into human milk has been reported as follows:

Treatment conditions Dose × Frequency × Duration; Route; No. of patients; Lactation stage	Concentration (mg/l)		Milk/ plasma ratio	Maximum observed milk conc. (mg/l)	Absolute dose to infant (mg/kg/day)		Ref.
	Milk	Plasma			Ave	Max	
1000 mg × 1/d × 1 d; i.v.; 18; ?	0.52 (ave)	–	–	2.38	–	0.36	(1)
1000 mg × 1/d × 1 d; i.v.; 5, ?	0.43 (ave)	–	–	0.84	–	0.13	(2)
1000 mg × 1/d × 1 d; i.v.; 7, ?	0.54 (ave)		–	0.74	–	0.11	(3)

The milk concentrations are average values based on area measurements and the maximum milk concentrations are the highest values recorded in an individual. The limit of detection was 0.32 mg/l.

RELATIVE DOSE IN MILK

The amount of ceftizoxime which a suckling infant would ingest is a maximum of 0.4% (2.38 × 180/1000)* of the weight-adjusted maternal single dose.

DATA ON THE INFANT

No data are available in breast-fed infants.

ASSESSMENT AND RECOMMENDATIONS

The risk to the suckling infant of administering ceftizoxime to its mother is low on the basis that the that the quantity of drug that passes into milk is small. Breast-feeding may be regarded as safe.

* An explanation of the calculation (s) appears on pp. 71–72.

REFERENCES

1. Matsuda S, Shimizu T, Ichinoe K, Cho N, Noda K, Ninomiya et al (1988) Pharmacokinetic and clinical studies of ceftizoxime in the perinatal period. *Jpn. J. Antibiot., 41*, 1129–1141.
2. Cho N, Fukunaga K, Kunii K, Tezuka K, Kobayashi I (1988) Studies on ceftizoxime in perinatal period. *Jpn. J. Antibiot., 41*, 1142–1154.
3. Ito K, Izumi K, Takagi H, Yokoyama Y, Tamaya T, Baba Y, Hayasaki M (1988) Pharmacokinetic and clinical studies of ceftizoxime in obstetrical and gynaecological field (2). *Jpn. J. Antibiot., 41,* 1155–1163.

CEFTRIAXONE

GENERAL

Ceftriaxone is a cephalosporin antibiotic that is poorly absorbed from the adult gastrointestinal tract and is given i.m. or i.v. It is 90% bound to plasma proteins; 55% of the drug is excreted in the urine and much of the remainder appears in the bile. The plasma half-life is 6 h.

EVALUATION OF DATA

Passage of ceftriaxone into human milk has been reported as follows:

Treatment conditions: Dose × Frequency × Duration; Route; No. of patients; Lactation stage	Concentration (mg/l) Milk	Concentration (mg/l) Plasma	Milk/plasma ratio	Maximum observed milk conc. (mg/l)	Absolute dose to infant (mg/kg/day) Ave	Absolute dose to infant (mg/kg/day) Max	Ref.
1000 mg × 1/d × 1 d; i.v.; 10; 3 d	0.49 (ave)	16.3	0.03	–	0.06	–	(1)
1000 mg × 1/d × 1 d; i.m.; 10; 3 d	0.88 (ave)	15.8	0.06	–	0.08	–	(1)
1000 mg × 1/d × 1 d; i.v.; 12; colostrum	0.58 (ave)	–	–	2.25	–	0.34	(2)
1000 mg × 1/d × 1 d; i.v.; 5; colostrum	0.47 (ave)	–	–	0.93	–	0.14	(3)

The milk and serum concentration-time profiles were defined and the Table quotes average values for the group (1) based on areas under serum concentration-time curves. Milk concentrations were fairly constant for 2–20 h after dosing but serum concentrations fell during this time. The average milk to serum ratio thus does not reflect this difference. The mean milk half-life was 17.3 h after im and 12.8 h after iv dosing. These relatively long half lives indicate that steady-state concentrations in milk would be significantly higher than those quoted above and would be achieved only after 1.5–3 days. References (2, 3) give average values in milk for the group based on area measurements and the maximum milk concentration is the highest value recorded in an individual.

RELATIVE DOSE IN MILK

The amount of ceftriaxone which a suckling infant would ingest in a feed is on average 0.2% (0.88 × 180/1000)* of the weight-adjusted maternal single dose (1). The dose to the infant would be less than this estimate if ceftriaxone is incompletely absorbed from its gastrointestinal tract.

DATA ON THE INFANT

No data are available for breast-fed infants.

* An explanation of the calculation (s) appears on pp. 71–72.

ASSESSMENT AND RECOMMENDATIONS

Only single dose data are available, but the risk to the suckling infant of administering ceftriaxone to its mother would appear to be low on the basis that the quantity of drug that passes into milk is small. Breast-feeding may be regarded as safe.

REFERENCES

1. Kafetzis DA, Brater DC, Fanourgakis JE, Voyatzis J, Georgakopoulos P (1983) Ceftriaxone distribution between maternal blood and fetal blood and tissues at parturition and between blood and milk postpartum. *Antimicrob. Agents Chemother., 23*, 870–873.
2. Hirabayashi K, Okada E (1988) Pharmacokinetic and clinical studies on ceftriaxone in the perinatal period. *Jpn. J. Antibiot., XLI-2,* 216–224.
3. Cho N, Fukunaga K, Kunii K, Deguchi K (1988) Bacteriological, pharmacokinetic and clinical studies on the use of ceftriaxone in perinatal period. *Jpn. J. Antibiot., XLI-1*, 180–195.

CEFUROXIME

GENERAL

Cefuroxime is a cephalosporin antibiotic. It is administered i.v. as the sodium salt and orally as cefuroxime axetil, an ester prodrug which is rapidly hydrolysed in the intestinal mucosa and blood to cefuroxime. The drug is 30% bound to plasma proteins and is excreted in the urine. The plasma half-life is 75 min.

EVALUATION OF DATA

Secretion of cefuroxime into human milk has been reported as follows:

Treatment conditions Dose × Frequency × Duration; Route; No. of patients; Lactation stage	Concentration (mg/l)		Milk/ plasma ratio	Maximum observed milk conc. (mg/l)	Absolute dose to infant (mg/kg/day)		Ref.
	Milk	Plasma			Ave	Max	
500 mg x 1 x 1/d; p.o.; 1; ?	0.74	–	–	1.05	–	0.16	(1)

The milk concentrations quoted are average values for samples taken from an infected breast 30–90 min after an oral dose; the value for the uninfected breast was 0.32 mg/l (max. 0.59 mg/l).

RELATIVE DOSE IN MILK

The concentration of cefuroxime that a suckling infant would ingest would be at maximum of 0.4% (1.05 × 180/500) of the weight-adjusted maternal single dose.

DATA ON THE INFANT

No data are available from breast-fed infants.

ASSESSMENT AND RECOMMENDATIONS

Only single dose data are available but the risk to the suckling infant of administering cefuroxime to its mother is low on the basis that the quantity of drug that passes into milk is small. Breast-feeding may be regarded as safe.

REFERENCE

1. Nakamura T, Hashimoto I, Sawada Y, Mikami J (1987) Clinical studies on cefuroxime axetil in acute mastitis. *Jpn. J. Antibiot., XL-2,* 340–348.

CHLORAMPHENICOL

GENERAL

Chloramphenicol is an antimicrobial drug. It is well absorbed following oral administration to the adult and is 60% bound to plasma proteins. The plasma half-life is 4 h. Chloramphenicol is inactivated in the liver by conjugation with glucuronic acid or by reduction to aryl amines. Deficiency in glucuronide conjugation is the cause of potentially lethal circulatory collapse (grey syndrome) in neonates. Adverse effects of chloramphenicol also include bone marrow depression, which is dose-dependent, and idiosyncratic aplastic anaemia.

EVALUATION OF DATA

Passage of chloramphenicol into human milk has been reported as follows:

Treatment conditions Dose × Frequency × Duration; Route; No. of patients; Lactation stage	Concentration (mg/l) Milk	Plasma	Milk/ plasma ratio	Maximum observed milk conc. (mg/l)	Absolute dose to infant (mg/kg/day) Ave	Max	Ref.
3200 mg/d × 2.25 d; p.o.; 1; ?	25, 16	49, 26	0.51, 0.62	25.0	–	–	(1)
1000 mg × 1/d × 1 d; p.o.; 8; 4–16 d	2.67	–	–	14.20	4.01	2.13	(2)
500 mg × 1/d × 1 d; p.o.; 4;4 d	1.43	2.83	0.51	3.24	0.22	0.49	(3)
500 mg × d/d × 2 d;	1.86 (24 h)	2.87 (24 h)	0.65	–	–	–	(3)
p.o.; 5; 4–6 d	1.62 (48 h)	1.20 (48 h)	1.35	–	–	–	
250 mg × 4/d × 7–10 d; p.o ; 5; 7–10 d	1.36–2.32	–	–	5.2	–	–	(4)
500 mg × 4/d × 7–10 d; p.o.; 5; 7–10 d	2.95–5.15	–	–	7.2	0.43	1.08	(4)
500 mg × 1/d × 1 d; p.o.; 2–3; 5–5 d	2.88	3.94	0.73	4.2	0.43	0.63	(5)

Reference (1) reports 2 pairs of milk and blood samples taken from a patient successive days of treatment. The milk concentration-time profile is defined in reference (2); the table gives the mean value based on area measurements for the group but the maximum milk concentration is the highest value recorded in an individual. Reference (3) gives concentration-time profiles over 8 h after a single dose and these were concurrent. The half-life of chloramphenicol was 1.77 h in milk and 1.90 h in plasma. This reference also gives milk and plasma concentrations 24 h and 48 h after commencing repeated dosing, i.e. when steady-state dosing conditions may be assumed. Reference (4) reports, in the first column, the average minimum and maximum milk concentrations during therapy with chloramphenicol; the highest milk concentration recorded in any individual is given in the fourth column. These analyses were performed by a chemical method which gave values on average 49% higher than a microbiological assay. Reference (5) defines the concentration-time profiles over 6 h after dosing. The table gives average values for the group based on area measurements but the maximum milk concentration is the highest value recorded in an individual.

RELATIVE DOSE IN MILK

The amount of chloramphenicol which a suckling infant would ingest in a day is on average 1.3–2.3% (2.95 × 900/2000)–(5.15 × 900/2000)* (4) and at maximum 3.2% (7.2 × 900/2000)* (4) of the weight-adjusted maternal daily dose. A suckling infant would ingest in a feed at maximum 2.6% (14.2 × 180/1000)* of a maternal single dose (2).

DATA ON THE INFANT

Vomiting and refusal to feed have been reported in a series of 50 breastfeeding neonates whose mothers were being treated with chloramphenicol (6).

ASSESSMENT AND RECOMMENDATIONS

Although the quantity of chloramphenicol that an infant would receive in milk is but a small fraction of the weight-related maternal dose, metabolic inactivation of chloramphenicol by the neonate is slow. Adverse effects in infants have been associated with its use by breast-feeding mothers. The risk to the suckling infant of administering chloramphenicol to its mother is considered significant on the basis of the inherent pharmacological and toxicological properties of this drug. A mother who is receiving chloramphenicol should not breast-feed.

REFERENCES

1. Smadel JE, Woodward TE, Ley HL, Lewthwaite R (1949) Chloramphenicol (chloromycetin) in the treatment of tsutsugamushi disease (scrub typhus). *J. Clin. Invest., 28,* 1196–1215.
2. Prochazka J, Havelka J, Hejzlar M (1964) Excretion of chloramphenicol by human milk. *Cas. Lek. Cesk., 103*, 378–80.
3. Plomp TA, Thiery M, Maes RAA (1983) The passage of thiamphenicol and chloramphenicol into human milk after single and repeated oral administration. *Vet. Hum. Toxicol., 25*, 167–72.
4. Havelka J, Hejzlar M, Popov V, Viktorinova D, Prochazka J (1968) Excretion of chloramphenicol in human milk. *Chemotherapy, 13*, 204–211.
5. Matsuda S (1984) Transfer of antibiotics into maternal milk. *Biol. Res. Pregnancy Perinatol., 5*, 57–60.
6. Havelka J, Frankova A (1972) Contribution to the question of side effects of chloramphenicol therapy in newborns. *Cesk. Pediatr., 27*, 31–33.

* An explanation of the calculation (s) appears on pp. 71–72.

CHLOROQUINE

GENERAL

Chloroquine is used for the prophylaxis and treatment of malaria. It is rapidly and almost completely absorbed from the adult gastrointestinal tract. The drug is 60% bound to plasma proteins but is highly bound to certain tissues, notably the retina. Chloroquine is widely distributed in body fluids and tissues (distribution volume 200 l/kg). It undergoes hepatic metabolism to desethylchloroquine and approximately half the dose appears unchanged in urine. The half-life of elimination from plasma is 30–60 days (see also hydroxychloroquine, p. 375.

EVALUATION OF DATA

Passage of chloroquine into human milk has been reported as follows:

Treatment conditions Dose × Frequency × Duration; Route; No. of patients; Lactation stage	Concentration (mg/l) Milk	 Plasma	Milk/ plasma ratio	Maximum observed milk conc. (mg/l)	Absolute dose to infant (mg/kg/day) Ave	 Max	Ref.
600 mg (base) × 1/d × 1 d; p.o.; 3; 2–5 d	0.06 (0.012)	0.02 (0.01)	2.86	–	–		(1)
600 mg (base) × 1/d × 1 d; p.o.; 5; mature milk	3.97 max 1.18 ave	(1.19) (saliva)		3.97	0.18	0.6	(2)
600 mg (base) × 1/d × 1 d; p.o.; 11; ?	–	–	6.6 (1.5)	4.4		0.66	(3)

The milk and plasma figures in (1) are average values based on area measurements; values for desmethylchloroquine appear in parentheses. The milk figures in (2) are average values for the group studied. The maximum milk concentration quoted in (3) is an average value. All chloroquine figures refer to the base.

RELATIVE DOSE IN MILK

The relative dose estimate for a single dose used elsewhere in this text is less appropriate to apply to a slowly eliminated drug such as chloroquine for which the usual intervals between doses may be long. Reference (1) reports that on average 0.58 mg of chloroquine would be recovered in milk during the study period if 1 litre of milk were produced per day: this represents 1.2% (0.58 x 60 x 100/600 x 5) of the maternal single dose corrected for infant (5 kg) and maternal (60) kg weights. Alternatively, the 600 mg dose may be regarded as a weekly dose, equivalent to 86.7 mg/day. On this basis a suckling infant would ingest on average 0.8% (0.06 + 0.012 × 900/85.7)* (1) to 12.3% (1.18 × 900/85.7)* (2) of the weight-

* An explanation of the calculation (s) appears on pp. 71–72.

adjusted maternal daily dose.(Note that the latter calculation does not take into account a contribution from desethylchloroquine). Chloroquine is commonly given once weekly for malaria prophylaxis, under which conditions a greater percentage of the drug may be expected to be recovered from milk as steady-state dosing conditions are reached.

DATA ON THE INFANT

Chloroquine (1.24 μg/kg) and desethylchloroquine (0.14 μg/kg) were observed in 12–24 h urine of 4 neonates breast-fed by mothers who received chloroquine. No adverse effects were reported.

ASSESSMENT AND RECOMMENDATIONS

The amount of chloroquine estimated to be received by the suckling infant is on average low to moderate but would be greater under steady-state conditions of dosing; data on more mothers are required to define the range of milk concentrations when these conditions apply. Nevertheless, extensive experience with chloroquine in lactating women without evident adverse effects in their infants suggests that this drug is compatible with breast-feeding when used for prophylaxis and treatment of malaria (personal communication, R.G. Hendrickse, School of Tropical Medicine, University of Liverpool, UK).

REFERENCES

1. Edstein MD, Veenendaal JR, Newman K, Hyslop R (1986) Excretion of chloroquine, dapsone, and pyrimethamine in human milk. *Br. J. Clin. Pharmacol., 22,* 733–735.
2. Ette EI, Essien E, Ogonor JI, Brown-Awala JI (1987) Chloroquine in human milk. *J. Clin. Pharmacol., 27,* 499–502.
3. Ogunbona FA, Onyeji CO, Bolaji O, Toriniro EA (1987) Excretion of chloroquine and desethylchloroquine in human milk. *Br. J. Clin. Pharmac., 23,* 473–476.
4. Witte AMC, Klever HJH, Brabin BJ, Eggelte TA, Van der Kaay HJ, Alpers MP (1990) Field evaluation of the use of ELISA to detect choroquine and its metabolites in blood, urine and breast-milk. *Trans. Royal Soc. Trop. Med. Hyg., 84,* 521–525.

CHLORTETRACYCLINE

GENERAL

Chlortetracycline is an antibiotic drug. About 55% of the dose is absorbed from the adult gastrointestinal tract and 50–60% is bound to plasma proteins. Unlike most other tetracyclines, chlortetracycline is eliminated largely by passage into the bile. The plasma half-life is 4 h. Tetracyclines bind to calcium and, being widely distributed in body fluids and tissues, are deposited at sites of new bone formation and recent calcification, including developing teeth. Dental staining and occasionally dental hypoplasia may result if exposure is prolonged.

EVALUATION OF DATA

Passage of chlortetracycline into human milk has been reported as follows:

Treatment conditions	Concentration (mg/l)		Milk/ plasma ratio	Maxi- mum observed milk conc. (mg/l)	Absolute dose to infant (mg/kg/day)		Ref.
Dose × Frequency × Duration; Route; No. of patients; Lactation stage	Milk	Plasma			Ave	Max	
500 mg × 4/d × 3–4 d; p.o.; 8; ?	1.25	4.13	0.30	2.0	–	–	(1)

A single pair of milk and serum samples was taken at an unstated interval after dosing, i.e. the concentration-time profiles were not defined. Steady-state conditions of dosing were probably achieved.

RELATIVE DOSE IN MILK

The amount of chlortetracycline which a suckling infant would ingest in a day is on average 0.6% (1.25 × 900/2000)* and at maximum 0.9% (2.0 × 900/2000)* of the weight-adjusted maternal daily dose (1). The dose to the infant would be less than these estimates if chlortetracycline is incompletely absorbed from its gastrointestinal tract, e.g. by binding to calcium in milk.

DATA ON THE INFANT

No data are reported in the study quoted.

ASSESSMENT AND RECOMMENDATIONS

The data suggest that the risk to the suckling infant of administering chlortetracy-

* An explanation of the calculation (s) appears on pp. 71–72.

cline to its mother is low on the basis that the quantity of drug that passes into milk is small. The generally accepted practice now is to avoid therapy with tetracyclines in children but it seem unlikely that adverse effects would occur in a suckling infant whose mother receives, for example, a 1-week course of chlortetracycline.

REFERENCES

1. Guilbeau JA, Schoenbach EB, Schaub IG, Latham DV (1950) Aureomycin in obstetrics: therapy and prophylaxis. *J. Am. Med. Assoc., 143*, 520–526.

CIPROFLOXACIN

GENERAL

Ciprofloxacin is a fluoroquinolone antimicrobial drug with a wide spectrum of activity. It is rapidly absorbed after oral administration (bioavailability approximately 70%); food delays but does not prevent absorption. Plasma protein binding is 30%. Excretion is 70% renal and the remainder is converted to active metabolites by the liver. The plasma half-life is 4 h. Arthropathy has developed in weight-bearing joints in immature animals exposed to quinolones, and in the hip and knee joints of adolescents (1).

EVALUATION OF DATA

Passage of ciprofloxacin into human milk has been reported as follows:

Treatment conditions Dose × Frequency × Duration; Route; No. of patients; Lactation stage	Concentration (mg/l)		Milk/ plasma ratio	Maximum observed milk conc. (mg/l)	Absolute dose to infant (mg/kg/day)		Ref.
	Milk	Plasma			Ave	Max	
500 mg × 1 × 1; p.o.; 1; 17 d	1.99–3.02	–	–	3.02	–	0.45	(2)
750 mg × 12 h × 36 h; p.o.; 10; ?	3.79 (2 h)	2.06 (2 h)	1.7–2.13	3.79	–	0.57	(4)
500 mg × 1/d × 10 d; p.o.; 1; 3 months	0.98 (8 h)	0.21 (8 h)	4.7 (8 h)		–		(5)

Reference (1) gives milk values for ciprofloxacin over 4–16 after taking the drug. Co-administration of ferrous sulphate may have reduced the bioavailability of ciprofloxacin in this case (3). In reference (4) samples were taken for 2–24 h after the last dose and the maximum values are quoted. Reference (5) gives values at 8 h after the last dose.

RELATIVE DOSE IN MILK

A suckling infant would ingest in a day at maximum 2.2 % (3.79 × 900/1500)* of the weight-adjusted maternal daily dose.

DATA ON THE INFANT

The infant in reference (5) was breast-fed exclusively. No adverse effects were observed and ciprofloxacin was undetectable in the infant's serum (concentration <0.03 mg/l).

* An explanation of the calculation (s) appears on pp. 71–72.

ASSESSMENT AND RECOMMENDATIONS

The estimated quantity of ciprofloxacin that is ingested by the suckling infant is low but animal and human data suggest that some quinolones cause arthropathy. Since an alternative microbial can normally be found it is recommended that a breast-feeding mother should not be given ciprofloxacin.

REFERENCES

1. Alfaham A, Holt ME, Goodchild MC (1987) Arthropathy in a patient with cystic fibrosis taking ciprofloxacin. *Br. Med. J., 295*, 699.
2. Cover DL, Mueller BA (1990) Ciprofloxacin penetration into human breast milk: a case report. *DICP, Ann. Pharmacother., 24,* 703–704.
3. Polk RE, Healy DP, Sahai J, Drwal L, Racht E (1989) Efect of ferrous sulphate and multivitamins with zinc on absorption of ciprofloxacin in normal volunteers. *Antimicrob. Agents Chemother., 33*, 1841–1844.
4. Giamarellou H, Kolokythas E, Petrikkos G (1989) Pharmacokinetics of three newer quinolones in pregnant and lactating women. *Am. J. Med., 87 (suppl. 5A),* 49S-51S.
5. Gardner DK, Gabbe SG, Harter C (1992) Simultaneous concentrations of ciprofloxacin in breast milk and in serum in mother and breast-fed infant. *Clin. Pharm., 11*, 352–354.

CLINDAMYCIN

GENERAL

Clindamycin is an antibiotic drug. It is almost completely absorbed from the adult gastrointestinal tract and is 90% bound to plasma proteins. Clindamycin is extensively metabolised to products that retain significant antimicrobial activity; only about 10% of a dose is excreted unchanged in the urine. The plasma half-life is 2 h.

EVALUATION OF DATA

Passage of clindamycin into human milk has been reported as follows:

Treatment conditions Dose × Frequency × Duration; Route; No. of patients; Lactation stage	Concentration (mg/l)		Milk/ plasma ratio	Maximum observed milk conc. (mg/l)	Absolute dose to infant (mg/kg/day)		Ref.
	Milk	Plasma			Ave	Max	
150 mg × 3/d × 7 d; p.o.; 5; 1–2 weeks	<5 (pre-dose) <5-3.1 (post-dose)	6.0	0.23	3.1	–	–	(1)
150 mg × 1/d × 1 d; p.o.; 2–3; ?	0.66	1.82	0.36	1.2	0.1	0.18	(2)

Reference (1) reports mothers who received clindamycin for puerperal anaerobic sepsis. Steady-state dosing conditions were achieved. The concentration-time curve in a 6 h dose interval was defined in serum but not in milk for which samples were taken only before dosing and at the end of the dose interval. The table gives the range of milk and the average serum concentrations. Peak serum concentrations were very variable indicating differences in absorption but there was a significant correlation between the area under the serum concentration-time curve (and hence the average serum concentration) and the milk concentration at the end of the dose interval. The milk to serum ratio was calculated on this basis. Reference (2) defined the concentration-time profiles for 6 h after the dose; the peak occurred in serum at 1 h but at 4 h in milk. The table gives average values based on area measurements but the maximum milk concentration is the highest value recorded in an individual. In a further report (3) maximum milk clindamycin concentrations of 2.1–3.8 mg/l were recorded in 2 mothers who received 600 mg 6 hourly; when the dose was reduced to 300 mg p.o. the maximum concentration was 1.8 mg/l.

RELATIVE DOSE IN MILK

The amount of clindamycin that a suckling infant would ingest in a feed is at maximum 1.4% (1.2 × 180/150)* of the weight-adjusted maternal single dose (1). The amount the infant would ingest in a day is at maximum 6.2% (3.1 × 900/450)* of the weight-adjusted maternal daily dose (2). The lowest recommended single dose for a child is 3 mg/kg and a suckling infant would ingest in a feed at maxi-

* An explanation of the calculation (s) appears on pp. 71–72.

mum 3.1% (3.1 × 3/3)* of this (1). It is not known if these amounts of clindamycin have any effect on the infant's bowel flora.

DATA ON THE INFANT

A child who was breast-fed while the mother received clindamycin and gentamycin passed 2 grossly bloody stools but was otherwise well. Breast-feeding was discontinued and the stools became negative to testing for blood within 24 h (4).

ASSESSMENT AND RECOMMENDATIONS

The estimated quantity of clindamycin that is ingested by the suckling infant is small but bloody diarrhoea has been recorded in an infant who was exposed to the drug in breast milk. Since an alternative microbial can normally be found it is recommended that a breast-feeding mother should avoid clindamycin.

REFERENCES

1. Steen B, Rane A (1982) Clindamycin passage into human milk. *Br. J. Clin. Pharmac., 13*, 661–664.
2. Matsuda S (1984) Transfer of antibiotics into maternal milk. *Biol. Res. Preg., 5*, 57–60.
3. Smith JA, Morgan JR, Rachlis AR, Papsin FR (1975) Clindamycin in human breast milk. *Can. Med. Ass. J., 112,* 806.
4. Mann CF (1980) Clindamycin and breast-feeding. *Pediatrics, 66,* 1030.

CYCLOSERINE

GENERAL

Cycloserine is an anti-tuberculosis drug but is normally reserved for resistant mycobacteria because of its toxic effects on the central nervous system. It is absorbed from the adult gastrointestinal tract, is not appreciably bound to plasma proteins and is eliminated in the urine. The plasma half-life is 20 min.

EVALUATION OF DATA

Passage of cycloserine into human milk has been reported as follows:

Treatment conditions Dose × Frequency × Duration; Route; No. of patients; Lactation stage	Concentration (mg/l) Milk	 Plasma	Milk/ plasma ratio	Maximum observed milk conc. (mg/l)	Absolute dose to infant (mg/kg/day) Ave	 Max	Ref.
250 mg × 4/d × ?; p.o.; 5; ?	13.4	18.8	0.71	19.0	2.01	2.85	(1)

A single pair of milk and blood samples was taken from each patient, i.e. the concentration-time profile was not defined. The milk concentration quoted is the average for the group and the maximum concentration is the highest value recorded in an individual.

RELATIVE DOSE IN MILK

The amount of cycloserine that a suckling infant would ingest in a day is on average 12.1% (13.4 × 900/1000)* and at maximum 17.1% (19 × 900/1000)* of the weight-adjusted maternal daily dose (1).

DATA ON THE INFANT

No data are reported in the study quoted.

ASSESSMENT AND RECOMMENDATIONS

Only limited data are available but the risk to the suckling infant of administering cycloserine to its mother should be regarded as unacceptable on the basis that the

* An explanation of the calculation (s) appears on pp. 71–72.

quantity of drug that passes into milk is significant and the toxic effects that are associated with its use. Breast-feeding should be regarded as unsafe.

REFERENCES

1. Morton RF, McKenna MH, Charles E (1955–56) Studies on the absorption, diffusion and excretion of cycloserine. *Antibiot. Ann., 3,* 169–172.

DAPSONE

GENERAL

Dapsone is a sulphone that is used for malaria prophylaxis and to treat leprosy and dermatitis herpetiformis. It is slowly but completely absorbed from the adult gastrointestinal tract. Dapsone is 73% bound to plasma proteins and is metabolised to monoacetyldapsone; only 15% is recovered unchanged in the urine. The plasma half-life is 24 h. Adverse effects of dapsone include haemolytic anaemia.

EVALUATION OF DATA

Passage of dapsone into human milk has been reported as follows:

Treatment conditions	Concentration (mg/l)		Milk/ plasma ratio	Maximum observed milk conc. (mg/l)	Absolute dose to infant (mg/kg/day)		Ref.
Dose × Frequency × Duration; Route; No. of patients; Lactation stage	Milk	Plasma			Ave	Max	
50 mg × 1/d × LT; p.o.; 1;41 d	1.09 (N.D.)	1.62 (0.74)	0.67	–	–	–	(1)
100 mg × 1/d x 1 d; p.o.; 3; 2–5 d	0.152	0.446	0.34	–	0.23	–	(2)

L.T., long term. N.D., not detected. Reference (1) reports a case in which dapsone was used to treat dermatitis herpetiformis in a lactating woman aged 25 y. A single pair of milk and plasma samples was taken. The figure in brackets refers to monoacetyldapsone. The ratio of monoacetyldapsone to dapsone was consistent with rapid acetylator phenotype in both mother and infant (see below). The mother had a mild haemolytic anaemia with a haematocrit of 37.5% and reticulocyte count of 2.8%. In reference (2) milk and blood samples were collected for 52–124 h after the dose. The table gives average values based on the areas under the respective concentration-time curves.

RELATIVE DOSE IN MILK

The amount of dapsone that a suckling infant would ingest in a day is 19.6% (1.09 × 900/50)* of the weight-adjusted maternal daily dose of dapsone (1). Reference (2) reports that on average 0.58 mg of dapsone would be recovered in milk during the study period if 1 l of milk were produced per day: this represents 9.6% of the maternal single dose corrected for infant and maternal weights. Dapsone is commonly given once weekly for malaria prophylaxis (in combination with pyrimethamine), under which conditions a greater percentage of the drug may be expected to be recovered from milk once steady-state dosing conditions are reached.

* An explanation of the calculation (s) appears on pp. 71–72.

DATA ON THE INFANT

The infant's serum contained dapsone 0.44 mg/l and monoacetyldapsone 0.20 mg/l. The infant had a haemolytic anaemia, indicated by a haematocrit of 37.0% and a reticulocyte count of 2.4% (normal for age 0.2–0.8%) (1).

ASSESSMENT AND RECOMMENDATIONS

The quantity of dapsone that passes into milk after a single dose to the mother suggests the suckling infant would ingest a significant amount of the drug under steady-state conditions of dosing. Data from a case report are consistent with this view and furthermore haemolytic anaemia, a recognised adverse effect of dapsone, occurred in the baby. Breastfeeding should be regarded as unsafe.

REFERENCES

1. Sanders SW, Zone JJ, Flotz RL, Tolman KG, Rollins DE (1982) Haemolytic anaemia induced by dapsone transmitted through breast milk. *Ann. Int. Med., 90,* 465–466.
2. Edstein MD, Veenendaal JR, Newman K, Hyslop R (1986) Excretion of chloroquine, dapsone and pyrimethamine in human milk. *Br. J. Clin. Pharmacol., 2,* 733–735.

DEMECLOCYCLINE

GENERAL

Demeclocycline is a tetracycline antibiotic. Its availability from the adult gastrointestinal tract is 66% and 75% is bound to plasma proteins. Demeclocycline is excreted primarily in the urine and the plasma half-life is 15 h. Tetracyclines bind to calcium and, being widely distributed in body fluids and tissues, are deposited at sites of new bone formation and recent calcification, including developing teeth. Dental staining and occasionally dental hypoplasia may result if exposure is prolonged.

EVALUATION OF DATA

Passage of demeclocycline into human milk has been reported as follows:

Treatment conditions — Dose × Frequency × Duration; Route; No. of patients; Lactation stage	Concentration (mg/l)		Milk/ plasma ratio	Maximum observed milk conc. (mg/l)	Absolute dose to infant (mg/kg/day)		Ref.
	Milk	Plasma			Ave	Max	
300 mg × 2/d × ?; p.o.; 7; >5 d	0.51	0.93	0.55	0.61	0.08	0.09	(1)
600 mg × 2/d × ?; p.o.; 4; >5 d	0.49	1.21	0.41	2.4	0.07	0.36	(1)
900 mg × 2/d × ?; p.o.; 5; >5 d	0.66	1.11	0.60	1.0	0.1	0.15	(1)

Concentration-time profiles are defined in the reference (1) and peak drug concentrations occurred 3–4 h after dosing in colostrum and serum. The paper gives data on a range of doses and a selection of these are shown in the table which gives average values for paired milk and serum concentrations at intervals up to 12 h. The maximum milk concentrations are the highest values recorded in individuals. Three days following discontinuation of treatment demeclocycline was still present in milk but none was detectable in serum.

RELATIVE DOSE IN MILK

The amount of demeclocycline that a suckling infant would ingest in a day is on average 0.8% (0.51 × 900/600)* and at maximum 2.4% (2.4 × 900/900)* of the weight-adjusted maternal daily dose (1). The dose to the infant would be less than these estimates if demeclocycline is incompletely absorbed from its gastrointestinal tract, e.g. by binding to calcium in milk.

* An explanation of the calculation (s) appears on pp. 71–72.

DATA ON THE INFANT

No data are available.

ASSESSMENT AND RECOMMENDATIONS

The data suggest that the risk to the suckling infant of administering demeclocycline to its mother is low on the basis that the quantity of drug that passes into milk is small. The generally accepted practice now is to avoid therapy with tetracyclines in children but it seem unlikely that adverse effects would occur in a suckling infant whose mother receives, for example, a 1-week course of demeclocycline.

REFERENCES

1. Von Kobyletzki D, Strauchg D. Zur frage der diaplazentaren Passage und Ausscheidung mit der Muttermilch von Demethylchlortetracyclin (1964). *Z. Geburtsh. Gynakol., 461*, 292–305.

DOXYCYCLINE

GENERAL

Doxycycline is a tetracycline antibiotic. Its systemic availability after oral administration to the adult exceeds 90% and protein binding is 80–95%. Urinary excretion accounts for 35% of the dose, the remainder appearing in the bile and faeces in an active form. The plasma half-life is 12–22 h. Tetracyclines bind to calcium and, being widely distributed in body fluids and tissues, are deposited at sites of new bone formation and recent calcification, including developing teeth. Dental staining and occasionally dental hypoplasia may result if exposure is prolonged.

EVALUATION OF DATA

Passage of doxycycline into human milk has been reported as follows:

Treatment conditions Dose × Frequency × Duration; Route; No. of patients; Lactation stage	Concentration (mg/l) Milk	 Plasma	Milk/ plasma ratio	Maximum observed milk conc. (mg/l)	Absolute dose to infant (mg/kg/day) Ave	 Max	Ref.
200 mg × 1/d × 1 d + 100 mg 24 h later; p.o.; 15; 15 30 d	0.77 (3 h) 0.38 (24h)	2.42 (3 h) 1.05 (24 h)	0.32–0.36	1.4 (3 h) 0.85 (24 h)	0.12	0.21	(1)

Milk and serum samples were taken only at the stated times after the last dose of doxycycline, i.e. the concentration-time profiles were not defined. Steady-state dosing conditions were not achieved. The concentrations quoted are average values for the group and the maximum milk concentration is the highest value recorded.

RELATIVE DOSE IN MILK

The data are assumed to describe a single dose administration. Thus the amount of doxycycline which a suckling infant would ingest in a feed is at maximum 0.8% (1.4 × 180/300)* of the weight-adjusted maternal dose (1). The dose to the infant may be less than this estimate if doxycycline is incompletely absorbed from its gastrointestinal tract, e.g. by binding to calcium in milk.

DATA ON THE INFANT

No data are reported in the study quoted.

* An explanation of the calculation (s) appears on pp. 71–72.

ASSESSMENT AND RECOMMENDATIONS

The estimated amount of drug received by the infant would be greater if steady-state conditions had been reached. Nevertheless the risk to the suckling infant of administering doxycycline to its mother is low on the basis that the quantity of drug that passes into milk is small. The generally accepted practice now is to avoid therapy with tetracyclines in children but it seems unlikely that adverse effects would occur in a suckling infant whose mother receives, for example, a 1-week course of doxycycline.

REFERENCE

1. Morganti G, Ceccarelli G, Ciaffi G (1968) Concentrazioni comparative di un antibiotico tetraciclinico nel siero e nel latte materno. *Antibiotica, 214,* 216–223.

EPICILLIN

GENERAL

Epicillin is an antibiotic with a spectrum of activity that is similar to that of ampicillin. It is absorbed from the adult gastrointestinal tract, is 40–60% bound to plasma proteins and has a plasma half-life of 1 h.

EVALUATION OF DATA

Passage of epicillin into human milk following repeated oral dosing has been reported as follows:

Treatment conditions Dose × Frequency × Duration; Route; No. of patients; Lactation stage	Concentration (mg/l)		Milk/ plasma ratio	Maximum observed milk conc. (mg/l)	Absolute dose to infant (mg/kg/day)		Ref.
	Milk	Plasma			Ave	Max	
500 mg × 4/d × 54 h; p.o.; 11; 0–14 weeks	0.16	0.89	0.18	0.17	0.02	0.03	(1)

Steady-state conditions of dosing may be assumed. The table gives average values based on the areas under the milk and serum concentration-time curves the over 6 h. The maximum milk concentration is also an average value.

RELATIVE DOSE IN MILK

The amount of epicillin which a suckling infant would ingest in a day is on average 0.07% (0.16 × 900/200)* and at maximum 0.08% (0.17 × 900/2000)* of the weight-adjusted maternal daily dose (1).

DATA ON THE INFANT

No data are reported in the study quoted.

ASSESSMENT AND RECOMMENDATIONS

The risk to the suckling infant of administering epicillin to its mother is negligible on the basis that the quantity of drug that passes into milk is small. Breastfeeding should be regarded as safe.

* An explanation of the calculation (s) appears on pp. 71–72.

REFERENCES

1. Mischler TW, Corson SL, Larranaga A, Bolognese RJ, Neiss ES, Vukovich RA (1978) Cephradine and epicillin in body fluids of lactating and pregnant women. *J. Reprod. Med., 21*, 130–136.

ERYTHROMYCIN

GENERAL

Erythromycin is a macrolide antibiotic. It is incompletely absorbed from the adult gastrointestinal tract, is 80% bound to plasma proteins and is eliminated largely in the bile and faeces. The plasma half-life is 1.5 h.

EVALUATION OF DATA

Passage of erythromycin into human milk has been reported as follows:

Treatment conditions Dose × Frequency × Duration; Route; No. of patients; Lactation stage	Concentration (mg/l)		Milk/plasma ratio	Maximum observed milk conc. (mg/l)	Absolute dose to infant (mg/kg/day)		Ref.
	Milk	Plasma			Ave	Max	
500 mg × 1/d × 1 d; p.o.; 2–3; 5–7 d	1.0	2.09	0.48	1.4	0.15	0.21	(1)

The table gives average values based on the areas under the milk and plasma concentration-time curves for 6 h. The maximum milk concentration is the highest value recorded in an individual.

RELATIVE DOSE IN MILK

A suckling infant would ingest in a feed at maximum 0.5% (1.4 × 180/500)* of the weight-adjusted maternal single dose (1).

DATA ON THE INFANT

No data are available on the infants in the quoted study. Pyloric stenosis was reported in an infant who breast-fed while her mother received erythromycin for mastitis; a review of 122 infants who underwent pyloromyotomy for hypertrophic pyloric stenosis found that 6 had received erythromycin to treat infection (2).

ASSESSMENT AND RECOMMENDATIONS

The risk to the suckling infant of administering a single dose of erythromycin to its mother is low on the basis that the quantity of drug that passes into milk is small,

* An explanation of the calculation (s) appears on pp. 71–72.

and is unlikely to increase significantly during, for example, a 1-week course of therapy. Breastfeeding may be regarded as safe.

REFERENCES

1. Matsuda T (1984) Transfer of antibiotics into maternal milk. *Biol. Res. Preg., 5*, 57–60
2. Stang H (1986) Pyloric stenosis associated with erythromycin ingested through breast-milk. *Minnesota Medicine, 69,* 669–670.

FLUCONAZOLE

GENERAL

Fluconazole is a triazole drug that is used to treat fungal infections. It is well absorbed from the adult gastrointestinal tract and is 11% bound to plasma proteins. About 80% of a dose is excreted unchanged in the urine and the remainder is metabolised. The half-life in plasma is 30 h.

EVALUATION OF DATA

Passage of fluconazole into human milk has been reported as follows:

Treatment conditions: Dose × Frequency × Duration; Route; No. of patients; Lactation stage	Concentration (mg/l): Milk	Concentration (mg/l): Plasma	Milk/plasma ratio	Maximum observed milk conc. (mg/l)	Absolute dose to infant (mg/kg/day): Ave	Absolute dose to infant (mg/kg/day): Max	Ref.
150 mg × 1/d × 1 d; p.o.; 1; 12 weeks	2.93 (max.) 1.80 (ave.)	6.42 (max.) 2.40 (ave.)	0.75	2.93	0.27	0.44	(1)

Plasma and milk samples were taken for 48 h after the dose; the table gives the value at 2 h (max.) and average values calculated from the areas under the concentration-time curves to 48 h.

RELATIVE DOSE IN MILK

The amount of fluconazole that a suckling infant would ingest in a day is on average 10.8% (1.8 × 900/150)* of the weight-adjusted maternal dose (1).

DATA ON THE INFANT

No data are available.

ASSESSMENT AND RECOMMENDATIONS

Data from a single mother suggests that there is risk to the suckling infant of administering fluconazole to its mother is significant on the basis that the quantity of drug that passes into milk. When fluconazole is given in repeated doses, the mother should not breast-feed but when the drug is used in a single dose, resumption of

* An explanation of the calculation (s) appears on pp. 71–72.

breast-feeding after avoidance for 4 days (as in Ref. (1)) would not expose the infant to significant risk.

REFERENCE

1. Force RW (1995) Fluconazole concentrations in breast milk. *Pediatr. Inf. dis. J., 14,* 235–236.

HEXAMINE

GENERAL

Hexamine (methenamine) is a urinary antiseptic but it is not widely prescribed, and little is known about its pharmacokinetics.

EVALUATION OF DATA

Passage of hexamine into human milk has been reported as follows:

Treatment conditions Dose × Frequency × Duration; Route; No. of patients; Lactation stage	Concentration (mg/l)		Milk/ plasma ratio	Maximum observed milk conc. (mg/l)	Absolute dose to infant (mg/kg/day)		Ref.
	Milk	Plasma			Ave	Max	
1000 mg × 1/d × 1 d; p.o.; 6; ?	8.6 (2–3 h)	9.2	0.93	9.8	1.3	1.5	(1)
	3.7 (6–7 h)	3.3	1.12	3.6	–	–	

The table gives average values for paired milk and plasma samples in 2 women at the times stated.

RELATIVE DOSE IN MILK

A suckling infant would ingest in at feed at maximum 1.8% (9.8 × 180/1000)* of the weight-adjusted maternal single dose (1).

DATA ON THE INFANT

None are recorded.

ASSESSMENT AND RECOMMENDATIONS

The risk to the suckling infant of administering hexamine to the mother is low on the basis that the quantity that enters milk is small. Breast-feeding may be regarded as safe.

REFERENCES

1. Allgen LG, Holmberg G, Persson B, Sarbo B (1979) Biological fate of methamine in man. *Acta Obstet. Gynecol. Scand.*, *58*, 287–293.

* An explanation of the calculation (s) appears on pp. 71–72.

ISONIAZID

GENERAL

Isoniazid is used in standard anti-tuberculosis regimens. It is well absorbed from the adult gastrointestinal tract and is negligibly bound to plasma proteins. In the liver N-acetylisoniazid is formed at a rate that is genetically controlled. The plasma half-life is 0.5–2 h in fast acetylators and 2–6.5 h in slow acetylators, i.e. acetylation rate is bimodally distributed.

EVALUATION OF DATA

Passage of isoniazid into human milk has been reported as follows:

Treatment conditions: Dose × Frequency × Duration; Route; No. of patients; Lactation stage	Concentration (mg/l) Milk	Plasma	Milk/plasma ratio	Maximum observed milk conc. (mg/l)	Absolute dose to infant (mg/kg/day) Ave	Max	Ref.
300 mg × 1/d × 1 d; p.o.; 1; mature milk	16.6 (3.76)	–	2.0 at 2 h	16.6	–	2.49	(1)
5–10 mg/kg × 2/d × 1 d; p.o.; 3; ?	1–11	–		11	–	1.65	(2)

In reference (1) milk and plasma concentrations were measured for 24 h after the dose of isoniazid. The value quoted was the maximum and was achieved at 3 h. The figure in parentheses refers to the acetylated metabolite. In (2) the women received 5 and 10 mg/kg on separate occasions; the range of maximum milk concentrations is given.

RELATIVE DOSE IN MILK

A suckling infant would ingest in a feed a maximum of 12.2% ((16.6 + 3.76) × 180/300)* of the weight-adjusted maternal single dose (1). Alternatively, an infant would receive 6.1% ((16.6 + 3.76) × 3/10 of the recommended child's dose of 10 mg/kg.

DATA ON THE INFANT

No data are reported.

ASSESSMENT AND RECOMMENDATIONS

A significant amount of isoniazid may pass into breast milk but the data currently

* An explanation of the calculation (s) appears on pp. 71–72.

available do not permit a clear recommendation to be made. Any risk will be increased if the suckling infant is a slow acetylator of isoniazid.

REFERENCES

1. Berlin CM, Lee C (1979) Isoniazid and acetylisoniazid disposition in human milk, saliva and plasma. *Fed. Proc., 38*, 426.
2. Snider DE, Powell KE (1984) Should women taking antituberculosis drugs breast-feed? *Arch. Intern. Med., 144*, 589–590.

IVERMECTIN

GENERAL

Ivermectin is an antiparasitic drug that is used as a single dose treatment. It is readily absorbed from the gastrointestinal tract, is extensively metabolised and the plasma half-life is 12 h.

EVALUATION OF DATA

Passage of ivermectin into human milk has been reported as follows:

Treatment conditions Dose × Frequency × Duration; Route; No. of patients; Lactation stage	Concentration (μg/l)		Milk/ plasma ratio	Maximum observed milk conc. (μg/l)	Absolute dose to infant (μg/kg day)		Ref.
	Milk	Plasma			Ave	Max	
150 μg/kg × 1 × d × 1 d; p.o.; 4; ?	9.9 (20.6)	22.6 (40.0)	0.51 (0.39–0.57)	22.6	1.49	3.09	(1)

The report provides plasma and milk concentration-times curves and these are not concurrent. The values quoted are means values for the group and the concentration figures in parentheses are the maximum recorded in individual.

RELATIVE DOSE IN MILK

Assuming a maternal weight of 60 kg, and thus a maternal dose of 9000 μg (150 μg/kg × 60 kg), the amount of ivermectin that a suckling infant would ingest in a feed is on average 0.2% (9.9 × 180/9000)* and at maximum 0.4% (20.6 × 180/9000)* of the weight-adjusted maternal single dose.

DATA ON THE INFANT

No data are available.

ASSESSMENT AND RECOMMENDATIONS

The risk to the suckling infant of administering ivermectin to its mother is low on the basis that the quantity of milk that passes into milk is small. Breast-feeding may be regarded as safe.

* An explanation of the calculation (s) appears on pp. 71–72.

REFERENCES

1. Ogbuokiri JE, Ozumba BC, Okonkwo PO (1994) Ivermectin levels in human breast milk. *Eur. J. Clin. Pharmacol., 46*, 89–90.

KANAMYCIN

GENERAL

Kanamycin is an aminoglycoside antibiotic. It is poorly absorbed from the gastrointestinal tract and is administered i.m. injection or by i.v. infusion. Kanamycin does not bind to plasma proteins and is eliminated by the kidney. The plasma half-life is 3 h.

EVALUATION OF DATA

Passage of kanamycin into human milk has been reported as follows:

Treatment conditions Dose × Frequency × Duration; Route; No. of patients; Lactation stage	Concentration (mg/l)		Milk/ plasma ratio	Maxi-mum observed milk conc. (mg/l)	Absolute dose to infant (mg/kg/day)		Ref.
	Milk	Plasma			Ave	Max	
1000 mg × 1/d × 1 d; i.m.; 4; ?	–	–	–	18.4	–	2.76	(1)
1000 mg × 1/d × 1 d; i.m.; 2–3; 5–7 d	0.25	29.2	0.009	0.8	0.038	0.12	(2)

Concentration-time profiles were defined in references (1) and (2) and were not concurrent. Kanamycin appeared in milk within 30 min of the i.m. injection and after 8 h the concentration in milk exceeded that in blood (1). In reference (2) the maximum concentration was reached in serum at 1 h and in milk at 6 h after injection. The table gives average values based on area measurements but the maximum milk concentration was the highest value recorded in an individual.

RELATIVE DOSE IN MILK

The data from reference (1) suggests that the amount of kanamycin that a suckling infant would ingest in a feed is at maximum 3.3% (18.4 × 180/1000)* of the weight-adjusted maternal single dose. More recent findings indicate that an infant would ingest at maximum 0.1% (0.8 × 180/1000)* of the weight-adjusted maternal single dose (2). The dose to the infant would be less than these estimates if kanamycin is incompletely absorbed from its gastrointestinal tract.

DATA ON THE INFANT

No adverse effects are reported in the studies quoted.

* An explanation of the calculation (s) appears on pp. 71–72.

ASSESSMENT AND RECOMMENDATIONS

Single dose data suggest that the quantity of kanamycin ingested by a suckling infant is small. Milk and serum concentration-time profiles however are not concurrent and higher milk concentrations are to be anticipated after repeated doses. Furthermore, elimination of aminoglycosides by the neonate is slow. A mother who is receiving kanamycin regularly should avoid suckling a neonate but could probably breast-feed an older child with safety.

REFERENCES

1. Chyo N, Sunada H, Nohara S (1962) Clinical studies of kanamycin applied in the field of obstetrics and gynecology. *Asian Med. J., 5,* 265–275.
2. Matsuda S (1984) Transfer of antibiotics into human milk. *Biol. Res. Preg., 5,* 57–60.

KETOCONAZOLE

GENERAL

Ketoconazole is an imidazole drug used to treat fungal infections. It is incompletely absorbed from the adult gastrointestinal tract, undergoes presystemic metabolism and 99% is bound to plasma proteins. The plasma half-life is 6–10 h.

EVALUATION OF DATA

Passage of ketoconazole into human milk has been reported as follows:

Treatment conditions	Concentration (mg/l)		Milk/ plasma ratio	Maximum observed milk conc. (mg/l)	Absolute dose to infant (mg/kg/day)		Ref.
Dose × Frequency × Duration; Route; No. of patients; Lactation stage	Milk	Plasma			Ave	Max	
200 mg/d × 10 d; p.o.; 1; 1 month	0.22 (max.) 0.068 (ave.)	–	–	–	0.01	0.03	(1)

The concentration-time profile was defined in milk. The table gives the maximum figure (achieved at 3.25 h) and the average value based on the area measurement.

RELATIVE DOSE IN MILK

The amount of ketoconazole that a suckling infant would ingest in a day is on average 0.3% (0.068 × 900/200)* and at maximum 1.0% (0.22 × 900/200)* of the weight-adjusted maternal daily dose (1).

DATA ON THE INFANT

No data are available.

ASSESSMENT AND RECOMMENDATIONS

Data from one mother suggests that the risk to the suckling infant of administering ketoconazole to its mother is low on the basis that the quantity of drug that passes into milk is small. Breast-feeding can probably be regarded as safe.

* An explanation of the calculation (s) appears on pp. 71–72.

REFERENCE

1. Moretti ME, Ito S, Koren G (1995) Disposition of maternal ketoconazole in breast milk. *Am. J. Obstet. Gynecol., 173*, 1625–1626.

LINCOMYCIN

GENERAL

Lincomycin is an antibiotic that is used against anaerobic organisms. Only 25% of an oral dose is absorbed from the adult gastrointestinal tract and 85% is bound to plasma proteins. Lincomycin is extensively metabolised in the liver and the metabolites are excreted in bile. The plasma half-life is 5 h. Adverse effects associated with this drug include antibiotic-associated colitis.

EVALUATION OF DATA

Passage of lincomycin into human milk has been reported as follows:

Treatment conditions Dose × Frequency × Duration; Route; No. of patients; Lactation stage	Concentration (mg/l)		Milk/plasma ratio	Maximum observed milk conc. (mg/l)	Absolute dose to infant (mg/kg/day)		Ref.
	Milk	Plasma			Ave	Max	
500 mg × 4/d × 3 d; p.o.; 10; ?	1.28	1.32	1.11	2.4	0.192	0.360	(1)

A single pair if milk and blood samples was taken from each mother 6 h after the 12th dose of lincomycin, i.e. the concentration-time profiles were not defined. The table gives the averages for the group but the maximum milk concentration is the highest value recorded in an individual.

RELATIVE DOSE IN MILK

The amount of lincomycin that a suckling infant would ingest in a day is on average 0.6% (1.28 × 900/2000)* and at maximum 1.1% (2.4 × 900/2000)* of the weight-adjusted maternal daily dose (1). The dose to the infant would be less than these estimates if lincomycin is incompletely absorbed from its gastrointestinal tract.

DATA ON THE INFANT

No data are reported in the study quoted. Bloody diarrhoea has been recorded in an infant who was exposed to the closely-related drug, clindamycin, in breast milk (see p. 136).

* An explanation of the calculation (s) appears on pp. 71–72.

ASSESSMENT AND RECOMMENDATIONS

The estimated quantity of lincomycin that is ingested by the suckling infant is small but bloody diarrhoea has been recorded in an infant who was exposed to the closely related drug, clindamycin, in breast milk. Since an alternative microbial can normally be found it is recommended that a breast-feeding mother should avoid lincomycin.

REFERENCE

1. Medina A, Fiske N, Hjelt-Harvey I, Brown CD, Prigot A (1963) Absorption, diffusion, and excretion of a new antibiotic, lincomycin. *Antimicrob. Agents Chemother.*, 189–196.

MEFLOQUINE

GENERAL

Mefloquine is used for the prophylaxis and treatment of malaria. Some 75–80% is absorbed from the adult gastrointestinal tract and >98% is bound to plasma proteins. Mefloquine is excreted predominantly in the bile and faeces, about half as metabolites. The half-life in plasma is 21 days.

EVALUATION OF DATA

Passage of mefloquine into human milk has been reported as follows:

Treatment conditions Dose × Frequency × Duration; Route; No. of patients; Lactation stage	Concentration (mg/l)		Milk/ plasma ratio	Maximum observed milk conc. (mg/l)	Absolute dose to infant (mg/kg/day)		Ref.
	Milk	Plasma			Ave	Max	
250 mg (base) × 1/d × 1; p.o.; 2; 2–58 d	0.07	0.48	0.15	–	0.01	–	(1)

The milk and plasma concentration-time profiles were defined. The table gives average values for both subjects based on area measurements over 0–96 h.

RELATIVE DOSE IN MILK

The system for calculating the relative dose to the infant used elsewhere in this book is inappropriate to apply to a drug such as mefloquine which has a long half-life and is administered weekly. A relative dose may be expressed in the following way. The data in (1) allows a calculation of an average absolute daily dose received by the infant over the first 4 days, i.e. 0.01 mg/kg per day (see table). As mefloquine is administered weekly, the average weight-adjusted maternal daily dose is 0.6 mg/kg per day (250/60 × 7). Thus the infant would receive 1.7% (0.01 × 100/0.6) of the weight-adjusted maternal daily dose over this initial period. A mean accumulation factor of 4.9 for mefloquine (3) indicates that the relative dose would be 8.3% (1.7 × 4.9) at steady-state.

DATA ON THE INFANT

Normal development to 2 years was reported in the infants of 20 women treated with mefloquine prior to delivery (2).

ASSESSMENT AND RECOMMENDATIONS

Limited data suggest that the risk to the suckling infant of administering is low on the basis that the quantity of drug that passes into milk is small. Evidence also indicates normal development of infants exposed to mefloquine in utero. Breastfeeding is probably safe but more data are required before a firm recommendation can be made.

REFERENCES

1. Edstein MD, Veenendaal JR, Hyslop R (1988) Excretion of mefloquine in human breast milk. *Chemotherapy, 34*, 165–169.
2. Nosten F, Karbwang J, White NJ, Honeymoon K, Bangchang NA, Bunnag D, Harinasuta T (1990) Mefloquine antimalarial prophylaxis in pregnancy: dose finding and pharmacokinetic study. *Br. J. Clin. Pharmacol., 30*, 79–85.
3. Mimica I, Fry W, Eckert G, Schwartz DE (1983) Multiple-dose kinetic study of mefloquine in healthy male volunteers. *Chemotherapy, 29,* 184–187.

METRONIDAZOLE

GENERAL

Metronidazole is an antimicrobial agent that is active against protozoa and anaerobic bacteria including those commonly found in the female genital tract. The drug is often used to treat pelvic or vaginal infection. Metronidazole is well absorbed from the adult gastrointestinal tract. Plasma protein binding is 10% and the drug is eliminated in the urine, partly unchanged and partly as metabolites. The plasma half-life varies with age, being 6 h in adults, 11 h in new-born infants (7) and 25–75 h in premature babies. Large doses of metronidazole are carcinogenic in rodents and the drug is mutagenic in bacteria although large-scale studies have failed to discover oncogenic effects in humans (2–4)

EVALUATION OF DATA

Passage of metronidazole into human milk has been reported as follows:

Treatment conditions Dose × Frequency × Duration; Route; No. of patients; Lactation stage	Concentration (mg/l) Milk	 Plasma	Milk/ plasma ratio	Maximum observed milk conc. (mg/l)	Absolute dose to infant (mg/kg/day) Ave	 Max	Ref.
200 mg × 3/d × 1–9 d; p.o.; 11; 0–22 d	5.7 (2.1)	5.0 (1.7)	1.14 (1.24)	12.2 (3.8)	0.9 (0.3)	1.8 (0.6)	(5)
400 mg × 3/d × 1–9 d; p.o.; 11; 0–22 d	14.4 (3.5)	12.5 (3.2)	1.15 (1.09)	18.0 (6.3)	2.2 (0.5)	2.7 (1.0)	(5)
2.0 g × 1/d × 1 d; p.o.; 3; 6–14 weeks	15.5	–	–	45.8	2.33	6.87	(6)
400 mg × 3/d × LT; p.o.; 6; ?	13.5	15.0	0.9	–	2.0	–	(7)
400 mg × 3/d × 3–4 d; p.o.; 12; ?	15.5 (2 h) 9.07 (8 h)	17.5 (2 h) 9.9 (8 h)	0.91 (2 h) 0.96 (8 h)	15.5 (ave.)	–	–	(10)

LT, long term; figures for an hydroxy metabolite of metronidazole appear in parentheses. Reference (5) reports on lactating mothers who received metronidazole for puerperal endometritis. Each woman gave 1–2 milk and plasma samples 20–240 min after a dose. The concentration-time profile was defined in one mother. The quoted milk concentrations are mean values for the group and the maximum concentrations are the highest values recorded in individuals. Reference (6) describes a study in which metronidazole was given to lactating women with trichomoniasis and milk was collected for the next 48 h. The concentration-time profile shows that the peak milk concentration occurred 2–4 h after dosing. The milk concentration quoted is the average based on the area calculation and the maximum milk value is the mean in the 3 women for the 2 h samples.

RELATIVE DOSE IN MILK

A suckling infant would ingest in a day on average 11.7% ((5.7 + 2.1) × 900/600)* and 13.4% ((14.4 + 3.5) × 900/1200)* of the two weight-adjusted maternal daily doses quoted in reference (5); the corresponding maximum values would be 24.0% ((12.2 + 3.8) × 900/600)* and 18.2% ((18.0 + 6.3) × 900/1200)*. Note that the metabolite has been included in the calculation. A suckling infant would ingest in a feed at maximum 4.1% (45.8 × 180/2000)* of the weight-adjusted maternal single dose. The metabolite is not included in this calculation. The recommended child's dose of metronidazole is 7.5 mg/kg 8 hourly. A suckling infant would ingest in a day on average 11.9% ((14.4 + 3.5) × 15/7.5 × 3)* and at maximum 16.2% ((18.0 + 6.3) × 15/7.5 × 3)* of this (5).

DATA ON THE INFANT

Heisterberg and Branebjerg (5) found concentrations of metronidazole in infant plasma to be 16.0% and 19.2% of those in maternal plasma on the 600 mg/day and 1200 mg/day doses respectively. Total clearance of metronidazole by the infant was approximately 60% of maternal clearance by body weight and 24% by surface area, independent of dosage. Diarrhoea and secondary lactose intolerance were reported in a suckling infant whose mother received metronidazole (8) but no adverse effects were recorded in the studies quoted above (5,6) or in an earlier work (9).

ASSESSMENT AND RECOMMENDATIONS

The risk to the suckling infant of administering metronidazole to its mother appears to be significant on the basis of the quantity of drug that passes into milk. Potential adverse effects of the drug must also give cause for concern for its use by nursing mothers. When metronidazole is used in repeated doses, it is probably advisable to discontinue breast-feeding, especially if the infant is premature. When metronidazole is given as a single large dose, the amount of drug ingested by the infant depends on the length of time between maternal dosing and infant feeding. Exposure of the infant to the drug may be limited by avoiding breast-feeding in the 12–24 h following dosing.

REFERENCES

1. Jager-Roman E, Doyle PE, Baird-Lambert J, Cvejic M, Buchannan N (1982) Pharmacokinetics and tissue distribution of metronidazole in the newborn infant. *J. Pediatr., 100,* 651–654.
2. Beard CM, Noller KL, O'Fallon WM, Kurland LT, Dockerty MB (1979) Lack of evidence for cancer due to use of metronidazole. *N. Engl. J. Med., 301*, 519–522.

* An explanation of the calculation (s) appears on pp. 71–72.

3. Friedman GD (1980) Cancer after metronidazole. *N. Engl. J. Med., 302*, 519–520.
4. Goldman P. Metronidazole: proven benefit and potential risks (1980) *Johns Hopkins Med. J., 147*, 1–9.
5. Heisterberg L, Branebjerg PE (1983) Blood and milk concentrations of metronidazole in mothers and infants. *J. Perinat. Med., 11,* 114–120.
6. Erickson SH, Oppenheim GL, Smith GH (1981) Metronidazole in breast milk. *Obstet. Gynecol., 57,* 48–50.
7. Amon I, Amon K. (1983) Wirkstoffkonzentrationen von Metronidazol bie Schwangeren und postpartal. Fortschritte der antimikrobiellen und antineoplastischen. *Chemotherapie, Band 2–4*, 605–612.
8. Clements CJ (1980) Metronidazole and breast-feeding. *N. Z. Med. J., 92*, 329.
9. Gray MS, Kane PO, Squires S (1961) Further observations on metronidazole (Flagyl). *Br. J. Vener. Dis., 37*, 278–279.
10. Passmore CM, McElnay JC, Rainey EA, D'Arcy PF (1988) Metronidazole excretion in human milk and its effect on the suckling neonate. *Br. J. Clin. Pharmacol., 26*, 45–51.

MINOCYCLINE

GENERAL

Minocycline is a tetracycline antibiotic. It is rapidly and almost completely absorbed from the adult gastrointestinal tract, is 80–95% bound to plasma proteins and is excreted mainly in the bile and faeces. The plasma half life is 12–16 h. Tetracyclines bind to calcium and, being widely distributed in body fluids and tissues, are deposited at sites of new bone formation and recent calcification, including developing teeth. Dental staining and occasionally dental hypoplasia may result if exposure is prolonged.

EVALUATION OF DATA

Passage of minocycline into human milk has been reported as follows:

Treatment conditions Dose × Frequency × Duration; Route; No. of patients; Lactation stage	Concentration (mg/l) Milk	 Plasma	Milk/ plasma ratio	Maximum observed milk conc. (mg/l)	Absolute dose to infant (mg/kg/day) Ave	 Max	Ref.
200 mg × 1/d × 1 d; p.o.; 1; ?	0.6	5.6	0.12	0.8	0.9	0.12	(1)

Milk and serum concentration-time profiles were defined over 12 h after dosing. The table gives the average values and the maximum milk concentration is the highest single value recorded. The total drug recovered in milk in this time was 16.3 μg.

RELATIVE DOSE IN MILK

The amount of minocycline that a suckling infant would ingest in a feed is at maximum 0.7% (0.8 × 180/200)* of the weight-adjusted maternal single dose (1).

DATA ON THE INFANT

No data are reported in the study quoted.

ASSESSMENT AND RECOMMENDATIONS

Single dose data suggest that the risk to the suckling infant of administering minocycline to its mother is low on the basis that the quantity of drug that passes into

* An explanation of the calculation (s) appears on pp. 71–72.

milk is small. The generally accepted practice now is to avoid therapy with tetracyclines in children but it seem unlikely that adverse effects would occur in a suckling infant whose mother receives, for example, a 1-week course of minocycline.

REFERENCES

1. Mizuno S, Takata M, Sano S, Ueyama T (1969) Studies on minocycline. *Jpn. J. Antibiot., 22,* 473–479.

NALIDIXIC ACID

GENERAL

Nalidixic acid is an antimicrobial agent used for the prophylaxis and treatment of infections of the urinary tract. The drug is 93% bound to plasma proteins and 80% of a single oral dose is eliminated in the urine within 8 hours. In adults the plasma half-life is 1.5 h.

EVALUATION OF DATA

Excretion of nalidixic acid in human milk has been reported as follows:

Treatment conditions Dose × Frequency × Duration; Route; No. of patients; Lactation stage	Concentration (mg/l) Milk	 Plasma	Milk/ plasma ratio	Maximum observed milk conc. (mg/l)	Absolute dose to infant (mg/kg/day) Ave	 Max	Ref.
2.0 g × 1/d × 1 d; p.o.; 13; 3–8 d	0.64	–	0.06	1.3	0.1	0.2	(1)

Nalidixic acid was taken by lactating mothers who did not nurse their babies on the day of the study. All available milk was collected at intervals for 24 h. The milk concentration of 0.64 mg/l was the mean value for the first 4 h after dosing. Negligible amounts of nalidixic acid were present in the 16–24 h sample. The milk to serum ratio was based on the concentration in milk in the 4–7 h collection and a blood sample taken at 7 h.

RELATIVE DOSE IN MILK

The estimated amount of nalidixic acid ingested by the infant per feed was on average 0.03% (0.32 × 180/2000) and at maximum 0.06% (0.64 × 180/2000)* of the weight-adjusted maternal dose in this study.

DATA ON THE INFANT

Rarely, haemolytic anaemia is associated with the use of nalidixic acid in patients who are deficient in glucose-6-phosphate dehydrogenase (G6PD). Haemolytic anaemia has been reported in a breast-feeding infant whose mother was taking nalidixic acid but on testing after recovery, the infant was found not to be G6PD deficient (2).

* An explanation of the calculation (s) appears on pp. 71–72.

Antimicrobial drugs, pp.75–203

ASSESSMENT AND RECOMMENDATIONS

If a suckling infant is not deficient in G6PD, then the risk to it of administering nalidixic acid to its mother is negligible on the basis that the quantity of drug that passes into milk is small. Breast-feeding such an infant may be regarded as safe. If a suckling infant is G6PD deficient, then the risk to it of administering nalidixic to its mother is unacceptable, for haemolysis may be provoked by very small amounts of the drug. In communities in which the prevalence of G6PD deficiency is high, nalidixic acid should not be given to a breast-feeding woman unless her infant is known not to be enzyme deficient.

REFERENCES

1. Traeger A, Peiker G (1980) Excretion of nalidixic acid via mother's milk. *Arch. Toxicol., 4 Suppl.*, 388–390.
2. Belton EM, Vaughn Jones R (1965) *Lancet, i*, 691.

NITROFURANTOIN

GENERAL

Nitrofurantoin is an antimicrobial agent used only for the treatment and prevention of urinary tract infection. The drug is well absorbed from the adult gastrointestinal tract and although plasma concentrations are low, it is effectively concentrated in the urine where about 45% of a dose appears unchanged. The plasma half-life is 30 min.

EVALUATION OF DATA

Passage of nitrofurantoin into human milk has been reported as follows:

Treatment conditions: Dose × Frequency × Duration; Route; No. of patients; Lactation stage	Concentration (mg/l) Milk	Concentration (mg/l) Serum	Milk/plasma ratio	Maximum observed milk conc. (mg/l)	Absolute dose to infant (mg/kg/day) Ave	Absolute dose to infant (mg/kg/day) Max	Ref.
100 mg × 4/d × 1/d (see below); p.o.;9; ?	0.4	1.35	0.3	0.5	0.06	0.08	(1)

Nine mothers received nitrofurantoin 100 mg by mouth every 6 h for one day and the following morning 5 received nitrofurantoin 100 mg and 4 received 200 mg; milk and serum samples were obtained 2 h later. Thus the concentration-time profiles were not defined. Nitrofurantoin could be quantified in milk from 2 of the mothers who received the higher dose but in no other milk samples. The milk and plasma concentrations quoted are the average values from these 2 patients, and the maximum concentration is the highest value recorded in an individual. Another study (2) failed to detect nitrofurantoin in 20 milk samples from mothers who took 100 mg 4 times a day for 3 or 4 days; the limit of sensitivity of the assay was 2.0 mg/l.

RELATIVE DOSE IN MILK

The amount of nitrofurantoin that a suckling infant would ingest in a day is on average 0.7% (0.4 × 900/500)* and at maximum 0.9% (0.5 × 900/500)* of the weight-adjusted daily dose received by the 2 mothers whose data are quoted (1). The maternal dose of 500 mg refers to the amount of drug taken by these mothers in the 24 h prior to the collection of milk samples.

DATA ON THE INFANT

Nitrofurantoin may cause haemolytic anaemia in patients with glucose-6-phosphate

* An explanation of the calculation (s) appears on pp. 71–72.

dehydrogenase (G6PD) deficiency but there are no reports of this condition being caused by ingestion of the drug in breast milk.

ASSESSMENT AND RECOMMENDATIONS

If a suckling infant is not deficient in G6PD, then the risk to it of administering nitrofurantoin to its mother is negligible on the basis that the quantity of drug in milk is small. Breast-feeding such an infant may be regarded as safe. If a suckling infant is G6PD deficient, then the risk to it of administering nitrofurantoin to its mother is unacceptable, for haemolysis may be provoked by very small amounts of the drug. In communities in which the prevalence of G6PD deficiency is high, nitrofurantoin should not be given to a breast-feeding woman unless her infant is known not to be enzyme deficient.

REFERENCES

1. Varsano I, Fischl J, Sochet SB (1973) The excretion of orally ingested nitrofurantoin in human milk. *J. Pediatr., 82*, 886–887.
2. Hosbach RE, Foster RB (1967) The absence of nitrofurantoin from human milk. *J. Am. Med. Ass., 202*, 1057.

PHENOXYMETHYLPENICILLIN

GENERAL

Phenoxymethylpenicillin is sufficiently acid-stable to be given by mouth. It may be used to treat mastitis caused by penicillin-susceptible bacteria. About 60% of an oral dose is absorbed from the gastrointestinal tract and 80% is bound to plasma proteins. Phenoxymethylpenicillin is partly metabolised by the liver and partly excreted in the urine. The elimination half life is 0.5 h.

EVALUATION OF DATA

Passage of phenoxymethylpenicillin into human milk has been reported as follows:

Treatment conditions	Concentration (mg/l)		Milk/ plasma ratio	Maximum observed milk conc. (mg/l)	Absolute dose to infant (mg/kg/day)		Ref.
Dose × Frequency × Duration; Route; No. of patients; Lactation stage	Milk	Serum			Ave	Max	
2640 mg/d × 7 d; p.o.; 7; 10–131 d	0.21–1.55	–	0.86	1.55	–	0.23	(1)[1]
2650 mg/d × 7 d; p.o.; 7; 10–131 d	0.30–.25	–	1.05	1.25	–	0.19	(1)[2]
2650 mg/d × 7 d; p.o.; 4; 21–330 d	0.28–0.50	3.0–6.6	0.12–0.18	0.50	–	0.08	(1)[3]

Serum and milk concentration-time profiles were defined during a dose interval and were concurrent. The table gives the range of milk values for mastitic[1], non-mastitic[2] (from unaffected breast) and controls[3] (volunteers without mastitis). Higher peak concentrations were achieved in mastitic milk but there was no significant differences in the areas under the milk concentration-times curves.

RELATIVE DOSE IN MILK

A suckling infant would ingest at maximum 0.5% (1.55 × 900/2640)* of the weight adjusted maternal daily dose.

DATA ON THE INFANT

Of the twelve infants whose mothers had mastitis, seven were normal, three had loose stools and one had a rash on the buttocks.

* An explanation of the calculation (s) appears on pp. 71–72.

ASSESSMENT AND RECOMMENDATIONS

The risk to the suckling infant of administering phenoxymethylpenicillin to its mother is low on the basis that the quantity of drug that passes into milk is small. Breast-feeding may be regarded as safe.

REFERENCE

1. Matheson I, Samseth M, Loberg R, Faegri A, Prentice A (1988) Milk transfer of phenoxymethylpencillin during puerperal mastitis. *Br. J. Clin. Pharmacol., 25*, 33–40.

PRAZIQUANTEL

GENERAL

Praziquantel is a systemically-acting anthelmintic drug. It is well absorbed from the adult gastrointestinal tract, is 80% bound to plasma proteins and distributes widely to body tissues. It is inactivated by metabolism; the plasma half-life of the parent drug is 1.5 h, and of its total metabolites 4 h.

EVALUATION OF DATA

Passage of praziquantel into human milk has been reported as follows:

Treatment conditions Dose × Frequency × Duration; Route; No. of patients; Lactation stage	Concentration (mg/l) Milk	 Plasma	Milk/plasma ratio	Maximum observed milk conc. (mg/l)	Absolute dose to infant (mg/kg/day) Ave	 Max	Ref.
3160 mg × 1/d × 1 d; p.o.; 5; ?	0.136	0.429	0.32	0.94	0.02	0.14	(1)
3600 mg × 1/d × 1 d; p.o.; 5; ?	0.135	0.548	0.25	1.68	0.02	0.25	(1)

In the first part of the study (upper line) a single dose was administered and in the second part (lower line) 3 equal doses were administered 4 h apart. The table gives average values based on areas under the milk and plasma concentration-time curves for 12 h (first study) and 26 h (second study). The maximum milk concentrations were the highest values recorded in individuals. The report defines the profiles in milk and plasma and these were concurrent. The milk concentration was negligible 24–26 h after either dose.

RELATIVE DOSE IN MILK

If the second part of the study is regarded as a single-dose administration, a suckling infant would ingest in a feed at maximum 0.1% (1.68 × 180/3600)* of the weight-adjusted maternal dose (1).

DATA ON THE INFANT

No data are available.

ASSESSMENT AND RECOMMENDATIONS

The risk to the suckling infant of administering a single dose of praziquantel to its

* An explanation of the calculation (s) appears on pp. 71–72.

mother is low on the basis that the quantity of drug that passes into milk is small. Breastfeeding may be regarded as safe.

REFERENCES

1. Pütter J, Held F (1979) Quantitative studies on the occurrence of praziquantel in milk and plasma of lactating mothers. *Eur. J. Drug. Metab. Pharmacokinet., 4,* 193–198.

PYRAZINAMIDE

GENERAL

Pyrazinamide is an antituberculosis drug which is part of standard combination drug regimens. In adults pyrazinamide is completely absorbed from the adult gastrointestinal tract and 50% is bound to plasma proteins; it is metabolised in the liver, only 1% appearing unchanged in the urine. The half-life in plasma is 10–24 h.

EVALUATION OF DATA

Passage of pyrazinamide into human milk has been reported as follows:

Treatment conditions Dose × Frequency × Duration; Route; No. of patients; Lactation stage	Concentration (mg/l) Milk	Concentration (mg/l) Plasma	Milk/ plasma ratio	Maximum observed milk conc. (mg/l)	Absolute dose to infant (mg/kg/day) Ave	Absolute dose to infant (mg/kg/day) Max	Ref.
1.0 g × 1/d × 1 d; p.o.; 1; ?	1.5 (3 h)	42.0 (2 h)	–	1.5	–	0.23	(1)

The milk and plasma concentrations are single maximum values obtained at the times stated but the concentration-time profiles are not reported. The half-life of elimination of pyrazinamide from milk was 9.0 h. The available data suggest a very low milk to plasma ratio. Pyrazinamide is used for long term therapy and higher milk and plasma concentrations are to be anticipated under steady-state conditions of dosing.

RELATIVE DOSE IN MILK

The amount of pyrazinamide that a suckling infant would ingest in a feed is at maximum 0.27% (1.5 × 180/1000)* of the weight-adjusted maternal single dose (1).

DATA ON THE INFANT

No data are available.

ASSESSMENT AND RECOMMENDATIONS

The only data available is a single dose study of a single case. This suggests that the risk to the suckling infant of administering pyrazinamide to its mother is low on

* An explanation of the calculation (s) appears on pp. 71–72.

the basis that the quantity of drug that passes into milk is small. More evidence is required before a recommendation can be made about breast-feeding.

REFERENCES

1. Holdiness MR (1984) Antituberculous drugs and breast-feeding. *Arch. Int. Med., 144*, 1888.

PYRIMETHAMINE

GENERAL

Pyrimethamine is used to prevent and treat malaria. It is well absorbed from the adult gastrointestinal tract, 87% bound to plasma proteins and is extensively metabolised. The plasma half-life is 85 h.

EVALUATION OF DATA

Passage of pyrimethamine into human milk has been reported as follows:

Treatment conditions: Dose × Frequency × Duration; Route; No. of patients; Lactation stage	Concentration (μg/l): Milk	Concentration (μg/l): Plasma	Milk/plasma ratio	Maximum observed milk conc. (μg/l)	Absolute dose to infant (μg/kg day): Ave	Absolute dose to infant (μg/kg day): Max	Ref.
12.4 mg × 1/d × 1 d; p.o.; 3; 2–5 d	24.7	48.5	0.5	–	3.7	–	(1)

Milk and blood samples were collected for 217–227 h after the dose. The table gives average values based on the areas under the milk and plasma concentration-time curves.

RELATIVE DOSE IN MILK

The relative dose estimate for a single dose used elsewhere in this text is less appropriate to apply to a slowly eliminated drug such as pyrimethamine for which the usual intervals between doses may be long. The authors report that on average 0.23 mg of pyrimethamine would be recovered in milk during the study period if 1 l of milk were produced per day: this represents 22.1% (0.23 × 60 100/12.5 × 5) of the maternal single dose corrected for infant (5 kg) and maternal (60 kg) weights (1). Alternatively, the 12.5 mg dose may be regarded as a weekly dose, equivalent to 1.786 mg/d. On this basis a suckling infant would ingest in a day 12.5% (24.7 × 900/1786)* of the weight-adjusted maternal daily dose. Pyrimethamine is commonly given once weekly for malaria prophylaxis (in combination with dapsone or sulfadoxine), under which conditions a greater percentage of the drug may be expected to be recovered from milk as steady-state dosing conditions are reached.

* An explanation of the calculation (s) appears on pp. 71–72.

DATA ON THE INFANT

No data are available.

ASSESSMENT AND RECOMMENDATIONS

The calculations indicate that the suckling infant would receive a moderate amount of pyrimethamine, and this would be greater under steady-state conditions of dosing. Data on more mothers are required to define the range of milk concentrations when these conditions apply. Nevertheless, extensive experience with pyrimethamine in lactating women without evident adverse effects in their infants suggests that the use of this drug is compatible with breast-feeding (personal communication, R.G. Hendrickse, School of Tropical Medicine, University of Liverpool, UK).

REFERENCES

1. Edstein MD, Veenendaal JR, Newman K, Hyslop R (1986) Excretion of chloroquine, dapsone and pyrimethamine in hyman milk. *Br. J. Clin. Pharmac.*, *22*, 733–735.

QUININE

GENERAL

Quinine is used to treat severe and complicated falciparum malaria. It is administered by intravenous infusion or by mouth as the dihydrochloride, hydrochloride, bisulphate or sulphate salt. Quinine is rapidly and almost completely absorbed from the adult gastrointestinal tract, is 80% bound to plasma proteins and is extensively metabolised, <20% passing unchanged into the urine. Its most serious adverse effects are disturbance of cardiac rhythm and allergy causing thrombocytopenia and asthma.

EVALUATION OF DATA

The excretion of quinine into human milk has been reported as follows:

Treatment conditions Dose × Frequency × Duration; Route; No. of patients; Lactation stage	Concentration (mg/l) Milk	 Plasma	Milk/ plasma ratio	Maximum observed milk conc. (mg/l)	Absolute dose to infant (mg/kg/day) Ave	 Max	Ref.
8.3 mg/kg (base) × 3/d × 1–2 d; i.v. infusion; 5; 1–10 d	0.5–8.0 (ave 3.4)	2–23	0.11–0.32 (ave. 0.21)	8.0	0.51	1.2	(1)
? × ? × 1–10 d; p.o.; 25; ?	0.5–3.6 (ave. 2.6)		0.11–0.53 (ave. 0.31)	3.6	0.39	0.54	(1)

The mothers were treated for malaria. A single pair of milk and blood samples was collected, after 2–7 doses in those who received quinine by i.v. infusion, and after 1–10 days in those who received quinine orally.

RELATIVE DOSE IN MILK

The amount of quinine that a suckling infant would ingest in a day is at maximum 4.8% (8.0 × 900/1494)* of the weight-adjusted maternal daily dose for quinine administered by i.v. infusion; such patients are likely to be too ill to consider breast-feeding. The corresponding value for quinine given orally is 2.2% (3.6 × 900/1494)* and such patients may be able to breastfeed.

DATA ON THE INFANT

No data are reported in (1).

* An explanation of the calculation (s) appears on pp. 71–72.

ASSESSMENT AND RECOMMENDATIONS

The risk to the suckling infant of administering quinine to its mother appears to be low on the basis that the quantity of drug that passes into the milk is small and treatment is usually for a short period. Breast-feeding would appear to be safe unless there is allergy in which case even small quantities of quinine may provoke reactions such as thrombocytopenia and asthma.

REFERENCES

1. Phillips RE, Looareesuwan S, White NJ, Silamut K, Kietinun S, Warrell DA (1986) Quinine pharmacokinetics and toxicity in pregnant and lactating women with falciparum malaria. *Br. J. Clin. Pharmacol., 21*, 677–683.

ROXITHROMYCIN

GENERAL

Roxithromycin is a macrolide antibiotic with actions and uses similar to those of erythromycin. It is well absorbed from the adult gastrointestinal tract and is 90% bound to plasma proteins. Some 10% is excreted unchanged in urine, and the remainder in the faeces. The plasma half life is 10 h.

EVALUATION OF DATA

Passage of roxithromycin into human milk has been reported as follows:

Treatment conditions	Concentration (mg/l)		Milk/ plasma ratio	Maximum observed milk conc. (mg/l)	Absolute dose to infant (mg/kg/day)		Ref.
Dose × Frequency × Duration; Route; No. of patients; Lactation stage	Milk	Plasma			Ave	Max	
300 mg × 1/d × 1 d; p.o.; 10, >1 month	0.26	5.95	0.04	–	–	–	(1)

The milk and plasma values are averages based on area measurements. The half life of roxithromycin in this study was 7.1 h in plasma and 4.5 h in milk.

RELATIVE DOSE IN MILK

The amount of roxithromycin which a suckling infant would ingest in a feed is on average 0.2% (0.26 × 180/300)* of the weight-adjusted maternal single dose (1).

DATA ON THE INFANT

No data are available.

ASSESSMENT AND RECOMMENDATIONS

The risk to the suckling infant of administering roxithromycin to its mother is small on the basis of the quantity that passes into milk. Breast-feeding may be regarded as safe.

REFERENCE

1. Lassman HB, Puri SK, Ho I, Sabo R, Mezzino MJ (1988) Pharmacokinetics of roxithromycin (RU 965). *J. Clin. Pharmacol.*, *28*, 141–152.

* An explanation of the calculation (s) appears on pp. 71–72.

STIBAMINE GLUCOSIDE

GENERAL

Pentavalent antimony (Sb_v) as sodium stibogluconate is used to treat leishmaniasis. It is administered by slow i.v or deep i.m. injection. Some 80% of a dose is recovered in the urine on 24 h. Elimination from the plasma is biphasic, the half-life of the initial phase being 2 h and that of the subsequent phase 76 h. In high dose cardiac, renal or hepatic toxicity may occur.

EVALUATION OF DATA

Passage of antimony in milk has been reported as follow:

Treatment conditions	Concentration (mg/l)		Milk/ plasma ratio	Maximum observed milk conc. (mg/l)	Absolute dose to infant (mg/kg/day)		Ref.
Dose × Frequency × Duration; Route; No. of patients; Lactation stage	Milk	Serum			Ave	Max	
1400 mg × 1/d × 14 d; i.v.; 1; 8 weeks	0.7–3.5	0.1–85	0.36(4 h) 5 (23 h)	3.5	–	0.53	(1)

Milk and serum concentrations of antimony were measured on the 5th and 14th day after daily administration of stibamine glucoside. The table gives the peak value for milk concentration (3.5 mg/l) and that before the next dose(0.7 mg/l). Milk concentrations exceeded those in serum for much of the dose interval.

RELATIVE DOSE IN MILK

As sodium stibogluconate (mol. wt. 393) was administered but antimony (mol. wt. 122) was assayed a factor of 3.2 (393/122) is introduced into the equation. A suckling infant would ingest on a day at maximum 7.2% (3.5 × 900 × 3.2/1400)* of the weight-adjusted maternal daily dose. This estimate assumes complete absorption of antimony by the infant. Experiments in rodents suggest that antimony is not absorbed from the gastrointestinal tract (1).

DATA ON THE INFANT

The infant in the above study was formula fed once treatment commenced. No data are therefore available.

* An explanation of the calculation (s) appears on pp. 71–72.

ASSESSMENT AND RECOMMENDATIONS

Data from one subject suggest that the risk to the suckling infant of administering stibamine glucoside to its mother is low on the basis that the quantity of drug that passes into milk is small and may not be absorbed by the infant. Stibamine glucoside is, however, a toxic substance and breast-feeding is best avoided until further data become available, but may be acceptable if safe artificial infant nutrition is not readily accessible.

REFERENCE

1. Berman JD, Melby PC, Neva FA (1989) Concentration of Pentostam® in human breast milk. Trans. *Royal Soc. Med. Hyg.*, *83*, 784–785.

SULBACTAM

GENERAL

Sulbactam is an irreversible inhibitor of β-lactamase. It possesses little intrinsic antimicrobial activity but enhances that of other antibiotics, e.g. ampicillin and cephalosporins, when it is administered with these drugs. Sulbactam is poorly absorbed from the gastrointestinal tract and is given by i.v. infusion as the sodium salt or orally as the pro-drug sultamicillin. The pharmacokinetics of sulbactam are similar to those of ampicillin; the plasma half-life is 1 h.

EVALUATION OF DATA

Passage of sulbactam into human milk has been reported as follows:

Treatment conditions Dose × Frequency × Duration; Route; No. of patients; Lactation stage	Concentration (mg/l) Milk	 Plasma	Milk/plasma ratio	Maximum observed milk conc. (mg/l)	Absolute dose to infant (mg/kg/day) Ave	 Max	Ref.
500–1000 mg × 6 h × ?; i.v. infusion; 11; 1–5 d	0.52 (ave)	0.3–106.7		2.8	–	0.42	(1)

Sulbactam was administered with cephalothin. There was no apparent difference in milk concentrations between the 500 mg and 1000 mg doses. The milk values quoted were collected over 8 h after i.v. infusion of sulbactam.

RELATIVE DOSE IN MILK

A suckling infant would receive a maximum of 1.0% (2.8 × 180/500)* of the weight-adjusted maternal single dose.

DATA ON THE INFANT

No data are reported.

ASSESSMENT AND RECOMMENDATIONS

The risk to the suckling infant of administering sulbactam to its mother is low on the basis that the quantity of drug that passes into milk is small. Breast-feeding may be regarded as safe.

* An explanation of the calculation (s) appears on pp. 71–72.

REFERENCE

1. Foulds G, Miller RD, Knirsch AK, Thrupp LD (1985) Sulbactam kinetics and excretion into breast milk in postpartum women. *Clin. Pharmacol. Ther.*, *38*, 692–696.

SULFAMETHOXAZOLE

GENERAL

Sulfamethoxazole is a sulphonamide antimicrobial. It is well absorbed from the adult gastrointestinal tract, 65% is bound to plasma proteins and 20–50% is excreted unchanged in the urine. In adults the plasma half-life is 11 h. Sulfamethoxazole is usually given in a fixed-ratio combination with trimethoprim as co-trimoxazole. Sulphonamide drugs are capable of displacing unconjugated bilirubin from plasma albumin and the free bilirubin may enter the infant brain to cause encephalopathy (kernicterus).

EVALUATION OF DATA

Passage of sulfamethoxazole into human milk has been reported as follows:

Treatment conditions	Concentration (mg/l)		Milk/ plasma ratio	Maxi-mum observed milk conc. (mg/l)	Absolute dose to infant (mg/kg/day)		Ref.
Dose × Frequency × Duration; Route; No. of patients; Lactation stage	Milk	Plasma			Ave	Max	
0.8 g × 2/d × 5 d; p.o.; 40; 0–10 d	4.45	† (see below)	† (see below)	–	0.67	–	(1)
1.2 g × 2/d × 5 d; p.o.; 10; 0–10 d	5.43	† (see below)	† (see below)	–	0.82	–	(1)

The mothers received tablets of Septrin (Burroughs Wellcome), each containing sulfamethoxazole 400 mg and trimethoprim 80 mg. All patients had bacterial infections; therapy began within 5 days of delivery and lasted at least 5 days. Blood and milk samples were collected daily for 5 days and the figures quoted are the means of these. The mean sulfamethoxazole milk concentration for both groups was 4.71 mg/l and the corresponding plasma concentration was 49.06 mg/l; the milk to plasma concentration ratio calculated on this basis is 0.1†.

RELATIVE DOSE IN MILK

The amount of sulfamethoxazole that a suckling infant would ingest in a day is on average 2.5% (4.45 × 900/1600)* of the lower and 2.0% (5.34 × 900/2400)* of the higher weight-adjusted maternal daily dose used in the study (1).

DATA ON THE INFANT

No data were reported in the study quoted.

* An explanation of the calculation (s) appears on pp. 71–72.

ASSESSMENT AND RECOMMENDATIONS

The risk to the suckling infant of administering sulfamethoxazole to its mother appears to be low on the basis that the quantity of drug that passes into milk is small. As a general rule, however, a women who is breast-feeding should avoid sulphonamide drugs, especially if her infant is a neonate, because of the danger of displacing bilirubin from albumin (above).

REFERENCES

1. Miller RD, Salter AJ (1973) The passage of trimethoprim/sulphamethoxazole into breast milk and its significance. In: *Proceedings of the 8th International Congress of Chemotherapy. Athens: International Congress of Chemotherapy, 1,* 687–691.

SULFAMETHOXYPYRIDAZINE

GENERAL

Sulfamethoxypyridazine is a long acting sulphonamide antimicrobial. It is absorbed from the adult gastrointestinal tract and 85% is bound to plasma proteins. About 20% of a single dose is excreted in the urine in 24 h, partly as the parent drug and partly as the acetylated metabolite. The plasma half-life is 42 h

EVALUATION OF DATA

Passage of sulfamethoxypyridazine into human milk has been reported as follows:

Treatment conditions Dose × Frequency × Duration; Route; No. of patients; Lactation stage	Concentration (mg/l) Milk	 Plasma	Milk/ plasma ratio	Maxi-mum observed milk conc. (mg/l)	Absolute dose to infant (mg/kg day) Ave	 Max	Ref.
2.0 g × 1/d × 1 d + 1.0 g/d × ?; p.o.; 3; ?	15.6	101.2	0.15	27.0	2.34	4.05	(1)

An initial dose of 2.0 g was given to each mother, then 1.0 g/day. The milk and serum concentrations are average values and the maximum milk concentration is the highest value recorded in an individual. Sulfamethoxypyridazine has a long half-life and it is not known if steady state conditions of dosing were achieved.

RELATIVE DOSE IN MILK

The amount of sulfamethoxypyridazine that a suckling infant would ingest in a day is on average 14.0% (15.6 × 900/1000)* and at maximum 24.3% (27.0 × 900/1000)* of the weight-adjusted maternal daily dose (1).

DATA ON THE INFANT

The concentrations of sulfamethoxypyridazine in the infants' serum were 1.0 and 3.0 mg/l (1). Haemolytic anaemia has been reported in breastfeeding infants whose mothers took sulfamethoxypyridazine (2, 3).

ASSESSMENT AND RECOMMENDATIONS

The risk to the suckling infant of administering sulfamethoxypyridazine to its mother is unacceptable on the basis that the quantity of drug that passes into milk is

* An explanation of the calculation (s) appears on pp. 71–72.

large and adverse effects have been reported in infants who ingested the drug in breast milk. Breastfeeding should be regarded as unsafe.

REFERENCES

1. Sparr RA, Pritchard JA (1958) Maternal and newborn distribution and excretion of sulfamethoxypyridine (Kynex). *Obstet. Gynecol., 12*, 131–134.
2. Harley JD, Robin H (1962) 'Late' neonatal jaundice in infants with glucose-6-phosphate dehydrogenase deficient erythrocytes. *Aust. Ann. Med., 11*, 148.
3. Brown AK, Cevik N (1965) Haemolysis and jaundice in the newborn following maternal treatment with sulfamethoxypyridazine (Kynex). *Pediatrics, 36*, 742–744.

TETRACYCLINE

GENERAL

Tetracycline is broad spectrum antibiotic. About 80% of a dose is absorbed from the adult gastrointestinal tract and 60% is bound to plasma proteins. Tetracycline is eliminated mainly by the kidney but also partly in the bile. The plasma half-life is 9 h. Tetracyclines bind to calcium and, being widely distributed in body fluids and tissues, are deposited at sites of new bone formation and recent calcification, including developing teeth. Dental staining and occasionally dental hypoplasia may result if exposure is prolonged.

EVALUATION OF DATA

Passage of tetracycline into human milk has been reported as follows:

Treatment conditions Dose × Frequency × Duration; Route; No. of patients; Lactation stage	Concentration (mg/l) Milk	 Plasma	Milk/ plasma ratio	Maximum observed milk conc. (mg/l)	Absolute dose to infant (mg/kg/day) Ave	 Max	Ref.
500 mg × 4/d × 3 d; p.o.; 5; ?	1.14	1.92	0.59	2.58	0.17	0.39.	(1)
275 mg × 1/d × 1 d; i.v.; 6; ?	1.25	0.98	1.28	2.51	0.19	0.38	(2)
150 mg × 1/d × 1 d; p.o.; 3,; 5–7 d	0.56	0.97	0.58	1.20	0.08	0.18	(3)

Reference (1) reports single pairs of milk and serum samples taken on the 2nd, 3rd and 4th days after starting tetracycline. The table gives the average of all samples and the maximum milk concentration was the highest individual value recorded. Reference (2) defines the concentration-time profiles over 24 h; these were concurrent and the maximum concentration occurred at 4 h. The table gives average values for the group based on area measurements. Concentration-time profiles were also concurrent over 6 h in reference (3) and maximum concentrations occurred at 2–4 h. Average values are given in the table and the maximum milk concentration is the highest value recorded in an individual.

RELATIVE DOSE IN MILK

The amount of tetracycline that a suckling infant would ingest in a day is on average 0.5% (1.14 × 900/2000)* and at maximum 1.2% (2.58 × 900/2000)* of the weight-adjusted maternal daily dose (1). A suckling infant would ingest in a feed at maximum 1.6% (2.51 × 180/275)* of the maternal single dose (2). The dose to the

* An explanation of the calculation (s) appears on pp. 71–72.

infant would be less than these estimates if tetracycline is incompletely absorbed from its gastrointestinal tract, e.g. by binding to calcium in milk.

DATA ON THE INFANT

Tetracycline was not found in serum samples taken from nursing infants on the 2nd, 3rd and 4th days after the mother commenced a course of tetracycline, the limit of detection being 0.05 mg/l (1). A similar conclusion is reported in reference (2).

ASSESSMENT AND RECOMMENDATIONS

The data suggest that the risk to the suckling infant is low on the basis that the quantity of drug that passes into milk is small. Additionally, permanent incisor calcification begins at 3–5 months of age when breast-feeding may have ceased. The widely accepted practice now is to avoid therapy with tetracyclines in children but it appears unlikely that adverse effects would occur in a suckling infant whose mother receives, for example, a 1-week course of tetracycline.

REFERENCES

1. Posner AC, Prigot A, Konicoff NG (1954–1955) Further observations on the use of tetracycline hydrochloride in prophylaxis and treatment of obstetric infections. In: *Antibiotics Annual*, pp 594–598. Medical encyclopedia, New York.
2. Graf von H, Riemann S (1959) Untersuchungen uber die konzentration von pyrrolidino-methyl-tetracyclin in der muttermilch. *Dtsch. Med. Wochenschr.*, *84*, 1694–1696.
3. Matsuda S (1984) Transfer of antibiotics into maternal milk. *Biol. Res. Pregnancy Perinatol.*, *5*, 57–60.

THIAMPHENICOL

GENERAL

Thiamphenicol has a broad spectrum antibacterial activity similar to chloramphenicol. It is well absorbed from the adult gastrointestinal tract and is excreted largely unchanged in the urine. In this respect thiamphenicol differs from chloramphenicol which is inactivated largely by glucuronide conjugation (deficient performance of this metabolic reaction is the cause of potentially lethal grey syndrome in neonates, see p. 127). The plasma half-life of thiamphenicol is 2 h.

EVALUATION OF DATA

Passage of thiamphenicol into human milk has been reported as follows:

Treatment conditions	Concentration (mg/l)		Milk/ plasma ratio	Maxi- mum observed milk conc. (mg/l)	Absolute dose to infant (mg/kg/day)		Ref.
Dose × Frequency × Duration; Route; No. of patients; Lactation stage	Milk	Plasma			Ave	Max	
500 mg × 1/d × 1 d; p.o.; 7; 4 d	2.16	3.64	0.2–1.43	3.65	–	0.55	(1)
500 mg × 7 hourly × 2 d; p.o.; 5; 4 d	1.86	2,87	0.65–1.35	2.43	–	0.37	(1)

In the single dose study (upper line of the table) the milk and plasma figures are mean peak values for the group. The repeated dose study (lower line) can be taken to represent steady-state conditions; the milk and plasma samples were taken 24 h after dosing commenced, i.e. 3 h after the third 500 mg dose which probably represents peak concentration for the group. For both parts of the study, the maximum milk concentrations are the highest values recorded in individuals.

RELATIVE DOSE IN MILK

A suckling infant would receive in a feed a maximum of 1.3% (3.65 × 180/500)* of the weight-adjusted maternal single dose. Under steady-state conditions an infant would receive in a day at maximum 1.5% (2.43 × 900/1500) of the weight-adjusted maternal daily dose.

DATA ON THE INFANT

No data are reported.

* An explanation of the calculation (s) appears on pp. 71–72.

ASSESSMENT AND RECOMMENDATIONS

The quantity of thiamphenicol excreted in breast milk is low. Immature renal capacity to clear the drug, however, may lead to accumulation in the neonate and thiamphenicol, like chloramphenicol, may cause dose-related marrow toxicity. On the basis of its inherent toxic effects, therefore, it is recommended that the risk to the suckling infant of administering thiamphenicol to its mother is unacceptable.

REFERENCE

1. Plomp TA, Thiery M, Maes RAA (1983) The passage of thiamphenicol and chloramphenicol into human milk after single and repeated oral administration. *Vet. Hum. Toxicol., 25,* 167–172.

TICARCILLIN

GENERAL

Ticarcillin is a semi-synthetic penicillin with a broad spectrum of activity that includes *Pseudomonas aeruginosa*. It is not absorbed from the adult gastrointestinal tract and is administered i.m. or by i.v. injection or infusion. Ticarcillin is 65% bound to plasma proteins and 80% of the drug is excreted in the urine. The plasma half-life is 1 h.

EVALUATION OF DATA

Passage of ticarcillin into human milk has been reported as follows:

Treatment conditions	Concentration (mg/l)		Milk/ plasma ratio	Maximum observed milk conc. (mg/l)	Absolute dose to infant (mg/kg/day)		Ref.
Dose × Frequency × Duration; Route; No. of patients; Lactation stage	Milk	Serum			Ave	Max	
1.0 g × 1/d × 1 d; i.v.; 5; ?	Trace	–	–	Trace	–	–	(1)
1.0 g × 1/d × 1 d; i.m.; 2–3; 5–7 d	Trace	6.03	–	Trace	–	–	(2)
5.0 g × 3/d × ?; i.v.; 10; ?	2.0–2.25	–	–	–	0.34	–	(3)

The serum concentration in reference (2) is based on the area calculation over 6 h after dosing. Reference (3) does not give details of milk concentrations but indicates the average values obtained on the stated dosage schedule.

RELATIVE DOSE IN MILK

The amount of ticarcillin which a suckling infant would ingest in a day is on average 0.1% (2.25 × 900/15000)* of the weight-adjusted maternal daily dose (3).

DATA ON THE INFANT

No data are reported.

ASSESSMENT AND RECOMMENDATIONS

Only single dose data are available, but the risk to the suckling infant of adminis-

* An explanation of the calculation (s) appears on pp. 71–72.

tering ticarcillin to its mother is low on the basis that the quantity of drug that passes into milk is small. Breast-feeding may be regarded as safe.

REFERENCES

1. Cho N, Nakayama T, Uehara K, Kunii K, Takeda J, Matsuzaki H, Fujiyama T (1977) Laboratory and clinical evaluation of ticarcillin in the field of obstetrics and gynecology. *Chemotherapy (Tokyo), 25*, 2911–2923.
2. Matsuda S (1984) Transfer of antibiotics into maternal milk. *Biol. Res. Preg., 5,* 57–60.
3. von Kobyletzki D, Dalhoff A, Lindemeyer H, Primavesi CA (1983) Ticarcillin serum and tissue concentrations in gynecology and obstetrics. *Infection, 11*, 144–149.

TINIDAZOLE

GENERAL

Tinidazole is an antimicrobial agent used for anaerobic bacterial and protozoal infections, often in the puerperium. It is an imidazole, like metronidazole but tinidazole has a longer plasma half-life (13 h). In adults tinidazole is absorbed from the gastrointestinal tract and is not significantly bound to plasma proteins. Tinidazole is eliminated in the urine mostly in the unchanged form.

EVALUATION OF DATA

Passage of tinidazole into human milk has been reported as follows:

Treatment conditions Dose × Frequency × Duration; Route; No. of patients; Lactation stage	Concentration (mg/l)		Milk/ plasma ratio	Maximum observed milk conc. (mg/l)	Absolute dose to infant (mg/kg/day)		Ref.
	Milk	Serum			Ave	Max	
0.5 g × 1/d × 1 d; i.v.; 24; 1–3 d	2.30	2.36	0.98	5.8	0.345	0.870	(1)
1.6 g × 1/d × 1 d; i.v.; 5; 1–4 d	–	–	0.62–1.39	–	–	–	(2)

The women reported in reference (1) received tinidazole as an i.v. infusion lasting 20 min at caesarean section. Blood and milk samples were collected for 96 h but were quantifiable only up to 72 h; the analysis is therefore of colostrum. The concentration-time profiles were concurrent with maximum concentrations at 12 h. The table gives the average milk and plasma concentrations over the period 0–72 h based on area calculations. The maximum concentration quoted is the average for the group. Steady-state conditions of dosing were not attained. Presently recommended adult dosages of tinidazole exceed the 500 mg used in this study and vary between 800 mg/day i.v. for anaerobic infection and 2.0 g p.o. as a single dose for urogenital trichomoniasis. Use of the latter schedules would expose infants to greater absolute doses of tinidazole than those estimated here. In reference (2) an infusion of tinidazole was given over 1.5 h. Blood samples were taken every 8 h and milk was collected by emptying the breasts at 4 h intervals for 96 h. The average serum half-life of tinidazole was 11.4 h. There was a close correlation between the serum and milk concentrations of tinidazole in individual patients; the table gives their range of milk to serum ratios. After 72 h the milk tinidazole concentration exceeded 0.5 mg/l in only one mother. The total amounts of tinidazole recovered in milk of the 5 mothers over the 96 h were 926, 26, 94, 53 and 33 μg.

RELATIVE DOSE IN MILK

The data in reference (1) may be treated either as a single or as a daily dose. The single dose assumption estimates that a suckling infant would ingest in a feed at maximum 2.1% (5.8 × 180/500)* of the weight-adjusted maternal single dose (1). The daily dose assumption estimates that an infant would ingest in a day on average 4.1% (2.3 × 900/500)* and at maximum 10.4% (5.8 × 900/500)* of the weight-adjusted maternal daily dose (1).

DATA ON THE INFANT

No data are reported.

ASSESSMENT AND RECOMMENDATIONS

When tinidazole is administered to a nursing mother as a single dose i.v. infusion, her infant may be exposed to a significant amount of the drug unless breast-feeding is delayed. The available information indicates that an infant who breast-feeds 72 h after infusion ingests minimal amounts of tinidazole.

REFERENCES

1. Mannisto PT, Karhunen K, Koskela O, Suikkari A-M, Mattila J, Haataja H (1983) Concentrations of tinidazole in breast milk. *Acta Pharmacol. Toxicol., 53,* 254–256.
2. Evaldson GR, Lindgren S, Nord CE, Rane AT (1985) Tinidazole milk excretion and pharmacokinetics in lactating women. *Br. J. Clin. Pharmacol., 19,* 503–507.

* An explanation of the calculation (s) appears on pp. 71–72.

TOBRAMYCIN

GENERAL

Tobramycin is an aminoglycoside antibiotic. It is poorly absorbed from the adult gastrointestinal tract and is administered by i.m. or i.v. injection. Binding of tobramycin to plasma proteins is negligible and it is eliminated unchanged in the urine. The plasma half-life is 2 h. Aminoglycosides are in general excreted more slowly by the neonate.

EVALUATION OF DATA

Passage of tobramycin into human breast milk has been reported as follows:

Treatment conditions	Concentration (mg/l)		Milk/ plasma ratio	Maximum observed milk conc. (mg/l)	Absolute dose to infant (mg/kg/day)		Ref.
Dose × Frequency × Duration; Route; No. of patients; Lactation stage	Milk	Plasma			Ave	Max	
80 mg × 1/d × 1 d; i.m.; 5; ?	–	–	–	0.52	–	0.08	(1)

The data quoted are for one woman, only trace quantities of tobramycin being detected on the other four.

RELATIVE DOSE IN MILK

The amount of tobramycin that a suckling infant would ingest in a feed is at maximum 1.2% (0.52 x 180/80)* of the weight-adjusted maternal single dose (1). The dose to the infant may be less than this estimate if tobramycin is incompletely absorbed from its gastrointestinal tract.

DATA ON THE INFANT

No adverse effects were reported in the study quoted.

ASSESSMENT AND RECOMMENDATIONS

The quantity of tobramycin estimated to be ingested by the infant is a small proportion of the single dose to the mother. There are no data on which to base an estimate of the amount ingested by the infant under steady-state conditions at an appropriate maternal dose. In common with other aminoglycosides, tobramycin may be eliminated more slowly by the infant, especially the neonate, in which it may thus accumulate. Use of tobramycin is best avoided when breast-feeding a neonate but is probably safe when the infant is older.

REFERENCES

1. Takase Z, Shirafuji H, Uchida M, Kanemitsu M (1975) Laboratory and clinical studies on tobramycin in the field of obstetrics and gynecology. *Chemotherapy (Tokyo), 23*, 1399–1402.

TRIMETHOPRIM

GENERAL

Trimethoprim is an antimicrobial drug. It is completely absorbed from the adult gastrointestinal tract, is 45% bound to plasma proteins and 70% is excreted unchanged in the urine, the remainder as metabolites. The half-life in plasma is 10 h. Trimethoprim is used either alone or, less commonly, in a fixed-ratio combination with a sulphonamide, e.g. sulfamethoxazole.

EVALUATION OF DATA

Passage of trimethoprim into human milk has been reported as follows:

Treatment conditions: Dose × Frequency × Duration; Route; No. of patients; Lactation stage	Concentration (mg/l)		Milk/ plasma ratio	Maxi-mum observed milk conc. (mg/l)	Absolute dose to infant (mg/kg/day)		Ref.
	Milk	Plasma			Ave	Max	
160 mg × 2/d × 5 d; p.o.; 40; 0–10 d	1.96	† (see below)	† (see below)	–	0.29	–	(1)
240 mg × 2/d ×5 d; p.o.; 10; 0–10 d	2.00	† (see below)	† (see below)	–	0.30	–	(1)

The mothers received tablets of Septrin (Burroughs Wellcome) each containing trimethoprim 80 mg and sulfamethoxazole 400 mg. All patients had bacterial infections; therapy began within 5 days of delivery and lasted at least 5 days. Blood and milk samples were collected daily for 5 days and the figures quoted are the means of these. The mean trimethoprim milk concentration for both groups was 1.97 mg/l and the corresponding plasma concentration was 1.57 mg/l; the milk to plasma concentration ratio calculated on this basis is 1.26†.

RELATIVE DOSE IN MILK

The amount of trimethoprim that a suckling infant would ingest in a day is on average 5.5% (1.96 × 900/320)* of the lower and 3.8% (2.0 × 900/480)* of the higher weight-adjusted maternal daily dose used in the study (1).

DATA ON THE INFANT

No data are reported.

ASSESSMENT AND RECOMMENDATIONS

The risk to the suckling infant of administering trimethoprim to its mother is low

* An explanation of the calculation (s) appears on pp. 71–72.

on the basis that the quantity of drug that passes into milk is small. Breast-feeding may be regarded as safe.

REFERENCES

1. Miller RD, Salter AJ (1973) The passage of trimethoprim/sulphamethoxazole into breast milk and its significance. In: *Proceedings of the 8th International Congress of Chemotherapy. Athens: International Congress of Chemotherapy, 1,* 687–691.

ACETAZOLAMIDE

GENERAL

Acetazolamide is a carbonic anhydrase inhibitor that is used for lowering intraocular pressure in glaucoma, to relieve premenstrual fluid retention and occasionally for epilepsy. It is well absorbed from the adult gastrointestinal tract, is >80% bound to plasma proteins and passes unchanged into the urine. Its plasma half-life is 4 h.

EVALUATION OF DATA

Passage of acetazolamide into breast milk has been reported as follows:

Treatment conditions Dose × Frequency × Duration; Route; No. of patients; Lactation stage	Concentration (mg/l) Milk	 Plasma	Milk/ plasma ratio	Maximum observed milk conc. (mg/l)	Absolute dose to infant (mg/kg/day) Ave	 Max	Ref.
500 mg × 2/d × 4–5 d; p.o.; 1; 10–11 d	1.7 (1.3–2.1)	5.8 (5.2–6.4)	–	2.1	0.26	0.32	(1)

Steady-state conditions of dosing may be assumed. The concentration-time profiles were not defined. The milk concentration was the mean of 4 samples and the plasma concentration was the mean of 3 samples taken 1–9 h after a dose. The maternal plasma concentration was less than that previously reported and may reflect the relative youth of the mother (18 y) since age is positively correlated with the steady-state plasma concentration of acetazolamide (2).

RELATIVE DOSE IN MILK

A suckling infant would ingest in a day on average 1.5% (1.7 × 900/1000)* and at maximum 1.9% (2.1 × 900/1000)* of the weight-adjusted maternal daily dose of acetazolamide (1).

DATA ON THE INFANT

Plasma concentrations measured in the 10 day old infant, 4 and 5 days after the mother started to take acetazolamide and 2–12 h after breast-feeding gave values of 0.2–0.6 mg/l. These were 6% of those in the mother and were considered by the authors to be high relative to the estimated dose received by the infant and probably reflect the infant's immature kidney function. During collection of the blood, spe-

* An explanation of the calculation (s) appears on pp. 71–72.

cial care was taken to avoid haemolysis which would have caused spuriously high figures. The infant exhibited no adverse clinical effects.

ASSESSMENT OF DATA

This case report suggests that the risk to the suckling infant of administering acetazolamide to its mother is low on the basis that the quantity of drug that passes into milk is small. If exposure to the drug is prolonged then an infant may accumulate acetazolamide because of immature renal function and the effects of this are not known.

REFERENCES

1. Soderman P, Hartvig P, Fagerlund C (1984) Acetazolamide excretion into human breast milk. *Br. J. Clin. Pharmacol., 17*, 599–600.
2. Alm A, Berggen L, Hartvig P, Roosdrop M (1982) Monitoring acetazolamide treatment. *Acta Ophthalmol., 60*, 107–116.

AMIODARONE

GENERAL

Amiodarone is a cardiac antidysrhythmic drug. In the adult it is well absorbed from the gastrointestinal tact, is 96% bound to plasma proteins and is noted for having an exceptionally large distribution volume (62 l/kg) and long plasma half-life (52 days, after chronic dosing). The drug is extensively metabolised to products that include desethylamiodarone (DA). Amiodarone contains 39% iodine by weight and its use in pregnancy has been limited by the possibility of adverse effects from placentally transferred iodine.

EVALUATION OF DATA

Passage of amiodarone into human milk has been reported as follows:

Treatment conditions — Dose × Frequency × Duration; Route; No. of patients; Lactation stage	Concentration (mg/l)		Milk/ plasma ratio	Maxi-mum observed milk conc. (mg/l)	Absolute dose to infant (mg/kg/day)		Ref.
	Milk	Plasma			Ave	Max	
400 mg/d × LT; p.o.; 1;6 weeks	2.8–16.4 (1.1–6.5)	–	–	16.4 (6.5)	–	2.5 (1.0)	(1)
400 mg × LT;p.o.; 1;9 weeks	3.7–14.6 (1.2–5.7)	1.6 (1.5)	–	14.6 (5.7)	–	2.2 (0.9)	(1)
400 mg/d × LT;p.o.; 1;4 weeks	3.7 (1.0)	0.6 (0.2)	6 (5)	–	0.55 (0.15)	–	(2)

LT = long term. The figures in parentheses refer to desmethylamiodarone. The 27 year old woman in (1) was treated with amiodarone for life-threatening dysrhythmias during pregnancy and lactation. The concentrations quoted are the ranges of up to 7 samples collected on 2 days during treatment at the stated times after delivery. Steady-state conditions of dosing are assumed to apply.

RELATIVE DOSE IN MILK

The amount of amiodarone and its principal metabolite DA that a suckling infant would ingest in a day is at maximum 51.5% (16.4 + 6.5 × 900/400)* of the weight-adjusted maternal daily dose(1).

DATA ON THE INFANT

Plasma concentrations of amiodarone in the infant were, at 6 weeks 0.4 (DA 0.25)

* An explanation of the calculation (s) appears on pp. 71–72.

mg/l, and at 9 weeks 0.4 (DA 0.15) mg/l (1). The infant was exposed to amiodarone for the last month of fetal life and was noted to have a bradycardia at birth, although its thyroid function was normal. In (2) the concentration of amiodarone and desmethylamiodarone were less than 0.1 and 0.05 mg/l respectively.

ASSESSMENT AND RECOMMENDATIONS

The first case report indicates that the risk to the suckling infant of administering amiodarone to its mother may be significant because the quantity of drug that passes into milk is substantial. Despite the low concentrations of amiodarone and its metabolites recorded in (2) breast-feeding should be regarded as unsafe until further data are available.

REFERENCES

1. McKenna WJ, Harris L, Rowland E, Whitelaw A, Storey G, Holt D (1983) Amiodarone therapy during pregnancy. *Am. J. Cardiol., 51*, 1231–1233.
2. Stunge P, Frandsen J, Andreasen F (1988) Amiodarone during pregnancy. *Eur. Heart J., 9,* 106–109.
3. Plomp TA, Vulsma T, de Vijlder JJ (1992) Use of amiodarone during pregnancy. *Eur. J. Obstet. Gynecol. Reprod. Biol., 43*, 201–207.

ATENOLOL

GENERAL

Atenolol is a β_1-selective adrenoceptor blocking drug. Atenolol is absorbed from the adult gastrointestinal tract, 5% bound to plasma proteins and eliminated by the kidneys. The plasma half-life is 6–9 h. Unwanted effects of β-blockade that are relevant to the infant include the possibility of delayed recovery from hypoglycaemia, for the maintenance of blood glucose during fasting by sympathetic-mediated hepatic glycogenolysis may be impaired.

EVALUATION OF DATA

Passage of atenolol into human milk has been reported as follows:

Treatment conditions Dose × Frequency × Duration; Route; No. of patients; Lactation stage	Concentration (mg/l) Milk	 Plasma	Milk/ plasma ratio	Maximum observed milk conc. (mg/l)	Absolute dose to infant (mg/kg/day) Ave	 Max	Ref.
100 mg × 1/dx LT; p.o.; 4;4–12 d	0.93	0.44	1.1–3.1	2.13	0.14	0.32	(1)
100 mg × 1/dx 7 d; p.o.;1; 1 month	–	–	–	1.7	–	0.26	(2)
100 mg × 1/dx ?; p.o.5; ?	0.63	0.71(blood)	1.3	1.04	0.10	0.16	(3)
50–100 mg × 1/dx ?; p.o.; 7; ?	–	–	1.5–6.8	–	–	–	(4)
50 mg × 2/dx ?; p.o.; 1; 10 d	0.47	–	–	–	–	–	(5)

LT = long term. Reference (1) defines concentration-time profiles during a dose interval under steady-state conditions and indicates that the values in milk and plasma are not concurrent. The table gives average values calculated from the area under the concentration-time curve and the maximum milk concentration is the highest value recorded in an individual. Reference (2) reports that the milk to plasma ratio was 3.6 after a single dose of atenolol 50 mg and 2.9 at steady-state conditions on thisdose. The concentrations quoted in ref (3) are average values in the 5 women of samples obtained 2 h after an oral dose of atenolol; the maximum milk concentration is the highest value reported in an individual. The milk to plasma ratios quoted in reference (4) are calculated from the areas under the concentration-time curves under steady-state dosing conditioins.

RELATIVE DOSE IN MILK

The amount of atenolol that a suckling infant would ingest in a day is on average 8.4% (0.93 × 900/100)* (3) and at maximum 19.2% (2.13 × 900/100)* (1) of the weight-adjusted maternal daily dose.

* An explanation of the calculation (s) appears on pp. 71–72.

DATA ON THE INFANT

Serum concentrations in a 2-week old infant who was suckled by his mother while she received atenolol 100 mg/day were undetectable on two occasions and 0.07 mg/l on a third occasion (4). Atenolol could not be detected in the plasma of an infant who had ingested milk containing atenolol 0.018 mg/l 4 h previously (2), the detection limit of the assay being 0.01 μg/l. He suckled for 5 weeks during which his mother received atenolol and showed no signs of respiratory depression, hypoglycaemia, lethargy or bradycardia. No signs of beta-blockade were observed in the suckling infants of 5 mothers who received atenolol (3). The infant reported in (5) had serum concentrations of 2.01 mg/l 48 h, and 0.14 mg/l 72 h after breast-feeding was discontinued. This infant suffered from hypothermia and bradycardia at the age of 5 d.

ASSESSMENT AND RECOMMENDATIONS

The risk to the suckling infant of administering atenolol to its mother may be significant because of the quantity of drug that passes into milk. Furthermore, certain inherent pharmacological properties of beta β-blockers, for example recovery from hypoglycaemia during fasting, give reason for caution when a drug of this class is administered to its mother. Breast-feeding is best regarded as unsafe and an alternative β-blocker should be used.

REFERENCES

1. Kulas J, Lunell NO, Rosing U, Steen B, Rane A (1984) Atenolol and metoprolol. A comparison of their excretion into breast milk. *Acta Obstet. Gynecol. Scand., Suppl., 118,* 65–69.
2. White WB, Andreoli JW, Wong SH, Cohn RD (1984) Atenolol in human plasma and breast milk. *Obstet. Gynecol., 63, Suppl. 3,* 42–44S.
3. Thorley KJ, McAinsh J (1983) Levels of the beta-blockers atenolol and propranolol in the breast milk of women treated for hypertension in pregnancy. *Biopharmaceut. Drug Dispos., 4,* 229–301.
4. Liedholm H, Melander A, Bitzen P-O, Helm G, Lonnerholm G, Mattiasson I, Nilsson B, Wahlin-Boll E (1981) Accumulation of atenolol and metoprolol in human milk. *Eur. J. Clin. Pharmacol., 20,* 229–231.

BENAZEPRIL

GENERAL

Benazepril is a long acting angiotensin converting enzyme (ACE) inhibitor used to treat hypertension. Benazepril is a prodrug that is extensively hydrolysed in vivo to the active metabolite benazeprilat. Both benazepril and its metabolite are highly bound to serum protein (approx 95%) and the distribution volume if benazepril is 8.7 l. The plasma half-life of benazepril is <1 h. ACE inhibitors are regarded as fetotoxic and are contraindicated in pregnancy.

EVALUATION OF DATA

Passage of benazepril into human milk has been reported as follows:

Treatment conditions Dose × Frequency × Duration; Route; No. of patients; Lactation stage	Concentration (ng/l) Milk	 Plasma	Milk/ plasma ratio	Maximum observed milk conc. (ng/l)	Absolute dose to infant (ng/kg day) Ave	 Max	Ref.
20 mg × 1/d × 3 d; p.o.;9; >1 month	0.15 (1.38)	14.03 (135.6)	0.01 (0.01)	0.92 (2.12)	0.02 (0.21)	0.14 (0.32)	(1)

The data in the table were obtained in normotensive volunteers on day 3 of treatment, i.e. before steady-state was achieved. The average benazepril concentrations quoted in the table were obtained from the areas under the concentration-time curves for milk and plasma. The figures in brackets refer to benazeprilat.

RELATIVE DOSE IN MILK

The amount of benazepril and benazeprilat that a suckling infant would ingest in a day is on average 0.00007% ((0.15 + 1.38) × 900/20 000 000)* and at maximum 0.00014% ((0.92 + 2.12) × 900/20 000 000)* of the weight-adjusted maternal daily dose of benazepril HCl (1).

DATA ON THE INFANT

No data are available.

ASSESSMENT AND RECOMMENDATIONS

The risk to the suckling infant of administering benazepril to its mother is low on

* An explanation of the calculation (s) appears on pp. 71–72.

the basis that the quantity of drug that passes into milk is minute. Breast-feeding is presumed to be safe but the effects of benazepril in infants, especially neonates, are little known and the baby should be observed carefully if a decision is taken to use the drug.

REFERENCES

1. Kaiser G, Ackermann R, Dieterle W, Fleiss PM (1989) Benazepril and benazeprilat in human plasma and breast milk. *IV World Conference on Clinical Pharmacology and Therapeutics, July.*

BETAXOLOL

GENERAL

Betaxolol is a β_1-selective adrenoceptor blocking drug. It is absorbed from the adult gastrointestinal tract, 50% bound to plasma proteins and is metabolised in the liver. The plasma half-life in adults is 17 h and 15–40 h in neonates (1). Unwanted effects of β-blockade that are relevant to the infant include the possibility of hypoglycaemia, for the maintenance of blood glucose during fasting by sympathetic-mediated hepatic glycogenolysis may be impaired.

EVALUATION OF DATA

Passage of betaxolol into human milk has been reported as follows:

Treatment conditions	Concentration (μg/l)		Milk/ plasma ratio	Maximum observed milk conc. (μg/l)	Absolute dose to infant (μg/kg/day)		Ref.
Dose × Frequency × Duration; Route; No. of patients; Lactation stage	Milk	Plasma			Ave	Max	
10 mg/d × 1–2 d; p.o.; 2; 1 d	7.8–48	2.6–15	3.0–3.2	48	–	7.2	(1)

This study was part of larger study in 28 women and their neonates on the perinatal pharmacokinetics of betaxolol. Milk and blood was analysed at 24, 48, and 72 h after delivery but only the 24 h values are reported here. The last dose was given 3 and 26 h prior to delivery. Both mothers also received dihydralazine.

RELATIVE DOSE IN MILK

The amount of betaxolol that a suckling infant would ingest in a day is at maximum 4.3% (48 × 900/10 000)* (1) of the weight-adjusted maternal daily dose.

DATA ON THE INFANT

Betaxolol half-life in neonates was negatively correlated with gestational age indicating slower elimination in premature infants (1). No data are available on effects of betaxolol ingested in milk.

ASSESSMENT AND RECOMMENDATIONS

The risk to the suckling infant of administering betaxolol to its mother appears to

* An explanation of the calculation (s) appears on pp. 71–72.

be low since the quantity of drug that passes into milk is small. Breast-feeding is probably safe but certain inherent pharmacological properties of β-blockers, for example recovery from hypoglycaemia during fasting, give reason for caution and special observation of the suckling infant when betaxolol is administered to its mother.

REFERENCES

1. Morselli PL, Boutroy MJ, Bianchetti G, Zipfel A, Boutroy JL, Vert P (1990) *Eur. J. Clin. Pharmacol., 38,* 477–483.

CAPTOPRIL

GENERAL

Captopril is an angiotensin converting enzyme (ACE) inhibitor used to treat hypertension and cardiac failure. In the adult it is absorbed from the gastrointestinal tract, is 30% bound to plasma proteins and about 50% is excreted unchanged by the kidney; elimination may thus be prolonged where renal function is reduced or is immature. The plasma half-life is 2 h. ACE inhibitors are regarded as fetotoxic and are contraindicated in pregnancy.

EVALUATION OF DATA

Passage of captopril into human milk has been reported as follows:

Treatment conditions Dose × Frequency × Duration; Route; No. of patients; Lactation stage	Concentration (μg/l) Milk	 Plasma	Milk/ plasma ratio	Maximum observed milk conc. (μg/l)	Absolute dose to infant (μg/kg/day) Ave	 Max	Ref.
100 mg × 3/d × 3 d; p.o.12; ?	2.9	133.4	0.03	4.7	0.44	0.71	(1)

The data in the table were obtained in normotensive volunteers under steady-state conditions of dosing and the concentration-time profiles were defined. The average concentrations quoted in the table were obtained by dividing the areas under the concentration-time curves (0–8 h) for milk (22.9 μg/l.h) and for blood (1067 μg/l.h) by 8. The maximum milk concentration was the average for the group.

RELATIVE DOSE IN MILK

The amount of captopril that a suckling infant would ingest in a day is on average 0.009% (2.9 × 900/300 000)* and at maximum 0.014% (47 × 900/300 000)* of the weight-adjusted maternal daily dose (1).

DATA ON THE INFANT

No data are available.

ASSESSMENT AND RECOMMENDATIONS

The risk to the suckling infant of administering captopril its mother is low on the

* An explanation of the calculation (s) appears on pp. 71–72.

basis that the quantity of drug that passes into milk is small. Nevertheless effects of captopril in infants, especially neonates, are little known and the baby ought to be observed carefully if a decision is taken to administer the drug to a nursing mother.

REFERENCES

1. Devlin RG, Fleiss PN (1981) Captopril in human blood and breast milk. *J. Clin. Pharmacol.*, *21*, 110–113.

CHLOROTHIAZIDE

GENERAL

Chlorothiazide is a diuretic that is used for mild oedema and arterial hypertension. Its main effect occurs within 4–6 h of dosing. Chlorothiazide is absorbed from the adult gastrointestinal tract, is 95% bound to plasma proteins and is eliminated mainly in the urine. The plasma half-life is 1.5 h.

EVALUATION OF DATA

Passage of chlorothiazide into human milk has been reported as follows:

Treatment conditions: Dose × Frequency × Duration; Route; No. of patients; Lactation stage	Concentration (mg/l): Milk	Concentration (mg/l): Plasma	Milk/plasma ratio	Maximum observed milk conc. (mg/l)	Absolute dose to infant (mg/kg/day): Ave	Absolute dose to infant (mg/kg/day): Max	Ref.
500 mg × 1/d × 1 d; p.o.; 11; 5.5 months	<1	<1	–	–	–	–	(1)

Blood and milk samples were taken 1, 2 and 3 h after ingestion of chlorothiazide. Diuresis was noted in the first 4 h.

RELATIVE DOSE IN MILK

A suckling infant would ingest in a feed <0.4% (1 × 180/500)* of the weight-adjusted maternal single dose (1).

DATA ON THE INFANT

No data are reported.

ASSESSMENT AND RECOMMENDATIONS

The risk to the suckling infant of administering chlorothiazide to its mother is low on the basis that the quantity of drug that passes into milk is small. Breast-feeding may be regarded as safe, but note that thiazide diuretics can suppress lactation (2).

* An explanation of the calculation (s) appears on pp. 71–72.

REFERENCES

1. Werthmann MW, Krees SV (1972) Excretion of chlorothiazide in human breast milk. *J. Paediatr., 81*, 781–783.
2. Healy M (1961) Suppressing lactation with oral diuretics. *Lancet*, *i*, 1353–1354.

CHLORTALIDONE

GENERAL

Chlortalidone (chlorthalidone) is a diuretic that is used for mild oedema and arterial hypertension. A single dose acts for 48–72 h. Chlortalidone is well absorbed from the adult gastrointestinal tract, is 75% bound to plasma proteins and is eliminated mainly in the urine. The plasma half-life is 44 h.

EVALUATION OF DATA

Passage of chlortalidone into human milk has been reported as follows:

Treatment conditions	Concentration (mg/l)		Milk/ plasma ratio	Maximum observed milk conc. (mg/l)	Absolute dose to infant (mg/kg/day)		Ref.
Dose × Frequency × Duration; Route; No. of patients; Lactation stage	Milk	Plasma			Ave	Max	
50 mg × 1/d × LT; p.o.; 9; 3d	0.37	6.34	0.062	0.86	0.056	0.129	(1)

LT, long term. The mothers received chlortalidone for toxaemia of pregnancy and drug administration was continued for 3 days after parturition. The milk and blood concentrations are average values from single paired samples in the mothers. The maximum concentration quoted is the highest recorded in an individual. Steady-state conditions of dosing had probably been attained.

RELATIVE DOSE IN MILK

A suckling infant would ingest in a day on average 6.7% (0.37 × 900/50)* and at maximum 15.5% (0.86 × 900/50)* of the weight-adjusted maternal daily dose (1).

DATA ON THE INFANT

No data are reported.

ASSESSMENT AND RECOMMENDATIONS

The risk to the suckling infant of administering chlortalidone to its mother may be significant on the basis of the quantity of drug that passes into milk. Breast-feeding

* An explanation of the calculation (s) appears on pp. 71–72.

should probably be regarded as unsafe. Note also that thiazide diuretics, to which chlortalidone is structurally related, may suppress lactation (2).

REFERENCES

1. Mulley BA, Parr GD, Pau WK, Rye RM, Mould JJ, Siddle NC (1982) Placental transfer of chlortalidone and its elimination in maternal milk. *Eur. J. Clin. Pharmacol.*, *13*, 129–131.
2. Healy M (1961) Suppressing lactation with oral diuretics. *Lancet.*, *i*, 1353–1355.

CLONIDINE

GENERAL

Clonidine is an α-adrenoreceptor stimulating agent that is used in the treatment of hypertension. It has high oral bioavailability and passes rapidly into the central nervous system. Some 45% of the drug is excreted unchanged by the kidneys and the remainder is metabolised to inactive products. The plasma half-life is 14 h in adults.

EVALUATION OF DATA

Passage of clonidine into human milk has been reported as follows:

Treatment conditions: Dose × Frequency × Duration; Route; No. of patients; Lactation stage	Concentration (μg/l)		Milk/plasma ratio	Maximum observed milk conc. (μg/l)	Absolute dose to infant (μg/kg/day)		Ref.
	Milk	Plasma			Ave	Max	
242–292 μg/d × LT; p.o.; 9;							(1)
1–5 d	1.8	1.2	1.5	–	–	–	
10–14 d	2.7	0.8	3.4	–	0.41	–	
45–60 d	2.8	0.5	3.6	–	–	–	
37.5 μg × 2/d × LT; p.o.; 1; 4 weeks	0.6	0.33	1.8	–	0.09	–	(2)

LT, long term. Study (1) was undertaken in mothers who received clonidine for hypertension during pregnancy. Steady-state dosing conditions had been achieved. Data represent average concentrations in the lactation periods indicated but there is no information about the time of sampling in relation to dose. In (2) milk and plasma samples were collected 1 and 2.5 h respectively after the dose,.

RELATIVE DOSE IN MILK

The amount of clonidine that a suckling infant would ingest in a day is on average 6.0% (2.1 × 900/314)* (1) and at maximum 7.9% (2.7 × 900/309)* (1) of the weight-adjusted maternal daily dose. The average daily intake is estimated as 6.8% (0.57 × 900/75) in (2).

* An explanation of the calculation (s) appears on pp. 71–72.

DATA ON THE INFANT

The infants in (2) underwent neurological examination and were normal. The clonidine concentrations in infant serum in (1) varied between averages of 0.6, 0.4, and 0.3 μg/l in the respective study period (see Table). Although the clonidine concentrations were close to therapeutic levels hypotension was not observed in any of the infants. The plasma in the infant in (2) did not contain any detectable clonidine. This may be explained by the lower maternal dose.

ASSESSMENT AND RECOMMENDATIONS

The risk to the suckling infant of administering clonidine to its mother is low but not negligible on the basis that the quantity of drug that passes into milk are sufficient to give subtherapeutic levels in the infant. Breast-feeding should be avoided during clonidine treatment until further data and experience is available.

REFERENCES

1. Hartikainen-Sorri AL, Heikkinen JE, Koivisto M (1987) Pharmacokinetics of clonidine during pregnancy and nursing. *Obstet. Gynecol.*, *69*, 598–600.
2. Bunjes R, Schaefer C, Holzinger D (1993) Clonidine and breast-feeding. *Clin. Pharm.*, *12*, 178–179.

DIGOXIN

GENERAL

Digoxin is a cardiac glycoside that is used to treat certain dysrhythmias and cardiac failure. In the adult digoxin is 60–85% absorbed from the gastrointestinal tract and 30% bound to plasma proteins. Digoxin is elimated in the kidneys by glomerular filtration, and 60–90% appears unchanged in the urine. The half-life in plasma is 36 h and appears to be similar in neonates (2). In pregancy, when the glomerular filtration rate rises, the steady-state plasma concentration is usually somewhat lower than in non-pregnant women.

EVALUATION OF DATA

Passage of digoxin into human milk has been reported as follows:

Treatment conditions	Concentration (μg/l)		Milk/ plasma ratio	Maximum observed milk conc. (μg/l)	Absolute dose to infant (μg/kg/day)		Ref.
Dose × Frequency × Duration; Route; No. of patients; Lactation stage	Milk	Plasma			Ave	Max	
250 μg × 1/d × LT; p.o.; 2; 14 d	0.41	0.51	0.8	0.61	0.06	0.09	(1)
	0.78	0.87	0.9	0.96	0.12	0.14	
250 μg × 1/d × LT; 11; 3–7 d	0.64	1.09	0.59	–	0.1	–	(2)
750 μg × 1/d × LT; p.o.;1; 7 d	1.9	2.1	0.91	1.9	0.29	0.29	(3)
500 μg × 1/d × 1 d; i.v.;11; weaning	–	–	0.62	–	–	–	(4)

LT, long term. In reference (1) the data for the two mothers appear separately in the upper and lower rows. The milk concentration-time profile was defined in each and the table gives the average milk concentration based on the area under the concentration-time curve; the milk to plasma ratio was calculated from a single pair of samples. Reference (2) gives the mean values for samples obtained daily between the 3rd and 7th days postpartum. Reference (3) gives only a single estimate of digoxin in milk and plasma. All these studies were conducted under steady-stateconditions of dosing. Reference (4) reports a single dose study and gives only an approximate estimate of the equilibrium between milk and blood.

RELATIVE DOSE IN MILK

The amount of digoxin that a suckling infant would receive in aday is on average 2.3% (0.64 × 900/250)* (2) and at maximum 3.5% (0.96 × 00/250)* (1) of the weight-adjusted maternal daily dose.

* An explanation of the calculation (s) appears on pp. 71–72.

DATA ON THE INFANT

On the fourteenth day after delivery when breast-feeding had been established, digoxin could not be detected in the plasma of either infant reported in reference (1), the limit of detection being 0.1 μg/l. In reference (3) the infant had a serum digoxin concentration of 0.2 μg/l, 7 days after delivery.

ASSESSMENT AND RECOMMENDATIONS

The risk to the suckling infant of administering digoxin to its mother is low in the basis that the quantity of drug that passes into milk is small. Breast-feeding may be considered safe.

REFERENCES

1. Loughnan PM (1978) Digoxin excretion in human breast milk. *J. Pediatr., 92*, 1019–1020.
2. Chan V, Tse TF, Wong V (1978) Transfer of digoxin across the placenta and into breast milk. *Br. J. Obstet. Gynaecol., 85*, 605–609.
3. Finley JP, Waxman MB, Wong PY, Lickrish GM (1979) Digoxin excretion in human milk. *J. Pediatr.,* 94, 339–340.
4. Reinhardt D, Richter O, Genz T, Potthoff S (1982) Kinetics of the translactal passage of digoxin from breast-feeding mothers to their infants. *Eur. J. Pediatr., 138*, 49–52.

DILEVALOL

GENERAL

Dilevalol is a β-adrenoceptor blocking drug and is the *R,R* isomer of labetalol. It is used in arterial hypertension. The plasma half-life is 9 h. Unwanted effects of β-blockade that are relevant to the infant include the possibility of hypoglycaemia, for the maintenance of blood glucose during fasting by sympathetic-mediated hepatic glycogenolysis may be impaired.

EVALUATION OF DATA

Passage of dilevalol into human milk has been reported as follows:

Treatment conditions	Concentration (μg/l)		Milk/ plasma ratio	Maxi- mum observed milk conc. (μg/l)	Absolute dose to infant (μg/kg/day)		Ref.
Dose × Frequency × Duration; Route; No. of patients; Lactation stage	Milk	Plasma			Ave	Max	
400 mg × 1/d × 1 d; p.o.; 6; ?	16 (25)	30 (237)	0.46	149 (155)	2.4 (3.8)	22.4 (23.3)	(1)

Both unchanged and 'total' dilevalol (assumed to dilevalol plus metabolites) were measured. The values for 'total' dilevalol appear in brackets. The milk and plasma concentration-time curves were concurrent. The milk/plasma ratio of 0.46 is based on areas under the plasma concentration-time curves; that based on the C_{max} values was 0.3.

RELATIVE DOSE IN MILK

The amount of 'total' dilevalol that a suckling infant would ingest in a day is on average 0.06% (25 × 900/400 00) and at maximum 0.35% (155 × 900/400000)* (1) of the weight-adjusted maternal single oral dose. Only 0.007% of the maternal single dose was secreted into breast milk over a 48 h period.

DATA ON THE INFANT

No data are available.

ASSESSMENT AND RECOMMENDATIONS

The risk to the suckling infant of administering dilevalol to its mother is low on the basis that the quantity of a single dose of dilevalol that passes into milk is small.

* An explanation of the calculation (s) appears on pp. 71–72.

Studies on milk excretion during maintenance treatment are required fully to assess the risk to the nursed infant.

REFERENCES

1. Radwanski E, Nagabhushan N, Affrime MB, Perentesis G, Symchowicz S, Patrick JE (1988) Secretion of dilevalol in breast milk. *J. Clin. Pharmacol.*, *28*, 448–453.

DILTIAZEM

GENERAL

Diltiazem is a calcium-channel blocking drug that is used in the management of angina pectoris and hypertension. In the adult diltiazem is well absorbed from the gastrointestinal tract and systemic availability by the oral route is 44%. It is 80% bound to plasma proteins and undergoes extensive metabolism in the liver. The plasma half-life is 4 h.

EVALUATION OF DATA

Passage of diltiazem into human milk was reported by Okada et al. (1) in a 40 year old puerperal woman. On the 14th day after delivery she began taking diltiazem 60 mg/6 h by mouth for premature ventricular contractions and samples were taken during the 4th day of treatment. The report does not quote concentrations but supplies an illustration which indicates that the milk and serum concentration-time profiles of diltiazem during 3 doses over 20 h were similar and suggests that the milk to serum ratio is close to unity. The milk concentrations of diltiazem ranged between 150–230 μg/l.

RELATIVE DOSE IN MILK

The amount of diltiazem that a suckling infant would ingest in a day is at maximum 0.9% (23 × 900/240 000)* of the weight-adjusted maternal daily dose (1).

DATA ON THE INFANT

No data are available.

ASSESSMENT AND RECOMMENDATIONS

The data from a single case report suggest that the risk to the suckling infant of administering diltiazem to its mother is low because the quantity of drug that passes into milk is small. More information is required before a general recommendation can be made about the safety of diltiazem in breast-feeding women.

REFERENCES

1. Okada M, Inoue H, Nakamura Y, Kishimoto M (1985) Excretion of diltiazem in human milk. *N. Engl. J. Med*, *312*, 992–993.

* An explanation of the calculation (s) appears on pp. 71–72.

DISOPYRAMIDE

GENERAL

Disopyramide is a cardiac antidysrhythmic drug. It is well absorbed from the adult gastrointestinal tract; binding to plasma proteins is dose-dependent and varies between 35–95%. The drug is excreted partly unchanged and part is metabolised in the liver; a metabolite *N*-monodesalkyldisopyramide (NMD) is pharmacologically active. The plasma half-life of is 6 h.

EVALUATION OF DATA

Passage of disopyramide into human milk has been reported as follows:

Treatment conditions: Dose × Frequency × Duration; Route; No. of patients; Lactation stage	Concentration (mg/l) Milk	Concentration (mg/l) Plasma	Milk/plasma ratio	Maximum observed milk conc. (mg/l)	Absolute dose to infant (mg/kg/day) Ave	Absolute dose to infant (mg/kg/day) Max	Ref.
200 mg × 3/d × 28 d; p.o.; 1; 5 d	3.9 (3.2)	4.0 (0.5)	0.9 (5.6)	5.7 (4.8)	0.589 (0.48)	0.86 (0.72)	(1)
100 mg × 5/d × LT; p.o.; 116 d	1.7	3.9	0.4	–	0.25	–	(2)
200 mg × 2/d × LT; p.o.; 1; 2 months	0.58 (pre-dose) 0.99 (3.5 h)	1.26 (pre-dose) 0.53 (3.5 h)	0.46 (pre-dose) 0.53 (3.5 h)	0.99	–	0.149	(3)
450 mg × 3/d × LT; p.o.; 12 weeks	2.6–4.4 (9.6–12.3)	3.1–4.0 (1.5–2.2)	1.06 (6.24)	4.4 (12.3)	0.563 (1.62)	0.66 (1.85)	(4)

LT, lomg term. The figures in brackets refer to the metabolite NMD.The milk and plasma concentrations quoted in reference (1) are the average of samples taken over 24 days and the maximum value is the highest concentration recorded in that time. The data in reference (2) are a single pair of milk and blood samples collected 3 h after a dose of disopyramide. Two pairs of milk and blood samples, taken at the times stated, are reported in reference (3). All studies were conducted under steady-state conditions of dosing. In (4), paired maternal serum and breast milk samples were obtained at 0, 2, 4 and 8 h after disopyramide.

RELATIVE DOSE IN MILK

The amount of disopyramide and its metabolite NMD that a suckling infant would ingest in a day is on average 10.7% (3.9 + 3.2 × 900/600)* and at maximum 15.9% (5.7 + 4.8 × 900/600)*of the weight-adjusted maternal daily dose (1).

* An explanation of the calculation (s) appears on pp. 71–72.

DATA ON THE INFANT

Plasma concentrations of disopyramide in the baby in reference (3) were 0.14 mg/l before and 0.10 mg/l both 1 and 2.5 h after suckling. The plasma concentration in the baby in reference (1) was 0.5 mg/l, and disopyramide was below the limit of detection (0.5 mg/l) in the plasma of the baby in reference (2). The effective plasma concentration of disopyramide in the adult is >3.0 mg/l. No adverse effects were reported in the infants.

ASSESSMENT OF DATA

There may be a risk to the suckling infant when disopyramide is administered to its mother because the quantity of drug that passes into milk is significant. Breast-feeding should be avoided.

REFERENCES

1. Barnett DB, Hudson SA, McBurnley A (1982) Disopyramide and its N-monodesalkyl metabolite in breast milk. *Br. J. Clin. Pharmacol.*, *14*, 310–312.
2. MacIntosh D, Buchanan N (1985) Excretion of disopyramide in human breast milk. *Br. J. Clin. Pharmacol. 21,* 553.
3. Hoppu K, Neuvonen P, Korte T (1986) Disopyramide and breast-feeding. *Br. J Clin. Pharmacol.*, *21*, 553.
4. Ellsworth AJ, Horn JR, Raisys VA, Miyagawa LA, Bell JL (1989) Disopyramide and N-monodesalkyl disopyramide in serum and breast milk. *Ann. Pharmacother.*, *23,* 56–57.

FLECAINIDE

GENERAL

Flecainide is a cardiac antidysrhythmic drug. It is well absorbed from the adult gastrointestinal tract and is 40 % bound to plasma proteins. About 75% is metabolised and the remainder is excreted unchanged. The plasma half-life is 20 h. Prodysrhythmic effects of flecainide have been a cause for concern.

EVALUATION OF DATA

Passage of flecainide into human milk has been reported as follows:

Treatment conditions	Concentration (mg/l)		Milk/plasma ratio	Maximum observed milk conc. (mg/l)	Absolute dose to infant (mg/kg/day)		Ref.
Dose × Frequency × Duration; Route; No. of patients; Lactation stage	Milk	Plasma			Ave	Max	
100 mg × 2/d × LT; p.o.;11; 1–6 d	0.27–1.53	0.16–0.445	2.6–3.7	1.53	–	0.23	(1)
100 mg × 2/d × LT; p.o.;1; 5–7 d	0.89–1.09	0.50–0.57	1.6–2.2	1.09	–	0.16	(2)

LT, long term. Study (1) was conducted for 5.5 days and apparent steady-state dosing was achieved in most cases by day 4. In study (2) the mother was also continuously treated with sotalol.

RELATIVE DOSE IN MILK

The amount of flecainide that a suckling infant would receive in a day is at maximum 6.9% (1.53 × 900/200)* (1) or 4.9% (1.09 × 900/200)* (3) of the weight-adjusted maternal daily dose.

DATA ON THE INFANT

No data were obtained from the infants in the evaluated studies but flecainide has been used in infants as young as 5 days of age to treat resistant dysrhythmias (3).

ASSESSMENT AND RECOMMENDATIONS

The studies were carried under steady-state conditions of dosing. These indicate that the risk to the suckling infant of administering flecainide to its mother is low

* An explanation of the calculation (s) appears on pp. 71–72.

on the basis that the quantity of drug that passes into milk is small. Breast-feeding would thus be regarded as safe.

REFERENCES

1. McQuinn RL, Pisani A, Wafa S, Chang SF, Miller AM, Frappel JM, Chamberlain GVP, Camm AJ (1990) Flecainide excretion in human breast milk. *Clin. Pharmacol. Ther.,48*, 262–267.
2. Wagner X, Jouglard J, Moulin M, Miller AM, Petitjean J, Pisapia A (1990) Coadministration of flecainide acetate and sotalol during pregnancy: Lack of teratogenic effects, passage across the placenta, and excretion in human breast milk. *Am. Heart J., 119*, 700–702.
3. Perry JC, McQuinn RL, Smith RT, Gothing C, Fredell P, Garson A (1989) Flecainide acetate for resitant arrhythmias in the young: efficacy and pharmacokinetics. *J. Am. Coll. Cardiol., 14*, 185–189.

HYDRALAZINE

GENERAL

Hydralazine is a vasodilator drug that is used to treat arterial hypertension. It is rapidly absorbed from the adult gastrointestinal tract and is acetylated in the liver; systemic avaialbility after oral administration is about 30% in rapid acetylators and about 50% in slow acetylators. Hydralazine is 87% bound to plasma proteins. It is excreted mainly as metabolites in the urine. The plasma half-life is 2–8 h.

EVALUATION OF DATA

Passage of hydralazine into human milk has been reported as follows:

Treatment conditions: Dose × Frequency × Duration; Route; No. of patients; Lactation stage	Concentration (mg/l)		Milk/ plasma ratio	Maxi-mum observed milk conc. (mg/l)	Absolute dose to infant (mg/kg/day)		Ref.
	Milk	Plasma			Ave	Max	
50 mg × 3/d× LT; p.o.; 1; 2 months	0.12	0.17	0.93	0.13	0.018	0.019	(1)

LT, long term. Hydralazine has in the past been assayed by a method that co-determined acid labile hydrazones; the true hydralazine represented only a minor fraction of the total estimated concentration (2). In the evaluated report (1), gas liquid chromatography which measures only hydralazine was used. The study was undertaken under steady-state conditions and blood and milk samples were collected simultaneously 0.5 and 2 h after dosing.

RELATIVE DOSE IN MILK

The amount of hydralazine that a suckling infant would ingest in a day is at maximum 0.8% (0.13 × 900/150)* of the weight-adjusted maternal daily dose (1).

DATA ON THE INFANT

The literature gives no relevant information on the effects in the infant.

ASSESSMENT AND RECOMMENDATIONS

This case report suggests that the risk to the suckling infant of administering hydralazine to its mother is low because the quantity of drug that passes into milk is small. Breast-feeding would appear to be safe, but more information is needed.

* An explanation of the calculation (s) appears on pp. 71–72.

REFERENCES

1. Liedholm H, Wahlin-Boll E, Hansson A, Ingemarsson I, Melander A. (1982) Transplacental passage and breast milk concentrations of hydralazine. *Eur. J. Clin. Pharmacol.*, *21*, 417–419.
2. Zak SB, Lucas G, Gilleran TG (1977) Plasma levels of real and 'apparent' hydralazine in man and rat. *Drug Metab. Dispos.*, *5*, 116–121.

HYDROCHLOROTHIAZIDE

GENERAL

Hydrochlorothiazide is a diuretic that is used for mild oedema and arterial hypertension. Its main effect occurs within 4–6 h of dosing. The drug is well absorbed from the adult gastrointestinal tract and is 64% bound to plasma proteins. Hyrdochrorothiazide is eliminated mainly in the urine and the plasma half-life is 2.5 h.

EVALUATION OF DATA

Passage of hydrochlorothiazide into human milk has been reported as follows:

Treatment conditions — Dose × Frequency × Duration; Route; No. of patients; Lactation stage	Concentration (mg/l)		Milk/plasma ratio	Maximum observed milk conc. (mg/l)	Absolute dose to infant (mg/kg/day)		Ref.
	Milk	Plasma			Ave	Max	
50 mg × 1/d × LT; p.o.; 1; 28 d	0.08	–	–	0.12	0.012	0.018	(1)

LT, long term. The concentration-time profiles were defined over 24 h and were not concurrent; the milk concentration was highest 5–9 h after the dose. The milk concentration is the average value; the maximum concentration quoted here is estimated from a graph in the report. Steady-state dosing conditions are assumed to apply.

RELATIVE DOSE IN MILK

A suckling infant would ingest in a day on average 1.4% (0.08 × 900/50)* and at maximum 2.2% (0.12 × 900/50)* of the weight-adjusted maternal daily dose of hydrochlorothiazide (2).

DATA ON THE INFANT

No data are reported.

ASSESSMENT AND RECOMMENDATIONS

The risk to the suckling infant of administering hydrochlorothiazide to its mother is low on the basis that the quantity of drug that passes into milk is small. Breastfeeding may be regarded as safe, but note that thiazide diuretics can suppress lactation (2).

* An explanation of the calculation (s) appears on pp. 71–72.

REFERENCES

1. Miller ME, Cohn RD, Burghart PH (1982) Hydrochlorothiazide disposition in a mother and her breast-fed infant. *J. Paediatr.*, *101*, 789–791.
2. Healy M (1961) Suppressing lactation with oral diuretics. *Lancet, i,* 1353–1354.

LABETALOL

GENERAL

Labetalol is a non-selective β-adrenoceptor blocking drug which also has α-adrenoceptor blocking properties. It is used in arterial hypertension including the hypertension of pregnancy. Labetalol is well absorbed from the adult gastrointestinal tract but because of extensive first-pass metabolism its systemic availability is 20%. It is 50% is bound to plasma proteins. Labetalol is almost completely metabolised in the liver and the products are excreted in the urine and in the bile; the plasma half-life is 5 h. Unwanted effects of β-blockade that are relevant to the infant include the possibility of hypoglycaemia, for the maintenance of blood glucose during fasting by sympathetic-mediated hepatic glycogenolysis may be impaired.

EVALUATION OF DATA

Passage of labetalol into human milk has been reported as follows:

Treatment conditions Dose × Frequency × Duration; Route; No. of patients; Lactation stage	Concentration (mg/l) Milk	 Plasma	Milk/ plasma ratio	Maximum observed milk conc. (mg/l)	Absolute dose to infant (mg/kg/day) Ave	 Max	Ref.
330 mg/d × LT; p.o.; 4; 3 d	0.029	0.064	0.45	–	0.004	–	(2)
400 mg/d × LT; p.o. ; 11; 3d	0.027	0.123	0.22	–	0.004	–	(2)
600 mg/d × LT; p.o.; 6; 7 d	0.039	0.135	0.29	–	0.006	–	(2)
600 mg/d × LT; p.o.; 2; 7d	0.127	0.084	1.51	0.223	0.019	0.034	(1)
700 mg/d × LT; p.o.; 2; 7 d	0.046	0.158	0.29	–	–	–	(2)
800 mg/d × LT; p.o.; 1; 7d	0.043	0.174	0.25	–	-	–	(2)
1200 mg/d × LT; p.o.; 1; 7 d	0.432	0.512	0.84	0.662	0.065	0.099	(1)

LT, long term. The studies report on mothers who received labetalol for hypertension during pregnancy. All the patients breast-fed the irinfants except the mother who took labetalol 1200 mg. In reference (1) the concentration–time profiles were defined and were not concurrent. The milk concentration frequently exceeded that in plasma and the peak milk concentration occurred 2–3 h after dosing. Average milk and plasma concentrations are given based on area calculations but the maximum milk concentration is the highest value recorded in an individual. In reference (2) the milk and plasma concentrations are average values based on single samples. Both studies were conducted under steady-state conditions of dosing.

RELATIVE DOSE IN MILK

The average milk concentration of the mothers quoted in the table for reference (2) was 0.037 mg/l and the average dose they received was 566 mg/d. Based on these data the amount of labetalol that a suckling infant would ingest in a day is on average 0.06% (0.037 × 900/566)* and at maximum 0.33% (0.223 × 900/600)* (1) of the weight-adjusted maternal daily dose.

DATA ON THE INFANT

Labetalol concentrations of 18 and 21 μ/1 were found in plasma of one infant (1). No adverse effects of labetalol were reported in the infants in the studies quoted.

ASSESSMENT AND RECOMMENDATIONS

The risk to the suckling infant of administering labetalol to its mother is low on the basis that the quantity of drug that passes into milk is small. Breast-feeding may be regarded as safe.

REFERENCES

1. Lunell N-O, Kulas J, Rane A (1985) Transfer of labetalol into amniotic fluid and breast milk in lactating women. *Eur. J. Clin. Pharmacol.*, *28*, 597–599.
2. Michael CA (1979) Use of labetalol in the treatment of severe hypertension during pregnancy. *Br. J. Clin. Pharmacol.*, *8*, 211S–215S.

* An explanation of the calculation (s) appears on pp. 71–72.

MEPINDOLOL

GENERAL

Mepindolol is a non-selective β-adrenoceptor blocking drug. It is absorbed from the adult gastrointestinal tract, is 40–60% bound to plasma proteins and its plasma half-life is 4 h. Unwanted effects of β-blockade that are relevant to the infant include the possibility of delayed recovery from hypoglycaemia, for the maintenance of blood glucose during fasting by sympathetic-mediated hepatic glycogenolysis may be impaired.

EVALUATION OF DATA

Passage of mepindolol into human milk has been reported as follows:

Treatment conditions Dose × Frequency × Duration; Route; No. of patients; Lactation stage	Concentration (μg/l)		Milk/plasma ratio	Maximum observed milk conc. (μg/l)	Absolute dose to infant (μg/kg/day)		Ref.
	Milk	Plasma			Ave	Max	
20 mg × 1/d × 1 d; p.o.;5; 3 d	17	38	0.45	34	3	5	(1)
20 mg × 1/d × 5 d; p.o.; 5; 8 d	28	53	0.52	95	4	14	(1)

Milk and plasma samples were taken 2 and 6 h after dosing, i.e. the concentration-time profile was not defined. The table gives average values for the group for these times but the maximum milk concentration is the highest value recorded in an individual. The measurements on the 5th day probably represent steady-state dosing conditions.

RELATIVE DOSE IN MILK

Mepindolol sulphate 20 mg is equivalent to 16.8 mg of the free base which was assayed in milk and a factor of 0.84 (16.8/20.0) has been introduced into the calculation. The amount of mepindolol that a suckling infant would ingest in a feed is at maximum 0.4% (34 × 180/20 000 × 0.84)* of the weight-adjusted maternal single dose (1). A suckling infant would ingest in a day on average 1.5% (28 × 900/20 000 × 0.84)* and at maximum 5.1% (95 × 900/20 000 × 0.84)* of the weight-adjusted maternal daily dose (1).

* An explanation of the calculation (s) appears on pp. 71–72.

DATA ON THE INFANT

Plasma mepindolol concentrations in the newborn babies were below the detection limit (1 μg/l) 4 h after dosing on the 1st and 5th days, except for one baby in whom concentrations of 2 and 5 μg/l were found at these times. No drug-related effects were observed in the infants.

ASSESSMENT AND RECOMMENDATIONS

This short-term study suggests that risk to the suckling infant of administering mepindolol to its mother is low because the amount of drug that passes into milk is small. Certain inherent pharmacological properties of β-blockers, for example recovery from hypoglycaemia during fasting, give reason for caution. Furthermore mepindolol is a drug of high potency and until there is satisfactory evidence to the contrary, a breast-feeding mother should use an alternative β-blocker.

REFERENCES

1. Krause W, Stopelli I, Milia S, Rainer E (1982) Transfer of mepindolol to newborns by breast-feeding mothers after single and repeated daily doses. *Eur. J. Clin. Pharmacol., 22*, 53–55.

METHYLDOPA

GENERAL

Methyldopa is used in the treatment of arterial hypertension. After oral administration to adults systemic availability is 25%. In the plasma less than 20% is bound to proteins. Methyldopa appears rapidly in the urine, 60–70% as the unchanged compound and the remainder as conjugates. The plasma half-life is 2 h but may be 9–20 h in neonates (1).

EVALUATION OF DATA

Passage of methyldopa into human milk has been reported as follows:

Treatment conditions Dose × Frequency × Duration; Route; No. of patients; Lactation stage	Concentration (mg/l)		Milk/ plasma ratio	Maxi-mum observed milk conc. (mg/l)	Absolute dose to infant (mg/kg/day)		Ref.
	Milk	Plasma			Ave	Max	
250–1500 mg × LT; p.o.; 8; ?	0.17 (0.26)	0.37	0.46	–	0.03	–	(2)
250 mg × 3–4/d × LT; p.o.; 3; 30–60 h	0.1 (0.35)	–	–	–	0.02(0.05)	–	(3)
500 mg x 4/d x LT; p.o.; 1; 30–60 h	0.2 (0.9)	0.2 (0.5)	–	–	0.03(0.14)	–	(3)
500 mg × 1/d ×LT; p.o.; 2 1, 3, 8 weeks	0.19, 0.05	0.69, 0.29	0.28, 0.17	0.66, 0.2	0.03, 0.01	0.10,0.03	(4)
1000 mg × 1/d × LT; p.o.; 1; 8 weeks	0.44	2.08	0.21	1.14	0.07	0.17	(4)

LT = long term. The studies were undertaken in mothers who received methyldopa for hypertension during pregnancy. Steady-state dosing conditions may be assumed to apply. References (2) and (3) quote the averages of single milk and plasma samples. The figures in brackets refer to conjugates of methyldopa. The concentration–time profiles were defined in reference (4) and were not concurrent; the the peak milk concentration occurred 6 h after dosing. The milk and plasma concentrations are average values for unchanged methyldopa and were obtained by dividing the area under the concentration-time curve by the corresponding time interval. The values for unchanged methyldopa were 37% of those for the total (free plus conjugated) drug.

RELATIVE DOSE IN MILK

The amount of methyldopa that a suckling infant would ingest in a day is on average 1.6% (0.17 + 0.26 × 900/250)* (2) and at maximum 3.2% (0.66 x 900/500 x 0.37)* (4) of the weight-adjusted maternal daily dose.

* An explanation of the calculation (s) appears on pp. 71–72.

DATA ON THE INFANT

No information is avaiable.

ASSESSMENT AND RECOMMENDATIONS

The risk to the suckling infant of administering methyldopa to its mother is low on the basis that the quantity of drug that passes into milk is small. Breast-feeding may be regarded as safe.

REFERENCES

1. Jones HMR, Cummings AJ, Setchell KDR, Lawson AM (1979) A study ofthe disposition of alpha-methyldopa in newborn infants following its administration to the mother for the treatment of hypertension during pregnancy. *Br. J. Clin. Pharmacol.*, *8*, 433–440.
2. Hoskins JA, Holliday SB (1982) Determination of alpha-methyldopa and methyldopate in human breast milk and plasma by ion-exchange chromatography using electrochemical detection. *J. Chromatogr.*, *230*, 162–167.
3. Jones, HMR, Cummings, AJ (1978) A study of the transfer of alpha-methyldopa to the human foetus and newborn infant. *Br. J. Clin. Pharmacol.*, *6*, 432–434.
4. White WB, Andreoli JW, Cohn RD (1985) Alpha-methyldopa disposition in mothers with hypertension and in their breast-frd infants. *Clin. Pharmacol. Therap.*, *37*, 387–390.

METOPROLOL

GENERAL

Metoprolol is a β_1-selective adrenoceptor blocking drug. It is well absorbed from the adult gastrointestinal tract but systemic availability is 40% due to first pass metabolism by the liver. It is 10% bound to plasma proteins. Metoprolol is extensively metabolised in the liver. The plasma half-life in adults is 3 h but it is longer in neonates. Unwanted effects of β-blockade that are relevant to the infant include the possibility of delayed recovery from hypoglycaemia, for the maintenance of blood glucose during fasting by sympathetic-mediated hepatic glycogenolysis may be impaired.

EVALUATION OF DATA

Passage of metoprolol into human milk has been reported as follows:

Treatment conditions Dose × Frequency × Duration; Route; No. of patients; Lactation stage	Concentration (μg/l) Milk	 Plasma	Milk/ plasma ratio	Maximum observed milk conc. (μg/l)	Absolute dose to infant (μg/kg/day) Ave	 Max	Ref.
50 mg × 2/d × LT; p.o.; 3; 4–60 d	75	26	2.0–3.1	200	11	30	(1)
50 mg × 2/d × LT; p.o.; 3; ?	–	–	3.4	422	–	60	(2)
100 mg × 2/d × LT; p.o.6; ?	–	–	3.4	457	–	70	(2)
50–100 mg × 2/d × LT; p.o.8; 7 d	–	–	2.8	670	–	100	(3)
100 mg × 1–2/d × 4 d; p.o.;3; 4 months	–	–	3.6	360	–	54	(4)

LT, long term. Reference (1) defined the concentration-time profiles; the values in milk exceeded those in plasma. The table gives average concentrations based on the area calculations but the maximum milk concentration is the highest value recorded in an individual. Data based on single samples 2 h (2) and at varying times after dosing (3) are also presented. The maximum milk concentrations are the highest values recorded in individuals. Steady-state dosing conditions may be taken to apply to all studies.

RELATIVE DOSE IN MILK

The amount of metoprolol that a suckling infant would ingest in a day is on average 0.7% (75 × 900/100 000)* (1) and at maximum 3.2% (360 × 900/100 000)* (4) of the weight-adjusted maternal daily dose.

* An explanation of the calculation (s) appears on pp. 71–72.

DATA ON THE INFANT

There are no reports in the literature of adverse effects of metoprolol ingested in milk. The infant capillary blood concentration after suckling varied mainly between 0.5 and 2.9 μg/l but one infant, whose mother was a poor metaboliser of metoprolol, had a blood concentration of 45.0 μg/l (3).

ASSESSMENT AND RECOMMENDATIONS

The risk to the suckling infant of administering metoprolol to its mother appears to be low because the quantity of drug that passes into milk is small. A proportion of the population (about 10% in Northern Europe) metabolise metoprolol at a slow rate and metoprolol would be more likely to produce effects if the infant or its mother (or both) were slow metabolisers. Breast-feeding may be regarded as generally safe but a special awareness should be maintained of the possibility of drug effects in the infant.

REFERENCES

1. Kulas J, Lunell, NO, Rosing U, Steen P, Rane A. (1984) Atenolol and metoprolol. A comparison of their excretion in human breast milk. *Acta Obstet. Gynecol. Scand., Suppl. 118,* 65–69.
2. Sandström B, Regårdh CG (1980) Metoprolol excretion into breast milk. *Br. J. Clin. Pharmac., 9,* 518–519.
3. Lindeberg S, Sandström B, Lundborg P, Regårdh CG. (1984) Disposition of the adrenergic blocker metoprolol in the late pregnant woman, the amniotic fluid, the cord blood and the neonate. *Acta Obstet. Gynecol. Scand., Suppl. 118*, 61–64.
4. Liedholm H, Melander A, Bitzen P-O, Helm G, Lönnerholm G, Mattiasson I, Nilsson B, Wahlin-Boll E (1981) Accumulation of atenolol and metoprolol in human milk. *Eur. J. Clin. Pharmac.,20*, 229–231.

MEXILETINE

GENERAL

Mexiletine is a cardiac antidysrhythmic drug used in ventricular tachyarrhythmias that are resistant to lignocaine. The drug is well absorbed from the adult gastrointestinal tract, is 70% bound to plasma proteins and the distribution volume is 9 l/kg. The plasma half-life is 9–12 h and the action of the drug is terminated mainly by metabolism, only 10% being eliminated unchanged in the urine.

EVALUATION OF DATA

Passage of mexiletine into human milk has been reported as follows:

Treatment conditions Dose × Frequency × Duration; Route; No. of patients; Lactation stage	Concentration (mg/l)		Milk/plasma ratio	Maximum observed milk conc. (mg/l)	Absolute dose to infant (mg/kg/day)		Ref.
	Milk	Plasma			Ave	Max	
200 mg × 3/d × LT; p.o.; 1; 2–5 d	0.94	0.72	1.45	0.96	–	0.14	(1)

LT, long term. Twelve paired milk and blood samples were obtained at intervals over 108 h. The concentration-time profiles were concurrent. The milk and blood concentrations quoted are the mean peak values. The milk/plasma ratio is a mean value. The patient also received propranolol 20 mg × 3/day.

RELATIVE DOSE IN MILK

The amount of mexiletine that a suckling infant would ingest in a day is at maximum 1.4% (0.96 × 900/600)* of the weight-adjusted maternal daily dose.

DATA ON THE INFANT

An infant who was exposed to mexiletine during pregnancy and breast-feeding was in good health at 10 months (2).

ASSESSMENT AND RECOMMENDATIONS

The data from a single case report suggest that the risk to the suckling infant of administering mexiletine to its mother is low because the quantity of drug that

* An explanation of the calculation (s) appears on pp. 71–72.

passes into milk is small. Nevertheless more information is required before a general recommendation can be made about the safety of mexiletine in breast-feeding women.

REFERENCES

1. Lewis AM, Johnston A, Patel L, Turner P (1981) Mexiletine in human blood and breast milk. *Postgrad. Med. J.*, *57*, 546–547.
2. Lownes HE, Ives TJ (1987) Mexiletine use in pregnancy and lactation. *Am. J. Obstet. Gynec.*, *157*, 446–447.

MINOXIDIL

GENERAL

Minoxidil is a potent vasodilator that is used to treat resistant hypertension. It is well absorbed from the adult gastrointestinal tract and is negligibly bound to plasma proteins. The action of minoxidil is terminated mainly by metabolism in the liver and the plasma half-life is 3 h.

EVALUATION OF DATA

Passage of minoxidil into human milk has been reported asfollows:

Treatment conditions: Dose × Frequency × Duration; Route; No. of patients; Lactation stage	Concentration (μg/l)		Milk/ plasma ratio	Maximum observed milk conc. (μg/l)	Absolute dose to infant (μg/kg/day)		Ref.
	Milk	Plasma			Ave	Max	
5 mg × 2/d × LT (but see comment below) p.o.; 1; 2 months	11	15	0.88	42	1.7	6.3	(1)

LT, long term. The patient also received propranolol 40 mg 2/d and frusemide 40 mg × 2/d for hypertension. On the morning of the study the patient received minoxidil 7.5 mg and the table gives average values for 5 estimates over 12 h thereafter.

RELATIVE DOSE IN MILK

The amount of minoxidil that a suckling infant would ingest in aday is on average 1.3% (11 × 900/7500)* and at maximum 5.0% (42 × 900/7500)* of the weight-adjusted maternal daily dose (1).

DATA ON THE INFANT

The mother took minoxidil throughout pregnancy and for 2 months while breast-feeding. No abnormality was noted in the infant.

ASSESSMENT AND RECOMMENDATIONS

The risk to the suckling infant of administering minoxidil to its mother is low on the basis that the quantity of drug that enters milk is small. However no general

* An explanation of the calculation (s) appears on pp. 71–72.

recommendation can be made because the available evidence is limited to a single case.

REFERENCES

1. Valdivieso A, Valdes G, Spiro TE, Westerman RL (1985) Minoxidil in breast milk. *Ann. Int. Med.*, *102*, 135.

NADOLOL

GENERAL

Nadolol is a non-selective β-adrenoceptor blocking drug. It is absorbed from the adult gastrointestinal tract and 30% is bound to plasma proteins. Nadolol is eliminated unchanged by the kidneys. The plasma half-life is 12–24 h. Unwanted effects of β-blockade that are relevant to the infant include the possibility of delayed recovery from hypoglycaemia, for the maintenance of blood glucose during fasting by sympathetic-mediated hepatic glycogenolysis may be impaired.

EVALUATION OF DATA

Passage of nadolol into human milk has been reported as follows:

Treatment conditions Dose × Frequency × Duration; Route; No. of patients; Lactation stage	Concentration (mg/l)		Milk/ plasma ratio	Maximum observed milk conc. (mg/l)	Absolute dose to infant (mg/kg/day)		Ref.
	Milk	Plasma			Ave	Max	
80 mg × 1/d × 5 d; p.o.; 12; >1 month	0.357	0.077	4.6	0.443	0.054	0.067	(1)

The concentration-time profiles were defined over the period of the study and were not concurrent, the maximum concentration in milk occurring later than in serum. Steady-state conditions of dosing applied. Following the final dose the half-life of elimination was 22 h from both milk and serum. The concentrations quoted are average values for the group. As the mothers took nadolol either at the time of weaning or did not breast-feed, no infant was exposed to the drug in milk.

RELATIVE DOSE IN MILK

A suckling infant would ingest in a day on average 4.0% (0.357 x 900/80)* and at maximum 5.0% (0.443 × 900/80)* of the weight-adjusted maternal daily dose (1).

DATA ON THE INFANT

No information is available.

ASSESSMENT AND RECOMMENDATIONS

The risk to the suckling infant of administering nadolol to its mother would appear

* An explanation of the calculation (s) appears on pp. 71–72.

to be low on the basis that the quantity of drug that passes into milk is small. Certain inherent pharmacological properties of β-blockers, for example recovery from hypoglycaemia during fasting, give reason for caution and special observation of the suckling infant when nadolol is administered to its mother.

REFERENCES

1. Devlin RG, Duchin KL, Fleiss PM (1981) Nadolol in human serum and breast milk. *Br. J. Clin. Pharmacol.*, 12, 393–396.

NIFEDIPINE

GENERAL

Nifedipine is a calcium antagonist used principally for the treatment of hypertension and angina. It is well absorbed from the adult gastrointestinal tract and is 95% bound to plasma proteins. Nifedipine is almost completely metabolised. The plasma half life is 2–6 h.

EVALUATION OF DATA

Passage of nifedipine into human milk has been reported as follows:

Treatment conditions: Dose × Frequency × Duration; Route; No. of patients; Lactation stage	Concentration (μg/l): Milk	Concentration (μg/l): Plasma	Milk/plasma ratio	Maximum observed milk conc. (μg/l)	Absolute dose to infant (μg/kg/day): Ave	Absolute dose to infant (μg/kg/day): Max	Ref.
10 mg × 4/d (capsules) × LT; p.o.; 1; ?	7–46 (2–22)	9–43 (4–15)	1.0	46 (22)	–	6.9 (3.3)	(1)

LT, long term. The study was performed after a 20 mg test dose during LT treatment and steady-state conditions can be assumed to apply. Milk and plasma concentration-time profiles were concurrent. Data for the pyridine metabolite appear in brackets.

RELATIVE DOSE IN MILK

The amount of nifedipine and its pyridine metabolite that a suckling infant would receive in a day is at maximum 1.5% ((46 + 22) × 900/40 000)* (1) of the weight-adjusted maternal daily dose.

DATA ON THE INFANT

No data are available.

ASSESSMENT AND RECOMMENDATIONS

The risk to the suckling infant of administering nifedipine to its mother is low on the basis that the quantity of drug that passes into milk is small but no general recommendation can be made as only a single case is reported.

* An explanation of the calculation (s) appears on pp. 71–72.

REFERENCES

1. Penny WJ, Lewis MJ (1989) Nifedipine is excreted in human milk. *Eur. J. Clin. Pharmacol., 36,* 427–428.

NITRENDIPINE

GENERAL

Nitrendipine is a long-acting calcium antagonist used for the treatment of hypertension and angina. It is well absorbed after oral administration but is subject to extensive first-pass metabolism and systemic availability is only 15%. Nitrendipine is 98% protein bound. The plasma half life is 10–22 h.

EVALUATION OF DATA

Passage of nitrendipine into human milk has been reported as follows:

Treatment conditions: Dose × Frequency × Duration; Route; No. of patients; Lactation stage	Concentration (μg/l) Milk	Concentration (μg/l) Plasma	Milk/plasma ratio	Maximum observed milk conc. (μg/l)	Absolute dose to infant (μg/kg/day) Ave	Absolute dose to infant (μg/kg/day) Max	Ref.
10 mg × 1/d × 1 d; p.o.; 3; >3 months	5.2 (9.3)	7.7 (17.1)	0.67 (0.54)	6.5	–	–	(1)
10 mg × 2/d × 5 d; p.o.; 2; >3 months	3.5 (4.5)	12.5 (20.1)	0.28 (0.22)	5.5 (6.6)	0.53 (0.68)	0.83 (0.99)	(1)

The first part of the study reports the results of single dose administration. The second part reports on short-term dosing at steady-state in 2 of the 3 subjects. The milk and plasma concentration-time curves were concurrent. Average milk and plasma values are quoted. The figures in brackets refer to the pyridine metabolite of nitrendipine. The drug was measured by a capillary gas chromatographic method using an electron capture detector and the detection limit and coefficient of variation were satisfactory for the purpose.

RELATIVE DOSE IN MILK

Using the data derived from steady-state conditions, the amount of nitrendipine and its pyridine metabolite that a suckling infant would receive in a day is on average 0.4% (3.5 + 4.5 × 900/20 000)* and at maximum 0.6% (5.5 + 6.6 × 900/20 000)* (1) of the weight-adjusted maternal daily dose.

DATA ON THE INFANT

No data are available.

ASSESSMENT AND RECOMMENDATIONS

The risk to the suckling infant of administering nitrendipine to its mother is low on

* An explanation of the calculation (s) appears on pp. 71–72.

the basis that the quantity of drug that passes into milk is small. Breast-feeding may be considered safe.

REFERENCES

1. White WB, Yeh SH, Krol GJ (1989) Nitrendipine in human plasma and breast milk. *Eur. J. Clin. Pharmacol., 36,* 531–534.

OXPRENOLOL

GENERAL

Oxperenolol is a non-selective β-adrenoceptor blocking drug. In the adult oxprenolol is completely absorbed from the gastrointestinal tract and 80% is bound to plasma proteins. It is extensively metabolised such that only 5% is excreted unchanged in the urine. The plasma half-life is 2–3 h. Unwanted effects of β-blockade that are relevant to the infant include the possibility of delayed recovery from hypoglycaemia, for the maintenance of blood glucose during fasting by sympathetic-mediated hepatic glycogenolysis may be impaired.

EVALUATION OF DATA

Passage of oxprenolol into human milk has been reported as follows:

Treatment conditions	Concentration (mg/l)		Milk/ plasma ratio	Maximum observed milk conc. (mg/l)	Absolute dose to infant (mg/kg/day)		Ref.
Dose × Frequency × Duration; Route; No. of patients; Lactation stage	Milk	Plasma			Ave	Max	
80 mg × 2/d × 1–17 d; p.o ; 9; <4 – >8 d	0.128	0.430	0.29	0.374	0.019	0.056	(1)
160 mg × 2/d 3–5 d; p.o.;3; <4 – >8 d	0.158	0.709	0.21	0.324	0.024	0.049	(1)
320 mg × 2/d × 2 d; p.o.; 1; <4 – >8 d	0.470	1.104	0.43	0.437	–	0.071	(1)
80 mg × 3/d × LT; p.o.;9; 3–6 d	0.116	0.427	0.45	0.402	0.174	0.060	(2)

LT, long term. Both studies were of hypertensive patients. Neither study defined the concentration-time profiles. In reference (1), milk was collected from patients in whom full milk flow was established, either in the mid-morning or mid-afternoon. The milk and plasma concentrations are arithmetical mean values, the milk to plasma ratios are geometric mean values and the maximum milk concentrations are the highest values recorded in individuals. Steady-state dosing conditions were probably not established in all the patients. In study (2) samples were collected 0.5–5.0 h after ingestion of oxprenolol. The milk and plasma concentrations and the milk:plasma ratios are average values and the maximum concentration is the highest value recorded in an individual.

RELATIVE DOSE IN MILK

The amount of oxprenolol that a suckling infant would ingest in a day is on average 0.7% (0.128 × 900/160)* (1) and at maximum 1.5% (0.402 × 900/240)* (2) of the weight-adjusted maternal daily dose.

* An explanation of the calculation (s) appears on pp. 71–72.

DATA ON THE INFANT

No drug effects were reported in the infants (1,2).

ASSESSMENT AND RECOMMENDATIONS

The risk to the suckling infant of administering oxprenolol to its mother appears to be low on the basis that the quantity of drug that passes into milk is small. Breast-feeding is probably safe but certain inherent pharmacological properties of β-blockers, for example recovery from hypoglycaemia during fasting, give reason for caution and special observation of the suckling infant when oxprenolol is administered to its mother.

REFERENCES

1. Fidler J, Smith V, de Swiet M (1983) Excretion of oxprenolol and timolol in breast milk. *Br. J. Obstet. Gynecol., 90*, 961–965.
2. Sioufi A, Hillion D, Lumbroso P, Wainer R, Olivier-Martin M, Schoeller JP, Colussi D, Leroux F, Mangoni P (1984) Oxprenolol placental transfer, plasma concentrations in newborns and passage into breast milk. *Br. J. Clin. Pharmacol., 18*, 453–456.

PENTOXIFYLLINE

GENERAL

Pentoxifylline (oxpentifylline) is a methylxanthine that is used to treat intermittent claudication due to chronic obstructive arterial disease, and sometimes to relieve the symptoms of Raynaud's syndrome; it is believed to lower blood viscosity by increasing erythrocyte flexibility. Pentoxifylline is readily absorbed from the gastrointestinal tract and is extensively metabolised in the liver. The half life is 2 h.

EVALUATION OF DATA

Passage of pentoxifylline into human milk has been reported as follows:

Treatment conditions Dose × Frequency × Duration; Route; No. of patients; Lactation stage	Concentration (mg/l)		Milk/plasma ratio	Maximum observed milk conc. (mg/l)	Absolute dose to infant (mg/kg/day)		Ref.
	Milk	Plasma			Ave	Max	
400 mg/d × 1 d; p.o.; 5; > 6 weeks	0.036 –	0.044 (0.95)	0.87	0.074 (0.97)	0.005	0.011	(1)

The 5 subjects were at the point of weaning when the study was performed and had abstained from xanthine-containing foods and beverages for at least 1 day prior to the dose of pentoxifylline. The table gives average milk and plasma values from samples obtained 4 h after the dose; the maximum milk concentration is the average value for the group measured at 2 h. The report also quotes concentrations of 3 metabolites and summed maximum values for these, whether occurring at 2 h or 4 h, appear in brackets.

RELATIVE DOSE IN MILK

The amount of pentoxifylline that an infant would ingest in a feed is at maximum of 0.5% (0.074 + 0.97 × 180/400)* of the weight-adjusted maternal single dose (1).

DATA ON THE INFANT

No data are available.

ASSESSMENT AND RECOMMENDATIONS

The risk to the suckling infant of administering pentoxifylline to its mother is low on the basis that the quantity of drug that passes into milk is small. Breast-feeding

* An explanation of the calculation (s) appears on pp. 71–72.

following occasoinal doses may be regarded as safe but there are no data on which to base a recommendation following chronic dosing.

REFERENCE

1. Witter FR, Smith RV (1985) The excretion of pentoxifylline and its metabolites into human breast milk. *Am. J. Obstet. Gynaecol.*, *151*, 1094–1097.

PROCAINAMIDE

GENERAL

Procainamide is a cardiac antidysrhythmic drug. It is rapidly and almost completely absorbed from the adult gastrointestinal tract and 15% is bound to plasma proteins. About 55% of the drug is excreted unchanged in the urine; the remainder is metabolised and the acetylated product, N-acetylprocainamide (NAPA), is pharmacologically active. The plasma half-life of procainamide is 3–4 h but was 13.5 h in one neonate (1); the half-life of NAPA is 6–9 h.

EVALUATION OF DATA

Passage of procainamide into human milk has been reported as follows:

Treatment conditions: Dose × Frequency × Duration; Route; No. of patients; Lactation stage	Concentration (mg/l): Milk	Concentration (mg/l): Plasma	Milk/plasma ratio	Maximum observed milk conc. (mg/l)	Absolute dose to infant (mg/kg/day): Ave	Absolute dose to infant (mg/kg/day): Max	Ref.
500 mg × 4/d × LT; p.o.; 1; ?	5.4 (3.5)	1.1 (1.6)	4.3 (3.8)	10.2 (5.0)	0.81 (0.52)	1.53 (0.75)	(2)

The figures in brackets refer to the metabolite NAPA. The milk and serum concentrations are mean values for 6 samples collected over 15 h during 6 hourly dosing; the maximum milk concentration quoted is the highest individual value recorded. Steady-state dosing conditions were probably attained.

RELATIVE DOSE IN MILK

The amount of procainamide and its metabolite NAPA that a suckling infant would ingest in a day is on average 4.0% (5.4 + 3.5 × 900/2000)* and at maximum 6.1% (10.2 + 3.4 × 900/2000)*of the weight-adjusted maternal daily dose.

DATA ON THE INFANT

No data are available.

ASSESSMENT OF DATA

The risk to the suckling infant of administering procainamide to its mother appears to be low because the quantity of drug that passes into milk is small, but the data

* An explanation of the calculation (s) appears on pp. 71–72.

refer to only one case. Furthermore procainamide is slowly eliminated from the neonate (1). In the absence of adequate data as to its safety, breast-feeding whilst taking procainamide is probably inadvisable.

REFERENCES

1. Lima JJ, Kuritzky PM, Schentag JJ, Jusko WJ (1978) Fetal uptake and neonatal disposition of procainamide and its acetylated metabolite: a case report. *Pediatrics*, *61*, 491–493.
2. Pittard III WB, Glazier H (1983) Procainamide excretion in human milk. *J. Pediatr.*, *102*, 631–633.

PROPRANOLOL

GENERAL

Propranolol is a non-selective β-adrenoceptor blocking drug. It is absorbed from the adult gastrointestinal tract but systemic availability is 30–40% due to first-pass metabolism by the liver. It is 90–96% bound to plasma proteins and its action is terminated by metabolism in the liver. The plasma half-life is 4 h. Unwanted effects of β-blockade that are relevant to the infant include the possibility of delayed recovery from hypoglycaemia, for the maintenance of blood glucose during fasting by sympathetic-mediated hepatic glycogenolysis may be impaired.

EVALUATION OF DATA

Passage of propranolol into human milk has been reported as follows:

Treatment conditions: Dose × Frequency × Duration; Route; No. of patients; Lactation stage	Concentration (μg/l) Milk	Concentration (μg/l) Plasma	Milk/plasma ratio	Maximum observed milk conc. (μg/l)	Absolute dose to infant (μg/kg/day) Ave	Absolute dose to infant (μg/kg/day) Max	Ref.
20 mg × 2/d × LT; p.o.; 1; 3–6 d	8	17	0.5	20	1	3	(1)
1.16–2.61 mg/kg/d × LT; p.o.; 3; 1 week	35 (10)	0.052 (100)	0.85 (0.10)	75 (20)	5 (2)	11	(2) (3)
40 mg × 1/d × 1 d; p.o.; 1; 6–7 weeks	6	13	0.5	–	–	–	(3)
40 mg × 4/d × 2 d; p.o.; 18 weeks	–	–	0.64	–	–	–	(3)
240 mg/d × 30 d; p.o.; 1; 3 months	–	–	–	0.064	–	0.01	(3)
40 mg × 2/d × LT; p.o.; 5; ?	27	0.054 (blood)	0.5	36	4	5	(4)

LT, long term. Reference (1) gives the average of paired milk and plasma samples obtained on the 4th and 6th days after delivery; the maximum milk concentration was recorded on the 3rd day. Milk and plasma concentrations were measured on 4 occasions 2–8 h after the last dose of propranolol in reference (2). The table gives average values. Figures in brackets refer to propranolol glucuronide. The maximum milk concentration is the highest value recorded in an individual. The mean half-ife of elimination of propranolol from milk was 6.5 h compared to 2.6 h from plasma. Reference (3) defined the concentration-time profiles after a single dose and under steady-state conditions of dosing. The peak concentration occurred 3 h after dosing in milk and plasma. Reference (4) reports paired milk and blood samples taken 2 h after a dose. The table gives average values and the maximum milk concentration is the highest value recorded in an individual.

RELATIVE DOSE IN MILK

The amount of propranolol that a suckling infant would ingest in a day is on average 0.3% (27 × 900/80 000)* (4) and at maximum 0.4% (36 × 900/80 000)* (4) of the weight-adjusted maternal daily dose.

DATA ON THE INFANT

No signs of beta-blockade were observed in the infants reoprted in references (3) and (4).

ASSESSMENT AND RECOMMENDATIONS

The risk to the suckling infant of administering propranolol to its mother is low on the basis that the quantity of drug that passes into milk is small. Breast-feeding is probably safe but certain inherent pharmacological properties of β-blockers, for example recovery from hypoglycaemia during fasting, give reason for caution and special observation of the suckling infant when propranolol is administered to its mother.

REFERENCES

1. Taylor EA, Turner P (1981) Antihypertensive therapy with propranolol during pregnancy and lactation. *Postgrad. Med. J.*, *57*, 42–43.
2. Smith MT, Livingstone I, Hooper WD, Eadie MJ, Triggs EJ (1983) Propranolol, propranolol glucuronide, and naphthoxylactic acid in breast milk and plasma. *Therapeut. Drug Monit.*, *5*, 87–93.
3. Bauer JH, Pape B, Zajicek J, Groshong T (1979) Propranolol in human plasma and breast milk. *Am. J. Cardiol.*, *43*, 860–862.
4. Thorley KJ, McAinsh J (1983) Levels of the beta-blockers atenolol and propranolol in the breast milk of women treated for hypertension in pregnency. *Biopharm. Drug Dispos.*, *4*, 299–301.

* An explanation of the calculation (s) appears on pp. 71–72.

SOTALOL

GENERAL

Sotalol is a non-selective β-adrenoceptor blocking drug. It is absorbed from the adult gastrointestinal tract and is excreted largely unchanged in the urine. The plasma half-life is 7–18 h. Unwanted effects of β-blockade that are relevant to the infant include the possibility of delayed recovery from hypoglycaemia, for the maintenance of blood glucose during fasting by sympathetic-mediated hepatic glycogenolysis may be impaired.

EVALUATION OF DATA

Passage of sotalol into human milk has been reported as follows:

Treatment conditions — Dose × Frequency × Duration; Route; No. of patients; Lactation stage	Concentration (mg/l) Milk	Plasma	Milk/ plasma ratio	Maximum observed milk conc. (mg/l)	Absolute dose to infant (mg/kg/day) Ave	Max	Ref.
200–800 mg/d × LT; p.o.; 5; 1 week	10.5	2.3	5.4 (range 2.2–8.8)	20.2	1.58	3.03	(1)
240 mg/d × LT; p.o.; 1; 5 d	3.9	0.72	5.5	–	0.58	–	(2)
160 mg/d × LT; p.o.; 1; 105 d	2.8	0.97	2.8	–	0.41	–	(2)
80 mg × 2/d × LT; p.o.; 1; 5–7 d	4.4–5.0	1.4–1.6	2.8–3.6	5	–	0.75	(3)

LT, long term. The mothers received sotalol for hypertension during pregnancy. The table gives average milk and plasma values for 20 paired samples, i.e. the concentration-time profile was not defined. The maximum milk concentration was the highest value recorded in an individual. Steady-state dosing conditions were attained. Average milk concentrations for pre- and postfeed are given in (2). The mother in study (3) also received flecainid continuously.

RELATIVE DOSE IN MILK

The mean daily dose of sotalol administered to 12 patients, of whom only 5 breastfed, was 433 mg. On this basis the amount of sotalol that a suckling infant would ingest in a day is on average 21.8% (10.5 × 900/433)* and at maximum 42.0% (20.2 × 900/433)* of the weight-adjusted maternal daily dose (1). The calculations based on the data in (2) and (3) are broadly in accord with these findings.

* An explanation of the calculation (s) appears on pp. 71–72.

DATA ON THE INFANT

The infant whose mother produced the highest milk concentration of sotalol (20.2 mg/l) was monitored for 8 h during which he breast-fed twice. Bradycardia did not occur. The infant reported in (2) developed normally and did not demonstrate bradycardia. Normal development was reported at one year in the infant reported in (3).

ASSESSMENT AND RECOMMENDATIONS

The risk to the suckling infant of administering sotalol to its mother is significant on the basis of the quantity of drug that passes into milk. Furthermore, certain inherent pharmacological properties of β-blockers, for example recovery from hypoglycaemia during fasting, give reason for caution. Despite the apparent absence of effects in some infants breast-feeding is best regarded as unsafe and an alternative β-blocker should be used.

REFERENCES

1. O'Hare MF, Murnaghau GA, Russel CJ, Leahey WJ, Varma PMPS, McDevitt DG (1980) Sotalol as a hypotensive agent in pregnancy. *Br. J. Obstet. Gynaecol., 87*, 814–820.
2. Hackett LP, Wojnar-Horton RE, Dusci LJ, Ilett KF, Roberts MJ (1990) Excretion of sotalol in breast milk. *Br. J. Clin. Pharmacol., 29*, 277–278.
3. Wagner X, Jouglard J, Moulin M, Miller AM, Petitjean J, Pisapia A (1990) Coadministration of flecainide acetate and sotalol during pregnancy: lack of teratogenic effects, passage across the placenta, and excretion in human breast milk. *Am. Heart. J., 119,* 700–702.

SPIRONOLACTONE

GENERAL

Spironolactone is a potassium-sparing diuretic that acts by antagonising the action of aldosterone on the distal renal tubule. It is used in the management of cardiac failure, ascites and primary aldosteronism. Spironolactone is absorbed from the adult gastrointestinal tract and is metabolised to canrenone which is responsible for much of its biological action. Spironolactone is 98% bound to plasma proteins. The half-life of parent spironolactone is 1.3 h and that of canrenone is 17 h. Potential human metabolic products of spironolactone are carcinogenic in rodents.

EVALUATION OF DATA

Passage of canrenone into human milk, after administration of spironolactone, has been reported as follows:

Treatment conditions: Dose × Frequency × Duration; Route; No. of patients; Lactation stage	Concentration (μg/l)		Milk/plasma ratio	Maximum observed milk conc. (μg/l)	Absolute dose to infant (μg/kg/day)		Ref.
	Milk	Plasma			Ave	Max	
25 mg × 4 d × LT; p.o.1; 17 d	104 (2 h) 47 (14.5 h)	144 (2 h) 92 (14.5 h)	0.72 0.51	104	–	16	(1)

LT, long term. The dose refers to spironolactone, the milk and plasma concentrations refer to canrenone. The value at 2 h was assumed to be the maximum, but the concentration-time profile was not defined.

RELATIVE DOSE IN MILK

If it is assumed that the biological activity of spironolactone (mol. wt. 417) is all due to canrenone (mol. wt. 340), then the amount of canrenone that a suckling infant would ingest in a day is at maximum equivalent to 1.2% (104 × 900 x 417/100 000 × 340)* of the weight-adjusted maternal daily dose of spironolactone (1).

DATA ON THE INFANT

No data are available.

* An explanation of the calculation (s) appears on pp. 71–72.

ASSESSMENT AND RECOMMENDATIONS

Limited data suggests that the risk to the suckling infant of administering spironolactone to its mother is low on the basis that the quantity of drug that passes into milk is small. Nevertheless, an alternative potassium-sparing diuretic should be used while the issue of the possible carcinogenicity of this drug remains unresolved.

REFERENCE

1. Phelps DL, Karim A (1977) Spironolactone: relationship between concentrations of dethioacetylated metabolite in human serum and milk. *J. Pharm. Sci., 66*, 1203.

TIMOLOL

GENERAL

Timolol is a non-selective β-adrenoceptor blocking drug. In adults, timolol is absorbed from the gastrointestinal tract and < 10% is bound to plasma proteins. The drug is extensively metabolised and only about 20% is excreted unchanged by the kidney. The plasma half-life is 4–5 h. Unwanted effects of β-blockade that are relevant to the infant include the possibility of delayed recovery from hypoglycaemia, for the maintenance of blood glucose during fasting by sympathetic-mediated hepatic glycogenolysis may be impaired.

EVALUATION OF DATA

Passage of timolol into human milk has been reported as follows:

Treatment conditions Dose × Frequency × Duration; Route; No. of patients; Lactation stage	Concentration (μg/l) Milk	Concentration (μg/l) Plasma	Milk/ plasma ratio	Maximum observed milk conc. (μg/l)	Absolute dose to infant (μg/kg/day) Ave	Absolute dose to infant (μg/kg/day) Max	Ref.
5 mg × 3/d × 1–25 d; p.o.;8; < 4 - > 8 d	16	16	0.80	55	2	8	(1)
10 mg × 3/d × 1–25; p.o.;3; < 4 - > 8 d	41	37	0.83	88	6	13	(1)
0.25 mg × 2/d × LT; eye drops; 9 weeks	0.5 5.6	0.15 0.93	3.33 6.02	–	–	–	(2)

LT, long term. Milk was collected from hypertensive mothers in whom full milk flow was established, either in the mid-morning or mid-afternoon, about 2 h after the dose. The concentration-time profiles were not defined and steady-state dosing was not attained in all patients. The milk and plasma concentrations are arithmetical means, the milk to plasma ratios are geometric means and the maximum milk concentrations are individual values (1). In reference (2), a nursing woman applied timolol maleate 0.5% twice daily to her right eye. The milk sample that contained timolol 0.5 μg/l was obtained 12 h and the sample that contained 5.6 μg/l was obtained 1.5 h after instillation of timolol.

RELATIVE DOSE IN MILK

The amount of timolol that a suckling infant would ingest in a day is on average 1.2% (41 × 900/30 000)* and at maximum 3.3% (55 × 900/15 000)* of the weight-adjusted maternal daily dose (1).

* An explanation of the calculation (s) appears on pp. 71–72.

DATA ON THE INFANT

No effects of timolol were reported in the infants (1,2).

ASSESSMENT AND RECOMMENDATIONS

The risk to the suckling infant of administering timolol to its mother appears to be low on the basis that the quantity of drug that passes into milk is small. Breast-feeding is probably safe but certain inherent pharmacological properties of β-blockers, for example recovery from hypoglycaemia during fasting, give reason for caution and special observation of the suckling infant when timolol is administered to its mother.

REFERENCES

1. Fidler J, Smith V, de Swiet M (1983) Excretion of oxprenolol and timolol in breast milk. *Br. J. Obstet. Gynecol.*, *90*, 961–965.
2. Lustgarten JS, Podos SM (1983) Topical timolol and the nursing mother. *Arch. Ophthalmol.*, *101*, 1381–1382.

VERAPAMIL

GENERAL

Verapamil is a calcium-channel blocking drug which is used for patients with cardiac dysrythmias, angina pectoris and arterial hypertension. In adults the drug is almost completely absorbed from the gastrointestinal tract but its bioavaiability is low due to pre-systemic metabolism in the liver. Its products include norverapamil which has 20% of the pharmacological activity of the parent compound. Verapamil is 90% bound to plasma proteins. The plasma half-life at steady-state is 5 h.

EVALUATION OF DATA

Passage of verapamil into human milk has been reported as follows:

Treatment conditions Dose × Frequency × Duration; Route; No. of patients; Lactation stage	Concentration (mg/l) Milk	 Plasma	Milk/ plasma ratio	Maximum observed milk conc. (mg/l)	Absolute dose to infant (mg/kg/day) Ave	 Max	Ref.
80 mg × 3/d × 5 weeks; p.o.; 1;3–5 d	–	–	0.23	–	–	–	(1)
120 mg × 3/d × 3 d; p.o.;1; 8 weeks	0.11–0.21 (0.05–0.07)	0.16–0.36 (0.12–0.26)	0.54–0.94	0.21 (0.07)	–	0.03 (0.01)	(2)
80 mg × 4/d × 4 d; p.o.1; 2 weeks	–	–	–	0.3	–	0.05	(3)
80 mg × 3/d × 4 weeks; p.o.1; 3 months	0.03 (0.01)	0.04 (0.06)	0.6 (0.16)	0.08 (0.02)	0.005 (0.002)	0.01 (0.003)	(4)

Data from reference (1) indicate that the milk and plasma concentration–time profiles were not concurrent over 65 h. Reference (2) quotes the range of concentrations before and 4 h after dosing. The figures in brackets refer to the metabolite, norverapamil. Reference (3) indicates that the milk and plasma concentration–time profiles of verapamil were similar and reference (4) shows that the profiles of verapamil and norverapamil were concurrent in milk and plasma. Peak drug concentrations occurred about 1 h after dosing. All studies were conducted under steady-state conditions of dosing.

RELATIVE DOSE IN MILK

The amount of verapamil and norverapamil that a suckling infant would ingest in a day is at maximum 0.4–1.1% (0.08 + 0.02 × 900/240 – 0.3 × 900/240)* of the weight-adjusted maternal daily dose (3,4).

* An explanation of the calculation (s) appears on pp. 71–72.

DATA ON THE INFANT

The concentration of verapamil in serum was 2.1 μg/l in the infant reported in reference (1) and was less than 1.0 μg/l in the infant reported in reference (2).

ASSESSMENT OF DATA

The risk to the suckling infant of administering verapamil to its mother is low on the basis that the quantity of drug that passes into milk is small. Breast-feeding may be regarded as safe.

REFERENCES

1. Andersen HJ (1983) Excretion of verapamil in human breast milk. *Eur. J. Clin. Pharmacol.,25*, 279–280.
2. Miller MR, Withers R, Bhamra R, Holt DW (1986) Verapamil and breast-feeding. *Eur. J. Clin. Pharmacol., 30*, 125–126.
3. Inoue H, Unno N, Ou M-C, Iwama Y, Sugimoto T (1984) Level of verapamil in human milk. *Eur. J. Clin. Pharmacol., 26*, 657–658.
4. Andersson P, Bondesson K, Mattiasson I, Johansson BW (1987) Concentrations of verapamil and norverapamil in human milk. *Eur. J. Clin. Pharmacol., 31*, 625–628.

AZATHIOPRINE

GENERAL

Azathioprine is an antimetabolite drug that is used mainly as an immunosuppressant in renal transplantation, rheumatoid arthritis, and lupus erythematosus. It is absorbed from the adult gastrointestinal tract and converted in the liver to 6-mercaptopurine (6-MP) which has similar actions. The plasma half-life of azathioprine is 10 min and of 6-MP is 50 min.

EVALUATION OF DATA

Data on two renal allograft patients are reported; both were studied under steady-state conditions of dosing (1). The first patient breast-fed her infant and, 2 weeks after delivery, milk was collected before and at intervals for 12 h after her daily dose of azathioprine 75 mg by mouth. The milk concentration-time profile defined two peak milk concentrations of 6-MP, 2 h and 8 h after azathioprine, and these were 3.4 and 4.5 μg/l respectively. This patient also received methylprednisolone 6 mg/day. The concentrations of IgA in her breast milk were similar to those obtained in normal controls. The second patient decided not to breast-feed, but agreed to supply breast secretions on the 7th day after delivery, every 2 h between 2 and 12 h after her daily dose of azathioprine 25 mg by mouth. The peak concentration of 6-MP was 18 µg/l and was observed 2 h after azathioprine; the higher concentration in this patient may be explained by the fact that she was not breast-feeding.

RELATIVE DOSE IN MILK

The calculation refers only to the mother who breast-fed her infant. As azathioprine (mol. wt. 277) was administered but 6-MP (mol. wt. 152) was assayed in milk a factor of 1.8 (= 277/152) is included in the calculation. On this basis a suckling infant would ingest in a day at maximum 0.1% ($0.0045 \times 900 \times 1.8/75$)* of the weight-adjusted maternal daily dose of azathioprine (1).

DATA ON THE INFANT

The infant who was breast-fed had a normal haemoglobin concentration and leukocyte and platelet counts and remained in the 75th percentile for height and weight during the first 3 months of life. Grekas et al. (2) reported 2 infants breast-fed by mothers receiving azathioprine 75 and 100 mg/day. Milk concentrations of azathio-

* An explanation of the calculation (s) appears on pp. 71–72.

prine were not measured but their infants had normal blood cell counts, no increase in the incidence of infection and above average growth rates.

ASSESSMENT AND RECOMMENDATIONS

Data on 2 infants suggest that the quantity of azathioprine that passes into milk is small, and short-term observations on 3 infants did not reveal adverse drug effects. In general, however, if bottle feeding is feasible, women should refrain from breast-feeding whilst taking cytotoxic drugs on the grounds that such agents are inherently toxic.

REFERENCES

1. Coulam CB, Moyer TP, Jiang NS, Zincke H (1982) Breast-feeding after renal transplantation. *Transplant Proc., 14,* 605–609.
2. Grekas DM, Vasiliou SS, Lazarides, AN (1984) Immunosuppressive therapy and breast-feeding after renal transplantation. *Nephron, 37*, 68.

CISPLATIN

GENERAL

Cisplatin is a platinum-containing cytotoxic drug which has an alkylating action; it also causes immunosuppression. After intravenous administration, cisplatin disappears from plasma in a biphasic manner with a terminal half-life of 58–73 h. It is extensively bound to plasma proteins. Cisplatin is concentrated in liver, kidneys and large and small intestines. It is excreted mainly in the urine.

EVALUATION OF DATA

Chemotherapy with doxorubicin and cisplatin was undertaken in a patient with an infant aged 7 months. Milk and plasma were sampled at intervals for 71 h after the start of cisplatin infusion (total dose 130 mg in the course of 26 h). Cisplatin was assayed by flameless atomic absorption spectrometry and the limit of detection was 0.1 mg/l. Cisplatin could not be detected in milk when the plasma concentration was at its peak of 3 mg/1, 24 h after the start of the infusion (1). Another patient received cisplatin 36 mg/d for 5 d; on the 3rd day of treatment, 30 min before the drug was infused the platinum content was 0.9 mg/l in milk and 0.8 mg/l in plasma (2).

RELATIVE DOSE IN MILK

As the molecular weight of cisplatin is 300.1 but platinum (molecular weight 195.1) was assayed, a factor of 1.54 (300.1/195.1) is introduced into the calculation. A suckling infant would ingest in a day 34.7% (0.9 × 900 × 1.54/36)* of the weight-adjusted maternal daily dose.

DATA ON THE INFANT

No data are available.

ASSESSMENT OF DATA

Cisplatin passes into breast milk in substantial quantities and is inherently toxic. A mother who is receiving cisplatin should not breast-feed.

* An explanation of the calculation (s) appears on pp. 71–72.

REFERENCES

1. Egan PC, Costanza ME, Dodion P, Egorin MJ, Bachur NR (1985) Doxorubicin and cisplatin excretion into human milk. *Cancer Treat. Rep.*, *69*, 1387–1389.
2. de Vries EGE, van der Zee AGJ, Uges DRA, Sleijfer Dth (1989) *Lancet, i,* 497, 798 (and personal communication).

CYCLOPHOSPHAMIDE

GENERAL

Cyclophosphamide is a nitrogen mustard analogue used for the treatment of cancer and for immunosuppression. Cyclophosphamide is absorbed from the adult gastrointestinal tract and is activated by hepatic metabolism. About 10% of cyclophosphamide and 60% of the active metabolite are bound to plasma proteins. Unchanged drug in urine amounts to 5–25% of a dose. The plasma half-life of cyclophosphamide is 9 h.

EVALUATION OF DATA

Wiernik and Duncan (1) reported the case of a 22-year-old woman with generalised lymphosarcoma who received cyclophosphamide 500 mg and vincristine 0.9 mg by rapid iv injection as single doses. Cyclophosphamide was identified by mass spectrometry in her breast milk 1–6 h after the injection but quantitative data were not given in this account.

RELATIVE DOSE IN MILK

No data are available.

DATA ON THE INFANT

A Nigerian woman experienced a recurrence of Burkitt lymphoma 3 weeks after giving birth. She was given cyclophosphamide 6 mg/kg i.v. daily for 3 days (total 300 mg) and continued breast-feeding. Between the first and third day's treatment, her baby's leucocyte count fell from 4800 to 3200 per mm^3 and the platelet count fell from 270 000 to 47 000 mm^3. These changes were ascribed to toxicity from cyclophosphsmide received in breast milk.

ASSESSMENT OF DATA

Cyclophosphamide passes into breast milk and is inherently toxic. A woman who is receiving cyclophosphamide should not breast-feed.

REFERENCES

1. Wiernick PH, Dunchan JH (1971) Cyclophosphamide in human milk. *Lancet, i*, 912.
2. Durodola JI (1979) Administration of cyclohosphamide during late pregnancy and early lactation: a case report. *J. Natl. Med. Assoc., 71*, 165–166.

CYCLOSPORIN

GENERAL

Cyclosporin is an immunosuppressant agent used for organ and marrow transplants. It is variably (20–50%) absorbed from the adult gastrointestinal tract, 90–95% bound to plasma proteins and extensively metabolised to products that are excreted in bile and faeces. The plasma half-life is 27 h.

EVALUATION OF DATA

Passage of cyclosporin into human milk has been reported as follows:

Treatment conditions Dose × Frequency × Duration; Route; No. of patients; Lactation stage	Concentration (μg/l) Milk	 Plasma	Milk/ plasma ratio	Maximum observed milk conc. (μg/l)	Absolute dose to infant (μg/kg/day) Ave	 Max	Ref.
325 mg/d × 1 d; p.o. 1; 7 d	16	52	0.31	–	–	–	(1)

The mother, who was not breast-feeding, gave single milk and plasma samples 22 h after a dose of cyclosporin.

RELATIVE DOSE IN MILK

Based on the only milk concentration available, the amount of cyclosporin that a suckling infant would ingest in a day is 0.04% (0.016 × 900/325)* of the weight-adjusted maternal daily dose.

DATA ON THE INFANT

No data are available.

ASSESSMENT AND RECOMMENDATIONS

The limited data available suggests that the quantity of cyclosporin that passes into breast milk is small. The inherently toxic of the drug, however, is reason to advise against allowing exposure of the infant to it through breast-feeding.

* An explanation of the calculation (s) appears on pp. 71–72.

REFERENCES

1. Flechner SM, Katz AR, Rogers AJ, Van Buren C, Kaban BD (1985) The presence of cyclosporin in body tissues and fluids during pregnancy. *Am. J. Kidney Dis., 5,* 60–63.

DOXORUBICIN

GENERAL

Doxorubicin is a cytotoxic drug that acts by forming a stable complex with DNA; it also has immunosuppressant properties. After an intravenous dose, doxorubicin is 75% bound to plasma proteins and is metabolised in the liver, the products being excreted mainly in bile and faeces. The metabolite doxorubicinol retains pharmacological activity. The plasma half-life of doxorubicin is 30 h.

EVALUATION OF DATA

Passage of doxorubicin and its metabolite, doxorubicinol into milk is reported as follows:

Treatment conditions	Concentration (μg/l)		Milk/ plasma ratio	Maximum observed milk conc. (μg/l)	Absolute dose to infant (μg/kg/day)		Ref.
Dose × Frequency × Duration; Route; No. of patients; Lactation stage	Milk	Plasma			Ave	Max	
90 mg × 1/d × 1 d; i.v. infusion, 15 min; 1; 7 months	–	821 (82)	1.2 (9.7)	131 (109)	–	20 (16)	(1)

The figures in parentheses refer to doxorubicinol. The areas under the plasma and milk concentration-time curves were defined but only peak concentrations are quoted in the report; these were achieved 24 h after dosing for both doxorubicin and doxorubicinol. Doxorubicin was detectable in milk for 72 h. The patient also received cisplatin.

RELATIVE DOSE IN MILK

The amount of doxorubicin and doxorubicinol that a suckling infant would ingest in a feed is at maximum 0.5% (0.131 + 0.109 × 180/90)* of the weight-adjusted maternal single dose and in a day is at maximum 2.4% (0.131 + 0.109 × 900/90)* of the weight-adjusted maternal daily dose(1).

DATA ON THE INFANT

No data are available.

* An explanation of the calculation (s) appears on pp. 71–72.

ASSESSMENT OF DATA

Doxorubicin and doxorubicinol pass into breast milk in small quantities. Nevertheless, these substances are inherent toxic and a mother who is receiving doxorubicin should not breast-feed.

REFERENCES

1. Egan PC, Costanza ME, Dodion P, Egorin MJ, Bachur NR (1985) Doxorubicin and cisplatin excretion into human milk. *Cancer Treat. Rep.*, *69*, 1387–1389.

HYDROXYUREA

GENERAL

Hydroxyurea is a cytotoxic agent used for myeloid leukaemia and solid tumours. It is well absorbed from the adult gastrointestinal tract, is widely distributed through body tissues, and is excreted largely unchanged in the urine. The plasma half-life is 4 h.

EVALUATION OF DATA

Passage of methotrexate into human milk has been reported as follows:

Treatment conditions	Concentration (mg/l)		Milk/ plasma ratio	Maximum observed milk conc. (mg/l)	Absolute dose to infant (mg/kg/day)		Ref.
Dose × Frequency × Duration; Route; No. of patients; Lactation stage	Milk	Plasma			Ave	Max	
500 mg× 3/d × 7 d; p.o.; 1; ?	6.1 (3.8–8.4)	–	–	8.4	0.92	1.26	(1)

Milk samples were collected 2 h after taking the last daily dose of hydroxyurea. The table gives the mean, and the range (in parentheses) of values on days 1, 3 and 4.

RELATIVE DOSE IN MILK

A suckling infant would ingest in a day at maximum 5.0% (8.4 × 900/1500)* of the weight-adjusted maternal daily dose (1).

DATA ON THE INFANT

The infant was weaned before hydroxyurea was commenced and no data are available.

ASSESSMENT OF DATA

Limited data indicate that when hydroxyurea is administered to a nursing mother the quantity of drug ingested by her suckling infant is small. Nevertheless hydroxyurea is inherently toxic and a woman who is receiving it should not breastfeed.

* An explanation of the calculation (s) appears on pp. 71–72.

REFERENCES

1. Sylvester RK, Lobell M, Teresi ME, Brundage D, Dubowy R (1987) Excretion of hydroxyurea into milk. *Cancer, 60*, 2177–2178.

METHOTREXATE

GENERAL

Methotrexate is a folic acid antagonist that is used as a cytotoxic and as an immunosuppressant agent. Bioavailability from the adult gastrointestinal tract is 65% and 50% is bound to plasma proteins. Most of a dose is excreted unchanged in the urine within 24 h. The plasma half-life is 7 h.

EVALUATION OF DATA

Passage of methotrexate into human milk has been reported as follows:

Treatment conditions	Concentration (μg/l)		Milk/ plasma ratio	Maximum observed milk conc. (μg/l)	Absolute dose to infant (μg/kg/day)		Ref.
Dose × Frequency × Duration; Route; No. of patients; Lactation stage	Milk	Plasma			Ave	Max	
22.5 mg × 1/d × 1 d; p.o.; 1; 1 month	2.56	81.8	0.02–0.08	2.73	0.38	0.41	(1)

The concentration-time profiles was defined for 12 h after the first dose and were not concurrent, the peak concentration being reached in milk at 10 h and in plasma at 6 h. The milk to plasma ratio is the range of 6 paired samples. The same dose repeated on the 2nd and 3rd days gave peak milk concentrations of 0.003 ug/l on each occasion. The cumulative excretion of methotrexate in the first 12 h after administration was 0.32 ug in milk and 4.3 mg in urine.

RELATIVE DOSE IN MILK

A suckling infant would ingest in a feed at maximum 0.02% (0.002 × 180/22.5)* of the weight-adjusted maternal single dose (1). The paediatric dose of methotrexate is 0.12 mg/kg and a suckling infant would ingest in a feed at maximum 0.05% (0.002 x 3/0.12)* or in a day 0.3% (0.002 × 15/0.12)* of this (1).

DATA ON THE INFANT

No data are avaialble.

ASSESSMENT OF DATA

Limited data indicate that when methotrexate is administered to a nursing mother

* An explanation of the calculation (s) appears on pp. 71–72.

the quantity of drug ingested by her suckling infant is small. Nevertheless methotrexate is inherently toxic and a woman who is receiving it should not breast-feed.

REFERENCES

1. Johns DG, Rutherford LD, Leighton PC, Vagel CL (1982) Secretion of methotrexate into human milk. *Am. J. Obstet. Gynaec.*, *112*, 978–980.

CARBETOCIN

GENERAL

Carbetocin is a synthetic analogue of oxytocin. Like oxytocin, carbetocin is administered by i.v. or i.m. injection but it acts for longer to prevent uterine atony and postpartum haemorrhage.

EVALUATION OF DATA

Passage of carbetocin into human milk has been reported as follows:

Treatment conditions Dose × Frequency × Duration; Route; No. of patients; Lactation stage	Concentration (ng/l)		Milk/ plasma ratio	Maximum observed milk conc. (ng/l)	Absolute dose to infant (ng/kg/day)		Ref.
	Milk	Plasma			Ave	Max	
70 μg/d × 1 d; i.m.; 5; 7–14 weeks	0.018	1.035	3.08	0.018	–	–	(1)

All the mothers had had normal vaginal deliveries. The table quotes the maximum milk and plasma concentrations which were attained within 3 h of drug administration.

RELATIVE DOSE IN MILK

A suckling infant would ingest in a feed at maximum 0.00005% (0.018 × 180/70 000)* of the weight-adjusted maternal single dose of carbetocin.

DATA ON THE INFANT

No data are available.

ASSESSMENT AND RECOMMENDATIONS

The risk to the suckling infant of administering carbetocin to its mother is negligible on the basis that the quantity of drug that passes into milk very small. Breastfeeding may be regarded as safe.

REFERENCES

1. Silcox J, Schulz P, Horbay GLA, Wassenaar W (1993) Transfer of carbetocin into human breast milk. *Obstet. Gynecol., 83,* 456–459.

* An explanation of the calculation (s) appears on pp. 71–72.

CARBIMAZOLE

GENERAL

Carbimazole inhibits the formation of thyroid hormones and is used to treat hyperthyroidism. It is absorbed from the adult gastrointestinal tract and is rapidly and completely transformed to methimazole, which is pharmacologically active. Methimazole is 40% bound to plasma proteins and its plasma half-life is 4 h.

EVALUATION OF DATA

Passage of methimazole into human milk after administration of carbimazole or methimazole has been reported as follows:

Treatment conditions: Dose × Frequency × Duration; Route; No. of patients; Lactation stage	Concentration (μg/l) Milk	Concentration (μg/l) Plasma	Milk/plasma ratio	Maximum observed milk conc. (μg/l)	Absolute dose to infant (μg/kg/day) Ave	Absolute dose to infant (μg/kg/day) Max	Ref.
2.5 mg[a] × 2/d × LT; p.o.; 1; ?	–	–	1.16	65	–	9.8	(1)
40 mg[b] × 1/d × 1 d; p.o.; 5; 2–6 weeks	182 (1 h) 83 (8 h)	253 (1 h) 89 (8 h)	0.98	182	–	27.3	(2)
40 mg[b] × 1/d × 1 d; p.o.; 4; 3–6 months	–	710	0.99	720	–	108	(3)
30 mg[b] × 1/d × 8–24 weeks; p.o.; 1; 8–24 weeks	43 (0–92)	–	–	92	–	–	(4)

[a]Methimazole; [b]carbomazole; LT, long term. In references (1–3) methimazole was measured in mothers' milk and plasma 8–10 h after dosing. The concentration-time profiles in milk and serum were were similar. The table gives average values at the times stated (2) and average peak concentrations (3). The mean total milk volume collected during 8 h was 225 ml and the mean methimazole content was 70 μg or 0.175% of the maternal dose (3). Reference (4) reports the mean and range of methimazole concentrations in milk in a patient who became hyperthyroid 2 months after giving birth to healthy twins; the dose of carbimazole was reduced as she became euthyroid. A milk to serum ratio of 1.05 was recorded after administration of ^{35}S-labelled carbimazole (5).

RELATIVE DOSE IN MILK

When carbimazole (mol. wt. 186) was administered but methimazole (mol. wt. 114) was assayed in milk a factor of 1.6 (=186/114) was introduced into the calculation. The amount of carbimazole that a suckling infant would ingest in a feed is at maximum 3.2% (0.72 × 180 ×/40)* of the weight-adjusted maternal single dose

* An explanation of the calculation (s) appears on pp. 71–72.

(3). A suckling infant would ingest in a day on average 2.1% (0.043 × 900 × 1.6/30)* (4) and at maximum 11.7% (0.065 × 900/5)* (1) of the weight-adjusted maternal daily dose. In the 24 h after administration of ^{35}S-labelled carbimazole, 0.47% of the dose was recovered in 320 ml of milk.

DATA ON THE INFANT

Plasma carbimazole was 45 μ/l and 53 μ/l in the twin infants of the mother reported in reference (4). These values are at the lower end of the range reported to cause thyroid suppression in adults with thyrotoxicosis (50–100 μ/l) (6) and the infants' thyroid stimulating hormone, thyroxine and triiodothyronine concentrations were normal throughout 1–16 weeks.

ASSESSMENT AND RECOMMENDATIONS

When carbimazole is administered to a lactating mother the estimated quantity of methimazole ingested by her infant in milk is small. Limited data suggest that the concentrations of methimazole attained in the infant do not suppress thyroid function provided the maternal dose of carbimazole does not exceed 30 mg/day. Nevertheless further data are required to establish whether carbimazole may safely be given to nursing mothers. Currently propylthiouracil (see p. 310) is preferred.

REFERENCES

1. Tegler L, Lindstrom B (1980) Antithyroid drugs in milk. *Lancet, ii*, 591.
2. Johansen K, Anderson AN, Kampmann JP, Hansen JM, Mortensen HB (1982) Excretion of methimazole in human milk. *Eur. J. Clin. Pharmacol., 23*, 339–341.
3. Cooper DS, Bode HH, Nath B, Saxe V, Maloof F, Ridgway EC (1984) Methimazole pharmacology in man: studies using a newly developed radioimmunoassay for methimazole. *J. Clin. Endocrinol. Metab., 58*, 473–479.
4. Rylance RY, Woods CG, Donnelly MC, Oliver JS (1987) Carbimazole and breast-feeding. *Lancet, i*, 928.
5. Low LCK, Lang J, Alexander WD (1979) Excretion of carbimazole and propylthiouracil in breast milk. *Lancet, ii*, 1011.
6. Low LKC, McCruden DC, Alexander WD, Hilditch TE, Skellern GG, Knight BI (1981) Intrathyroid binding rates and plasma methimazole concentrations in hyperthyroid patients on small doses of carbimazole. *Br. J. Clin. Pharmacol., 12*, 315–318.

CYPROTERONE ACETATE

GENERAL

Cyproterone acetate is a synthetic steroid that possesses both anti-androgenic and progestogenic properties. In females it may be used to treatment hyperandrogenic conditions, e.g. hirsutism, androgenic alopecia and, combined with ethinyl oestradiol, as an anti-acne preparation. It is well absorbed from the adult gastrointestinal tract and binds to albumin in plasma. Cyproterone acetate is metabolised and the products appear in bile and urine. The plasma half-life is 2 d.

EVALUATION OF DATA

Passage of cyproterone acetate into human milk has been reported as follows:

Treatment conditions	Concentration (μg/l)		Milk/plasma ratio	Maximum observed milk conc. (μg/l)	Absolute dose to infant (μg/kg/day)		Ref.
Dose × Frequency × Duration; Route; No. of patients; Lactation stage	Milk	Plasma			Ave	Max	
50 mg × 1/d × 1 d; p.o.; 6; ?	98	248	0.39	260	14.7	39	(1)

The milk and plasma concentrations quoted are average values 3 h after the dose. The maximum milk concentration is the highest single value noted in the six women studied.

RELATIVE DOSE IN MILK

The amount of cyproterone acetate that a suckling infant would ingest in a feed is at maximum 0.9% (0.26 × 180/50)* of the weight-adjusted maternal single dose.

DATA ON THE INFANT

No data are recorded.

ASSESSMENT AND RECOMMENDATIONS

Although the absolute and relative amounts of cyproterone acetate that pass into breast milk are small, its inherent pharmacological properties are such that there

* An explanation of the calculation (s) appears on pp. 71–72.

may be a risk of anti-androgenic effects in a suckling infant. Breast-feeding should be regarded as unsafe.

REFERENCES

1. Stoppeli I, Rainer E, Humpel M (1980) Transfer of cyproterone acetate to the milk of lactating women. *Contraception, 22*, 485–493.

ESTRADIOL

GENERAL

Estradiol (oestradiol) is a naturally-occurring oestrogen that is secreted by the ovary. It may be used for oestrogen replacement therapy, e.g. postmenopausal or after ovariectomy. Estradiol is available as oral and transdermal preparations. It is 98% bound to plasma proteins and is extensively metabolised. The plasma half-life is 1 h.

EVALUATION OF DATA

Passage of estradiol into human milk has been reported as follows:

Treatment conditions Dose × Frequency × Duration; Route; No. of patients; Lactation stage	Concentration (mg/l) Milk	 Plasma	Milk/ plasma ratio	Maxi- mum observed milk conc. (mg/l)	Absolute dose to infant (mg/kg/day) Ave	 Max	Ref.
50 mg × 1/d × 1 d;	0.4 (3 h)	1.8	0.2	1.0	0.06	0.15	(1)
vaginal; 3; ?	0.1 (11 h)	0.7	0.14	–	–	–	
100 mg × 1/d × 1 d;	0.18 (3 h)	2.5	0.07	0.3	0.018	0.04	(1)
vaginal; 3; ?	0.075 (23 h)	0.25	0.3	–	–	5	

Estradiol was given as a single pessary dose of 50 mg and 100 mg to 3 women. Samples of milk and plasma were obtained 3, 7, 11 and 23 h after the dose. The milk and plasma concentrations quoted are the averages for the 3 women and are taken from a figure in the report (1). The maximum milk concentrations quoted are the average maximum figures and were seen at 3 h (in 2 women) or at 7 h (1 woman) after dosing.

RELATIVE DOSE IN MILK

The amount of estradiol that a suckling infant would ingest in a feed is at maximum 0.004% (0.001 × 180/50)* of the weight-adjusted maternal single dose (1).

DATA ON THE INFANT

No data are recorded.

ASSESSMENT AND RECOMMENDATIONS

The risk to the suckling infant of administering estradiol to its mother is negligible

* An explanation of the calculation (s) appears on pp. 71–72.

on the basis that the quantity of drug that passes into milk is small. Breast-feeding may be considered safe.

REFERENCES

1. Nilsson S, Nygren KG, Johansson ED (1978) Transfer of oestradiol to human milk. *Am. J. Obstet. Gynaec., 13*, 653–657.

ETHINYLESTRADIOL

GENERAL

Ethinylestradiol (ethinyloestradiol) is a potent synthetic oestrogen that is widely used in combined oral contraceptive steroid preparations. Breast-feeding mothers may be taking ethinylestradiol as it is common practice is to start the drug 4–6 weeks post partum. It is absorbed from the adult gastriontestinal tract but only 40–60% is systemically availabile because of extensive gut wall metabolism. Ethinylestradiol is >95% bound to plasma proteins. It is primarily metabolised by direct conjugation with sulphate or glucuronide, or by ring hydroxylation followed by conjugation. The metabolites are inactive. Ethinylestradiol undergoes an entero-hepatic circulation. The plasma half-life is 5–16 h.

EVALUATION OF DATA

Passage of ethinylestradiol into human milk has been reported as follows:

Treatment conditions Dose × Frequency × Duration; Route; No. of patients; Lactation stage	Concentration (ng/l) Milk	 Plasma	Milk/ plasma ratio	Maximum observed milk conc. (ng/l)	Absolute dose to infant (ng/kg/day) Ave	 Max	Ref.
500 μg × 1/d × 1 d; p.o.; 4; ?	175	700	0.25	300	26	45	(1)
50 μg × 1/d × 1d; p.o.; 4; ?	<50	60	–	–	–	–	(1)

The concentration-time profiles were defined in milk (7–11 h) and plasma (23 h) and the table gives mean values. The maximum observed milk concentration is the average maximum figure for the four women studied. Ethinylestradiol was not detected in human milk after 50 ug by mouth, i.e. the order of dose used in oral contraceptive. One of the conjugated metabolites, ethinylestradiol sulphate, is usually present in human plasma at up to 20 times the concentration of ethinylestradiol itself. Very little ethinylestradiol sulphate is excreted in breast milk (2).

RELATIVE DOSE IN MILK

Ethinylestradiol is not detectable in human milk at standard therapeutic doses. A suckling infant would ingest in a feed at maximum 0.1% (0.3 × 180/500)* of the weight-adjusted large single maternal dose (1).

* An explanation of the calculation (s) appears on pp. 71–72.

DATA ON THE INFANT

Forty-eight breast-fed children of mothers who took oral contraceptives containing ethinyloestradiol 50 μg whilst lactating were compared with a matched control group: there were no differences between the groups in intellectual or psychological behaviour or in health records (3).

ASSESSMENT AND RECOMMENDATIONS

The risk to the suckling infant of administering a normal contraceptive dose of ethinylestradiol to its mother is low on the basis that the quantity of drug that enters milk is small. (See also 'Steroid contraception during lactation', p. 36.) Breastfeeding may be regarded as safe provided a low dose preparation is used.

REFERENCES

1. Nilsson S, Nygren KG, Johansson ED (1977) Ethinyloestradiol in human milk and plasma after oral administration. *Contraception, 17*, 131–139.
2. Klinger Von G, Claussen C, Schroeder S. (1977) Exkretion von Äthinyloestradiol sulphonat in der Frauenmilch. (1981) *Zentralbl. Gynakol., 103*, 91–95.
3. Nilsson S, Mellbin T, Hovander Y, Sundelin C, Valentin J, Nygren KG. (1986) Long-term follow-up of children breast-fed by mothers using oral contraceptives. *Contraception, 34*, 443–457.

ETYNODIOL

GENERAL

Ethynodiol (ethynidiol) diacetate is a progestogen that is mainly used as an oral contraceptive steroid combined with ethinyloestradiol. It is totally metabolised to norethisterone (see p. 305).

EVALUATION OF DATA

Passage of norethisterone into human milk after administeration of etynodiol diacetate has been reported as follows:

Treatment conditions	Concentration (μg/l)		Milk/ plasma ratio	Maximum observed milk conc. (μg/l)	Absolute dose to infant (μg/kg/day)		Ref.
Dose × Frequency × Duration; Route; No. of patients; Lactation stage	Milk	Plasma			Ave	Max	
500 μg × 1/d × LT; p.o.; 12; ?	0.13	0.87	0.15	0.57	0.020	0.086	(1)

LT, long term. Milk concentrations were measured at 4 h intervals over 2 days. The milk and plasma concentrations shown are average figures. The maximum milk concentration is the mean of the individual maximum concentrations over the first 12 h of the study.

RELATIVE DOSE IN MILK

As etynodiol diacetate (mol.wt. 385) was administered but norethisterone (mol. wt. 298) was assayed a factor of 1.3 (= 385/298) was introduced into the calculation. On this basis the amount of etiynodiol diacetate that a suckling infant would ingest in a day is on average 0.3% (0.13 × 900 × 1.3/500)* and at maximum 1.3% (57 × 900 × 1.3/500)* of the weight-adjusted maternal daily dose (1).

DATA ON THE INFANT

No effects on the infant were reported in the study quoted. Norethisterone was measurable in the infants' plasma, the highest concentration being 0.5 μg/l with a median figure of 0.1 μg/l. In no case this was ever more that 25% of the maternal concentration.

* An explanation of the calculation (s) appears on pp. 71–72.

ASSESSMENT AND RECOMMENDATIONS

The risk to the suckling infant of administering ethinodiol diacetate to its mother is low on the basis that the quantity of drug and of its main metabolite, norethisterone, that enters milk is small. Breast-feeding may be regarded as safe. (See also 'Steroid contraception during lactation', p. 36.)

REFERENCES

1. Cooke ID, Back DJ, Shroff NE (1985) Norethisterone concentrations in breast milk, and in infant and maternal plasma during ethynodiol diacetate administration. *Contraception, 31*, 611–621.

LEVONORGESTREL

GENERAL

Levonorgestrel is a potent progestogenic drug that is widely used in combined oral contraceptive steroids, and as a contraceptive on its own (the 'mini pill'). It was formerly known as d-norgestrel. Levonorgestrel is commonly started 4–6 weeks after delivery and thus may be taken by breast-feeding mothers. It is 97% bound in plasma to albumin and more specifically to sex hormone binding globulin. Levonorgestrel is primarily metabolised by ring reduction followed by hydroxylation or conjugation. These metabolites are believed not have pharmacological activity. The drug is excreted as conjugated metabolites in bile, faeces and urine. The half-life of the terminal exponential phase of elimination from plasma in adults is 4–16 h.

EVALUATION OF DATA

Passage of levonorgestrel into human milk has been reported as follows:

Treatment conditions Dose × Frequency × Duration; Route; No. of patients; Lactation stage	Concentration (ng/l) Milk	Plasma	Milk/ plasma ratio	Maximum observed milk conc. (ng/l)	Absolute dose to infant (mg/kg/day) Ave	Max	Ref.
150 μg × 1/d × LT; p.o.; 2; ?	180	3060	0.06	223	27	33	(1)
150 μg × 1/d × LT; p.o.; 4; ?	360	3500	0.10	400	56	60	(2)
50 μg × 1/d ×LT; p.o.; 4?	100	800	0.12	130	15	19	(2)
25 000 μg × 1/d × 1 d; i.m.; 4; ?	120	700	0.17	200	18	30	(2)
250 μg × 1/d × LT; p.o.; 5; ?	360	2600	0.14	2500	54	375	(3)
150 μg × 1/d × LT; p.o.; 5; ?	160	1200	0.13	1100	24	165	(3)
30 μg × 1/d × LT; p.o.; 5; ?	<30	270	–	–	–	–	(3)
30 μg × 1/d × LT; p.o.; 3;?	85	–	–	135	13	20	(4)
10 μg × 1/d × LT; IUD; 5; ?	56	207	0.27	144	8	22	(5)
30 μg × 1/d × LT; IUD; 5; ?	57	235	0.24	166	9	25	(5)
204 μg × 1/d × LT; implant;31; mature milk	120	690	0.17	311	18	47	(6)

LT, long term; IUD, intrauterine device. The milk and plasma concentrations of levonorgestrel are mean values from various studies. The maximum milk concentrations are the highest values reported in individuals in each study. The intrauterine devices (5,6) were designed to release levonorgestrel 10–30 μg/day.

RELATIVE DOSE IN MILK

The amount of levonorgestrel that a suckling infant would ingest in a day is on average 1.3% (0.36 × 900/250)* (2,3) to 2.6% (0.085 × 900/30)* (4) and at maximum 9% (2.5 × 900/250)* (3) of the weight-adjusted maternal daily dose. Note that the units quoted in the table are in ng/l and the calculations are in μg/l.

DATA ON THE INFANT

No effects have been recorded on neonates but Nilsson at al (3) found plasma concentrations of levonorgestrel in two infants to be less than 125 pg/ml when they breast-fed from mothers taking levonorgestrel 250 μg/day. This compares to average plasma concentrations of 2600 pg/ml in the mothers. In a 12 month study of infants who were breast-fed by mothers who had received a levonorgestrel 240 mg implant, there were no effects on infant growth or development (6). One case of breast enlargement is described in an 18 month old girl who was breast-fed and whose mother was taking combined contraceptive steroids including levonorgestrel. Breast enlargement subsided over 6 months once breast-feeding ceased (7). The case is an isolated one and the relationship to the contraceptive steroids is not established.

ASSESSMENT AND RECOMMENDATIONS

The risk to the suckling infant of administering levonorgestrel to its mother is low on the basis that the quantity of drug that passes into milk is small. Breast-feeding should be regarded as safe. (See also 'Steroid contraception during lactation', p. 36.)

REFERENCES

1. Saxena BM, Shrimanker K, Grudzinskas JG (1977) Levels of contraceptive steroids in breast milk and plasma of lactating womem. *Contraception, 16*, 605–613.
2. Toddywalla VS, Metha S, Virkar KD, Saxena BN (1980) Release of 19-nortestosterone type of contraceptive steroids through different drug delivery systems into serum and breast milk of lactating women. *Contraception, 21,* 217–222.
3. Nilsson S, Nygren KE, Johansson EDB (1977) D-Norgestrel concentrations in maternal plasma, milk and in child plasma during administration of oral contraceptives to nursing women. *Am. J. Obstet. Gynecol., 129*, 178–183.
4. Thomas MJ, Danutra V, Read GF, Hillier SG, Griffiths K. (1977) The detection and measurement of D-Norgestrel in human milk using Sephadex LH20 chromatography and radioimmunassay. *Steroids,* 30, 349–361.

* An explanation of the calculation (s) appears on pp. 71–72.

5. Heikkila M, Haukkamaa M, Luukkainen T (1982) Levonorgestrel in milk and plasma of breast-feeding women with a levonorgestrel releasing I.U.D. *Contraception, 25*, 41–49.
6. Diaz S, Herreros C, Juez G, Casado ME, Salvatierra AM, Miranda P, Peralta O, Croxatto HB (1985) Fertility regulation in nursing women. VII Influence of Norplant levonorgestrel implants upon lactation and infant growth. *Contraception, 32*, 53–74.
7. Madhavapeddi R, Ramachandran P (1985) Side effects of oral contraceptive use in lactating women - enlargement of breast in a breast-fed child. *Contraception, 32*, 437–443.

LYNESTRENOL

GENERAL

Lynestrenol is a potent progestogenic drug that is used in a few combined oral contraceptive steroid preparations. It is almost entirely converted to norethisterone in the body (see page 000).

EVALUATION OF DATA

Lynestrenol has not been widely studied but Van der Molen et al (1) examined the excretion of radioactivity in breast milk after [14^C] lynestrenol 5 mg by mouth. The total activity (not unchanged drug) in milk over a 5 day period was between 0.022% and 0.88% of the maternal dose. This is equivalent to 7.5 μg to a 5 kg child.

RELATIVE DOSE IN MILK

See above.

DATA IN THE INFANT

No data are reported.

ASSESSMENT AND RECOMMENDATIONS

Lynestrenol is metabolised to norethisterone which passes into milk in very small quantities (p. 305) and the quoted data with radiolabelled lynestrenol are compatible with this finding. The risk to the suckling infant of administering lynestrenol the mother would appear to be negligible. Breast-feeding may be regarded as safe. (See also 'Steroid contraception during lactation', p. 36.)

REFERENCES

1. Van der Molen HJ, Hart PG, Wijmenga HG (1969) Studies with 4–14^C lynestrenol in normal and lactating women. *Acta Endocrinol., 61,* 255–274.

MEDOXYPROGESTERONE

GENERAL

Medoxyprogesterone acetate is a synthetic progestogen that is widely used as a contraceptive agent in its own right. It is uaually given as a single depot injection about every three months (Depot Provera). The steroid is released steadily over the succeeding 12 weeks from the depot. Medoxyprogesterone acetate is lipid soluble and penetrates tissues. It is extensively metabolised by conjugation, and the inactive metabolites are excreted in the bile and the urine. The plasma half-life after oral dosing is about 30 h.

EVALUATION OF DATA

Passage of medoxyprogesterone acetate into human milk has been reported as follows:

Treatment conditions Dose × Frequency × Duration; Route; No. of patients; Lactation stage	Concentration (μg/l) Milk	 Plasma	Milk/ plasma ratio	Maximum observed milk conc. (μg/l)	Absolute dose to infant (μg/kg/day) Ave	 Max	Ref.
150 mg × 1/d × 1 d; i.m.; 7;?	1.03	1.36	0.76	2.29	0.16	0.34	(1)
150 mg × 1/d × 1 d; i.m.; 7;?	0.97	1.29	0.75	50.3	0.15	7.5	(2)
150 mg × 1/d × 1 d; i.m.; 6; ?	3.8	6.2	0.61	16.5	0.57	2.5	(3)

Medoxyprogesterone acetate is measured in biological samples as the free base. The milk and plasma concentrations quoted are average figures. The maximum observed milk concentrations are the highest individual values for references (1) and (3) and the mean peak concentration for reference (2).

RELATIVE DOSE IN MILK

The amount of medoxyprogesterone that a suckling infant would receive in a feed is at maximum 0.06% (0.0503 ×180/150)* of the weight-adjusted maternal single dose (2).

DATA ON THE INFANT

No data are recorded.

* An explanation of the calculation (s) appears on pp. 71–72.

ASSESSMENT AND RECOMMENDATIONS

The risk to the suckling infant of administering standard therapeutic doses of medoxyprogesterone acetate to its mother is negligible on the basis that the quantity of drug that enters milk is small. Breast-feeding may be regarded as safe. (See also 'Steroid contraception during lactation', p. 36.)

REFERENCES

1. Saxena NB, Shrimanker K, Grudzinskasn JG (1977) Level of contraceptive steroids in breast milk and plasma of lactating women. *Contraception, 16*, 605–613.
2. Koetswang S, Nukulkarn P, Fotherby K, Shrimanker K, Mangalam M, Towobola K (1982) Transfer of contraceptive steroids in milk of women using long-acting gestagens. *Contraception, 25*, 321–331.
3. Koetswang S (1977) Injected long-acting medoxyprogesterone acetate: effect on human lactation and concentrations in milk. *J. Med. Ass. Thailand, 60*, 57–60.
4. Jimenez J, Ochoa M, Soler MP, Portales P (1984) Long-term follow-up of children breast-fed by mothers receiving depot-medroxyprogesterone acetate. *Contraception, 30*, 523–533.

MEGESTROL

GENERAL

Megestrol acetate is a synthetic progesterone that is used on its own and in some combination contraceptive steroid preparations. It is absorbed from the adult gastrointestinal tract and is extensively bound in plasma to albumin and to sex hormone binding globulin. It is metabolised mainly by ring reduction followed by conjugation. The metabolites are thought to have no pharmacological activity. The plasma half-life is 15–20 h.

EVALUATION OF DATA

Passage of megestrol acetate into human milk has been reported as follows:

Treatment conditions: Dose × Frequency × Duration; Route; No. of patients; Lactation stage	Concentration (μg/l)		Milk/ plasma ratio	Maximum observed milk conc. (μg/l)	Absolute dose to infant (μg/kg/day)		Ref.
	Milk	Plasma			Ave	Max	
4 mg × 1/d × LT; p.o.; 5; ?	2.95	4.2	0.7	7.5	0.44	1.12	(1)

LT, long term. The concentrations in milk and plasma are average concentrations over 24 h. The maximum milk concentration is an average of the individual maximum concentrations reported. The study was conducted under steady-state conditions of dosing.

RELATIVE DOSE IN MILK

The amount of megestrol acetate that a suckling infant would ingest in a day is on average 0.7% (0.00295 × 900/4)* and at maximum 1.7% (0.0075 × 900/4)* of weight-adjusted maternal daily dose (1).

DATA ON THE INFANT

No data are recorded.

ASSESSMENT AND RECOMMENDATIONS

The risk to the suckling infant of administering megestrol acetate to its mother is

* An explanation of the calculation (s) appears on pp. 71–72.

low on the basis that the quantity of drug that enters milk is small. Breast-feeding may be regarded as safe. (See also 'Steroid contraception during lactation', p. 36.)

REFERENCES

1. Nilsson S, Nygren KG, Johansson EDB (1977) Megestrol acetate concentrations in plasma and milk during administration of an oral contraceptive containing 4 mg megestrol acetate to nursing women. *Contraception, 16*, 615–622.

METHYLERGOMETRINE

GENERAL

Methylergometrine is a derivative of the ergot alkaloid ergometrine. It has little vasoconstrictor activity but causes uterine contraction and its main use is immediately after delivery to prevent post partum haemorrhage. Methylergometrine is absorbed fom the adult gastrointestinal tract, is 35% bound to plasma proteins and is extensively metabolised. The plasma half-life is 0.5–2 h.

EVALUATION OF DATA

Passage of methylergometrine into human milk has been reported as follows:

Treatment conditions Dose × Frequency × Duration; Route; No. of patients; Lactation stage	Concentration (μg/l) Milk	 Plasma	Milk/ plasma ratio	Maximum observed milk conc. (μg/l)	Absolute dose to infant (μg/kg/day) Ave	 Max	Ref.
125 μg × 3/d × 5 d; p.o.; 8; 5 d	0.64	2.4	0.27	1.096	0.096	0.164	(1)

Methylergometrine was measured in milk and plasma, 1 and 8 h after drug administration on the last day of therapy. In four of the women, no methylergometrine was detected in the milk. The milk and plasma concentrations are the averages for 4 women 1 h after drug administration. The maximum milk concentration is the highest individual value reported.

RELATIVE DOSE IN MILK

The amount of methylergometrine that a suckling infant would ingest in a day is on average 1.5% (0.64 × 900/375)* and at maximum 3.1% (1.3 × 900/375)* of the weight adjusted maternal daily dose (1).

DATA ON THE INFANT

No data are recorded.

ASSESSMENT AND RECOMMENDATIONS

The risk to the suckling infant of administering methylergometrine to its mother is

* An explanation of the calculation (s) appears on pp. 71–72.

low on the basis that quantity that passes into milk the small. Breast-feeding may be regarded as safe.

REFERENCES

1. Erkkola R, Kanto J, Allonen H, Kleimola T, Mantyla R (1978) Excretion of methylergometrine (methylergonovine) into the human breast milk. *Int. J. Clin. Pharmacol., 16,* 579–580.

METHYLPREDNISOLONE

GENERAL

Methylprednisolone is a synthetic glucocorticoid that is used as an immunosuppressant, e.g. in patients receiving organ transplants or with immune disorders. It is well absorbed from the adult gastrointestinal tract and is extensively metabolised, less than 5% of the drug being excreted unchanged in the urine. The plasma half-life is 3 h.

EVALUATION OF DATA

Passage of methylprednisolone in human milk has been reported as follows:

Treatment conditions	Concentration (μg/l)		Milk/ plasma ratio	Maximum observed milk conc. (μg/l)	Absolute dose to infant (μg/kg/day)		Ref.
Dose × Frequency × Duration; Route; No. of patients; Lactation stage	Milk	Plasma			Ave	Max	
6 mg × 1/d × LT; p.o.; 1; 2–16 d	3	–	–	7.5	–	1.13	(1)

LT, long term. The mother received methylprednisolone following renal transplantation. The milk concentration is an average value during a dose interval and this and the maximum concentration are estimated from a graph (1). The milk concentration-time profile was defined during steady-state conditions of dosing.

RELATIVE DOSE IN MILK

The amount of methylprednisolone that a suckling infant would ingest in a day is on average 0.5% (3 × 900/6000)* and at maximum 1.1% (75 × 900/6000)* of the weight-adjusted maternal daily dose (1).

DATA ON THE INFANT

No data are available.

ASSESSMENT AND RECOMMENDATIONS

Data from one patient suggest that the risk to the suckling infant of administering methylprednisolone to its mother is low on the basis that the quantity of drug that

* An explanation of the calculation (s) appears on pp. 71–72.

passes into milk is small. Information on more subjects is required before a generally applicable recommendation can be made.

REFERENCES

1. Coulam CB, Moyer TP, Jiang NS, Zincke H (1982) Breast-feeding after renal transplantation. *Transplant. Proc., 14*, 605–609.

NORETHISTERONE

GENERAL

Norethisterone is a potent progestogenic drug that is widely used in combined oral contraceptive preparations, and as a contraceptive on its own (the 'mini-pill'). A common practice is to start the drug 4–6 weeks post partum and hence breast-feeding mothers are quite likely to be taking it. The drug is is extensively bound in plasma to albumin and more specificially to sex hormone binding globulin. Norethisterone is primarily metabolised by ring reduction followed by hydroxylation or conjugation. None of the metabolites is thought to have pharmacological activity. Conjugated metabolites are eliminated in bile, faeces and urine. The half-life of the terminal exponential phase of elimination from plasma is 4–16 h in adults.

EVALUATION OF DATA

Passage of norethisterone into human milk has been reported as follows:

Treatment conditions	Concentration (μg/l)		Milk/ plasma ratio	Maximum observed milk conc. (μg/l)	Absolute dose to infant (μg/kg/day)		Ref.
Dose × Frequency × Duration; Route; No. of patients; Lactation stage	Milk	Plasma			Ave	Max	
200 mg × 1/d × 1 d; i.m.; 10;?	0.23	0.9	0.26	8.0	0.035	1.2	(1)
200 mg × 1/d × 1 d; i.m.; 20; ?	0.15	0.6	0.25	4.0	0.023	0.6	(2)
40 mg × 1/d ×1 d; i.m.; 5; ?	0.15	–	–	0.24	0.023	0.036	(3)
25 mg × 1/d ×1 d; i.m.; 4; ?	0.3	1.20	0.25	0.40	0.045	0.06	(4)
1 mg × 1/d × LT; p.o.; 4; ?	2.0	7.5	0.27	3.0	0.30	0.45	(4)
0.35 mg × 1/d × LT; p.o.; 4; ?	0.4	2.5	0.16	0.6	0.06	0.09	(4)
0.35 mg × 1/d × LT; p.o.; 5; ?	0.5	2.8	0.18	1.36	0.075	0.20	(5)

LT, long term. The milk and serum concentration-time profiles were defined in these references and were concurrent. The table gives average values estimated from graphs in the reports. The maximum milk concentrations are mean maximum figures in reference (1) and the highest values recorded in individuals in the remaining references. When norethisterone was administered by im injection or by implant the milk and serum concentrations of the drug declined progressively from these maxima to about 0.1 μg/l over 5 (2), 7 (1) and 28 (3) weeks.

RELATIVE DOSE IN MILK

When norethisterone acetate (mol. wt. 359) was administered but norethisterone (mol.wt. 298) was assayed a factor of 1.2 (=359/298) is included in the calculation. On this basis a suckling infant would ingest in a day on average 2.2% (0.002 × 900 × 1.2/1)* (4) and at maximum 3.5% (0.00136 × 900/0.35)* (5) of the weight-adjusted maternal daily dose.

DATA ON THE INFANT

No data are recorded.

ASSESSMENT AND RECOMMENDATIONS

The risk to the suckling infant of administering norethisterone as a regular therapeutic dose to its mother is low on the basis that the quantity of drug that enters milk is small. The quantity of norethisterone that would be ingested during suckling in the first few weeks after a depot injection or insertion of an implant would be larger but is unlikely to represent a significantly increased risk. Breast-feeding should be regarded as safe. (See also 'Steroid contraception during lactation', p. 36.)

REFERENCES

1. Koetswang S, Nulkulkarn P, Fotherby K, Shrimanker K, Mangalam M, Towobola K (1982) Transfer of contraceptive steroids in milk of women using long-acting gestagens. *Contraception, 25*, 321–331.
2. Fotherby K, Towobola O, Muggeridge J, Elder MG (1983) Norethisterone levels in maternal serum and milk after intramuscular injection of norethisterone oenanthate as a contraceptive. *Contraception, 28*, 405–411.
3. Bhaskar A, Schulze PE, Acksteiner B, Laumas KR (1979) Quantitative analysis of norethindrone in milk using deuterated carrier and gas-chromatography mass spectrometry. *J. Steroid. Biochem., 11*, 1323–1328.
4. Toddywalla VS, Mehta S, Virkar KD, Saxena BN (1980) Release of 19-nortestosterone type of contraceptive steroids through different drug delivery systems into serum and breast milk of lactating women. *Contraception, 21*, 217–222.
5. Saxena BM, Shrimanker K, Grudzinskas JG (1977) Levels of contraceptive steroids in breast milk and plasma of lactating women. *Contraception, 16*, 605–613.

* An explanation of the calculation (s) appears on pp. 71–72.

NORETYNODREL

GENERAL

Noretynodrel (norethynodrel) is a potent synthetic progestogen that is used in a few combined oral contraceptive steroid preparations. It is extensively (probably totally) metabolised to norethisterone in the body.

EVALUATION OF DATA

Noretynodrel has not been extensively studied in its own right. Pincus et al. (1) found that after an oral dose of 14^{C} noretynodrel, less than 0.14% of radioactivity was excreted in breast milk over the following 24 h. In a similar study over 5 days, Laumas et al. (2) found a maximum of 1.5% of the dose in breast milk as total radioactivity. Much of the radioactivity will have been present in inactive metabolites.

ASSESSMENT AND RECOMMENDATIONS

Noretynodrel is largely metabolised to norethisterone which enters milk in very small quantities (see page 000) and the quoted data with radiolabelled norethynodrel are compatible with this finding. The risk to the suckling infant of administering noretynodrel to the mother would appear to be negligible. (See also 'Steroid contraception during lactation', p. 36.)

REFERENCES

1. Pincus G, Bialy G, Layne DS, Paniagua M, Williams KIH (1966) Radioactivity in the milk•of subjects receiving radioactive 19-norsteroids. *Nature (London)*, *212*, 924–925.
2. Laumas K, Malkani PK, Bhatnagar S,Laumas V (1967) Radioactivity in the breast milk of lactating women after oral administration of H^3-norethynodrel. *Am. J. Obstet. Gynaecol.*, *98*, 411–413.

PREDNISOLONE
PREDNISONE

GENERAL

Prednisolone and prednisone are potent synthetic glucocorticoids with some mineralocorticoid activity. Both are absorbed from the adult gastrointestinal tract and are 75–95% bound to plasma proteins. Prednisone is converted in the liver to the active metabolite, prednisolone and both drugs undergo extensive further metabolism. In adults the plasma half-life is 3 h but the half-life of biological activity is much longer (18–36 h).

EVALUATION OF DATA

Passage of prednisone and prednisolone into human milk has been reported as follows:

Treatment conditions Dose × Frequency × Duration; Route; No. of patients; Lactation stage	Concentration (μg/l) Milk	Plasma	Milk/plasma ratio	Maximum observed milk conc. (μg/l)	Absolute dose to infant (μg/kg/day) Ave	Max	Ref.
10–80 mg[a] × 1/d × LT; p.o.; 6; ?	62	390	0.16	317	9.3	47.6	(1)
10 mg[b] × 1/d × 1 d; p.o.; 1; ?	–	–	–	26.7[b] 1.6[a]	–	4.0[b] 0.24[b]	(2)

[a]Prednisolone; [b]prednisone; LT, long term. In reference (1), doses of prednisolone between 10 and 80 mg/day were given. The milk and plasma concentrations quoted are average figures. The maximum milk concentration is the highest value reported in an individual. In reference (2), the drug was given as prednisone but both prednisone and prednisolone were assayed in milk 2 h after the dose when maximum concentrations have been assumed. In a further report (4), 3 women received prednisolone 50 mg as a single i.m. injection and gave serum and milk samples over 6 h. The concentrations of prednisolone in milk were similar to expected unbound concentrations in serum, suggesting rapid and bidirectional exchange between serum and milk. The half-life of prednisolone was shorter in milk than in serum.

RELATIVE DOSE IN MILK

The amount of prednisolone that a suckling infant would ingest in a feed is at maximum 0.5% (26.7 + 1.6 × 180/10 000)* of the weight-adjusted maternal single dose (2). A suckling infant would ingest in a day on average 1.9% (62 × 900/30 000)* and at maximum 3.6% (0.317 × 900/80)* of the weight-adjusted

* An explanation of the calculation (s) appears on pp. 71–72.

maternal daily dose (1). In another study 7 lactating mothers received prednisolone 5 mg labelled with ^3H. Radioactivity in milk declined rapidly to reach a plateau after 36 h. The mean total recovery in 1 litre of milk during the 48 h after the dose was 0.14% (range 0.07–0.23%) (3).

DATA ON THE INFANT

No data are recorded.

ASSESSMENT AND RECOMMENDATIONS

The risk to the suckling infant of administering prednisone or prednisolone to its mother is low on the basis that the quantity of drug that enters milk is small. Breast-feeding may be regarded as safe.

REFERENCES

1. Ost L, Wettrell G, Bjorkheim I, Rane A (1985) Prednisolone excretion in human breast milk. *J. Paediatr., 106*, 1008–1011.
2. Katz FH, Duncan BR (1975) Entry of prednisone into human milk. *N. Engl. J. Med., 293,* 1154.
3. McKenzie SA, Selley JA, Agnew JE (1975) Secretion of prednisolone into breast milk. *Arch. Dis. Child., 50*, 894–896.
4. Greenbeger PA, Odeh YK, Frederiksen MC, Atkinson AJ (1993) Pharmacokinetics of prednisolone transfer to breast milk. *Clin. Pharmacol. Ther., 53*, 324–328.

PROPYLTHIOURACIL

GENERAL

Propylthiouracil is an antithyroid drug which acts by inhibiting the iodination of tyrosine. It is well absorbed from the adult gastrointestinal tract and is 75% bound to plasma albumin. Propylthiouracil is metabolised by oxidation and conjugation and the metabolites are excreted in bile. The plasma half-life is 2 h, but the half-life of biological activity is considerably longer.

EVALUATION OF DATA

Passage of propylthiouracil into human milk has been reported as follows:

Treatment conditions	Concentration (mg/l)		Milk/ plasma ratio	Maxi-mum observed milk conc. (mg/l)	Absolute dose to infant (mg/kg/day)		Ref.
Dose × Frequency × Duration; Route; No. of patients; Lactation stage	Milk	Plasma			Ave	Max	
400 mg × 1/d × 1 d; p.o.; 9; 1–8 months	0.6	5.8	0.09 (1.5 h) 0.13 (4.0 h)	0.7	0.09	0.11	(1)

The concentration-time profiles were defined for 4 h after the dose and were not concurrent as is shown by the milk to plasma ratio. The Table gives average milk and plasma and maximum milk concentrations.

RELATIVE DOSE IN MILK

The amount of propylthiouracil that a suckling infant would ingest in a feed is at maximum 0.3% (0.7 × 180/400)* of the weight-adjusted maternal single dose (1). The authors report that on average 99 μg or 0.025% of the dose was recovered in 184 ml of milk in the 4 h after the dose. Others found 0.077% of a 100 mg dose of radiolabelled propylthiouracil in 500 ml of milk collected from a woman during 24 h after administration (2).

DATA ON THE INFANT

Propylthiouracil has not been reported to have harmful effects in the few infants studied (1,3).

* An explanation of the calculation (s) appears on pp. 71–72.

ASSESSMENT AND RECOMMENDATIONS

The risk to the suckling infant of administering a single therapeutic dose of propylthiouracil to its mother is low on the basis that the quantity of drug that passes into milk is small. There are scant data on which to base a recommendation about infants of mothers taking repeated doses but a reasonable course is to advise that breast-feeding is safe provided the thyroid status of the infant is monitored regularly.

REFERENCES

1. Kampmann JP, Hansen JM, Johansen K, Helweg J (1980) Propylthiouracil in human milk. Revision of Dogma. *Lancet, i,* 736–737.
2. ow LCK, Lang J, Alexander WD (1979) Excretion of carbimazole and propylthiouracil in breast milk. *Lancet, ii,* 1011.
3. Cooper DS (1984) Antithyroid Drugs. *N. Engl. J. Med., 311,* 1353–1362.
4. McDougall IR, Bayer MF (1986) Should a woman taking propylthiouracil breast-feed? *Clin. Nucl. Med., 11,* 249–250.

THYROXINE

GENERAL

Thyroxine (tetraiodothyronine, T_4) is the main hormone secreted by the thyroid gland and is the precursor of triiodothyronine (T_3) which is the principal mediator of physiological effect. Both hormones absorbed from the adult gastrointestinal tract and are extensively bound to specific carrier plasma proteins. The effect of a single dose of T_4 lasts 2–3 weeks and that of T_3 lasts 1 week.

EVALUATION OF DATA

Passage of T_3 and T_4 into human milk has been reported as follows:

T_3 (μg/l)		Milk to serum ratio	T_4 (μg/l)		Ref.
Milk	Serum		Milk	Serum	
0.26–1.12	1.25–3.68	0.16–0.58	–	–	(1a)
0.59–1.11	1.31–1.90	0.39–0.65	–	–	(1b)
0.1 ± 0.09^s	–	–	<7	45–240	(1c)
–	–	–	<0.1	–	(2)
–	–	–	<1.0–4.0	–	(3)
–	–	–	0.71 ± 0.4^s	–	(4)
		(0.9–2.0)			
0.775 ± 0.21^s	–	–	<2.0	–	(5)

s, standard deviation. Reference (1) reports on 10 patients with Graves' disease 1–4 months after delivery (1a), 5 patients with Hashimoto's disease 1–3 months after delivery (1b) and a patient with Graves' disease, one with Hashimoto's disease and 3 normal subjects 6 days to 7 months after delivery (1c). Reference (2) gives data on 114 samples of milk collected from euthyroid subjects 1–8 weeks after delivery. Concentrations of T_3 were significantly higher in colostrum than in mature milk but T_4 was not detected in any sample. T_4 was assayed by gas chromatography-mass spectrometry in 4 women 17–39 days after delivery in reference (3). The data in reference (5) refer to mature milk which were not significantly different from those in colostrum.

RELATIVE DOSE IN MILK

The replacement dose of T_3 for adults is 60 μg/day, or 1 μg/kg/day, assuming a body weight of 60 kg. A suckling infant taking 0.15 l/kg/day of milk containing the average T_3 concentration of 0.1 μg/l (2) would ingest 0.015 μg/kg/day or 1.5% of the adult replacement dose. The normal replacement dose of T_4 for infants is 10 μg/kg/day. A suckling infant taking 0.15 l/kg/day of milk containing 0.71 μg/l(4) would ingest 0.1 μg/kg/day, ie 1.0% of the infant replacement dose.

DATA ON THE INFANT

No effects were reported in infants.

ASSESSMENT AND RECOMMENDATIONS

When an infant has normal thyroid function, its physiological feed-back mechanisms would be expected to adjust to thyroid hormone ingested in milk. The supply of T_3 and T_4 in breast milk is, however, insufficient for the biological needs of an infant without an active thyroid gland and if such an infant were wholly dependent for its nutrition on breast milk then development of its nervous system would be impared. T_3 or T_4 supplements should be given to an athyreotic infant that is breast-fed.

REFERENCES

1. Mizuta H, Amino N, Ichihara K, Harada T, Nose O, Tanizawa O, Miyai K (1983) Thyroid hormones in human milk and their influence on thyroid function of breast-fed babies. *Ped. Res., 17*, 468–471.
2. Sato T, Suzuki Y (1979) Presence of triiodothyronine, no detectable thyroxine and reverse triiodothyronine in human milk. *Endocrinol. Jpn., 26*, 507–13.
3. Moller B, Bjorkheim I, Falk O, Lantto O, Larsson A (1983) Identification of thyroxine in human breast milk by gas chromatography mass-spectrometry. *J. Clin. Endocrinol. Metab., 56*, 30–34.
4. Mallol J, Obregon, MJ, Morreale de Escobar G (1982) Analytical artifacts in radioimmunoassay of L-throxine in human milk. *Clin. Chem., 28*, 1277–1282.
5. Jansson L, Ivarsson S, Larsson I, Ekman R (1983) Tri-iodothyronine and thyroxine in human milk. *Acta Paediatr. Scand., 72,* 703–705.

TOLBUTAMIDE

GENERAL

Tolbutamide is an oral antidiabetic drug of the sulfonylurea group. It promotes hypoglycaemia by increasing insulin secretion and decreasing hepatic glycogenolysis and gluconeogenesis; the duration of action of a single dose is 6–12 h. Tolbutamide is almost completely absorbed from the adult gastrointestinal tract, is 96% bound to plasma proteins and is inactivated by metabolism. The plasma half-life is 5 h.

EVALUATION OF DATA

Passage of tolbutamide into human milk has been reported as follows:

Treatment conditions: Dose × Frequency × Duration; Route; No. of patients; Lactation stage	Concentration (mg/l): Milk	Concentration (mg/l): Plasma	Milk/plasma ratio	Maximum observed milk conc. (mg/l)	Absolute dose to infant (mg/kg/day): Ave	Absolute dose to infant (mg/kg/day): Max	Ref.
500 mg × 2/d × LT;	18 (No. 1)	45	0.4	18	–	2.7	(1)
p.o.; 2; 3 d	3 (No. 2)	35	0.09	–	–		

LT, long term. The mothers received tolbutamide throughout pregnancy and steady-state conditions of dosing may be assumed to apply. Milk and serum samples were taken once, 4 h after the dose, i.e. the concentration-time profile was not defined. Note the 4.4-fold difference in milk to plasma ratio between these two subjects.

RELATIVE DOSE IN MILK

A suckling infant would ingest in a day at maximum 16.2% (18 × 900/1000)* of the weight-adjusted maternal daily dose (1).

DATA ON THE INFANT

These were not reported in the study quoted (1).

ASSESSMENT AND RECOMMENDATIONS

Limited data suggest that the risk to the suckling infant of administering tolbutamide to its mother is significant because of the quantity of drug that passes into

* An explanation of the calculation (s) appears on pp. 71–72.

milk. Breast-feeding is probably best avoided until the milk and plasma profiles of tolbutamide are defined in nursing women.

REFERENCES

1. Moiel RH, Ryan JR (1967) Tolbutamide orinase in human breast milk. *Clin. Pediatr.*, 6, 480.

CIMETIDINE

GENERAL

Cimetidine inhibits secretion of gastric acid through its action as a histamine H_2-receptor antagonist; it is used for peptic ulcer and gastric hypersecretory conditions. Cimetidine is absorbed from the adult gastrointestinal tract, from which its bioavailability is 65–80%, is 20% bound to plasma proteins and its apparent distribution volume is 1–2 l/kg. Clearance is primarily by renal and to a lesser extent by hepatic processes. The plasma half-life in adults is 2 h. In 3 neonates the half-life of cimetidine was 1.1–2.2 h (2). Cimetidine decreases liver mixed function oxidase activity.

EVALUATION OF DATA

Passage of cimetidine into human milk has been reported as follows:

Treatment conditions Dose × Frequency × Duration; Route; No. of patients; Lactation stage	Concentration (mg/l) Milk	 Serum	Milk/ serum ratio	Maxi- mum observed milk conc. (mg/l)	Absolute dose to infant (mg/kg/day) Ave	 Max	Ref.
100 mg × 1/d × 1 d; p.o.; 12; 45 weeks	2.5	0.7	5.65	2.5	–	0.38	(1)
600 mg × 1/d × 1 d; p.o.; 12; 45 weeks	16.2	4.2	5.84	16.2		2.43	(1)
1200 mg × 1/d × 1 d; p.o.; 12; 45 weeks	37.2	9.6	5.83	37.2		5.58	(1)
400 mg × 1/d; p.o.;1; 6 months	–	–	1.7 (0.44–3.5)	4.0	–	–	(2)
200 mg × 3/d at night, × 3 d; p.o.; 1; 6 months	5.6	0.8	4.6–11.8	–	0.84	–	(2)

The milk and serum values quoted in (1) are means for the group. Areas under the concentration-time curves were defined and were not concurrent, with the maximum milk concentration occurring 1–2 h after that in serum. The quoted milk and serum ratios are based on area measurements and the mean values for all doses was 5.77. This exceeded by x 5.5 the value predicted by the model of Fleishaker et al. (3) which assumes that only free unionised drug equilibrates across the blood-milk barrier, and is indicative of active transport of drug into milk. Non-concurrence of milk and plasma concentration-time profiles was also noted in (2). The maximum concentration in milk of 4 mg/l is estimated from the graph in the paper. The same mother took part in the 3-day repeated-dose study. On day 4, samples were collected during the day just before each dose. The milk and plasma concentrations quoted are the average values for these times. Note the milk to plasma ratio varation from 4.6 to 11.8 with the latter reflecting accumulation of drug in milk 10 h after the final 400 mg dose the previous day.

RELATIVE DOSE IN MILK

A suckling infant would ingest in a feed at maximum 5.6% (37.2 × 180/1200)* of the weight-adjusted maternal single dose of cimetidine (1). A calculation based on the observed milk to serum ratio, the maternal oral clearance and assuming 0.15 l/kg/day to be ingested, indicated a relative dose of 6.7% at steady-state (1). The estimated amount of drug that an infant would ingest in a day is on average 5.0% (5.6 × 900/1000)* of the weight-adjusted maternal daily dose (2). The dose for infants is 20 mg/kg/d in 4 divided doses. A suckling infant would ingest in a feed 2.4% (4 × 3/5)* of the single dose for children, and in a day 4.2% (5.6 × 15/20)* of the daily dose for children (2). Note that the estimates of relative *daily* dose are based on milk samples taken just *before* each dose of cimetidine was taken and do not refer to the average concentration throughout the day, which may be expected to be higher than those quoted here.

DATA ON THE INFANT

No data are available.

ASSESSMENT AND RECOMMENDATIONS

The risk to the suckling infant of administering cimetidine to its mother appears to be low on the basis that the quantity of drug that passes into milk is small. Breast-feeding may be regarded as safe.

REFERENCES

1. Oo CY, Kuhn RJ, Desai N, McNamara PJ (1995) Active transport of cimetidine into human milk. *Clin. Pharmacol. Ther., 58,* 548–555.
2. Somogyi A, Gugler R (1979) Cimetidine excretion into breast milk. *Br. J. Clin. Pharmacol., 6,* 627–629.
3. Fleishaker JC, Desai N, McNamara PJ (1987) Factors affecting the milk to plasma drug concentration ratio in lactating women; physical interaction with protein and fat. *J. Pharmacol. Sci., 76,* 189–193.

* An explanation of the calculation (s) appears on pp. 71–72.

CISAPRIDE

GENERAL

Cisapride stimulates uppper gastrointestinal motility by promoting acetylcholine release in the gut wall. It is used to relieve gastro-oesophageal reflux and to accelerate gastric emptying. It is well absorbed fom the gastrointestinal tract, undergoes pre-systemic (55%), and further extensive metabolism in the liver. The half-life is 8 h.

EVALUATION OF DATA

Passage of cisapride into human milk has been reported as follows:

Treatment conditions	Concentration (μg/l)		Milk/plasma ratio	Maximum observed milk conc. (μg/l)	Absolute dose to infant (μg/kg/day)		Ref.
Dose × Frequency × Duration; Route; No. of patients; Lactation stage	Milk	Plasma			Ave	Max	
20 mg × 8 h × 4 d; p.o.; 10; 5 d	6.2	137	0.045	–	0.93	–	(1)

The table gives mean values for milk and plasma at 1 h after dosing, i.e. milk and plasma concentration-time profiles are not available. Steady-state conditions were achieved.

RELATIVE DOSE IN MILK

The amount of cisapride that a suckling infant would ingest in a feed based on the milk concentration 1 h after dosing is 0.3% (6.2 × 900/20 000)* of the weight-adjusted maternal daily dose.

DATA ON THE INFANT

No data are available.

ASSESSMENT AND RECOMMENDATIONS

The risk to the suckling infant of administering cisapride to its mother would appear to be low in the basis that the quantity of drug that passes into milk is small. Breast-feeding may be regarded as safe.

* An explanation of the calculation (s) appears on pp. 71–72.

REFERENCES

1. Hofmeeyer GJ, Sonnendecker EWW (1986) Secretion of the gastrokinetic agent cisapride in human milk. *Eur. J. Clin. Pharmacol., 30,* 735–736.

DOMPERIDONE

GENERAL

Domperidone is a dopamine D_2-receptor antagonist; it is used to relieve nausea and vomiting and has also been given to women with premature babies in order to stimulate serum prolactin secretion and thereby milk yield (1). Domperidone is absorbed from the adult gastrointestinal tract, is metabolised in the liver and is excreted in the bile, mainly as inactive metabolites. The plasma half-life is 7 h.

EVALUATION OF DATA

Passage of domperidone into human milk and plasma has been reported as follows:

Treatment conditions: Dose × Frequency × Duration; Route; No. of patients; Lactation stage	Concentration (μg/l): Milk	Concentration (μg/l): Plasma	Milk/plasma ratio	Maximum observed milk conc. (μg/l)	Absolute dose to infant (μg/kg/day): Ave	Absolute dose to infant (μg/kg/day): Max	Ref.
10 mg × 3/d × 4 d; p.o.; 2; 3–6 d	2.6	10.3	0.25	–	4	–	(1)
20 mg × 1/d × 1 d; p.o.;10; 1 week	0.24	8.0	–	1.1	–	–	(2)

Reference (1) reports the mean milk concentration in 30 samples collected during the 4 days of the study; the serum concentration is the mean of 5 samples taken 1.75–3 h after a dose. In reference (2), milk and serum were taken 2 h after the single dose of domperidone and are mean values for the 10 subjects. Milk was sampled again after 4 h and appears as the maximum milk concentration. Neither study defined the concentration-time profiles.

RELATIVE DOSE IN MILK

The amount of domperidone that a suckling infant would ingest in a day is on average 0.1% (0.0026 × 900/30)* of the weight-adjusted maternal daily dose (1). If the paediatric daily dose is assumed to be 0.9 mg/kg, then a suckling infant would ingest on average 0.001% (0.0026 × 15/30)* of this (1).

DATA ON THE INFANT

No data are available.

* An explanation of the calculation (s) appears on pp. 71–72.

ASSESSMENT AND RECOMMENDATIONS

The data show that when domperidone is given to a nursing woman, the quantity of drug ingested by her infant in milk is small. Breast-feeding would appear to be safe.

REFERENCES

1. Hofmeyr GJ, van Iddekinge B (1983) Domperidone and lactation. *Lancet*, *i*, 47.
2. Hofmeyr GJ, van Iddekinge B, Blott JA (1985) Domperidone: secretion in breast milk and effect on puerperal prolactin levels. *Br. J. Obstet. Gynaecol.*, *92*, 141–144.

MESALAZINE

GENERAL

Mesalazine (5-aminosalicylic acid) is the active component of sulfasalazine and is available as a drug in its own right. It is well absorbed from the adult gastrointestinal tract; its presentation in delayed-release and slow-release formulations is necessary to prevent absorption from the small bowel and deliver the drug to its desired site of action in the colon. Mesalazine is extensively metabolised and the plasma half-life is 1 h.

EVALUATION OF DATA

Passage of mesalazine in human milk has been reported as follows:

Treatment conditions Dose × Frequency × Duration; Route; No. of patients; Lactation stage	Concentration (mg/l) Milk	 Plasma	Milk/plasma ratio	Maximum observed milk conc. (mg/l)	Absolute dose to infant (mg/kg/day) Ave	 Max	Ref.
500 mg × 3/d	0.11	0.41	0.27	–	–	–	(1)
× ?; p.o.; 1; ?	(12.4)	(2.44)	(5.1)				
1000 mg × 3/d × ?;	No. 1: 0.1	No. 1:0.6	0.07	–	–	–	(2)
p.o.; 1; ; 1 week	No. 2: 0.1	No: 2:1.1	0.09				
	(No. 1:18.1	(No. 1:1.1	(16.5)				
	No. 2:12.3)	No.2: 1.8)	(6.8)				

In reference (1) a single pair of milk and blood samples was taken 5.25 h after the last dose of mesalazine. In reference (2) paired milk and blood sampleas were taken 7 d (No. 1) and 11 d (No. 2) after delivery, both 5 h after the last dose. In both studies, the figures in brackets refers to acetyl-5-aminosalicylic acid. A further woman received mesalazine 1 g/day; 5-aminosalicylic acid was not measurable in her milk and the concentration of acetyl-5-aminosalicylic acid was 2.2 mg/l (2).

RELATIVE DOSE IN MILK

The two studies give similar findings but neither allows an assessment of whether the samples represent average or maximum values. Nevertheless the quantity of mesalazine the an infant would ingest in a day may be calculated to be 7.5% (0.11 + 12.4 × 900/1500)* of the weight-adjusted maternal dose.

* An explanation of the calculation (s) appears on pp. 71–72.

DATA ON THE INFANT

Watery diarrhoea occurred in a breast-fed infant whose mother took mesalazine, ceased when the drug was discontinued and recurred on each of 4 occasions when it was readministered (3).

ASSESSMENT AND RECOMMENDATIONS

Limited data suggest that the quantity of mesalazine and its metabolite that passes into milk is just below the limit accepted in this text to signify safety on the basis of the weight-adjusted dose received by the infant. The drug has also been closely associated with causing diarrhoea in a breast-fed infant. Should a mother wish to breast-feed, a reasonable course would be to advise her to proceed but to discontinue if her infant develops diarrhoea.

REFERENCES

1. Jenss H, Weber P, Hartman F (1990) 5-aminosalicylic acid and its metabolite in breast milk during lactation. *Am. J. Gastroenterol., 85,* 331.
2. Klotz U, Harings-Kaim A (1993) Negligible excretion of 5-aminosalicylic acid in breast milk. *Lancet, 342,* 618–619.
3. Nelis GF (1989) Diarrhoea due to 5-aminosalicylic acid in breast milk. *Lancet, i,* 383.

METOCLOPRAMIDE

GENERAL

Metoclopramide is a dopamine D_2-receptor blocking drug. It acts both peripherally and centrally and is used for treatment of gastrointestinal dysfunction, notably nausea and vomiting. Metoclopramide is well absorbed from the adult gastrointestinal tract and is extensively metabolised in the liver. Glucuronide and sulphate metabolites and unchanged drug are cleared by the kidney. The plasma half-life is 5 h. Metoclopramide may cause dystonic reactions in children.

EVALUATION OF DATA

Passage of metoclopromide into human milk has been reported as follows:

Treatment conditions — Dose × Frequency × Duration; Route; No. of patients; Lactation stage	Concentration (mg/l) Milk	Plasma	Milk/plasma ratio	Maximum observed milk conc. (mg/l)	Absolute dose to infant (mg/kg/day) Ave	Max	Ref.
10 mg × 3/d × 3 weeks; p.o.;5; 17–23 d	0.051–0.157 (2 h)	0.017–0.293 (2 h)	0.52–0.157 4.06 (2 h)	0.157	0.016 per ref	0.024 per ref	(1)
10 mg × 3/d × 2 weeks; p.o.; 18; 10–14 weeks	0.02–0.125	(?)	(?)	0.125	0.005 per ref	0.013 per ref	(1)
10 mg × 1/d × 1 d; p.o.; 10; 7–10 d	0.126+0.042 (2 h)	0.069+0.030 (2 h)	1.84	–	0.019	–	(2)

Reference (1) reports a trial in which mothers were given metoclopramide to improve milk yield. The paper lists only the milk and plasma concentrations obtained 1–2 h after dosing and the range of these is presented in the table. The maximum milk concentration quoted is the highest value recorded in an individual. The full concentration-time profiles after a dose are shown graphically in two cases and indicate a lack of concurrence with reversal of the milk to plasma ratio. The paper gives enough data for calculation of a milk to plasma ratio and appreciation of a range. In reference (2), only mean ± sem milk and plasma concentrations are given. The milk to plasma ratio for both reports is >1 for some periods after dosing as is expected for a basic drug, but an average ratio cannot be derived without more kinetic profiles in additional subjects.

RELATIVE DOSE IN MILK

An infant suckling during the early puerperium would ingest in a day on average 3.3% (0.109 × 900/30)* and at maximum 4.7% (0.157 × 900/30)* of the weight-adjusted maternal daily dose (1). Here the average milk concentration (0.109 mg/l)

* An explanation of the calculation (s) appears on pp. 71–72.

is that for all 2 h samples and the maximum concentration (0.157 mg/l) is the highest 2 h sample. An infant suckling during the late puerperium would ingest in a day on average 1.5% (0.050 × 900/30)* and at maximum 3.8% (0.125 × 900/30)* of the weight-adjusted maternal daily dose. The paediatric single dose is 0.1 mg/kg for children up to 6 years of age. An infant suckling during the early puerperium would ingest in a feed at maximum 4.7% (0.157 × 3/0.1)* of the paediatric single dose and during the late puerperium the estimate would be 3.8% (0.125 × 3/0.1)* (1). The paediatric daily dose is 0.5 mg/kg. An infant suckling during the early puerperium would ingest in a day on average 3.3% (0.109 × 15/0.5) and at maximum 4.7% (0.157 × 15/0.5)* of this (1). During the late puerperium a suckling infant would ingest on average 1.5% (0.050 × 15/0.5)* and at maximum 3.8% (0.125 × 15/0.5)* of the paediatric daily dose (1). Reference (1) estimates the maximum dose in milk to be 24 and 13 μg/kg/d for the early and late puerperium respectively, as compared to the maximum recommended paediatric dose 500 μg/kg/d. Reference (2) calculates that the average intake of metoclopramide by the infant would not exceed 45 μg/kg/d.

DATA ON THE INFANT

Plasma metoclopramide concentrations of 0.021 (day 4) and 0.019 mg/l (day 14) were found in one infant; in all the other infants the concentrations were < 0.002 mg/l. Effects on nursing infants were not systematically studied (1). In a randomised, double-blind study, plasma thyrotropin, free thyroxine and prolactin did not differ between the infants of mothers who received metoclopramide for 3 weeks and those who received placebo (3).

ASSESSMENT AND RECOMMENDATIONS

The data suggest that when metoclopramide is administered to a nursing mother, the quantity of drug ingested by her infant in milk is small. Breast-feeding would appear to be safe.

REFERENCES

1. Kauppila A, Arvela P, Koivisto M, Kivinen S, Ylikorkala O, Pelkonen O (1983) Metoclopromide and breast-feeding: transfer into milk and the newborn. *Eur. J. Clin. Pharmacol.*, 25, 819–823.
2. Lewis PJ, Devenish C, Kahn, C (1980) Controlled trial of metoclopramide in the initiation of breast-feeding. *Br. J. Clin. Pharmacol.*, 9, 217–219.
3. Kauppila A, Anunti P, Kivinen S, Koivisto M, Ruokonen (1985) Metoclopramide and breast-feeding: efficacy and anterior pituitary responses of the mother and the child. *Eur. J. Obstet. Gynec. Reprod. Biol.*, *19*, 19–22.

NIZATIDINE

GENERAL

Nizatidine is a histamine H_2-receptor antagonist that is used to treat peptic ulcer and gastric hypersecretory conditions. More than 70% of an oral dose is absorbed from the gastrointestinal tract and plasma protein binding is 30%. The action of nizatidine is terminated mostly by renal excretion. The plasma half-life is 2 h.

EVALUATION OF DATA

Passage of nizatidine into human milk has been reported as follows:

Treatment conditions: Dose × Frequency × Duration; Route; No. of patients; Lactation stage	Concentration (mg/l): Milk	Concentration (mg/l): Plasma	Milk/plasma ratio	Maximum observed milk conc. (mg/l)	Absolute dose to infant (mg/kg/day): Ave	Absolute dose to infant (mg/kg/day): Max	Ref.
150 mg × 12/h 2.5 d; p.o.; 5; ?	–	1.59	1.0–4.9	–	–	–	(1)

Five postpartum lactating and five non-lactating women were studied, two initially as lactating and subsequently as non-lactating volunteers. The plasma concentration quoted is the mean maximum value. The table shows the variation in the milk:plasma ratio with time after dosing; the mean value at the time of maximum plasma concentration was taken from the graph in (1) to be unity, and a milk concentration of 1.59 mg/l is used to estimate the dose in milk (below).

RELATIVE DOSE IN MILK

The amount of nizatidine which a suckling infant would ingest in a day is at maximum 4.8% (1.59 × 900/300)* of the weight-adjusted maternal daily dose.

DATA ON THE INFANT

No data are available.

ASSESSMENT AND RECOMMENDATIONS

The risk to the suckling infant of administering nizatidine to its mother is low on the basis that the amount of drug that passes into milk is small. Breast-feeding would appear to be safe.

* An explanation of the calculation (s) appears on pp. 71–72.

REFERENCES

1. Obermeyer BD, Bergstrom RF, Callaghan JT, Knadler MP, Golichowski A, Rubin A (1990) Secretion of nizatidine into human brerast milk after single and multiple doses. *Clin. Pharmacol. Ther., 47*, 724–730.

RANITIDINE

GENERAL

Ranitidine is a histamine H_2-receptor antagonist that is used to treat peptic ulcer and gastric hypersecretory conditions. About 50% of an oral dose is absorbed and plasma protein binding is 15%. The action of ranitidine is terminated mostly by renal excretion and to a lesser extent by hepatic metabolism. The plasma half-life is 2 h.

EVALUATION OF DATA

Passage of ranitidine into human milk has been reported as follows:

Treatment conditions: Dose × Frequency × Duration; Route; No. of patients; Lactation stage	Concentration (mg/l): Milk	Concentration (mg/l): Plasma	Milk/plasma ratio	Maximum observed milk conc. (mg/l)	Absolute dose to infant (mg/kg/day): Ave	Absolute dose to infant (mg/kg/day): Max	Ref.
150 mg × 1/d × 1 d; p.o.; 6; 6–10 d	0.25–3.3 (2 h)	0.16–0.55 (2 h)	0.6–2.7 (2 h)	3.3	–	0.5	(1)
	0.39–3.0 (4 h)	0.28–0.37 (4 h)	1.1–10.2 (4 h)				
	<5–1.8 (8 h)	0.11–0.29 (8 h)	2.9–17.1 (8 h)				
150mg × 2/d × 3 d; p.o.; 1; 54 d	0.99 (pre-dose)	0.053 (pre-dose)	18.7 (pre-dose)	3.6	–	0.4	(2)
	0.72 (1.5 h)	0.106 (1.5 h)	6.8 (1.5 h)				
	2.61 (5.5 h)	0.309(5.5h)	8.4 (5.5 h)				
	1.57 (12 h)	0.066(12 h)	23.8 (12 h)				

Reference (1) does not give enough data points to describe a profile for ranitidine in milk and plasma. The concentrations and milk to plasma ratios quoted are the range of values and the maximum milk concentration is the highest value recorded in an individual. The milk to plasma ratio showed both dose interval and inter-individual variability. One patient showed marked accumulation of ranitidine in milk. In the case reported in reference (2) milk and serum were analysed just before and at the stated times after the first dose of ranitidine on the 3rd day of treatment. The concentration-time profile suggests accumulation of the drug in milk. The mean milk concentration derived from the area under the concentration-time curve was 1.79 mg/l. Neither study may have given data under steady-state dosing conditions for milk. The marked inter-individual variation and potential for accumulation of drug in milk require additional long-term studies on more women.

RELATIVE DOSE IN MILK

The calculation assumes that ranitidine hydrochloride (mol. wt. 350) was administered but that the free base (mol. wt. 314) was assayed and a factor of 1.1

(=350/314) is introduced. On this basis a suckling infant would ingest in a feed at maximum 4.4% (3.3 × 180 × 1.1/150)* of the weight-adjusted maternal single dose of ranitidine (1). Calculation from the multiple dose study indicates that an infant would ingest in a day on average 6.0% (1.79 × 900 × 1.1/300)* and at maximum 11.9% (3.6 900 1.1/300)* of the weight-adjusted maternal daily dose of ranitidine (2).

DATA ON THE INFANT

No data were reported.

ASSESSMENT AND RECOMMENDATIONS

The data in women given a single dose of an appropriate amount of ranitidine defined the milk and plasma concentration-time profiles. This showed that there was considerable inter-individual variation in the milk profile following a standard dose and that the drug may accumulate in milk. Reliable data for the milk profile under steady-state dosing conditions are not available. Breast-feeding is probably safe if, as does occur, use of ranitidine is occasional or limited to a single dose at night. There are no data on which to base a recommendation when ranitidine is used more frequently and long-term.

REFERENCES

1. Riley AJ, Crowley P, Harrison C (1981) Transfer of ranitidine to biological fluids: milk and semen. In: Misiewicz JJ, Wormsley KG (Eds), *The Clinical Use of Ranitidine,* pp 77–86. (Medicine Publishing Foundation Series, Vol 5.) Medicine Publishing Foundation, Oxford.
2. Kearns GL, McConnel Jr RF, Trang JM, Kluza RB (1985) Appearance of ranitidine in breast milk following multiple dosing. *Clin. Pharmacol.*, 4, 322–324.

* An explanation of the calculation (s) appears on pp. 71–72.

ROXATIDINE

GENERAL

Roxatidine is a histamine H_2-receptor antagonist that is used to treat peptic ulcer and gastric hypersecretory conditions. It is rapidly and almost completely absorbed from the adult gastrointestinal tract. The action of roxatidine is terminated mainly by renal excretion and to a lesser extent by hepatic metabolism. The plasma half-life is 5 h.

EVALUATION OF DATA

Passage of roxatidine into human milk has been reported as follows:

Treatment conditions Dose × Frequency × Duration; Route; No. of patients; Lactation stage	Concentration (mg/l) Milk	Plasma	Milk/ plasma ratio	Maxi-mum observed milk conc. (mg/l)	Absolute dose to infant (mg/kg/day) Ave	Max	Ref.
150 mg/d × 1/d; p.o.; 10; > 1month	(see below)	(see below)	1.0–3.4	–	–	–	(1)

Single dose data are reported. The concentration–time profile for plasma was taken from a different population of volunteers but was similar to the milk profile after the same dose. The table shows the variation in the milk:plasma ratio with time after dosing; the mean value at the time of maximum plasma concentration was taken from the graph in (1) to be unity, and a milk concentration of 4.5 mg/l is used to estimate the dose in milk (below).

RELATIVE DOSE IN MILK

The amount of roxatadine that an infant would ingest in a feed is at maximum 4.5% (4.5 × 180/150)* of the weight-adjusted maternal single dose.

DATA ON THE INFANT

No data are available.

ASSESSMENT AND RECOMMENDATIONS

The risk to the suckling infant of administering roxatidine to its mother is low on the basis that the amount of drug that passes into milk is small. Breast-feeding would appear to be safe.

* An explanation of the calculation (s) appears on pp. 71–72.

REFERENCES

1. Bender W, Brockmeier D (1989) Pharmacokinetic characteristics of roxatidine. *J. Clin. Gastroenterol., 11 (Suppl 1.),* S6–S19.

SENNA GLYCOSIDES

GENERAL

Senna is a stimulant or contact laxative of the anthraquinone group. In the gut, bacterial action on the glycoside liberates the active derivative which is partly absorbed; it acts by increasing peristalsis and by accumulation of ions and fluid in the colon. The action begins within 6–8 h of dosing. The oral dose is given only once a day.

EVALUATION OF DATA

Twenty-five mothers who had been breast-feeding for 2.5–15 months took a single dose of Senokot (containing sennosides A and B 8.602 mg) and gave breast milk at 0.5 h intervals for 6 h. Sennosides A and B were not found in breast milk. The lower limit of sensitivity of the assay was 0.34 mg/l. No plasma concentration data are available. Maternal and infants effects were observed for 24 h following senna. Loose stools were recorded in 15 mothers and 3 infants. When the mothers of these infants were rechallenged by giving double the original dose, senna was not found in their milk nor did loose stools occur in the nursed infants. Single or repeated doses of senna were effective in 50 breast-feeding women but bowel habit was unaffected in their infants who were observed from birth (2).

RELATIVE DOSE IN MILK

A suckling infant would ingest in a feed <7.1% (0.34 × 180/8.602)* of the weight-adjusted maternal single dose.

DATA ON THE INFANT

Data from references (1–3) suggest that administration of senna to nursing mothers does not affect bowel function in her infant. Study (4) reported a 17% incidence of diarrhoea among breast-feeding infants whose mothers took Senokot.

ASSESSMENT AND RECOMMENDATIONS

The dose of senna glycosides that passes into breast milk remains unknown. Nevertheless the risk of inducing diarrhoea in a suckling infant by administering senna glycosides to its mother appears to be negligible. Breast-feeding should be regarded as safe.

* An explanation of the calculation (s) appears on pp. 71–72.

REFERENCES

1. Werthmann Jr MW, Krees SV (1973) Quantitative excretion of Senokot in human breast milk. *Med. Ann.*, 42, 4–5.
2. Baldwin WF Clinical study of senna administration to nursing mothers: assessment of effects on infant bowel habits (1963) *Can. Med. Assoc. J.*, 89, 566–568.
3. Shelton MG (1980) Standardised senna in the management of constipation in the puerperium: a clinical trial. *S. Afr. Med. J.,* 57, 78–80.
4. Greenhalf JO, Leonard HSD (1980) Laxatives in the treatment of constipation in pregnant and breast-feeding mothers. *Practitioner*, 210, 259–263.

SULFASALAZINE

GENERAL

Sulfasalazine (sulphasalazine) (salazosulfapyridine) is used to induce and maintain remission in ulcerative colitis, and to suppress the disease process in Crohn's disease and rheumatoid arthritis. It is a chemical combination of sulfapyridine and 5-aminosalicylic acid, which components are separated by bacterial action in the colon. Most of the adverse effects of salazosulfapyridine are due to the sulfapyridine moiety. In adults salazosulfapyridine is absorbed from the intestinal tract as the unchanged drug and has a half-life in plasma of 8 h. Sulfapyridine is absorbed from the colon, is 10–45% bound to plasma proteins and has a plasma half-life of 8 h. Both salazosulfapyridine and sulfapyridine are excreted in the urine chiefly as acetlyated derivatives. 5-aminosalicylic acid appears only in very low concentrations in the plasma. Sulphonamide and salicylate drugs are capable of displacing unconjugated bilirubin from plasma albumin and in infants the free bilirubin may enter the brain to cause encephalopathy (kernicterus).

EVALUATION OF DATA

Passage of sulfasalazine and its metabolites in human milk have been reported as follows:

Treatment conditions: Dose × Frequency × Duration; Route; No. of patients; Lactation stage	Concentration (mg/l): Milk	Concentration (mg/l): Plasma	Milk/plasma ratio	Maximum observed milk conc. (mg/l)	Absolute dose to infant (mg/kg/day): Ave	Absolute dose to infant (mg/kg/day): Max	Ref.
0.5 g × 4/d × LT; p.o.; 3; 7 d	2.7 (10.3)	8.8 (19.8)	0.31 (0.54)	–	–	–	(1)
1–3 g/d × 2–3 weeks; p.o.; 12; 5–6 weeks	(see below)	(see below)	(0.45) (0.59 un–changed)	–	–	–	(2)
0.5 g × 4/5; 2 months; p.o.; 1; 4.5–6.5 months	(3.2–13.0)	(18.4–22.4)	(0.60–0.63)	(13.0)	–	(0.5–2.0)	(3)

LT, long term. Figures in brackets refer to sulfapyridine plus its metabolites unless otherwise stated. Reference (1) reports on mothers with ulcerative colitis who took sulfasalazine throughout pregnancy and the puerperium. The table gives average values based on single samples of blood and milk. Reintroduction of sulfasalazine treatment for mothers with ulcerative colitis or Crohn's disease after delivery is described in reference (2). Paired milk and plasma samples were collected on 31 occasions. The concentration of sulfasalazine was less than 1.0 mg/l (the limit of detection) in 26 milk samples the and in the remainder it was between 1.0–5.0 mg/l. Mothers who received sulfasalazine 2 g/day had milk concentrations of sulfapyridine and its metabolites in the range 5–15 mg/l but in those who received 3 g/day the concentrations were 20–35 mg/l (estimated from the figure in the report). The mother reported in reference (3) was studied in detail over a 2-month period. Milk and plasma concentration-time profiles during a dosing interval were defined. Sulfasalazine was not detected in her milk. The table gives the range of values. All quoted reports give data that refer to steady-state conditions of dosing.

RELATIVE DOSE IN MILK

According to the data in reference (1), the amount of sulfasalazine plus sulfapyridine and its metabolites which an infant would ingest in milk in a day is 5.9% ((2.7 +10.3) × 900/2000)* of the weight-adjusted maternal daily dose. The estimate from reference (2) for the same (2 g) daily dose would be similar. The maximum milk concentration noted in reference (2) for a mother on the 3 g daily dose is estimated to be 35 mg/l. An infant suckling at this concentration would receive in a day 10.5% (35 × 900/3000)* of the weight-adjusted maternal daily dose.

DATA ON THE INFANT

Random samples of urine collected from the infant contained 3.0–4.1 mg/l of sulfapyridine and its metabolites (1). Bloody diarrhoea was reported in an exclusively breast-fed infant whose mother was receiving long-term treatment for ulcerative colitis with sulfasalazine 3.0 g/d. The bloody diarrhoea resolved 48–72 h after the mother discontinued sulfasalazine (4).

ASSESSMENT AND RECOMMENDATIONS

The risk to the suckling infant of administering sulfasalazine to its mother appears to be low on the basis that the quantity of drug that passes into milk is small, specially when a standard dose of 2.0 g/day is given. Some mothers receiving sulfasalazine 3.0 g/day, however, achieve significant concentrations of sulfapyridine in milk. Bloody diarrhoea has been reported in a suckling infant whose mother was receiving this dose of sulfasalazine. Possible dangers associated with displacement of bilirubin from albumin by the components of sulfasalazine must also give cause for caution. Breast-feeding may be regarded as acceptable but the infant should be observed carefully if the drug is used in the higher dose.

REFERENCES

1. Azad Khan AK, Truelove SC (1979) Placental and mammary transfer of sulphasalazine. *Br. Med. J.*, 2, 1553.
2. Jarnerot G, Into-Malmberg M-B (1979) Sulphasalazine treatment during breast-feeding. *Scand. J. Gastroenterol.*, 14, 869–871.

* An explanation of the calculation (s) appears on pp. 71–72.

3. Berlin CM, Yaffe SJ (1980) Disposition of salicylazosulfapyridine (Azulfidine) and metabolites in human breast milk. *Dev. Pharmacol. Ther.*, 1, 31–39.
4. Branski D, Kerem E, Gross-Kieselstein, Hurvitz H, Litt R, Abrahamov A (1986) Bloody diarrhoea – a possible complication of sulphasalazine transferred through human breast milk. *J. Pediatr. Gastroent. Nutr.*, 5, 316–317.

ACENOCOUMAROL

GENERAL

Acenocoumarol (nicoumalone, acenocoumarin) is a coumarin anticoagulant. The drug is moderately lipid soluble, readily absorbed from the gastrointestinal tract and extensively bound (98%) to plasma proteins. Elimination is via the kidneys mainly as the unchanged drug. The plasma half-life in adults is 8 h.

EVALUATION OF DATA

Passage of acenocoumarol into human milk has been reported as follows:

Treatment conditions	Concentration (mg/l)		Milk/ plasma ratio	Maximum observed milk conc. (mg/l)	Absolute dose to infant (mg/kg/day)		Ref.
Dose × Frequency × Duration; Route; No. of patients; Lactation stage	Milk	Plasma			Ave	Max	
1–3 mg × 1/d × 5–10 d; p.o.; 20 5–10 d	<0.015	0.31 0.097	–	–	–	–	(1)

A high performance liquid chromatographic method with a detection limit of 12 μg/l (2) failed to identify acenocoumarol in any sample, even at the time of maximum serum concentration or at 6 thereafter. Maternal thrombotest values ranged from 5–24% (therapeutic range 6–12%).

RELATIVE DOSE IN MILK

A relative dose cannot be calculated as no acenocoumarol could be detected in milk.

DATA ON THE INFANT

Thrombotest values varied between 20–64%, which is in the normal range for neonates.

ASSESSMENT AND RECOMMENDATIONS

The risk to the suckling infant of administering acenocoumarol to its mother appears to be negligible on the basis that the drug was not detected in milk, despite the use of a sensitive assay method, and no effect was observed on the infant Thrombotest values. Breast-feeding may be regarded as safe.

REFERENCES

1. Houwert-de Jong M, Gerards LJ, Tatteroo-Templeman CAM, de Wolff FA (1981) May mothers taking acenocoumarol breast-feed their infants? *Eur. J. Clin. Pharmacol.*, *21*, 61–64.
2. de Wolff FA, Tatteroo-Templeman CAM, Edelbroek PM (1980) Determination of nanogram levels of the anticoagulant acenocoumarin by high-performance liquid chromatography. *J. Anal. Toxicol.*, *4*, 156–159.

PHENINDIONE

GENERAL

Phenindione is an indandione anticoagulant. It is absorbed from the adult gastrointestinal tract, is approximately 70% bound to plasma proteins and the plasma half-life is 5–10 h. Phenindione is eliminated in the urine.

EVALUATION OF DATA

Passage of phenindione into human milk has been reported as follows:

Treatment conditions: Dose × Frequency × Duration; Route; No. of patients; Lactation stage	Concentration (mg/l): Milk	Concentration (mg/l): Plasma	Milk/plasma ratio	Maximum observed milk conc. (mg/l)	Absolute dose to infant (mg/kg/day): Ave	Absolute dose to infant (mg/kg/day): Max	Ref.
25–75 mg × 1/d × 1 d; p.o.; 30; ?	0–5.0	-	-	5.0	-	0.75	(1)

Lactating women took phenindione as a single dose by mouth; the peak milk concentration occurred 3 h after later and was negligible 10 h after dosing. The table gives the range of values; the maximum milk concentration was the highest value recorded in an individual who took phenindione 50 mg.

RELATIVE DOSE IN MILK

A suckling infant would ingest in a feed at maximum 18.0% (5.0 × 180/50)* of the weight-adjusted maternal single dose used in this study (1).

DATA ON THE INFANT

An infant aged 5 weeks was breast-fed while his mother received phenindione 50 mg in the morning and 25–50 mg in the evening for pulmonary embolism. The infant developed a large scrotal haematoma following herniotomy and had abnormal blood coagulation tests which were corrected by administration of vitamin K (2).

ASSESSMENT AND RECOMMENDATIONS

The risk to the suckling infant of administering phenindione to its mother is unacceptable on the basis that the quantity of drug that passes into milk is significant

* An explanation of the calculation (s) appears on pp. 71–72.

and blood coagulation may be impaired. Breast-feeding should be regarded as unsafe.

REFERENCES

1. Goguel M, Noel G, Gillet J-Y, Girardel J-M, Muller P, Mayer G (1970) Therapeutique anticoagulante et allaitement. *Rev. Fr. Gynecol. Obstet.*, 65, 409–412.
2. Eckstein HB, Jack B (1970) Breast-feeding and anticoagulant therapy. *Lancet*, *i*, 672–673.

WARFARIN

GENERAL

Warfarin is a coumarin anticoagulant. It is well absorbed from the adult gastrointestinal tract, is 99% bound to plasma proteins and the apparent volume of distribution is 0.1 l/kg. Warfarin is extensively metabolised by the liver. It is administered as a racemic mixture, the plasma half-life of the *S*(–) form being 32 h and that of the *R*(+) form being 54 h.

EVALUATION OF DATA

Passage of warfarin into human milk has been reported as follows:

Treatment conditions Dose × Frequency × Duration; Route; No. of patients; Lactation stage	Concentration (mg/l) Milk	 Plasma	Milk/ plasma ratio	Maximum observed milk conc. (mg/l)	Absolute dose to infant (mg/kg/day) Ave	 Max	Ref.
2–12 mg × 1/d × 3–10 d; p.o.; 13; 3–10 d	< 0.025	2.01	–	–	–	–	(1)

Warfarin was assayed by a specific (gas-liquid chromatographic) method with a sensitivity limit of 0.025 mg/l and was detected neither in milk nor in infant plasma. The prothrombin time was prolonged in all the women who were studied. Other workers (2) also failed to detect warfarin in the milk of two mothers who were receiving warfarin and had prothrombin times in the therapeutic range.

RELATIVE DOSE IN MILK

No calculations can be made as warfarin was not detected in milk.

DATA ON THE INFANT

Prothrombin activity was within the normal range for the 4 babies aged 3–7 days in whom the test was performed (1) and in both infants whose mothers received warfarin for 56 and 130 days post-partum (2).

ASSESSMENT AND RECOMMENDATIONS

The risk to the suckling infant of administering warfarin to its mother is negligible on the basis that the drug cannot be detected in milk. Breast-feeding may be regarded as safe.

Haematological drugs, pp. 337–342

REFERENCES

1. Orme ML'E, Lewis PJ, de Sweit M, Serlin MJ, Sibeon R, Baty JD, Breckenridge AM (1977) May mothers given warfarin breast-feed their infants? *Br. Med. J.*, *1,* 1564–1565.
2. McKenna R, Cole ER, Vasan U (1983) Is warfarin sodium contraindicated in the lactating mother? *J. Pediatr.*, *103,* 325–327.

ACITRETIN

GENERAL

Acitretin is a synthetic aromatic derivative of retinoic acid used in the treatment of psoriasis and disorders of epithelial keratinisation. It is highly bound to plasma proteins and following long term therapy it has a terminal half-life of 47 h. Acitretin is partly metabolised to etretinate which has a half-life of 120 days and to a 13-*cis* metabolite. Acitretin is a known teratogen and pregnancy is contraindicated within 2 years exposure.

EVALUATION OF DATA

Passage of acitretin into human milk has been reported as follows:

Treatment conditions — Dose × Frequency × Duration; Route; No. of patients; Lactation stage	Concentration (μg/l) Milk	Serum	Milk/serum ratio	Maximum observed milk conc. (μg/l)	Absolute dose to infant (μg/kg/day) Ave	Max	Ref.
40 mg × 1/d × 9 d; p.o.; 1; 8 months	30–40	50 (100)	–	0.04	–	6	(1)

Values for the 13-*cis* metabolite appear in brackets. The figures in the table describe approximate steady-state conditions. The serum concentration is calculated from the area under the concentration-time curve; the milk values give the range of 11 measurements over days 3–9.

RELATIVE DOSE IN MILK

The amount of acitretin that a suckling infant would ingest in a day is on average 0.8% (35 × 900/40 000)* and at maximum 0.9% (40 × 900/40 000)* of the weight-adjusted maternal daily dose.

DATA ON THE INFANT

No data are available.

ASSESSMENT AND RECOMMENDATIONS

The quantity of acitretin that enters milk is a small proportion of the maternal dose. Exposure of the infant to acitretin by breast-feeding should nevertheless be re-

* An explanation of the calculation (s) appears on pp. 71–72.

garded as unsafe due to the inherent toxicity of this drug. Pregnancy or donation of blood should be avoided for 2 years after an adult is exposed to acitretin. In the absence of reliable data it seems reasonable that the same constraint should apply, i.e. that breast-feeding should not take place for two years after stopping acitretin.

REFERENCES

1. Rollman O, Pihi-Lundin I (1990) Acitretin excretion into human breast milk. *Acta Derm. Venereol. (Stockholm), 70*, 487–490.

CAFFEINE

GENERAL

Caffeine is a naturally-occurring xanthine derivative present in a variety of foodstuffs including coffee, tea and chocolate. It is well absorbed from the adult gastrointestinal tract, 36% bound to plasma proteins and extensively metabolised in the liver. The plasma half-life in adults is 4 h. In premature and new-born infants the half-life is 40–130 h (1,2) decreasing to 14 h in 3–5 month and 2.6 h and 5–6 month infants. Caffeine half-lives were longer in breast-fed than in formula fed infants (3).

EVALUATION OF DATA

Passage of caffeine into human milk has been reported as follows:

Treatment conditions Dose × Frequency × Duration; Route; No. of patients; Lactation stage	Concentration (mg/l)		Milk/ plasma ratio	Maximum observed milk conc. (mg/l)	Absolute dose to infant (mg/kg/day)		Ref.
	Milk	Plasma			Ave	Max	
150 mg × 1/d × 1 d; p.o.; 5; 4–12 months	1.58 (0.5 h)	3.05 (0.5 h)	0.52	2.41	–	0.36	(4)
150 mg × 5/d × 5 d; p.o.; 11; 11–127 d	8.0	–	–	28.6	–	–	(5)
26–35 mg × 12/d × 1 d; p.o.; 1; 5 months	0.78	1.69	0.15–0.63	1.15	0.12	0.17	(6)
146 mg × 1/d × 1 d; p.o.; 18; 4 d–19 weeks	0.82	–	0.76	2.25	–	–	(7)
66 – 90 mg/d × 3 d; p.o.; 40; 1.91–5.75 m	0.420 (ave)	–	–	2.13	–	–	(8)
100 mg × 1/d × 1 d; p.o.; 6; 3.5–17 weeks	2.45 (ave @ 1 h)	3.83) (ave @ 1 h)	0.70–0.81	6.15	–	–	(9)

The literature contains reports in which caffeine was administered to mothers as an exact amount of caffeine (4,5,9), studies in which the caffeine content of ingested coffee was measured (6–8) and reports of caffeine ingested in coffee when the precise intake of caffeine was not known (10). The milk and plasma concentrations quoted in reference (4) are average values at 0.5 h and the maximum milk concentration is the highest value recorded in an individual. The concentration-time profiles were defined and were concurrent. Reference (5) reports mothers who received decaffeinated coffee to which caffeine 150 mg per cup was added. A single milk sample was taken from each mother on the 5th day; the table gives the average concentration for the group and the maximum concentration was highest value reported in an individual. The mother described in reference (6) regularly took about 20 cups of coffee per day; in the reported study 12 drinks were taken during 11 h and the caffeine content of each drink was assayed. Average values for 8 milk and 2 plasma samples are given. In reference (7) the milk concentration and milk to plasma ratio was the average for the group. The milk and plasma concentration-time profiles were defined in one mother and were concurrent. The estimated quantity of caffeine ingested by the infants was 0.027–0.203 mg/kg/d. Samples of hind milk were collected throughout the day and the results are the average of the values found (8). Reference (9) gives good pharmacokinetic data for milk and plasma. In other studies, 15 mothers who drank up to 15 cups of coffee per day had an average concentration of caffeine in milk of about 4 mg/l and a maximum of 7.2 mg/l (10) and 9 mothers who took 750 mg per day had an average milk concentration of 4.3 mg/l and a maximum of 15.7 mg/l (11). In another study the mean milk to serum ratio, based on concentration-time curves from 5 mothers who took caffeine 200 mg, was 0.71 (12). This accords well with the above studies.

RELATIVE DOSE IN MILK

When caffeine sodium benzoate (50% caffeine) was administered but caffeine was assayed, a factor of 0.5 was introduced into the calculation. On this basis a suckling infant would ingest in a feed at maximum 5.8% (2.41 × 180/150 × 0.5)* of the weight-adjusted quantity of caffeine taken by the mother on a single occasion (6). An infant would ingest in a day on average 9.6% (8.0 × 900/750)* and at maximum 34.3% (28.6 × 900/750)* of the weight-adjusted quantity of caffeine taken by the mother per day (7). Using the concentrations reported in (11), and infant would ingest on average 5.2% (4.3 × 900/750)* and at maximum 18.8% (15.7 × 900/750 mg) of the weight adjusted maternal caffeine consumption.

DATA ON THE INFANT

Saliva caffeine concentrations in infants were < 0.05–0.75 mg/l (5). The infant of the mother reported in reference (6) was restless and irritable. One infant is described as 'having the jitters' while breast-feeding from his mother who drank large amounts of caffeine-containing drinks. No caffeine was detected in this infant's urine but the 'jitters' ceased when his mother stopped drinking excess caffeine (11). In other studies no caffeine was detected in infants' urine (10) or plasma (5) and there was no change in their heart rates and sleeping times (5). Infants however have been reported to absorb only a small proportion of the caffeine ingested (11) and this may contribute to the low incidence of reported side effects.

ASSESSMENT AND RECOMMENDATIONS

The risk to the suckling infant from maternal ingestion of caffeine is increased by slow elimination of the substance especially from the neonate. Synergistic effects may occur if the mother is also receiving a theophylline-containing medication. Breast-feeding may be regarded as safe when maternal caffeine intake is low but caffeine-related effects may occur in suckling infants whose mothers ingest large quantities (>8 cups of coffee per day) of the substance.

* An explanation of the calculation (s) appears on pp. 71–72.

REFERENCES

1. Parsons WD, Neims AH (1981) Prolonged half-life of caffeine in healthy term newborn infants. *J. Pediatr., 98,* 640–641.
2. Aldridge A, Aranda JV, Neims AH (1979) Caffeine metabolism in the newborn. *Clin. Pharmacol. Ther., 25,* 445–447.
3. Le Guennes JC, Billon B (1987) Delay in caffeine elimination in breast-fed infants. *Pediatrics, 79,* 264–268.
4. Tyrala EE, Dodson WE (1979) Caffeine secretion into breast milk. *Arch. Dis. Child, 54,* 787–789.
5. Ryu JE (1985) Caffeine in human milk and serum of breast-fed infants. *Dev. Pharmacol. Ther., 8,* 329–337.
6. Bailey DN, Welbert RT, Naylor AJ (1982) A study of salicylate and caffeine excretion in the breast milk of two nursing mothers. *J. Anal. Toxicol., 6,* 64–68.
7. Hildebrandt R, Gundert-Remy U (1983) Lack of pharmacological active saliva levels of caffeine in breast-fed infants. *Pediatr. Pharmacol., 3,* 237–244.
8. Blanchard J, Weber CW, Shearer L-E (1992) Methylxanthine levels in breast milk of lactating women of different ethnic and socioeconomic classes. *Biopharm. Drug Dis., 13,* 187–196.
9. Stavchansky S, Combs A, Sagraves R, Delgado M, Josh A (1988) Pharmacokinetics of caffeine in breast milk and plasma after single oral administration of caffeine to lactating mothers. *Biopharm. Drug Dis., 9,* 285–299.
10. Berlin CM, Denson HM, Daniel CH, Ward RM (1984) Disposition of caffeine in milk, saliva and plasma of lactating women. *Paediatrics., 73,* 59–63.
11. Rivera-Calimlim L (1977). Drugs in breast milk. *Drug Ther., 7,* 59–63.
12. Oo CY, Burgio DE, Kuhn RC, Desai N, McNamara PJ (1995) Pharmacokinetics of caffeine and its demethylated metabolites in lactation: predictions of milk to serum concentration ratios. *Pharmaceu.l Res., 12,* 313–316.

CANNABIS

GENERAL

Cannabis is an extract of the plant *Cannabis sativa*. The resin that is scraped off the plants is known as hashish and preparations that are smoked are called marihuana. The principal psychoactive component is tetrahyrdocannabinol (THC). Apart from their social use which is usually illegal, cannabinoids have been used to treat glaucoma and as antiemetics. Cannabis is poorly absorbed from the adult gastrointestinal tract and is 97% bound to plasma proteins. It is metabolised to 11-hydroxy-Δ^9-THC which is pharmacologically active and to 8,11-dehydroxy-Δ^9-THC which is inactive. The plasma half-life of THC is 20–36 h.

EVALUATION OF DATA

Passage of cannabis into human milk has been reported as follows:

Treatment conditions	Concentration (μg/l)		Milk/ serum ratio	Maximum observed milk conc. (μg/l)	Absolute dose to infant (μg/kg/day)		Ref.
Dose × Frequency × Duration; Route; No. of patients; Lactation stage	Milk	serum			Ave	Max	
1 pipe/d × LT; inhal.; 1; 7–8 months	105	–	–	–	–	–	(1)
7 pipes/d × LT; inhal.; 1; 7–8 months	340 (4)	–	–	–	–	–	(1)
	60.3 (1.1)	7.2 (2.5)	8.4 (0.4)	60.3 (1.1)		9.1	(1)

LT, long term. The figures in parentheses refer to 11-hydroxy-Δ^9-THC. The upper two lines of the table refer to random samples and the interval between smoking and sampling is not stated. The bottom line of the table gives concentrations 1 h after smoking.

RELATIVE DOSE IN MILK

A relative dose cannot be calculated as the quantity of cannabis taken by the mother is not known. As an illustration, however, 11 men who each smoked a single marihuana cigarette (mean THC content of 13 mg) had plasma THC concentrations in the range 33–118 μg/l (mean 77 μg/l) which includes the concentration recorded by the second mother (60.3 μg/l). On this basis the amount of cannabis to which the infant would be exposed in a feed is 0.8% (60.3 × 180/13 000)* of the THC content of a marihuana cigarette.

* An explanation of the calculation (s) appears on pp. 71–72.

DATA ON THE INFANT

Sixty-eight infants who were exposed to marijuana in maternal milk were matched with 68 infants who were not so exposed in respect of relevant factors including tobacco and alcohol use. Exposure to marijuana in milk was associated with a decrease in motor development at one month postpartum (3).

ASSESSMENT AND RECOMMENDATIONS

The estimate of the relative dose of cannabis to the suckling infant is low. Nevertheless, the possibility that cannabis ingested in milk may affect infant motor development strongly suggests that a mother who is exposed to the substance should not breast-feed.

REFERENCES

1. Perez-Reyes M, Wall ME (1982) Presence of Δ^9-tetrahydrocannabinol in human milk. *N. Engl. J. Med., 307,* 819–820.
2. Ohlsson A, Lindgren J-E, Wahlen A, Agurell S, Hollister LE, Gillespie HK (1890) Plasma delta-9-tetrahydrocannabinol concentrations and clinical effects after oral and intravenous administration and smoking. *Clin. Pharmacol. Ther., 28,* 409–416.
3. Astley S, Little RE (1990) Maternal marijuana use during lactation and infant development at one year. *Neurotoxicol. Teratol., 12*, 161–168.

DIATRIZOATE MEGLUMINE, DIATRIZOATE SODIUM

GENERAL

Meglumine and sodium salts of diatrizoic acid are water-soluble ionic contrast agents used for radiological imaging. Diatrizoate is poorly absorbed from the adult gastrointestinal tract, negligibly bound to plasma proteins and eliminated unchanged in the urine. The plasma half-life is 100 min.

EVALUATION OF DATA

A woman 7 weeks after delivery was given Urografin 370, 50 ml (a mixture of sodium and methylglutamine salts of diatrizoic acid and iodine 370 mg/ml; total weight of mixed salts 38.0 g) by rapid iv injection; milk samples were collected 6, 9, 13, and 16.5 h later. Diatrizoate could not be detected in these samples using a spectrophotometric technique which had a limit of sensitivity of 2 mg/l.

RELATIVE DOSE IN MILK

If the milk concentration was less than 2 mg/l, the amount of diatrizoate that a suckling infant would ingest in a feed would be less than 0.01% (2 × 180/29 000)* of the weight-adjusted maternal single dose (1).

DATA ON THE INFANT

No data are available.

ASSESSMENT OF DATA

Limited data suggests that the risk to the suckling infant of administering diatrizoate to its mother is low because the quantity of the contrast medium that passes into milk is small. Breast-feeding is probably safe.

REFERENCES

1. Fitz-John TP, Williams DG, Laker MF, Owen JP (1982) Intravenous urography during lactation. *Br. J. Radiol., 55,* 603–605.

* An explanation of the calculation (s) appears on pp. 71–72.

ETHANOL

GENERAL

Ethanol is widely available as a social drug. It is well absorbed from the adult gastrointestinal tract. The elimination kinetics of alcohol are zero order at concentrations encountered in social use and the average rate of ethanol metabolism in adults who are occasional drinkers is 6–8 mg/h. Ethanol is metabolised by oxidative pathways in the liver, and the products are excreted in the breath and urine.

EVALUATION OF DATA

Passage of ethanol into human milk has been reported as follows:

Treatment conditions Dose × Frequency × Duration; Route; No. of patients; Lactation stage	Concentration (mg/l)		Milk/plasma ratio	Maximum observed milk conc. (mg/l)	Absolute dose to infant (mg/kg/day)		Ref.
	Milk	Plasma			Ave	Max	
0.6 g/kg × 1/d × 1 d; p.o.; 12; 4–41 d	777 (1 h)	840 (1 h)	0.93	–		117	(1)
0.55 g/day; LT; p.o; 6; 3–7 months	84 (1 h)	90 (1 h)	0.93	116	12.6	17.4	(2)
29.8 g/day; LT; p.o.; 5; 3–7 months	274 (1 h)	261 (1 h)	0.95	410	41.1	61.5	(2)
0.3 g/kg × 1/d × 1 d; p.o.; 12; 25–216 d	630 (1 h)	–	–	–	–	94.5	(3)

The milk and plasma concentrations (1) in were the mean values at the times stated for all the subjects. The metabolite acetaldehyde was measured in plasma but was not detected in milk. Study (2) was carried out in Mexican Indian lactating women who regularly drank pulque, a beverage containing 3% ethanol. Peak milk and plasma concentrations were observed at 1 h (1–3).

RELATIVE DOSE IN MILK

A suckling infant would ingest in a feed at maximum 3.9% (777 × 180/600 × 60)* to 6.3% (630 × 180/300 × 60)* of the weight-adjusted quantity taken by the mother on a single occasion (1).

DATA ON THE INFANT

No cases of fetal alcohol syndrome were found in offspring of mothers who took alcohol during pregnancy and lactation (2). Infants consumed less milk following

* An explanation of the calculation (s) appears on pp. 71–72.

maternal ingestion of alcohol, a finding attributed to the sensory characteristics or the pharmacological actions of alcohol on the infant and/or mother (3). An infant at four months of age was found to have pseudo-Cushing's syndrome, thought to be due to his mother's ethanol intake (4). Ethanol ingested through breast milk has been reported to have a slight but significant effect on motor development, but not mental development, in breast-fed infants (5)

ASSESSMENT AND RECOMMENDATIONS

The risk to the suckling infant of a single drink of ethanol ingested by its mother is low on the basis that the quantity that passes into milk is small. Regular intake by breast-feeding women of even one alcoholic drink per day does appear to have an effect on infant development. Thus occasional partaking of alcohol may be safe but regular drinking should be regarded as unsafe.

REFERENCES

1. Kesäniemi YA (1974) Ethanol and acetaldehyde in the milk and peripheral blood of lactating women after ethanol administration. *J. Obstet. Gynaecol. Br. Commum., 81*, 84–86.
2. Flores-Huerta S, Hernandez-Montes H, Argote RM, Villalpando S (1992) Effects of ethanol consumption during pregnancy and lactation on the outcome and postnatal growth of the offspring. *Ann. Nutr. Metab., 36,* 121–128.
3. Mennella JA, Beauchamp GK (1991) The transfer of alcohol to human milk: Effect of flavor and the infant's behaviour. *N. Engl. J. Med.,* 325, 981–985.
4. Binkiewicz A, Robinson MJ, Senior B (1978) Pseudo-Cushings syndrome caused by alcohol in breast milk. *J. Paediatr., 93*, 965–967.
5. Little RE, Anderson KW, Ervin CH, Worthington-Roberts B, Clarren SK (1989) Maternal alcohol use during breast-feeding and infant mental and motor development at one year. *N. Engl. J. Med., 321*, 425–430.

FLUORESCEIN

GENERAL

Fluorescein is used in ophthalmology for its fluorescent properties, to study retinal blood flow and vascular permeability. It is given by i.v. injection, undergoes metabolism to a glucuronide and is eliminated by the kidneys. The plasma half-life is <1 h. Fluorescein may be used in children. A phototoxic reaction followed administration of fluorescein to a premature infant (1).

EVALUATION OF DATA

A 29-year-old woman developed acute loss of central vision shortly after premature delivery of twins. To elucidate the cause she received a 5 ml i.v. injection of 10% fluorescein sodium; the concentration of fluorescein in her breast-milk was 372 μg/l 6 h later and declined with a half-life of 62 h to 170 62 μg/l at 76 h (2).

RELATIVE DOSE IN MILK

A suckling infant would ingest in a feed at maximum 0.1 % (0.372 × 180/500)* of the weight-adjusted maternal single dose of fluorescein.

DATA ON THE INFANT

No data are available on fluorescein received by the infant in breast milk.

ASSESSMENT OF DATA

The data are confined to one case report and the long half-life of fluorescein in breast-milk is noted. The estimated quantity of fluorescein in a feed of breast-milk is orders of magnitude less than that which caused phototoxicity (1). Thus the risk to the suckling infant of administering fluorescein to its mother appears to be low on the basis that the quantity of drug that passes into milk is small. Breast-feeding is probably safe.

REFERENCES

1. Kearns GL, Williams BJ, Timmons OD (1985) Fluorescein phototoxicity in a premature infant. *J. Pediatr., 107,* 433–435.
2. Macguire AM, Bennett J (1988) Fluorescein elimination in human breast milk. *Arch. Ophthalmol., 106,* 718–719.

* An explanation of the calculation (s) appears on pp. 71–72.

IODAMIDE

GENERAL

Iodamide is a water-soluble ionic contrast medium used for radiological imaging. Its is rapidly and almost completely excreted in urine.

EVALUATION OF DATA

A woman 12 weeks after delivery was given Uromicro 340, 50 ml (a mixture of the sodium and methylglutamine salts of iodamide and iodine 340 mg/ml; total mixed salts 30.2 g) by rapid i.v. injection; milk samples were collected 4 and 9 h later. Iodamide could not be identified in these samples using a spectrophotometric technique that had a limit of sensitivity of 2 mg/l.

RELATIVE DOSE IN MILK

If the milk concentration was less than 2 mg/l, the amount of iodamide that a suckling infant would ingest in a feed would be less than 0.02% (2 × 180/350 × 50)* of the weight-adjusted maternal single dose of iodamide (1).

DATA ON THE INFANT

No data are available.

ASSESSMENT OF DATA

Limited data suggest that the risk to the suckling infant of administering iodamide to its mother is low because the quantity of drug that passes into milk is small. Breast-feeding is probably safe.

REFERENCES

1. Fitz-John TP, Williams DG, Laker MF, Owen JP (1982) Intravenous urography during lactation. *Br. J. Radiol.*, *55*, 603–605.

* An explanation of the calculation (s) appears on pp. 71–72.

IOHEXOL

GENERAL

Iohexol is a water-soluble non-ionic contrast medium used for radiological examinations. It is usually given i.v. or intra-arterially. Iohexol is not bound to plasma proteins and is excreted unchanged in urine within 24 h. Its plasma half-life is 2 h.

EVALUATION OF DATA

Passage of iohexol into human milk has been reported as follows:

Treatment conditions — Dose × Frequency × Duration; Route; No. of patients; Lactation stage	Concentration (mg/l) Milk	Plasma	Milk/plasma ratio	Maximum observed milk conc. (mg/l)	Absolute dose to infant (mg/kg/day) Ave	Max	Ref.
755 mg/kg × 1/d × 1 d; i.v.; 3; 1 week-14 months	24.6	–	–	35.0	3.7	–	(1)

Milk samples were taken 1.5, 3, 6, 24 and 48 h, and paired blood and milk samples 5, 15, 30 and 45 min after i.v. administration. The milk concentration quoted was the average calculated from the area under the milk concentration curve from 0–24 h. After 24 h the milk concentration was very low. The maximum concentration in milk was the average peak value for the three mothers and was observed 3–6 h after the contrast medium was given.

RELATIVE DOSE IN MILK

Assuming a maternal weight of 60 kg, the amount of iohexol that a suckling infant would ingest in a feed is at maximum 0.1% (35 × 180/755 × 60)* of the weight-adjusted maternal single dose. As iohexol would be used only once per day it is appropriate in this case also to estimate a daily dose. Thus a suckling infant would ingest in a day on average 0.5% (24.6 × 900/755 × 60)* and at maximum 0.7% (35 × 900/755 × 60)* of the weight-adjusted maternal daily dose. The infant dose is 1294 mg/kg and a suckling infant would receive at maximum 0.1% (35 × 3/1294)* of this in a feed (1).

DATA ON THE INFANT

Only one of the infants in the study was allowed to breast-feed and no notable effect was observed. Doses of up to 2 g/kg of iohexol have been given to infants weighing less than 6.5 kg (2).

* An explanation of the calculation (s) appears on pp. 71–72.

ASSESSMENT OF DATA

The risk to the suckling infant of administering iohexol to its mother is low on the basis that the quantity of drug that passes into milk is small and its absorption from the gastrointestinal tract is poor. Breast-feeding may be regarded as safe. Should hypersensitivity to iohexol be an issue, then the risk may be lessened by delaying breast-feeding for 24 h after the dose.

REFERENCE

1. Nielsen ST, Matheson I, Rasmussen JN, Skinnemoen K, Andrew E, Hafsahl G (1987) Excretion of iohexol and metrizoate in breast milk. *Acta Radiol.*, *28*, 523–526.
2. Jorulf H (1983) Iohexol compared with diatrizoate in pediatric urography. *Acta Radiol., Suppl. 366*, 42.

IOPANOIC ACID

GENERAL

Iopanoic acid is a lipid-soluble contrast medium used mainly to visualise the biliary tract. It is variably absorbed from the adult gastrointestinal tract and is 79% bound to plasma proteins. Iopanoic acid is conjugated with glucuronic acid in the liver and about 65% is excreted in the bile. Some 50% of the total dose is eliminated in 24 h.

EVALUATION OF DATA

Passage of iopanoic acid in human milk was reported by Holmdahl (1) in mothers undergoing cholecystography who received on average 2940 mg of iodine in the contrast medium. Milk production during normal suckling for up to 29 h was estimated by weighing the babies and measuring the expressed milk; the content of iodine in milk reached a maximum after about 15 h an on average 17.0 mg (range 6.7–29.9 mg) was recovered.

RELATIVE DOSE IN MILK

Assuming an infant weight of 5 kg and a maternal weight of 60 kg, the amount of iodine ingested by the infants was on average 6.9% (17 × 60 × 100/294 × 5)* of the weight-adjusted maternal dose.

DATA ON THE INFANT

Iopanoic acid was given to 21 mothers who breast-fed their infants. No reactions to the contrast medium were observed (1).

ASSESSMENT OF DATA

The risk to the suckling infant of administering iopanoic acid to its mother appears to be low on the basis that the quantity of contrast medium that passes into milk is small. Breast-feeding is proabaly safe but exposure of the infant may be limited by delaying breast-feeding for 24 h.

REFERENCES

1. Holmdahl KH (1956) Cholecystography during lactation. *Acta Radiol.*, *45*, 305–307.

* An explanation of the calculation (s) appears on pp. 71–72.

METRIZAMIDE

GENERAL

Metrizamide is a water-soluble non-ionic contrast medium used mainly for myelography. After intra-thecal or subarachnoid administration metrizamide is absorbed into the blood and the unchanged substance is excreted rapidly in the urine. The plasma half-life is 10 h (1).

EVALUATION OF DATA

Passage of metrizamide into human milk has been reported following cervical myelography (1). Metrizamide 5.06 g was injected into the subarachnoid space of a 38-year-old woman and milk, blood and urine samples were collected from her at intervals for 48 h. The blood concentration of metrizamide reached a peak of 32.9 mg/l at 6 h after dosing and was 2.7 mg/l at 48 h. By 24 h 68% of the dose of metrizamide had been recovered in the urine. The milk concentration-time profile was not defined but the cumulative excretion of metrizamide in milk increased linearly with time and amounted to 1.1 mg by 44.3 h. The volume of milk collected from the mother was not stated.

RELATIVE DOSE IN MILK

If the volume of milk that contained 1.1 mg of metrizamide represented normal infant requirements during the period of collection and the maternal and infant weights are assumed to be 60 kg and 5 kg respectively, then the total ingested by a suckling infant would be 0.3% (1.1 × 60 × 100/5060 × 5)* of the weight-adjusted maternal dose of metrizamide (1).

DATA ON THE INFANT

No data are available.

ASSESSMENT AND RECOMMENDATIONS

Limited data suggest that the risk to the suckling infant of administering metrizamide to its mother is low on the basis that the quantity of drug that passes into milk is small. Breast-feeding is probably safe.

REFERENCES

1. Ilett KF, Hackett LP, Paterson JW (1981) Excretion of metrizamide in milk. *Br. J. Radiol., 54,* 537–538.

* An explanation of the calculation (s) appears on pp. 71–72.

METRIZOIC ACID

GENERAL

Metrizoic acid is a water-soluble ionic contrast medium used for radiological examinations. It is given i.v. metrizoic acid does not bind significantly to plasma proteins and is excreted unchanged in the urine within 24 h of administration. The plasma half-life is 2 h.

EVALUATION OF DATA

Passage of metrizoic acid into human milk has been reported as follows:

Treatment conditions — Dose × Frequency × Duration; Route; No. of patients; Lactation stage	Concentration (mg/l)		Milk/ plasma ratio	Maximum observed milk conc. (mg/l)	Absolute dose to infant (mg/kg/day)		Ref.
	Milk	Plasma			Ave	Max	
37.7 g × 1/d × 1 d; i.v.; 2; 1 week-4 months	11.4	–	–	14	1.7	2.1	(1)

The values quoted were the averages for the 2 mothers. The milk concentration was derived from the area under the concentration-time curve for 24 h after dosing. The maximum milk concentration was attained 3–6 h after the dose.

RELATIVE DOSE IN MILK

A suckling infant would ingest in a feed at maximum 0.1% (14 × 180/37 700)* of the weight-adjusted maternal single dose of metrizoic acid (1).

DATA ON THE INFANT

No data are available.

ASSESSMENT OF DATA

The risk to the suckling infant of administering metrizoic acid to its mother is low on the basis that the quantity of drug that passes into milk is small and the contrast medium is poorly absorbed from the gastrointestinal tract. Nevertheless, exposure

* An explanation of the calculation (s) appears on pp. 71–72.

of the infant to metrizoic acid may be diminished by delaying nursing for 12 h after the injection. Breast-feeding may be regarded as safe.

REFERENCES

1. Nielsen ST, Matheson I, Rasmussen JN, Skinnemoen K, Andrew E, Hafsahl G (1987) Excretion of iohexol and metrizoate in breast milk. *Acta Radiol., 28,* 523–526.

NICOTINE

GENERAL

Nicotine is the addictive component of cigarette smoke and is rapidly absorbed from the lungs and buccal mucosa. It is available in patch and chewing gum formulations to assist persons who wish to give up the smoking habit. Nicotine is a relatively strong base that is poorly absorbed from the stomach at acid pH but is well absorbed from the intestine. It is 5% bound to plasma proteins. In the adult 85% is metabolised by the liver, and the plasma half-life is 75 min. One of the products is cotinine which has similar pharmacological actions to nicotine but a longer half-life (6–30 h). The presence of cotinine in the blood is frequently used to identify smokers. Infants born to mothers who smoke during pregnancy tend to have a lower birth weight and higher mortality than those born to non-smokers. Smokers wean their infants significantly earlier than non-smokers (1).

EVALUATION OF DATA

Passage of nicotine into human milk has been reported as follows:

Treatment conditions: No. of cigarettes smoked per day; no. of patients; Lactation stage	Concentration (μg/l) Milk	Concentration (μg/l) Plasma	Milk/plasma ratio	Maximum observed milk conc. (μg/l)	Absolute dose to infant (μg/kg/day) Ave	Absolute dose to infant (μg/kg/day) Max	Ref.
10–30; 9; ?	91	–	–	512	13.6	77.0	(2)
1–20; 10; 1–10 d	35	–	–	102	5.3	15.0	(3)
5–40; 23; 1–12 weeks	2–62	1–28	2.92	62	4.4	9.3	(4,5)
	(12–222)	(16–330)	(0.78)	(222)	(12.0)	(49.5)	

Most studies have been conducted in women smoking a defined number of cigarettes per day but the actual exposure of the mothers to nicotine has not been known. Plasma concentration-time profiles were defined in reference (4) and were concurrent, the half-life in serum being 81 min and in milk 95 min. The table gives the average (2,3) or the range (4,5) of concentrations of nicotine or cotinine (in brackets) in milk and plasma. The maximum observed milk concentrations are the highest values recorded in individuals.

RELATIVE DOSE IN MILK

Variation in the nicotine content of cigarettes and in smoking habits make for difficulty in estimating the daily exposure of mother to nicotine. Nevertheless, the data indicate that a 5 kg infant can receive up to 385 μg (77 × 5) of nicotine daily in breast milk (2). If the nicotine content of a cigarette is taken to be 10 mg (6) then a suckling infant would be exposed to the equivalent of 0.0385 of a cigarette per day;

adjusted for an assumed maternal weight of 60 kg the infant exposure is equivalent to 0.46 (0.0385 × 60/5) of a cigarette per day. Breast milk of mothers passively exposed to cigarette smoke has also been shown to contain nicotine (1–7 μg/l) and cotinine (2–10 μg/l) (7).

DATA ON THE INFANT

Nicotine and cotinine can be detected in very low concentrations in infant plasma and urine (5). The ratio of nicotine in the infant's plasma to that in maternal plasma was 0.06 (0.15 for cotinine). In children aged 18 months, the number of respiratory infections increased when the mother smoked and there was a decrease in breast-feeding duration (8).

ASSESSMENT AND RECOMMENDATIONS

The best advice for mothers wishing to breast-feed their infants is not to smoke.

REFERENCES

1. Anderson AN, Lund-Anderson C, Larsen JF, Christensen NJ, Legros JJ, Louis F, Angelo H, Molin J (1982) Supressed prolactin but normal neurophysin levels in cigarette smoking, breast-feeding women. *Clin. Endocrinol., 17*, 363–368.
2. Ferguson BB, Wilson DJ, Schaffner W (1976) Determination of nicotine concentrations in human milk. *Am. J. Dis. Child., 130.*, 837–839.
3. Trundle JI, Skellern GG (1983) Gas chromatographic determination of nicotine in human breast milk. *J. Clin. Hosp. Pharmacy, 8*, 289–293.
4. Luck W, Nau H (1984) Nicotine and cotinine concentrations in serum and milk of nursing mothers. *Br. J. Clin. Pharmacol., 18,* 9–15.
5. Luck W, Nau H (1984) Exposure of the foetus, neonate and nursed infant to nicotine and cotinine from maternal smoking. *N. Engl. J. Med., 311*, 672.
6. Benowitz NL, Hall SM, Herning RI, Jacob P, Jones RT, Osman A-L (1983) Smokers of low-yield cigarettes do not consume less nicotine. *N. Engl. J. Med., 309*, 139–142.
7. Hardee GE, Stewart T, Capomacchia AC (1983) Tobacco smoke xenobiotic compound appreance in mothers milk after involuntary smoke exposure. *Toxicol. Lett., 15, 109–112.*
8. Hakansson A, Carlsson B (1992) Maternal cigarette smoking and respiratory tract infections in infancy. *Scand. J. Prim. Health Care, 10,* 60–65.

AUROTHIOGLYCANIDE

GENERAL

Aurothioglycanide (sodium aurothiomalate) is a gold compound used in the management of rheumatoid arthritis; it is given by intramuscular injection. Aurothioglycanide is quickly absorbed and becomes bound to plamsa proteins. It is widely distributed in the body and may be detected in tissues for years after administration has ceased. Excretion in the urine accounts for 70%, and the remainder appears in the faeces. The initial half-life in plasma is 5 days and the terminal half-life is 250 days. Adverse effects may occur in bone marrow and kidney.

EVALUATION OF DATA

Passage of aurothiomalate into human milk has been reported as follows:

Treatment conditions	Concentration (mg/l)		Milk/ serum ratio	Maxi- mum observed milk conc. (mg/l)	Absolute dose to infant (mg/kg/day)		Ref.
Dose × Frequency × Duration; Route; No. of patients; Lactation stage	Milk	Serum			Ave	Max	
50 mg × 1/week × 12 –14 weeks; i.m.; 1; 16–18 weeks	0.021–0.065 (C_{SS} 0.041)	1.62–5.22 (C_{SS} 4.05)	0.007–0.014 (C_{SS} 0.01)	0.065	0.03	0.01	(1)
50 mg × 1/week × 7 weeks; i.m.; 1; 15 months	0.040, 0.022	–	–	0.04			(2)
10 mg × 1/month × 2 y; i.m., 1, 7–85 d	0.015–0.03	0.459–1.133	0.02–0.07	0.03		0.0045	(3)
50 mg over 11 days; i.m., 1; several weeks	<0.001–0.185	0.16–1.78		0.185		0.03	(4)
70 mg over 72 h; i.m.; 1; ?	<0.001–0.153	0.185–3.33	0.02–0.20 (ave. 0.1)	0.153		0.02	(4)

The milk and serum values quoted in (1) are the range recorded, and the concentration at steady-state (C_{SS}). Reference (2) gives two values 66 h and 7 days after gold injections. The range of milk and serum values for 19 days after an injection of aurothioglycanide 10 mg is quoted in (3). The values in (4) are considerably higher than in the other references and probably reflect 2 or 3 doses given over a short period. Data from (1), (3) and (4) indicate that the serum and milk concentration-time profiles are not concurrent.

RELATIVE DOSE IN MILK

If it is assumed that the maximum absolute dose to the infant of 0.0045 mg/kg/day (3) applied over 29 days (the time between doses) then the quantity ingested would have been 0.131 mg/kg (4.5 × 29). The 10 mg dose of aurothioglycanide given to the mother contains 4.6 mg of elemental gold which represents 0.077 mg/kg (assuming a maternal weight of 60 kg). The infant consequently would receive 170.1% (0.131 × 100/0.077) of the weight adjusted maternal dose. Using the C_{ss} value 0.041 mg/l and the weekly dosing regimen in reference (1), an infant would ingest in a day 11.2% (0.041 × 900/(50 × 0.46/7)* of the weight adjusted maternal daily dose.

DATA ON THE INFANT

Absorption of gold by the infant is shown by a serum concentration of 51 μg/l (3). No adverse effects are recorded in the infants reported in (1), (2) and (3) who were breast-fed throughout gold therapy. Transplacental passage of gold is indicated by the report of a mother who received aurothioglycanide 100 mg i.m. monthly throughout pregnancy and at birth had a venous gold concentration of 3.93 mg/l when the umbilical cord serum concentration was 2.25 mg/l (5). The infant had no obvious major or minor congenital abnormalities.

ASSESSMENT AND RECOMMENDATIONS

While the estimates from published case reports vary, it is clear that gold passes into breast milk in quantities greater than those observed for the majority of drugs. On the basis of quantitative exposure therefore, the risk to the suckling infant would be sufficient to advise against breast-feeding. It is also noted that three infants were exposed to gold in breast milk for considerable lengths of time, and one during pregnancy, without apparent adverse effects. This appears to be an instance where decision on whether or not to breast-feed should be resolved in the light of the circumstances relevant to the individual case.

REFERENCES

1. Rooney TW, Lorber A, Veng-Pedersen P, Herman RA, Meehan R, Hade J, Hade A, Furst DE (1987) Gold pharmacokinetics in breast milk and serum of a lactating women. *J. Rheumatol., 14,* 1120–1122.
2. Bell RAF, Dale IM (1976) Gold secretion in maternal milk. *Arthritis Rheum., 19,* 1374.
3. Bennett PN, Humphries SJ, Osborne JP, Clarke AK, Taylor A (1990) Use of sodium aurothiomalate during lactation. *Br. J. Clin. Pharmacol., 29,* 777–779.
4. Ostensen M, Skavdal K, Myklebust G, Tomassen Y, Aabakke J (1986) Excretion of gold into human breast milk. *Eur. J. Clin. Pharmacol., 31,* 251–252.
5. Cohen DL, Orzel J, Taylor A (1981) Infants of mothers receiving gold therapy. *Arthritis Rheum., 24,* 104–105.

* An explanation of the calculation (s) appears on pp. 71–72.

AZAPROPAZONE

GENERAL

Azapropazone has analgesic, anti-inflammatory and antipyretic properties. It is used in musculoskeletal and joint disorders. Due to its uricosuric properties, it is also used in the management of acute gout. Azapropazone is well absorbed from the adult gastrointestinal tract and is 99% bound to plasma proteins. Some 60–70% of the dose is excreted unchanged in the urine and the remainder undergoes hepatic metabolism. The plasma half-life is 13 h.

EVALUATION OF DATA

Passage of azapropazone into human breast milk has been reported as follows:

Treatment conditions	Concentration (mg/l)		Milk/ plasma ratio	Maximum observed milk conc. (mg/l)	Absolute dose to infant (mg/kg/day)		Ref.
Dose × Frequency × Duration; Route; No. of patients; Lactation stage	Milk	Plasma			Ave	Max	
600 mg × 2/d × 5–10 d; i.v.; 4; 4–6 d.	2.44 (ave.)	23.4–209	–	5.43	–	0.82	(1)

Azapropazone was administered for pain relief, e.g. after episiotomy. Steady-state condition of dosing were attained. The table gives the average drug concentration in all milk samples collected for 12 h after dosing. When aggregated, this represented 0.13% of the dose. The maximum concentration was the highest figure recorded for an individual.

RELATIVE DOSE IN MILK

A suckling infant would ingest in a day at a maximum of 4.1% (5.43 × 900/1200)* of the weight-adjusted maternal daily dose.

DATA ON THE INFANT

The infants in (1) were not breast-fed.

ASSESSMENT AND RECOMMENDATIONS

The risk to the suckling infant of administering azapropazone to its mother is low on the basis that the quantity of drug that passes into milk is small. Breast-feeding may be regarded as safe.

* An explanation of the calculation (s) appears on pp. 71–72.

REFERENCES

1. Bald R, Bernbeck-Betthäuser EM, Spahn H, Mutschler E (1990) Excretion of azapropazone in human breast milk. *Eur. J. Clin. Pharmacol.*, *39*, 271–273.

BACLOFEN

GENERAL

Baclofen is used to relieve muscle spasm and acts mainly in the spinal cord. It is structurally similar to gamma-aminobutyric acid. Baclofen rapidly absorbed from the adult gastrointestinal tract and 30% is bound to plasma proteins; a small proportion is metabolised but most of the drug is eliminated unchanged in the urine. The plasma half-life is 4 h.

EVALUATION OF DATA

Passage of baclofen into human milk has been reported as follows:

Treatment conditions — Dose × Frequency × Duration; Route; No. of patients; Lactation stage	Concentration (μg/l) Milk	Plasma	Milk/plasma ratio	Maximum observed milk conc. (μg/l)	Absolute dose to infant (μg/kg/day) Ave	Max	Ref.
20 mg × 1/d × 1 d; p.o.; 1; 14 d	11–134	12–312	0.25–1.8	134	–	20.1	(1)

The patient was a woman with spastic paraplegia. The concentration-time profiles were defined over 20–26 h and were not concurrent; the milk to plasma ratio ranged from 0.25 to 1.8 with reversal of the ratio occurring at about 8 h. The table gives the range of concentrations. After a single dose, 22 μg of baclofen were found in 26 h of milk collection made by complete emptying of breasts at each sampling such that 395 ml milk were produced. The data are not sufficient accurately to estimate the dose in milk during prolonged treatment.

RELATIVE DOSE IN MILK

A suckling infant would ingest in a feed at maximum 1.2% (0.134 × 180/20)* of the weight-adjusted maternal single dose of baclofen (1).

DATA ON THE INFANT

No data are available.

ASSESSMENT AND RECOMMENDATIONS

Baclofen was studied in one lactating woman, given a single dose of appropriate amount for one day. The findings indicate that the risk to the suckling infant of

* An explanation of the calculation (s) appears on pp. 71–72.

administering baclofen to its mother is low on the basis that the quantity of drug that passes into milk is small. Nevertheless the data are too limited to make a general recommendation about the safety of breast-feeding for baclofen is used long term and there is no information as to its concentrations in milk and plasma under steady-state conditions of dosing.

REFERENCES

1. Erikssons G, Swahn CF (1981) Concentrations of baclofen in serum and breast milk from a lactating woman. *Scand. J. Clin. Lab. Invest., 41,* 185–187.

COLCHICINE

GENERAL

Colchicine is used to relieve the pain of acute gout, and painful serositis in familial Mediterranean fever. It may act by inhibiting mitosis in granulocytes. Colchicine is rapidly absorbed from the gastrointestinal tract and found in high concentrations in leukocytes, kidneys, liver and spleen. It is partly deacetylated in the liver and both the parent drug and metabolite are excreted predominantly in the bile. The plasma half-life is 30 min. Colchicine may cause abdominal discomfort and diarrhoea; a more serious complication is bone marrow suppression.

EVALUATION OF DATA

Passage of colchicine in human milk has been reported as follows:

Treatment conditions Dose × Frequency × Duration; Route; No. of patients; Lactation stage	Concentration (μg/l) Milk	 Plasma	Milk/ plasma ratio	Maximum observed milk conc. (μg/l)	Absolute dose to infant (μg/kg/day) Ave	 Max	Ref.
0.6 mg x 2/d x LT; p.o.; 1; 16–21 d	2.5	1	–	2.5	–	0.375	(1)

LT, long term. The mother received colchicine for familial Mediterranean fever. The quoted milk concentration was taken 50 h and the serum concentration 45 h after colchicine and were the maximum values recorded. The concentration-time profiles were not defined.

RELATIVE DOSE IN MILK

A suckling infant would ingest in a day maximum of 1.9 % (2.5 × 900/1200)* of the weight adjusted maternal daily dose.

DATA ON THE INFANT

The baby was breast-fed without any supplements and showed no adverse effects in the first six months of life.

ASSESSMENT AND RECOMMENDATIONS

The risk to the suckling infant of administering colchicine to its mother is low on

* An explanation of the calculation (s) appears on pp. 71–72.

the basis that the quantity of drug that passes into milk is small. The infant in the case quoted apparently suffered no ill effects. Nevertheless colchicine does have a significant toxicity profile and the data are considered too limited to make a general recommendation about the safety of colchicine received by the breast-fed infant.

REFERENCES

1. Milunsky JM, Milusnsky A (1991) Breast-feeding during colchicine therapy for familial Mediterranean fever. *J. Pediatr., 119,* 164.

FLUFENISAL

GENERAL

Flufenisal (flufenamic acid) is a non-steroidal antiinflammatory drug; its mechanism of action is that of the other members of the group, i.e. inhibition of prostaglandin synthesis. It is absorbed from the adult gastrointestinal tract and is highly bound to plasma proteins. Flufenisal is extensively metabolised and the plasma half-life is 4 h.

EVALUATION OF DATA

Passage of flufenisal into human milk has been reported as follows:

Treatment conditions Dose × Frequency × Duration; Route; No. of patients; Lactation stage	Concentration (mg/l) Milk	 Plasma	Milk/ plasma ratio	Maximum observed milk conc. (mg/l)	Absolute dose to infant (mg/kg/day) Ave	 Max	Ref.
200 mg × 3/d × 4 d; p.o.; 10; early postpartum	0.054 (2 d) 0.055 (3 d) 0.055 (4 d)	3.23 (2 d) 2.96 (3 d) 6.41 (4 d)	0.008–0.019 (2–4 d)	0,.12	0.008	0.018	(1)

Milk and blood samples were collected 2 h after the first daily dose on days 2, 3 and 4., i.e. the concentration-time profiles were not defined. The table gives average milk and plasma concentrations for the group. The maximum milk concentration is the highest value recorded in an individual. The plasma concentrations showed a wide range on any given day of analysis. The milk to plasma ratio was less on day 4 than on the preceding days.

RELATIVE DOSE IN MILK

A suckling infant would ingest in a day on average 0.1% (0.055 × 900/600)* and at maximum 0.2% (0.12 × 900/600)* of the weight-adjusted maternal daily dose of flufenisal (1).

DATA ON THE INFANT

No data are available.

* An explanation of the calculation (s) appears on pp. 71–72.

ASSESSMENT AND RECOMMENDATIONS

Flufenisal was studied in ten lactating women given multiple doses of appropriate amount for 4 days. Studies after longer exposure to the drug are needed reliably to establish that steady-state conditions apply in milk. Nevertheless the risk to the suckling infant of administering flufenisal to its mother is low on the basis that the quantity of drug that passes into milk is small. Breast-feeding may be regarded as safe.

REFERENCES

1. Buchanan RA, Eaton CJ, Koeff ST, Kinkel AW (1969) The breast milk excretion of flufenamic acid. *Curr. Ther. Res., 11*, 533–538.

FLURBIPROFEN

GENERAL

Flurbiprofen is a non-steroidal anti-inflammatory drug and its mechanism of action is that of other members of the group, i.e. inhibition of prostaglandin synthesis. It is well absorbed from the adult gastrointestinal tract and 99% is bound to plasma proteins; 25% is excreted unchanged in the urine and the remainder is metabolised. The plasma half-life is 3 h.

EVALUATION OF DATA

The passage of flurbiprofen into human breast milk has been reported as follows:

Treatment conditions: Dose × Frequency × Duration; Route; No. of patients; Lactation stage	Concentration (mg/l)		Milk/plasma ratio	Maximum observed milk conc. (mg/l)	Absolute dose to infant (mg/kg/day)		Ref.
	Milk	Plasma			Ave	Max	
50 mg × 4/d × 9 doses; p.o.; 12; 3–5 d	0.06–0.07	–	0.008–0.013	0.07	–	0.011	(1)
100 mg x 1 x 1 d; p.o.; 10; > 1 month	0.09	15.0	0.013–0.028	0.09	–	0.014	(2)

In reference (1) milk samples were taken during dosing and for 36 h after. Flurbiprofen was detected in only 3 milk samples and the table gives values for an individual patient. The value in milk of 0.006 mg/l (2 h after the first dose) corresponded to a plasma concentration of 7.09 mg/l and that of 0.007 mg/l (immediately before the second dose) to a plasma concentration of 2.57 mg/l. No drug was detected in the remaining samples (detection limit <0.0025 mg/l). Steady-state dosing conditions were achieved. In (2) milk and plasma samples were taken for 48 h after flurbiprofen. The values in the table are the average maximum for the group and the milk to plasma values are the range. Flurbiprofen was detected in only half the samples collected and no drug was detected 24 h after the dose.

RELATIVE DOSE IN MILK

A suckling infant would ingest in a day at maximum 0.3 % (0.07 × 900/200)* of the weight-adjusted maternal daily dose (1) or 0.2% (0.09 × 180/100)* of weight-adjusted maternal single dose of flurbiprofen (2).

DATA ON THE INFANT

No data are reported.

* An explanation of the calculation (s) appears on pp. 71–72.

ASSESSMENT AND RECOMMENDATIONS

The risk to the suckling infant of administering flurbiprofen to its mother is low on the basis that the quantity of milk that passes into milk is small. Breast-feeding during the immediate post partum period may be regarded as safe.

REFERENCES

1. Smith IJ, Hinson JL, Johnson VA, Brown RD, Cook SM, Whitt RT, Wilson JT (1989) Flurbiprofen in post-partum women: plasma and breast milk disposition. *J. Clin. Pharmacol., 29,* 174–184.
2. Cox SR, Forbes BA (1987) Excretion of flurbiprofen into breast milk. *Pharmacotherapy, 7,* 211–215.

HYDROXYCHLOROQUINE

GENERAL

Hydroxychloroquine is a 4-aminoquinoline that is used principally for its immunosuppressant action; it is also an antimalarial. It is a weak base. Hydroxychloroquine is well absorbed from the adult gastrointestinal tract, is 50% bound to plasma proteins and is widely distributed in tissues. It undergoes partial hepatic metabolism and prolonged excretion in the urine. The plasma half-life is about 18 days. Adverse effects after repeated dosing include retinopathy. See also chloroquine, p. 129.

EVALUATION OF DATA

Passage of hydroxychloroquine into human milk has been reported as follows:

Treatment conditions Dose × Frequency × Duration; Route; No. of patients; Lactation stage	Concentration (mg/l) Milk	Concentration (mg/l) Plasma	Milk/ plasma ratio	Maximum observed milk conc. (mg/l)	Absolute dose to infant (mg/kg/day) Ave	Absolute dose to infant (mg/kg/day) Max	Ref.
400 mg × 1/d × 6 weeks; p.o.; 1; 9 months	1.4 (2 h)	–	5.5	1.46 (2 h)	–	0.22	(1)
	1.09 (9.5 h)						
	1.09 (14 h)	0.2 (1.76 in blood)					
	0.85 (17.7 h)	(15.5 h)					
200 mg × 2/d × 4 d; p.o.; 1; 8 weeks	0.003 (15–24 h)	–	–	0.01 (39–48 h)	–	–	(2)

Reference (1) reports on a lactating mother who received hydroxychloroquine for systemic lupus erythematosus. One blood sample and serial milk samples were collected. Milk concentrations were similar at sampling times 14 and 17.7 h after successive doses as is consistent with steady-state conditions of dosing for a drug with a long half-life. The mean milk concentration was 1.12 mg/l. The whole blood concentration greatly exceeded that for plasma indicating that hydroxychloroquine distributes extensively into erythrocytes. The milk to plasma ratio was calculated for samples taken at 14 and 15.5 h respectively; that for milk to whole blood at these times was 0.6. The patient reported in reference (2) received hydroxychloroquine when her rheumatoid arthritis relapsed 8 weeks after completion of her pregnancy. Concentrations of hydroxychloroquine in plasma rose much more rapidly after dosing than did those in milk: when the plasma concentration was just less than 100 μg/l, that in milk was 3.2 μg/l. The milk to plasma ratio was much less than unity after about 2.5 days (5 doses) which is substantially before the presumed time at which steady-state dosing conditions were achieved in plasma, i.e. 5× the half-life. These two papers present contrasting results to emphasise: 1. Estimates of drug in milk may be particularly erroneous for a base with a long half-life if only early dosing periods are examined. 2. The theoretical milk to plasma ratio for a base is approached under steady-state dosing conditions.

RELATIVE DOSE IN MILK

As hydroxychloroquine sulphate (mol.wt. 434) was administered but the free base (mol. wt. 336) was assayed in plasma a factor of 1.3 (434/336) was introduced into the calculation. Thus a suckling infant would ingest in a day on average 3.3% (1.12 × 900 × 1.3/400)* and at maximum 4.3% (1.46 × 900 × 1.3/400x)* of the weight-adjusted maternal daily dose of hydroxychloroquine sulphate (1).

DATA ON THE INFANT

No specific effects were studied (1,2).

ASSESSMENT AND RECOMMENDATIONS

Hydroxychloroquine was studied in two lactating women given multiple doses of appropriate amount for 4 days and 6 weeks. Collected samples allowed definition of the milk and plasma concentration-time profiles only for the patient studied for 4 days (2). In the other patient the milk to plasma ratio of hydroxychloroquine under steady-state dosing conditions was greater than unity, consistent with its basic nature (1). Although the estimated dose to the infant in milk was small, the immaturity of infant tissues and probable low clearance of the drug warrant avoidance of its use as an immunosuppressant in breast-feeding women until further kinetic and response studies can be undertaken. There are no data on hydroxychloroquine in doses appropriate for the prophylaxis or treatment of malaria (but see chloroquine pp. 129–130).

REFERENCES

1. Nation RL, Hackett LP, Dusci LJ, Ilett KF (1984) Excretion of hydroxychloroquine in human milk. *Br. J. Clin. Pharmaolc., 17,* 368–369.
2. Ostensen M, Brown ND, Chiang PK, Aarbakke J (1985) Hydroxychloroquine in human breast milk. *Eur. J. Clin. Pharmacol., 28,* 357–358.

* An explanation of the calculation (s) appears on pp. 71–72.

IBUPROFEN

GENERAL

Ibuprofen is a non-steroidal antiinflammatory drug and its mechanism of action is that of other members of this group, i.e. inhibition of prostaglandin synthesis. Ibuprofen is well absorbed from the adult gastrointestinal tract, 99% bound to plasma proteins and its action is terminated by metabolism. The plasma half-life is 2 h.

EVALUATION OF DATA

Twelve lactating mothers who had undergone caesarean section delivery received ibuprofen 400 mg 6 hourly for 5 doses on the 3rd to the 5th day after delivery for postoperative pain. Blood and milk samples were collected before and at 9 time points during 36 h after dosing. The elimination half-lives of the drug in plasma after the first and fifth doses were 1.78 and 1.47 h respectively. Ibuprofen could not be assayed in any milk sample, the limit of validation being 1.0 mg/l (1). A lactating mother was treated for 3 weeks with ibuprofen 400 mg × 2/day. Milk and serum samples were collected during 8 h after a first daily dose. The peak serum concentration reached 18.2 mg/l at 2 h after dosing, but no drug was found in 6 milk samples, the lower limit of detection being 0.5 mg/l (2). The pharmacokinetic profile described for the patients under steady-state dosing conditions is an appropriate approach. The findings are consistent with those predicted for an acidic, highly protein bound drug.

RELATIVE DOSE IN MILK

Ibuprofen was not detected in breast milk (1, 2).

DATA ON THE INFANT

No data are available.

ASSESSMENT AND RECOMMENDATIONS

Ibuprofen was given to lactating mothers in multiple doses of appropriate amount for 1.5–18 days. Collected samples did allow definition of the serum concentration-time profile but ibuprofen was not detected in milk. Thus the risk to the suckling infant of administering ibuprofen to its mother is negligible on the basis that the quantity of drug that passes into milk is insignificant. Breast-feeding may be regarded as safe.

REFERENCES

1. Townsend RJ, Benedetti TJ, Erickson SH, Cengiz C, Gillespie WR, Gschwend J, Albert KS (1984) Excretion of ibuprofen into breast milk. *Am. J. Obstet. Gynecol., 149*, 184–186.
2. Weibert RT, Townsend RJ, Kaiser DG, Naylor AJ (1983) Lack of ibuprofen secretion into human milk. *Clin. Pharmacol., 1,* 457–458.

INDOMETACIN

GENERAL

Indometacin (indomethacin) is a non-steroidal anti-inflammatory drug and its mechanism of action is that of other members of this group, i.e. inhibition of prostaglandin synthesis. It may be given to neonates to close a patent ductus arteriosus. Indometacin is rapidly absorbed from the gastrointestinal tract and 99% bound to plasma proteins. Less than 20% is excreted unchanged in the urine and the remainder is metabolised. The plasma half-life is 4 h adults and 15–30 h in neonates.

EVALUATION OF DATA

Passage of indometacin into human milk has been reported as follows:

Treatment conditions — Dose × Frequency × Duration; Route; No. of patients; Lactation stage	Concentration (mg/l) Milk	Plasma	Milk/plasma ratio	Maximum observed milk conc. (mg/l)	Absolute dose to infant (mg/kg/day) Ave	Max	Ref.
75–300 mg/d for >48 h; p.o. or p.r.; 16; <10 d	<0.02–0.115	<0.02–1.97	<0.01–0.70	0.115	0.01	0.02	(1)

In reference (1) milk and plasma samples were taken 0.7–22.6 h after a dose of indometacin. Pre- and post-feed milk concentrations were not significantly different and the table gives the range of average pre- and post-feed values, and also the range of milk to plasma ratios. In an equilibrium dialysis system the milk to plasma ratio was found to be <0.01 (2).

RELATIVE DOSE IN MILK

A suckling infant would receive at maximum 1.0% (0.115 × 900/100)* of the weight-adjusted maternal daily dose.

DATA ON THE INFANT

No adverse effects were reported in the infants; plasma indometacin was below the limit of detection (0.02 mg/l) in 6 and was 0.047 mg/l in one (1). Seizures in a seven-day-old breast-fed infant were attributed to maternal indometacin (3). Indometacin (50–6000 mg) given antenatally for preterm labour was associated with complications in the neonatal period (4).

* An explanation of the calculation (s) appears on pp. 71–72.

ASSESSMENT AND RECOMMENDATIONS

The risk to the suckling infant of administering indometacin post-partum to its mother is low on the basis that the quantity of milk that passes into milk is small. A low degree of exposure through breast-feeding is supported by data on infant plasma. Administration of indometacin during breast-feeding in the immediate post partum period appears to be safe. There are no data on infant exposure following longer term administration.

REFERENCES

1. Lebedevs TH, Wojnar-Horton RE, Yapp P, Roberts MJ, Dusci LJ, Hackett LP, Ilett KF (1991) Excretion of indomethacin in breast milk. *Br. J. Clin. Pharmacol., 32,* 751–754.
2. Beaulac-Baillargeon L, Allard G (1993) Distribution of indomethacin in human milk and estimation of its milk to plasma ratio in vitro. *Br. J. Clin. Pharmacol., 36*, 413–416.
3. Eeg-Olofsson O, Malmros I, Elwin CE, Steen B (1978) Convulsions in a breast-fed infant after maternal indomethacin. *Lancet, ii*, 215.
4. Norton ME, Merrill J, Cooper BAB, Kuller JA, Clyman RI (1993) Neonatal complications after the administration of indomethacin for preterm labour *N. Engl. J. Med., 329*, 1602–1607.

INDOPROFEN

GENERAL

Indoprofen is a non-steroidal antiinflammatory drug and its mechanism of action is that of the other members of the group, i.e. inhibition of prostaglandin synthesis. Indoprofen is rapidly and completely absorbed from the adult gastrointestinal tract, 99% bound to plasma proteins and is excreted in the urine mainly as the glucuronic acid conjugate and partly as the unchanged drug. The plasma half-life is 4 h.

EVALUATION OF DATA

Passage of indoprofen into human milk has been reported as follows:

Treatment conditions	Concentration (mg/l)		Milk/ plasma ratio	Maximum observed milk conc. (mg/l)	Absolute dose to infant (mg/kg/day)		Ref.
Dose × Frequency × Duration; Route; No. of patients; Lactation stage	Milk	Plasma			Ave	Max	
200 mg × 1/d × 1 d; p.o.; 3; early postpartum	Trace– 0.68 (2–48 h)	9.4– 12.4 (2 h)	0.07 (No 1) <1 (No 2) 0.006 (No 3)	0.681 (No 1, 2 h)	–	0.102	(1)
200 mg × 4/d × 2 d; p.o.; 4; early postpartum	Trace– 0.49 (2–50 h)	0.8–23.8 (2–50 h)		0.488 (No 4, 50 h)	–	0.07	(1)
	0.069 (2 h)	5.3	0.013				
	0.272 (26 h)	10.3	0.026				
	0.316 (50 h)	15.7	0.02				

The mothers received indoprofen 200 mg either as a single dose or 6 hourly for 9 doses. The table gives the range of milk and plasma concentration for the 3 subjects and their individual milk to plasma ratios (assessed only at 2 h) at the stated times and indicates the variation after the single dose. The table also shows the range and average milk and plasma concentrations at the stated times after repeated dosing. The milk to plasma ratio still showed variation but the average was 0.013–0.026. The data do not allow definition of the milk and plasma concentration-time profiles.

RELATIVE DOSE IN MILK

A suckling infant would ingest in a feed at maximum 0.6% (0.681 × 180/200)* of the weight-adjusted maternal single dose. A suckling infant would ingest in a day on average 0.4% (0.316 × 900/800)* and at maximum 0.6% (0.488 × 900/800)* of the weight-adjusted maternal daily dose (1).

* An explanation of the calculation (s) appears on pp. 71–72.

DATA ON THE INFANT

No data are reported.

ASSESSMENT AND RECOMMENDATIONS

The risk to the suckling infant of administering indoprofen to its mother is low on the basis that the quantity of drug that passes into milk is small. Breast-feeding should be regarded as safe for short term use. Indoprofen may be given to women on a long term basis and data on more subjects receiving prolonged dosing are needed to express the true interindividual variation in both milk concentration and milk to plasma ratio.

REFERENCES

1. Lakings DB, Lizarraga C, Haggerty WJ, Williamson MJ (1979) High performance liquid chromatograpic microdetermination of indoprofen in human milk. *J. Pharmacol. Sci., 68,* 1113–1116.

KETOROLAC

GENERAL

Ketorolac is a non-steroidal antiinflammatory drug and its mechanism of action is that of the other members of the group, i.e. inhibition of prostaglandin synthesis. It is rapidly absorbed from the adult gastrointestinal tract and 99% bound to plasma proteins. About half of a dose is excreted unchanged and the remainder as metabolites in the urine. The plasma half-life is 5 h.

EVALUATION OF DATA

Passage of ketorolac into human milk has been reported as follows:

Treatment conditions: Dose × Frequency × Duration; Route; No. of patients; Lactation stage	Concentration (μg/l): Milk	Concentration (μg/l): Plasma	Milk/plasma ratio	Maximum observed milk conc. (μg/l)	Absolute dose to infant (μg/kg/day): Ave	Absolute dose to infant (μg/kg/day): Max	Ref.
10 mg × 4/d × 2 d; p.o.; 10; 2–8 d	7.9	221, 363	0.015–0.037	7.9		1.19	(1)

The milk concentration was above the limit of detection (5 μg/l) in only 6 mothers mainly on the second day; the value quoted is the highest individual concentration quoted. The concentration-time profile was defined for plasma and the table quotes the average peak values on the first and second days.

RELATIVE DOSE IN MILK

As ketorolac tromethamine (mol. wt. 376) was administered but ketorolac base (mol. wt. 255) was assayed, a factor of 1.48 (376/255) is introduced into the calculation. A suckling infant would ingest in a day a maximum of 0.3% (7.9 × 1.48 × 900/40 000)* of the weight-adjusted maternal daily dose.

DATA ON THE INFANT

No data are available as the infants were not breast-fed.

ASSESSMENT AND RECOMMENDATIONS

The risk to the suckling infant of administering ketorolac to its mother is low on the basis that the quantity of drug that passes into milk is small. Breast-feeding should

* An explanation of the calculation (s) appears on pp. 71–72.

be regarded as safe for short term use. Ketorolac may be given to women on a long term basis and data on more subjects receiving prolonged dosing are needed to express the true interindividual variation in both milk concentration and milk to plasma ratio.

REFERENCES

1. Wischnik A, Manth SM, Lloyd J, Bullingham R, Thompson JS (1989) The excretion of ketorolac tromethamine into breast milk after multiple oral dosing. *Eur. J. Clin. Pharmacol., 36,* 521–524.

MEFECLORAZINE

GENERAL

Mefeclorazine (mefenamic acid) is a non-steroidal anti-inflammatory drug and its mechanism of action is that of other members of this group, i.e. inhibition of prostaglandin synthesis. It is well absorbed from the adult gastrointestinal tract, is 99% bound to plasma proteins and its action is terminated by metabolism in the liver. The plasma half-life is 4 h. Diarrhoea is a notable side effect.

EVALUATION OF DATA

Passage of mefeclorazine into human milk has been reported as follows:

Treatment conditions: Dose × Frequency × Duration; Route; No. of patients; Lactation stage	Concentration (mg/l) Milk	Plasma	Milk/plasma ratio	Maximum observed milk conc. (mg/l)	Absolute dose to infant (mg/kg/day) Ave	Max	Ref.
500 mg (stat.) +	0.17 (2 d)	0.95 (2 d)	0.18	–	0.026	–	(1)
250 mg × 3/d × 4 d;	0.13 (3 d)	0.97 (3 d)	0.13	–	0.020	–	
p.o.; 2–4 d	0.21 (4 d)	0.91 (4 d)	0.23	0.66 (4 d)	0.032	0.099	

Milk and plasma samples were collected 2 h after the morning dose on days 2, 3 and 4. On any study day, the milk concentrations varied about 5 fold between subjects. The figures shown are average values and the maximum concentration is the highest value attained by an individual on any study day. As the drug has a short half-life, steady-state dosing conditions were approximated during the study. Possibly because of this and the fixed sampling time at 2 h after a dose, the milk to plasma ratio average showed a narrow range on days 2–4.

RELATIVE DOSE IN MILK

A suckling infant would ingest on the 4th day on average 0.3% (0.21 × 900/750)* and at maximum 0.8% (0.66 × 900/750)* of the weight-adjusted maternal daily dose of mefeclorazine (1).

DATA ON THE INFANT

On the 4th day and 1 h following the afternoon nursing the mean plasma mefeclorazine concentration in the infants was 0.08 mg/l and their mean urine concentration was 9.8 mg/l.

* An explanation of the calculation (s) appears on pp. 71–72.

ASSESSMENT AND RECOMMENDATIONS

Samples from lactating women given multiple doses of appropriate amount for 4 days did not allow definition of the milk and plasma concentration-time profiles. The intrinsic pharmacological properties of this drug warrant observations on the nursing infant, at least during and one week after treatment of the mother to define the interdose kinetic profile and to estimate values applicable to the population in general. Nevertheless the present data suggest that the risk to the suckling infant of administering mefeclorazine to its mother is low on the basis that the quantity of drug that passes into milk is small. Breastfeeding is probably safe but additional studies are needed on the kinetic profile in nursing mothers.

REFERENCES

1. Buchanan RA, Eaton CJ, Koeff ST, Kinkel AW (1969) The breast milk excretion of mefenamic acid. *Cur. Ther. Res., 10,* 592–597.

NAPROXEN

GENERAL

Naproxen is a non-steroidal anti-inflammatory drug and its mechanism of action is that of other members of this group, i.e. inhibition of prostaglandin synthesis. It is completely absorbed from the adult gastrointestinal tract and is 99% bound to plasma proteins. The action of naproxen is terminated by hepatic metabolism; the plasma half-life is 14 h.

EVALUATION OF DATA

Passage of naproxen into human milk has been reported as follows:

Treatment conditions: Dose × Frequency × Duration; Route; No. of patients; Lactation stage	Concentration (mg/l): Milk	Concentration (mg/l): Plasma	Milk/ plasma ratio	Maximum observed milk conc. (mg/l)	Absolute dose to infant (mg/kg/day): Ave	Absolute dose to infant (mg/kg/day): Max	Ref.
250 mg × 2/d × LT; p.o.; 1; 5 months	–	–	–	1.25	–	0.19	(1)
375 mg × 2/d × 3 weeks; p.o.; 1; 6 months	–	–	–	2.37	–	0.36	(1)

LT, long term. The mother had received naproxen 250 mg × 2/day for 8 months; milk and urine samples were collected from her over two consecutive dosing intervals. The dose was then raised to 375 mg × 2/day and 3 weeks later milk and urine samples were taken for 12 h after the 1st dose of the day. The table quotes the maximum concentrations attained on each dose. The elimination half-life of naproxen measured by its appearance in urine was 7.8–8.8 h for the lower dose. Lines drawn through the two terminal data points of drug concentration in milk indicated half-lives of 22.8 and 23.8 h. These larger values suggest that naproxen may accumulate in milk

RELATIVE DOSE IN MILK

A suckling infant would ingest in a day at maximum 2.8% (2.37 × 900/750)* of the weight-adjusted maternal daily dose (1). The paediatric daily dose is 10 mg/kg/day and a suckling infant would ingest in a day at maximum 3.6% (2.37 × 15/10)* of this (1).

DATA ON THE INFANT

The infant's urine contained 0.47 mg of naproxen in a dose interval when the mother was receiving naproxen 375 mg × 12 h under steady-state dosing condi-

* An explanation of the calculation (s) appears on pp. 71–72.

tions. As recovery of naproxen in the mother's urine was only 48% of the dose she received, this may be an underestimate of the quantity of drug absorbed by the infant. Effects on the infant were not mentioned (1). A breast-fed infant whose mother took naproxen long term displayed prolonged prothrombin and increased platelet aggregation times (2).

ASSESSMENT AND RECOMMENDATIONS

Naproxen was studied in one lactating women under steady-state conditions of dosing with appropriate amounts of the drug. Collected samples did not allow definition of the milk and plasma concentration-time profiles and additional studies are needed to establish the milk to plasma ratio and the range of peak concentrations in milk. The limited data do, however, suggest that the risk to the suckling infant of administering naproxen to its mother is low on the basis that the quantity of drug that passes into milk is small. Breast-feeding is probably safe.

REFERENCES

1. Jamili F, Stevens DRS (1983) Naproxen in milk. *Drug Intell. Clin. Pharmacol., 17,* 910–911.
2. Fidalgo I, Correa R, Gomez Carrasco JA, Martinez Quiroga F (1989) Anemia aguda, rectorragia y hematuria asociadas a la ingestión de naproxén. *An. Esp. Pediatr., 30,* 317–319.

PIROXICAM

GENERAL

Piroxicam is a non-steroidal anti-inflammatory drug and its mechanism of action is that of other members of this group, i.e. inhibition of prostaglandin synthesis. It is well absorbed from the adult gastrointestinal tract, 99% bound to plasma proteins and metabolised in the liver. The plasma half-life is 30–60 h.

EVALUATION OF DATA

Passage of piroxicam into human milk has been reported as follows:

Treatment conditions — Dose × Frequency × Duration; Route; No. of patients; Lactation stage	Concentration (mg/l) Milk	Plasma	Milk/plasma ratio	Maximum observed milk conc. (mg/l)	Absolute dose to infant (mg/kg/day) Ave	Max	Ref.
20 mg × 1/d × 4 months; p.o.; 1; 7 months	0.06; 0.05	4.79; 5.85	0.013; 0.009	0.17	–	0.026	(1)
40 mg × 1/d × 2 d; p.o.; 1; 8 months	0.22 (0.11–0.18)	15.75	0.014	0.22	–	0.033	(1)
20 mg × 1/d × 52 d; p.o.; 4; > 52 d	0.073–0.102	3.4–5.02	0.02–0.03	0.141	–	0.02	(2)

Milk and serum concentrations were taken under steady-state dosing conditions from the first woman. The table gives paired values during two dose intervals; the maximum milk concentration is the highest value reported. The second woman received piroxicam for 2 days and milk and serum samples were taken 2 h after the second dose. The concentrations in brackets were taken 1.2 7 h after the first dose. Higher milk concentrations at 35.5 h and 26.3 h in the first and second cases respectively suggest late accumulation of piroxicam in milk (1). The milk concentration-time profile was defined in (2). The table gives the range of mean values for all subjects at steady-state; the value of 0.141 was the maximum observed in an individual.

RELATIVE DOSE IN MILK

If the second mother in reference (1) is regarded as having taken a single dose, then the weight-adjusted amount that a suckling infant would ingest in a feed 1.0% (0.22 × 180/40)* of this. Data from the first mother, who was under steady-state conditions of dosing, indicate that in a day a suckling infant would ingest on average 2.5% (0.055 × 900/20)* and at maximum 7.7% (0.17 × 900/20)* of the weight-adjusted maternal daily dose.

* An explanation of the calculation (s) appears on pp. 71–72.

DATA ON THE INFANT

Piroxicam could not be detected in the serum of the infant whose mother who took the drug for 4 months whilst breast-feeding (detection limit 0.02 μg/l) (1). Neither piroxicam nor its metabolites was found in the urine of one of the infants in reference (2). No adverse effects were observed in the infants.

ASSESSMENT AND RECOMMENDATIONS

The risk to the suckling infant of administering piroxicam to its mother is low on the basis that the quantity of drug that passes into milk is small. The long half-life of piroxicam indicates potential for accumulation on repeated dosing but neither parent drug nor metabolites was recovered in the urine of an exposed infant. Breast-feeding appears to be safe.

REFERENCES

1. Østensen M (1983) Piroxicam in human breast milk. *Eur. J. Clin. Pharmacol., 25,* 829–30.
2. Østensen M, Matheson I, Laufen H (1988) Piroxicam in breast milk after long-term therapy. *Eur. J. Clin. Pharmacol., 35*, 567–569.

SUPROFEN

GENERAL

Suprofen is a non-steroidal anti-inflammatory drug and its mechanism of action is that of other members of this group, i.e. inhibition of prostaglandin synthesis. Suprofen is absorbed from the adult gastrointestinal tract and is 99% bound to plasma proteins. The plasma half-life is 4 h.

EVALUATION OF DATA

Passage of suprofen into human milk has been reported as follows:

Treatment conditions	Concentration (mg/l)		Milk/ plasma ratio	Maximum observed milk conc. (mg/l)	Absolute dose to infant (mg/kg/day)		Ref.
Dose × Frequency × Duration; Route; No. of patients; Lactation stage	Milk	Plasma			Ave	Max	
200 mg × 1/d × 1 d; p.o.; 6; 6–11 months	0.06	4.8	0.013 (0.01–0.02)	0.232	–	–	(1)

Milk and blood samples were collected for 8 h after the dose of suprofen; the concentration-time profiles were defined and were concurrent. The table gives average milk and plasma values derived from the areas under the concentration-time curves (AUC). The milk to plasma ratio calculated from the AUC's was similar to that expected from physicochemical properties of the drug; the range during the period of dosing is shown in brackets. Extensive binding to plasma proteins (99%) and minimal binding to milk proteins (7–17%) may limit drug passage into milk. The design of the study is appropriate to describe disposition of a single dose of suprofen in milk and plasma.

RELATIVE DOSE IN MILK

A suckling infant would ingest in a feed at maximum 0.2% (0.232 × 180/200)* of the weight-adjusted maternal single dose (1).

DATA ON THE INFANT

These were not studied in the quoted report.

ASSESSMENT AND RECOMMENDATIONS

The risk to the suckling infant of administering a single dose of suprofen to its

* An explanation of the calculation (s) appears on pp. 71–72.

mother is low on the basis that the quantity of drug that passes into milk is small. Breast-feeding may be regarded as safe.

REFERENCES

1. Chaikin P, Chasin M, Kennedy B, Silverman BK (1983) Suprofen concentrations in human breast milk. *J. Clin. Pharmacol., 23*, 385–390.

TENOXICAM

GENERAL

Tenoxicam is a non-steroidal anti-inflammatory drug used widely in the treatment of rheumatic disorders. It is well absorbed from the gastrointestinal tract, is highly protein bound and is inactivated by metabolism. The half-life of elimination from plasma is 72 h.

EVALUATION OF DATA

The passage of tenoxicam into human breast milk has been reported as follows:

Treatment conditions	Concentration (mg/l)		Milk/ plasma ratio	Maxi- mum observed milk conc. (mg/l)	Absolute dose to infant (mg/kg/day)		Ref.
Dose × Frequency × Duration; Route; No. of patients; Lactation stage	Milk	Plasma			Ave	Max	
40 mg × 1/d × 1 d; p.o.; 6; 2–5 d	0.053 (0.077)	3.24	0.015	0.085 (0.116)	–	0.01 (0.02)	(1)

Figures for the hydroxy metabolite of tenoxicam appear in brackets. The milk and plasma concentration-time profiles appear in the report and are concurrent. The second and third columns of the table give the mean maximum values for the group; those in the fifth and seventh columns are the maximum values recorded in any individual. The milk to plasma values are based on area measurements. The plasma half-life in these lactating mothers was 39 h which is notably shorter than that quoted for non-lactating persons (72 h).

RELATIVE DOSE IN MILK

The amount of tenoxicam and its hydroxy metabolite that a suckling infant would ingest in a feed is at maximum 0.9% (0.085 + 0.116 × 180/40)* of the weight adjusted maternal single dose.

DATA ON THE INFANT

No data are available.

ASSESSMENT AND RECOMMENDATIONS

The risk to the suckling infant of administering a single dose of tenoxicam to its

* An explanation of the calculation (s) appears on pp. 71–72.

mother is low on the basis that the quantity of drug that passes into milk is small. Single or occasional doses would appear to be safe.

REFERENCE

1. Heintz RC, Stebler T, Lunell NO, Mueller S, Guentert TW (1993). Excretion of tenoxicam and 5′-hydroxy-tenoxicam into human milk. *J. Pharmacol. Med., 3,* 57–64.

ALPRAZOLAM

GENERAL

Alprazolam is a benzodiazepam derivative that is used in short courses principally for anxiety disorders. It is well absorbed from the adult gastrointestinal tract, is 75% bound to plasma proteins and is extensively metabolised in the liver. Pharmacological activity is ascribed to the parent drug with minimal contribution from metabolites. The plasma half-life in adults is 12 h.

EVALUATION OF DATA

Passage of alprazolam into human milk has been reported as follows:

Treatment conditions Dose × Frequency × Duration; Route; No. of patients; Lactation stage	Concentration (μg/l) Milk	Concentration (μg/l) Serum	Milk/serum ratio	Maximum observed milk conc. (μg/l)	Absolute dose to infant (μg/kg/day) Ave	Absolute dose to infant (μg/kg/day) Max	Ref.
0.5 mg × 1/d × 1 d; p.o.; 8; 6–28 weeks	3.70	8.88	0.36	3.70	–	0.56	(1)

The milk and serum values are mean maximum figures for the group. The concentration-time profiles were defined and were concurrent; the milk to plasma ratio is based on area measurements. The mean half-life of alprazolam in milk was 14.5 h.

RELATIVE DOSE IN MILK

A suckling infant would ingest in a feed at maximum 1.3% (3.7 × 180/500)* of the weight-adjusted maternal single dose of alprazolam.

DATA ON THE INFANT

None of the infants in (1) was breast-fed. Mild drowsiness which resolved despite continued exposure was reported in one of 5 infants whose mothers took alprazolam (2).

ASSESSMENT OF DATA

Single dose data indicate that the risk to the suckling infant of administering alprazolam to its mother is low on the basis that the quantity of drug that passes into

* An explanation of the calculation (s) appears on pp. 71–72.

milk is small. The relatively long half-life of the drug points to the possibility of drug effects in the infant on repeated dosing. Breast-feeding should be regarded as safe but the infant should be observed for sedation if repeated doses are given to the mother.

REFERENCES

1. Oo CY, Kuhn RJ, Desai N, Wright CE, McNamara PJ (1995) Pharmacokinetics in lactating women: prediction of alprazolam transfer into milk. *Br. J. Clin. Pharmacol., 40,* 231–235.
2. Anderson PO, McGiure G (1989) Neonatal alprazolam withdrawal; possible effects on breast-feeding. *Drug Intelligence Clin. Pharmacy, 23*, 614.

AMITRIPTYLINE (NORTRIPTYLINE)

GENERAL

Amitriptyline is a tricyclic antidepressant drug. It is absorbed from the adult gastrointestinal tract and is 95% bound to plasma proteins. Amitriptyline is extensively metabolised, principally by demethylation to nortriptyline which is pharmacologically active and both substances are further oxidised to metabolites that retain some biological activity. The plasma half-life of amitriptyline is 16 h; that of nortriptyline is 31 h but it may be 56 h in the new-born (1).

EVALUATION OF DATA

Passage of amitriptyline and nortriptyline into human milk has been reported as follows:

Treatment conditions Dose × Frequency × Duration; Route; No. of patients; Lactation stage	Concentration (μg/l) Milk	Plasma	Milk/plasma ratio	Maximum observed milk conc. (μg/l)	Absolute dose to infant (μg/kg/day) Ave	Max	Ref.
75 mg × 1/d × 2–10 weeks; p.o.; 1; 4 months	88 (69)	52 (64)	1.7 (1.1)	-	13 (10)	-	(2)
100 mg/d × LT; p.o.; 1; 6–8 weeks	143 (55)	112 (78)	1.35 (0.79)	-	22 (8)	-	(3)
nortriptyline 75–125 mg/d × LT; p.o.; 1 6–7 d	(180)	–	(0.87–2.03)	-	(27, 47)	-	(4)

LT, long term. The figures in brackets refer to nortriptyline. In references (2) and (3) the milk and plasma concentrations are the means of 2 samples taken 12–16 h after the daily dose of amitriptyline under steady-state conditions of dosing. The concentration-time profiles were not defined. Reference (4) gives concentration-time profiles which appeared concurrent. The milk concentration is the mean of 9 measurements.

RELATIVE DOSE IN MILK

A suckling infant would ingest in a day on average 1.9% (88 + 69 × 900/75000)* of the weight-adjusted maternal daily dose of amitriptyline and nortriptyline (2).

DATA ON THE INFANT

Amitriptyline and nortriptyline was <10 μg/l in the infants' plasma (2,3). No drug effects were noted in the infant in reference (2) and (4).

* An explanation of the calculation (s) appears on pp. 71–72.

ASSESSMENT OF DATA

The data suggest that when amitriptyline is administered to a nursing mother the risk to the suckling infant is low on the basis that the quantity of drug that passes into milk is small. A decision about the advisability of breast-feeding is probably best determined by the factors pertinent to the individual case. When the maternal dose is high, exposure to the infant to the drug may be reduced by limiting the number of feeds per day.

REFERENCES

1. Sjöquist F, Bergfors PG, Borgå O, Lind M, Ygge H (1972) Plasma disappearance of nortriptyline in a newborn infant following placental transfer from an intoxicated mother. *J. Paediatr., 80*, 496–500.
2. Brixen-Rasmussen L, Halgrener J, Jørgensen A (1982) Amitriptyline and nortriptyline excretion in human breast milk. *Psychopharmacology, 76*, 94–95.
3. Bader TF, Newman K (1980) Amitriptyline in human breast milk and the nursing infant's serum. *Am. J. Psychiatry, 137,* 855–856.
4. Matheson I, Skjæraasen J (1988) Milk concentrations of flupenthixol, nortriptyline and zuclopenthixol and between-breast differnces in two patients. *Eur. J. Clin. Pharmacol., 35*, 217–220.

AMOXAPINE

GENERAL

Amoxapine is an antidepressant drug that is structurally related to the tricyclics and to some tricyclic neuroleptics, e.g. loxapine and clozapine; amoxapine is the demethylated metabolite of loxapine. Amoxapine is well absorbed from the adult gastrointestinal tract, 90% bound to plasma proteins and extensively metabolised in the liver. The plasma half-life is 10 h.

EVALUATION OF DATA

Passage of amoxapine into human milk has been reported as follows:

Treatment conditions Dose × Frequency × Duration; Route; No. of patients; Lactation stage	Concentration (μg/l) Milk	 Plasma	Milk/plasma ratio	Maximum observed milk conc. (μg/l)	Absolute dose to infant (μg/kg/day) Ave	 Max	Ref.
250 mg/d × LT; p.o.; see below	<20 (140)	97 (380)	– –	– (170)	– –	– –	(1)

LT, long term. Figures in parentheses refer to the metabolite 8-OH-amoxapine. Amoxapine and its active metabolite 8-OH-amoxapine were measured in milk secretions from a patient who developed galactorrhea during treatment, i.e. she had not been pregnant and was not breast-feeding. Milk and serum concentrations were measured 45 min and 11.5 h after the dose.

RELATIVE DOSE IN MILK

The data are not referable to milk formed during breast-feeding and have not been used to calculate the infant dose.

DATA ON THE INFANT

No data are available.

ASSESSMENT AND RECOMMENDATIONS

Limited data suggest that the amount of amoxapine that passes into milk secretions during galactorrhoea, and by implication the quantity ingested by a suckling infant, would be small. More information is required, however, before a recommendation about breast-feeding can be made.

REFERENCES

1. Gelenberg A (1979) Amoxapine, a new antidepressant appears in human milk. *J. Nerv. Ment. Dis., 167*, 635–636.

BUTORPHANOL

GENERAL

Butorphanol is an opioid analgesic with mixed agonist/antagonist activity. The duration of action of a single dose is 2–4 h. Butorphanol is absorbed from the adult gastrointestinal tract and is highly bound to plasma proteins. It is excreted mainly by the kidneys and the plasma half life is 2.5–4 h.

EVALUATION OF DATA

Passage of butorphanol into human milk has been reported as follows:

Treatment conditions: Dose × Frequency × Duration; Route; No. of patients; Lactation stage	Concentration (μg/l) Milk	Concentration (μg/l) Plasma	Milk/plasma ratio	Maximum observed milk conc. (μg/l)	Absolute dose to infant (μg/kg/day) Ave	Absolute dose to infant (μg/kg/day) Max	Ref.
2 mg × 1/d × 1 d; i.m.; 6; <1 week	1.5 (0–2 h)	2.4 (1 h)	0.7	1.5	–	0.23	(1)
	0.7 (2–4 h)	1.1 (3 h)	0.8				
	0.3 (4–8 h)	0.5 (6.h)	0.7				
8 mg × 1/d × 1 d; p.o.; 6; <1 week	3.6 (0–3 h)	2.5 (1.5 h)	1.7	3.6	–	0.54	(1)
	1.8 (3–5 h)	1.2 (4 h)	1.7				
	1.1 (5–8 h)	0.6 (6.5 h)	2.2				

The data did not allow definition of the milk and plasma concentration-time profiles. Colostrum/milk was collected by emptying both breasts at the end of the stated intervals. The times in the table indicate hours after a dose and the concentrations quoted are average values for the group. The sampling period includes one half-life of butorphanol in milk and plasma and allows some estimate of the milk to plasma ratio. The calculations for the latter were consistent for each route: 0.7–0.8 i.m. and 1.7–2.2 p.o. The latter is similar to the theoretical ratio of 1.9 for a base.

RELATIVE DOSE IN MILK

As butorphanol tartrate (mol. wt. 478) was administered but butorphanol (mol. wt. 328) was assayed, a factor of 1.5 (478/328) has been introduced into the calculation. Thus a suckling infant would ingest in a feed at maximum 0.2% (1.5 × 180 × 1.5/2000)* and 0.1% (3.6 × 180 × 1.5/8000)* of the weight-adjusted maternal i.m. and p.o. doses respectively (1).

DATA ON THE INFANT

Respiratory depression was not observed in the infants of mothers who received

* An explanation of the calculation (s) appears on pp. 71–72.

butorphanol just prior to or after parturition. No data are available on breast-feeding infants as the mothers who took part in the study of butorphanol in milk (above) either did not nurse or suspended breast-feeding for 24 h (1).

ASSESSMENT AND RECOMMENDATIONS

Butorphanol was studied in 12 lactating women given single doses of appropriate amount for 1 day. The risk to the suckling infant of administering a single dose of butorphanol to its mother appears is low on the basis that the quantity of drug that passes into milk is small. Breast-feeding after occasional such doses would appear to be safe but there is a need for more prolonged studies of butorphanol in nursing mothers.

REFERENCES

1. Pittman KA, Smyth RD, Losada M, Zighelboim I, Maduska AL, Sunshine A (1980) Perinatal distribution of butorphanol. *Am. J. Obstet. Gynecol., 138,* 797–800.

CARBAMAZEPINE

GENERAL

Carbamazepine is effective for major and psychomotor epilepsy, and for trigeminal neuralgia. It is absorbed from the adult gastrointestinal tract and about 75% bound to plasma proteins. Carbamazepine is metabolised to carbamazepine-10,11-epoxide (CBZ-epoxide) which is effective for the treatment of trigeminal neuralgia, and probably also of epilepsy. The plasma half-life of carbamazepine is 15–35 h both in adults and in the newborn infants of carbamazepine-treated mothers (1). The plasma half-life of CBZ-epoxide in the newborn is similar (2).

EVALUATION OF DATA

Passage of carbamazepine into human milk has been reported as follows:

Treatment conditions	Concentration (mg/l)		Milk/ plasma ratio	Maxi- mum observed milk conc. (mg/l)	Absolute dose to infant (mg/kg/day)		Ref.
Dose × Frequency × Duration; Route; No. of patients; Lactation stage	Milk	Plasma			Ave	Max	
3–22 mg/kg/d × LT; p.o.; 4; 3–28 d	1.7 (0.39)	5.52 (1.03)	0.39 (0.49)	3.0 (0.80)	0.27 (0.06)	0.83 (0.16)	(2)
7.1–24.6 mg/kg/d × LT; p.o., 19; 2–75 d	2.5 (1.5)	7.1 (2.6)	0.4 (0.6)	3.6 (1.9)	0.38 (0.23)	0.72 (0.29)	(3)
5.8–7.3 mg/kg/d × LT; p.o.; 3; 2–35 d	1.6 (0.7)	2.7 (0.7)	0.6 (1.0)	1.8 (1.1)	0.24 (0.11)	0.27 (0.17)	(4)
8 mg/kg/d × LT; p.o.; 1; 2–30 d	1.6 (0.7)	2.8 (0.8)	0.6 (0.9)	1.8 (1.0)	0.24 (0.10)	0.26 (0.16)	(5)
1000 mg × 1/d × LT; p.o.; 1; 5 weeks	2.3	5.8	–	–	–	–	(6)
? × LT; p.o.; 3; 3–32 d	1.9	4.3	0.39	3.8	0.29	0.57	(7)
? x LT; p.o.; ?; ?	1.8	4.1	0.41	3.8	0.27	0.57	(8)

LT, long term. References (2–7) report average milk and serum values; the maximum milk concentrations are the highest figures recorded in individuals. Several patients were receiving other antiepilepsy drugs. No study defined the milk and plasma concentration-time profiles. Figures in brackets refer to CBX-epoxide.

RELATIVE DOSE IN MILK

A suckling infant would ingest in a day on average 3.6–4.1% (2.5 + 1.5 × 900/1000)–(1.6 + 0.7 × 900/500)* (3,4) and at maximum 5.0% (3.6 + 1.9 ×

* An explanation of the calculation (s) appears on pp. 71–72.

900/1000)* (3) of the weight-adjusted maternal daily dose of carbamazepine and CBZ-epoxide.

DATA ON THE INFANT

Reference (2) reports that serum carbamazepine in 12 nursed infants was usually in the range of 1.0 mg/l but was 4.7 mg/l in one infant; no adverse effects were reported. In another study the serum carbamazepine concentration in each of 7 infants was less that 1.5 mg/l 4–7 d after delivery (3). A breast-fed child was found to have a plasma carbamazepine concentration of 1.8 mg/l at 4 weeks of age (4) and a similar finding is recorded in reference (5). Poor weight gain which was related to a high incidence of vomiting and inadequate suckling was ascribed to antiepilepsy medication in general (8).

ASSESSMENT AND RECOMMENDATIONS

The risk to the suckling infant of administering carbamazepine to its mother appears to be low on the basis that the quantity of drug that passes into milk is small. Breast-feeding is probable safe but the infant should be closely observed for undue tiredness, poor suckling or vomiting; monitoring of plasma concentration may be helpful if there is diagnostic uncertainty or in any event if the maternal dose is high.

REFERENCES

1. Rane A, Bertilson L, Palmer L (1975) Disposition of placentally transferred carbamazepine (Tegretol) in the newborn. *Eur. J. Clin. Pharmacol., 8,* 283–284.
2. Kuhnz W, Jager-Roman E, Rating D, Deychl A, Kuhnze J, Helge H, Nau H (1983) Carbamazepine and carbamazepine-10,11-epoxide during pregnancy and the postnatal period in epileptic mothers and their nursed infants. Pharmacokinetics and clinical effects. *Pediatric Pharmacol., 3,* 199–208.
3. Froescher W, Eichelbaum M, Niesen M, Dietrich K, Rausch P (1984) Carbamazepine levels in breast milk. *Ther. Drug Monit., 6,* 266–271.
4. Pynnonen S, Kanto J, Sillanpaa M, Erkkola R. (1977) Carbamazepine: placental transport, tissue concentrations in foetus and newborn, and level in milk. *Acta Pharmacol. Toxicol., 41*, 244–253.
5. Pynnonen S, Sillanpaa M (1975) Carbamazepine and mothers milk. *Lancet, 2*, 563.
6. Niebyl J, Blake D, Freeman J, Luff R. Carbamazepine levels in•pregnancy and lactation. *Obstet. Gynecol., 53,* 139–40.
7. Kaneko S, Sato T, Suzuki K (1979) The levels of anticonvulsants in breast milk. *Br. J. Clin. Pharmacol., 7,* 624–626.
8. Kaneko S, Suzuki K, Sato T, Ogawa Y, Nomura Y (1982) The problems of antiepileptic medication in the neonatal period: is breast-feeding advisable? In: Janz D, Dam M, Richens A, Bossi L, Helge, H, Schmidt D, (Eds) *Pregnancy, Epilepsy and the Child*, pp 343–348, Raven Press, New York.

CLOMETHIAZOLE

GENERAL

Clomethiazole (chlormethiazole) is used as a sedative and anticonvulsant drug for various conditions, including pre-eclampsia and alcoholism. It may be given by mouth or iv. After oral administration clomethiazole is rapidly absorbed from the adult gastrointestinal tract and 65% is bound to plasma proteins. Clomethiazole is extensively metabolised; it is significantly extracted in first-pass through the liver. The blood half-life is 6 h.

EVALUATION OF DATA

Passage of clomethiazole into human milk has been reported as follows:

Treatment conditions	Concentration (mg/l)		Milk/ plasma ratio	Maximum observed milk conc. (mg/l)	Absolute dose to infant (mg/kg/day)		Ref.
Dose × Frequency × Duration; Route; No. of patients; Lactation stage	Milk	Plasma			Ave	Max	
1000 mg × 3–4/d × 3–5 d; p.o.; 4; 3–5 d	0.23	0.20	0.88	3.23 (1.3, mean) (0.2, mean)	0.04	0.49	(1)

The mothers received clomethiazole intravenously during labour and orally for 3–5 d after delivery. Milk and plasma concentrations were measured between 4 and 28 h following the last dose of clomethiazole and reflected steady-state dosing conditions. The concentration-time profiles were defined in one patient and were concurrent. The milk concentration quoted is the mean of all samples. The table also gives the highest individual milk concentration and mean maximum milk concentration. The milk to blood ratio is the mean of 14 paired samples.

RELATIVE DOSE IN MILK

The amount of clomethiazole that a suckling infant would ingest in a day is on average 0.1% (0.23 × 900/1800)* and at maximum 1.6% (3.23 × 900/1800)* of the weight-adjusted maternal daily dose (1). (The maternal dose used here takes account of the fact that clomethiazole edisylate 1000 mg is equivalent to 600 mg of the base.)

DATA ON THE INFANT

In 4–8 blood samples from each infant, clomethiazole was not detected in two of

* An explanation of the calculation (s) appears on pp. 71–72.

the infants, was detected once in one (0.006 mg/l) and twice in the other (0.009, 0.018 mg/l).

ASSESSMENT OF DATA

The risk to the suckling infant of administering clomethiazole to its mother is low on the basis that the quantity of drug that passes into milk is small. Breast-feeding may be regarded as safe.

REFERENCES

1. Tunstall ME, Campbell DM, Dawson BM, Jostell KG (1979) Chlormethiazole treatment and breast-feeding. *Br. J. Obstet. Gynaecol., 86*, 793–798.

CHLORPROMAZINE

GENERAL

Chlorpromazine is a phenothiazine drug that is used to treat psychoses. Chlorpromazine is readily absorbed from the adult gastrointestinal tract and is 90% bound to plasma proteins. It undergoes considerable pre-systemic metabolism which in part accounts for the wide intersubject variation that is observed in its plasma concentration after oral administration. Numerous active and inactive metabolites are formed. Chlorpromazine has a plasma half-life of 30 h.

EVALUATION OF DATA

Passage of chlorpromazine into human milk has been reported as follows:

Treatment conditions Dose × Frequency × Duration; Route; No. of patients; Lactation stage	Concentration (μg/l) Milk	 Plasma	Milk/ plasma ratio	Maximum observed milk conc. (μg/l)	Absolute dose to infant (μg/kg/day) Ave	 Max	Ref.
?; p.o.; 4; ?	7–98	16–52	–	98	–	15	(1)

The authors reported that chlorpromazine and its metabolite chlorpromazine sulfoxide were identified in all milk samples, that 7-hydroxychlorpromazine was present in milk from two mothers and that monodesmethylchlorpromazine was present in the milk from one. The table gives the ranges of chlorpromazine concentrations. The concentration-time profiles were not defined.

RELATIVE DOSE IN MILK

The relative dose in milk cannot be calculated as the maternal dose is not given in the report.

DATA ON THE INFANT

Two of the four mothers breast-fed their babies. One of these infants who had a chlorpromazine plasma concentration of 92 μg/l was reported to be drowsy and lethargic; the other who had a plasma concentration of 7 μg/l showed no adverse effects (1).

ASSESSMENT OF DATA

The limited data about the passage of chlorpromazine into breast milk do not allow an estimation of the quantity of drug ingested by the suckling infant but indicate that the concentrations of chlorpromazine in the infant's plasma are comparable to those in the mother. A decision about the advisability of breast-feeding is probably best determined by the factors pertinent to the individual case. When the maternal dose is high, exposure to the infant to the drug may be reduced by limiting the number of feeds per day.

REFERENCES

1. Wiles DH, Orr MW, Kolakowska T (1978) Chlorpromazine levels in plasma and milk of nursing mothers. *Br. J. Clin. Pharmacol., 5,* 272.

CLOBAZAM

GENERAL

Clobazam is an anxiolytic drug of the benzodiazepine group. It is absorbed from the adult gastrointestinal tract and is 90% bound to plasma proteins. Clobazam is extensively metabolised and its main metabolite, desmethylclobazam (DCZ), may accumulate during multiple dosing. The half-life in plasma is 20 h.

EVALUATION OF DATA

Passage of clobazam and DCZ into breast milk were investigated as follows:

Treatment conditions	Concentration (mg/l)		Milk/ plasma ratio	Maximum observed milk conc. (mg/l)	Absolute dose to infant (mg/kg/day)		Ref.
Dose × Frequency × Duration; Route; No. of patients; Lactation stage	Milk	Plasma			Ave	Max	
30 mg/d × 2 d; p.o.; 6; ?	0.125	0.418	0.36	0.330	0.019	0.050	(1)
30 mg/d × 5 d; p.o.; 6; ?	0.152	1.22	0.13	0.250	0.023	0.038	(1)

Six patients received clobazam 10 mg at 7 am and 20 mg at 3 pm daily by mouth for 5 days. Samples were taken 2 h after each dose, i.e. the concentration-time profiles were not defined. The milk concentrations refer to clobazam and DCZ combined since this assay was not specific for clobazam. The table gives average milk and plasma concentrations on the morning of the 2nd (upper line of table) and 5th (lower line) day of administration. The maximum milk concentrations are the highest values recorded in individuals. The milk to plasma ratio decreased from day 2 to day 5 possibly because DCZ accumulates in plasma.

RELATIVE DOSE IN MILK

A suckling infant would receive in a day on average 4.6% (0.152 × 900/30)* and at maximum 7.5% (0.25 × 900/30)* of the weight adjusted maternal daily dose of clobazam and DCZ (1). Almost the same dose would have been received on the 2nd as on the 5th day.

DATA ON THE INFANT

No data are available.

* An explanation of the calculation (s) appears on pp. 71–72.

ASSESSMENT AND RECOMMENDATIONS

The risk to the suckling infant of administering a short course of clobazam to its mother is low on the basis that the quantity of drug that passes into milk is small. The available data do not take into account the possibility that with long term dosing the metabolite DCZ may cause effects in the infant. Breast-feeding may be regarded as safe if the dose is low and the period of exposure is short.

REFERENCES

1. Hajdu P, Wernicke OA (1978) *Untersuchung zur Überprufung des Ubertritts von Frisium in die Muttermilch.* Internal Report, Hoechst.

CLONAZEPAM

GENERAL

Clonazepam is used to treat generalised and partial epileptic seizures. It augments the normal transmission of gamma-aminobutyric acid in the nervous system through specific benzodiazepine receptors. About 80 % of clonazepam is absorbed from the adult gastrointestinal tract and about 60% is bound to plasma proteins. The drug is completely metabolised. The plasma half-life is 29 h in adults.

EVALUATION OF DATA

Passage of clonazepam into human milk has been reported as follows:

Treatment conditions Dose × Frequency × Duration; Route; No. of patients; Lactation stage	Concentration (μg/l)		Milk/ plasma ratio	Maximum observed milk conc. (μg/l)	Absolute dose to infant (μg/kg/day)		Ref.
	Milk	Plasma			Ave	Max	
2 mg × 2/d × LT; p.o.; 1; 2–4 d	8.8–10.7	28.6–32.7	2.7	10.7	–	1.61	(1)

LT, long term. Reference (1) reports the range of concentrations in 5 milk and 6 plasma samples taken at specific times 2–4 days after the birth. The milk/plasma ratio quoted in the table relates to the only paired milk-plasma sample obtained 3 days after birth.

RELATIVE DOSE IN MILK

A suckling infant would ingest in a day at maximum 2.4% (10.7 × 900/4000)* of the weight-adjusted maternal daily dose of clonazepam.

DATA ON THE INFANT

No data are available.

ASSESSMENT AND RECOMMENDATIONS

Limited data suggest that the risk to the suckling infant of administering clonazepam to its mother is low on the basis that the quantity of drug in milk is small. Clonazepam, however, is normally used long-term and a general recommendation

* An explanation of the calculation (s) appears on pp. 71–72.

can be made only when experience and information with such usage becomes available.

REFERENCES

1. Söderman P, Matheson I (1988) Clonazepam in breast milk. *Eur. J. Pediatr., 147,* 212–213.

CLORPROTIXENE

GENERAL

Clorprotixene (chlorprothixene) is a thioxanthene neuroleptic drug with properties similar to chlorpromazine, but it is less sedative. It may also be used to treat anxiety and tension when benzodiazepines are ineffective. Clorprotixene is readily absorbed from the adult gastrointestinal tract and undergoes significant first-pass metabolism in the liver. The main metabolite is cloprotixene sulphoxide (CPX-SO) which is devoid of neuroleptic activity but may exert antimuscarinic effects. Cloprotixene is > 99% bound to plasma proteins and its plasma half-life is 9 h.

EVALUATION OF DATA

Passage of cloprotixene into human milk has been reported as follows:

Treatment conditions Dose × Frequency × Duration; Route; No. of patients; Lactation stage	Concentration (μg/l)		Milk/ plasma ratio	Maximum observed milk conc. (μg/l)	Absolute dose to infant (μg/kg/day)		Ref.
	Milk	Plasma			Ave	Max	
200 mg × 1/d × LT; p.o.; 1; 9 weeks (a)	16 (23)	10 (34)	1.6 (0.7)	31 (30)	2.4 (3.5)	4.7 (4.5)	(1)
200–400 mg × 1/d × 12 d; p.o.; 1; 6 weeks (b)	33 (17)	13 (34)	–	–	–	–	(1)

LT, long term. The mother (a) was studied under steady-state conditions of dosing. The milk and plasma profiles were defined over a 12 h period during which her baby suckled 3 times. The table gives average milk concentration and the maximum milk single concentration that was recorded. The mother (b) gave single milk and blood samples 30 h after her last dose of chlorprothixine. The figures in brackets refer to CPX-SO.

RELATIVE DOSE IN MILK

A suckling infant would ingest in a day on average 0.2% (0.016 + 0.023 × 900/200)* and at maximum 0.3% (0.031 + 0.030 × 900/200)* of the weight-adjusted maternal daily dose of cloprotixene and its metabolite CPX-SO (1).

DATA ON THE INFANT

No adverse effects were observed in the babies.

* An explanation of the calculation (s) appears on pp. 71–72.

ASSESSMENT OF DATA

There is wide inter-subject variation in plasma and thus probably also in milk concentration of cloprotixene. The limited information currently available, which suggests that the quantity of cloprotixene that passes into milk is small, must therefore be interpreted with caution. A decision about the advisability of breast-feeding is probably best determined by the factors pertinent to the individual case. When the maternal dose is high, exposure to the infant to the drug may be reduced by limiting the number of feeds per day.

REFERENCES

1. Matheson I, Evang A, Fredricson Overø K, Syversen G (1984) Presence of chlorprothixene and its metabolites in breast milk. *Eur. J. Clin. Pharmacol., 27*, 611–613.

CLORAZEPATE POTASSIUM

GENERAL

Clorazepate potassium is a benzodiazepine used in short courses for its anxiolytic and sedative properties. It is usually administered by mouth (not i.m. as in the report below) and is rapidly metabolised in the stomach to the active metabolite desmethyldiazepam (DDZ). The plasma half-life of DDZ is 30–90 h in adults but in neonates is 73–138 h (1).

EVALUATION OF DATA

Passage of clorazepate into human milk has been reported as follows:

Treatment conditions Dose × Frequency × Duration; Route; No. of patients; Lactation stage	Concentration (μg/l) Milk	Concentration (μg/l) Plasma	Milk/plasma ratio	Maximum observed milk conc. (μg/l)	Absolute dose to infant (μg/kg/day) Ave	Absolute dose to infant (μg/kg/day) Max	Ref.
20 mg × 1/d × 1 d; i.m.; 7; 2–4 d	10 (2 d) 9 (4 d)	56 (2 d) 41 (4 d)	0.18 (2 d) 0.22 (4 d)	16	–	2.4	(1)

The mothers received clorazepate potassium 0.5–12 h before delivery. The assay measured clorazepate plus DDZ. The table gives average concentrations in milk and plasma on the 2nd and on the 4th days after clorazepate potassium, i.e. the concentration-time profiles were not defined. The study was not conducted under steady-state conditions of dosing. The maximum milk concentration quoted is the highest value recorded in an individual; as the sample was taken 2 days after the injection of clorazepate potassium this does not represent the peak concentration in milk.

RELATIVE DOSE IN MILK

An infant suckling 2 days after the injection of clorazepate potassium would ingest in a feed at maximum 0.1% (16 × 180/20 000)* of the weight-adjusted maternal single dose (1).

DATA ON THE INFANT

Blood samples from the infants contained clorazepate plus DDZ in trace amounts to 9 μg/l; this includes drug received by placental transfer as well as in milk.

* An explanation of the calculation (s) appears on pp. 71–72.

ASSESSMENT OF DATA

This study suggests that the risk to the suckling infant of administering a single dose of clorazepate potassium to its mother is low because the quantity of drug that passes into milk is small. There are, however, no data on which to base a recommendation about repeated dosing and DDZ may accumulate in the new-born during prolonged administration. Occasional small doses of clorazepate potassium are probably safe during breast-feeding, but the infant should be observed, e.g. for undue sedation, during the first weeks postpartum and especially if it is premature.

REFERENCES

1. Rey E, Giraux P, d'Athis Ph, Turquais JM, Chavinie J, Olive G (1979) Pharmacokinetics of the placental transfer and distribution of chlorazepate and its metabolites in the feto-placental unit and in the neonate. *Eur. J. Clin. Pharmacol.*, *15*, 181–185.

CLOZAPINE

GENERAL

Clozapine is an atypical neuroleptic with a benzodiazepine structure. It is variably absorbed from the adult gastrointestinal tract, about 50% undergoes pre-systemic metabolism and it is 95% bound to plasma proteins. The plasma half-life is 12 h. Agranulocytosis is a serious risk with clozapine and restricts its use; the leukocyte count must be monitored during exposure to the drug.

EVALUATION OF DATA

Passage of clozapine into human milk has been reported as follows:

Treatment conditions Dose × Frequency × Duration; Route; No. of patients; Lactation stage	Concentration (μg/l) Milk	Concentration (μg/l) Plasma	Milk/plasma ratio	Maximum observed milk conc. (μg/l)	Absolute dose to infant (μg/kg/day) Ave	Absolute dose to infant (μg/kg/day) Max	Ref.
50 mg × 1/d × 9 weeks; p.o.; 1; 1 d;	63.5	14.7	4.3	–	9.5	–	(1)
100 mg × 1/d × 10 weeks; p.o.; 1; 1 week	115.6	41.7	2.8	–	17.3	–	(1)

Milk and plasma were collected 1 day and 1 week after delivery from one mother who did not breast-feed. The dose-sample interval is not stated.

RELATIVE DOSE IN MILK

The amount of clozapine that a suckling infant would ingest in a day is 1.1 % (63.5 × 900/50000)* of the weight-adjusted maternal daily dose (1).

DATA ON THE INFANT

No data are available.

ASSESSMENT OF DATA

Limited data suggest that when clozapine is administered to a nursing mother the quantity of drug that passes into milk is small. The inherent toxicity of the drug with risk of agranulocytosis suggests, however, that a mother who is receiving clozapine should not breast-feed.

REFERENCES

1. Barnas C, Bergant A, Hummer M, Fleischacker WW (1994) Clozapine concentration in maternal and fetal plasma, amniotic fluid and breast milk. *Am. J. Psychiatr., 151,* 945.

CODEINE

GENERAL

Codeine is an opioid drug that is used for mild to moderate pain, for diarrhoea, and to suppress cough. It is rapidly absorbed from the gastrointestinal tract, <25% is bound to plasma proteins and is extensively metabolised; the 0-demethylation product of codeine is morphine. The plasma half-life of codeine is 3–4 h.

EVALUATION OF DATA

Passage of codeine into human milk has been reported as follows:

Treatment conditions Dose × Frequency × Duration; Route; No. of patients; Lactation stage	Concentration (μg/l) Milk	Plasma	Milk/ plasma ratio	Maximum observed milk conc. (μg/l)	Absolute dose to infant (μg/kg/day) Ave	Max	Ref.
60 mg × 1/d × 1 d; p.o.; 2; 7–13 weeks	455 (16)	179	2.16	455	-	68.3	(1)

The 2 mothers each took a single tablet containing aspirin 454 mg, phenacetin 324 mg, caffeine 64 mg and codeine 60 mg. The milk and plasma values were similar in both mothers but the table gives only those for the one mother for whom actual concentrations are stated. These are maximum values, obtained 1 h after dosing; that for morphine is given in brackets.

RELATIVE DOSE IN MILK

The amount of codeine and morphine that a suckling infant would ingest in a single feed is at maximum 1.4% (455 + 16 × 180/60 000)* .

DATA ON THE INFANT

No data are available.

ASSESSMENT AND RECOMMENDATIONS

The risk to the suckling infant of administering codeine to its mother is low on the basis that the quantity of codeine and morphine that passes into milk is small. Breast-feeding after occasional doses may be regarded as safe.

* An explanation of the calculation (s) appears on pp. 71–72.

REFERENCES

1. Findlay JWA, DeAngelis RL, Kearney MF, Welch RM, Findlay JM (1981) Analgesic drugs in breast milk and plasma. *Clin. Pharmacol. Ther., 29,* 625–633.

DIAZEPAM

GENERAL

Diazepam is a benzodiazepine drug that is used principally for its anxiolytic, muscle relaxant and anticonvulsant properties. It is completely absorbed from the adult gastrointestinal tract and is metabolised in the liver; one of the principal metabolites, desmethyldiazepam (DDZ) retains pharmacological activity. Both diazepam and DDZ are >97% bound to plasma proteins. Diazepam has a plasma half-life of 20–100 h; in new-borns it is 31 h and in infants 10 h. Less than 1% is excreted unchanged in the urine. The half-life of DDZ is 30–90 h. In neonates conjugated DDZ may account for 70–80% of the urinary metabolites (1).

EVALUATION OF DATA

Passage of diazepam and desmethyldiazepam into human milk has been reported as follows:

Treatment conditions	Concentration (μg/l)		Milk/ plasma ratio	Maximum observed milk conc. (μg/l)	Absolute dose to infant (μg/kg/day)		Ref.
Dose × Frequency × Duration; Route; No. of patients; Lactation stage	Milk	Plasma			Ave	Max	
10 mg × 1/d × 6 d; p.o.; 4; 1–2 weeks	21 (35)	134 (131)	0.16 (0.27) (d 5)	43 (85)	3 (5)	6 (11)	(2)
10 mg × 3/d × 6 d; p.o.; 3; 1 week	78 (52)	60 (48)	0.13 (0.11) (d 6)	–	12 (8)	–	(3)
180–230 mg i.v. then 15 mg × 1/d × 3 d; p.o.; 2; 1 week	60 (60)	325 (435)	0.18 (0.15) (d 5)	90 (70)	9 (9)	13 (11)	(4)
2–10 mg/d × LT; p.o.; 1; 4 weeks	21 (21)	100 (200)	0.2 (0.1)	–	3 (3)	–	(5)
40 mg/d × LT; s p.o.; 1; 12 month	247 (133)	ca. 1000			0.20 (0.12)	307	(6)

LT, long term. The figures in parentheses refer to DDZ. Reference (2) gives mean concentrations 9 h after the single daily dose on the 5th day of treatment; the maximum milk concentration is the highest value recorded in an individual. Reference (3), reports mean milk and plasma concentrations taken on the 6th day of receiving diazepam. Reference (4) gives mean milk and plasma concentrations for the 3rd, 4th and 5th days after delivery, which was 1–3 days after administration of diazepam was started. In reference (5) diazepam 2 mg was taken by mouth 10 h before sampling on the 32nd day after delivery. None of the evaluated reports defined the milk or plasma concentration-time profiles and probably in none was steady-state dosing conditions attained. Reference (6) gives mean milk concentrations 4 and 5 d after the dose was reduced from 60 mg/d. None of the evaluated reports defined the concentration-time profiles and probably only (6) was conducted under steady-state conditions.

RELATIVE DOSE IN MILK

A suckling infant would ingest in a day on average 5.0% (21 + 35 × 900/10 000)* and at maximum 11.5% (43 + 85 × 900/10 000)* of the weight-adjusted maternal daily dose of diazepam and DDZ (2). If the paediatric oral dose of diazepam is assumed to be 0.5 mg/kg/day, then an infant would ingest on average 1.7% (21 + 35 × 15/500)* and at maximum 3.8% (43 + 85 × 15/500)* of this.

DATA ON THE INFANT

When diazepam was transferred only after birth in breast milk, adverse reactions were not reported, although infant plasma concentrations of diazepam and DDZ respectively amounted to 172 and 243 μg/l on the 4th day and 74 and 31 μg/l on the 6th day , i.e. values in the maternal range (3). Diazepam given to the mother during delivery and continued postpartum has been associated with lethargy, poor suckling and EEG abnormalities in the breast-fed neonate (7). DDZ may be detected up to 10 days postnatally in the new-born (8). The unbound fraction of diazepam and DDZ in plasma is increased in neonates, and the capacity for hydroxylation and glucuronidation of diazepam are limited at least in the first 4 days (7). DDZ may thus accumulate and it can depress respiration. A DDZ concentration of 46 μg/l was measured in a 32 day old infant whose mother had taken diazepam 2–10 mg daily throughout pregnancy and for a month postpartum; she reported infant sedation if she nursed within hours of taking diazepam (5). DDZ was 20 μg/l and diazepam < 5 μg/l in a 12-month-old infant whose mother withdrew (in stepwise mode) from diazepam 60–40 mg/d (6). The infant's plasma concentration was 2% of its mother's. No drug could be measured in the infant 8 d after cessation of diazepam and the infant showed no overt features of benzodiazepine intoxication.

ASSESSMENT OF DATA

Although the estimated quantities of diazepam and DDZ in milk are small, the evaluated studies do not adequately address the issue of accumulation to steady-state. Thus repeated doses of diazepam administered to a nursing mother may cause sedation in her infant, especially if diazepam is given before or during delivery or if the baby is premature. A mother who receives occasional small doses of diazepam can safely breast-feed but if administration is prolonged, the infant should be observed for drug effects, e.g. poor suckling or somnolence.

REFERENCES

1. Morselli PL (1977) Psychotropic drugs. In: Morselli PL (Ed) *Drug Disposition During Development*, pp 449–459. Spectrum, New York.

* An explanation of the calculation (s) appears on pp. 71–72.

2. Brandt R (1976)Passage of diazepam and desmethyldiazepam into breast milk. *Arzneimittelforschung, 26*, 454–457.
3. Erkkola R, Kanto J (1972) Diazepam and breast-feeding. *Lancet, I,* 1235–1236.
4. Sundsbak HP, Bredesen JE (1980) Diazepam i brystemelk. *Tidsskr. Nor. Laegefor., 100*, 582.
5. Wesson DR, Cambes S, Harkey M, Smith DE (1985) Diazepam and desmethyldiazepam in breast milk. *J. Psychoact. Drugs, 17,* 55–56.
6. Dusci LJ, Good SM, Hall RW, Ilett KF (1990) Excretion of diazepam and its metabolits in human milk during withdrawal from combination high dose diazepam and oxazepam. *Br. J. Clin. Pharmacol., 29*, 123–126.
7. Patrick HJ, Tilstone WJ, Reawey P (1972) Diazepam and breastfeeding. *Lancet, I,* 542–543.
8. Kanto J, Erkkola R (1974) Perinatal metabolism of diazepam. *Br. Med. J., 1,* 641–642.

DOSULEPIN

GENERAL

Dosulepin (dothiepin) is a tricyclic antidepressant drug. It is well absorbed from the adult gastrointestinal tract and 85% is bound to plasma proteins. Dosulepin undergoes extensive first-pass metabolism in the liver to produce its primary active metabolite, desmethyldosulepin (northiaden). The plasma half-life is 50 h.

EVALUATION OF DATA

Passage of dosulepin into human milk has been reported as follows:

Treatment conditions	Concentration (μg/l)		Milk/ plasma ratio	Maxi- mum observed milk conc. (μg/l)	Absolute dose to infant (μg/kg/day)		Ref.
Dose × Frequency × Duration; Route; No. of patients; Lactation stage	Milk	Plasma			Ave	Max	
25 mg × 3/d × LT; p.o.; 1; ?	11 (3 h)	33 (3 h)	3	–	–	–	(1)
300 mg over 6 d; p.o.;. 1; ?	10	10	–	–	–	–	(1)
25–225 mg/d × > 7 d; p.o.; 8; 0.13–12.5 months	5–475 3–73[a] 65–714[b] 27–400[c]	11–170 3–68[a] 58–682[b] 18–192[c]	0.78–1.59 0.85[a] 1.18[b] 1.86[c]	475 73[a] 714[b] 400[c]	–	71 11[a] 107[b] 60[c]	(2)

In reference (1) the first patient gave milk and plasma 3 h after a dose of dosulepin. The second patient gave samples after receiving dosulepin intermittently to a total of 300 mg over 6 days. Milk samples were obtained immediately before and after infant feeding and single plasma samples before or after feeding in reference (2). The table gives the range of values for dosulepin, nordosulepin (a), dosulepin–S-oxide (b), nordosulepin-S-oxide (c).

RELATIVE DOSE IN MILK

The data in (2) were calculated according to the formulae on pp. 71–72 and permit the following conclusions. A suckling infant would ingest on average 4.45% (comprising dosulepin 0.58%, nordosulepin 0.23%, dosulepin-S-oxide 2.47% and nordosulepin-S-oxide 1.17%) of the weight-adjusted maternal daily dose of dosulepin. The highest relative dose calculated for an individual in this group was 7.1%.

DATA ON THE INFANT

Dosulepin and its metabolites were below their minimum quantifiable concentrations in blood samples from 5 infants. No adverse drug effects were recorded in any of the 8 infants studied.

ASSESSMENT OF DATA

The limited information available suggests that when dosulepin is administered to a nursing mother the quantity of drug that passes into milk is small. A decision about the advisability of breast-feeding is probably best determined by the factors pertinent to the individual case. When the maternal dose is high, exposure to the infant to the drug may be reduced by limiting the number of feeds per day.

REFERENCES

1. Rees JA, Glass RC, Sporne GA (1976) Serum and breast milk concentrations of dothiepin. *The Practitioner, 217*, 686.
2. Ilett KF, Lebedevs TH, Wojnar-Horton RE, Yapp P, Roberts MJ, Dusci LJ, Hackett LP (1992) Excretion of dothiepin and its primary metabolites in breast milk. *Br. J. Clin. Pharmacol., 33*, 635–639.

DOXEPIN

GENERAL

Doxepin is a tricyclic antidepressant drug. It is readily absorbed from the adult gastrointestinal tract and 55–87% is demethylated in first-pass through the liver to form the primary metabolite, N-desmethyl-doxepin (DDP) which is pharmacologically active. Doxepin is 80% protein bound; DDP is 78% bound. The plasma half-life of doxepin is 8–25 h and of DDP is 33–81 h.

EVALUATION OF DATA

Passage of doxepin into human milk has been reported as follows:

Treatment conditions Dose × Frequency × Duration; Route; No. of patients; Lactation stage	Concentration (μg/l)		Milk/plasma ratio	Maximum observed milk conc. (μg/l)	Absolute dose to infant (μg/kg/day)		Ref.
	Milk	Plasma			Ave	Max	
150 mg × 1\d × LT; p. o.; 1; 2 months	60 (111)	46 (90)	1.08	–	9 (17)	–	(1)
25 mg × 3/5 × LT; p.o.; 1; 2 months	18 (9)	15 (57)	0.7 (0.16)	–	3 (1)	–	(2)

LT, long term. The figures in parentheses refer to DDP. Reference (1) reports means of 8 paired milk and plasma samples taken 17 h after the daily dose between days 7–99 after doxepin was started. In reference (2) the milk and plasma concentrations are means of 9 samples taken 0–6 h after doxepin. Both studies were conducted under steady-state conditions of dosing but neither defined the concentration-time profiles.

RELATIVE DOSE IN MILK

A suckling infant would ingest in a day on average 0.3–1.0% (0.018 + 0.009 × 900/75)-(0.060 + 0.111 × 900/150)* (1,2) of the weight-adjusted maternal daily dose of doxepin and DDP.

DATA ON THE INFANT

An 8-week-old infant whose mother had taken doxepin for 6 weeks was admitted to hospital with respiratory depression and sedation (2). The infant's serum contained doxepin 2.2 μg/l and DDP 58 μg/l; its urine contained DDP 39 μg/l. The mother was advised to breast-feed only at night while she continued her medication. Nine

* An explanation of the calculation (s) appears on pp. 71–72.

days later the infant's serum DDP concentration was 66 μg/l. Reference (1) reports that 43 days after therapy was started the infant's plasma contained no doxepin (detection limit 5 μg/l) and DDP was 15 μg/l. The authors found that the infant was not sedated and had normal motor development.

ASSESSMENT OF DATA

The data suggest that when doxepin is administered to a nursing mother the quantity of doxepin and N-desmethyldoxepin that is ingested by her infant in milk is small. N-desmethyl-doxepin may, however, accumulate in the infant. A decision about the advisability of breast-feeding is probably best determined by the factors pertinent to the individual case. When the maternal dose is high, exposure to the infant to the drug may be reduced by limiting the number of feeds per day.

REFERENCES

1. Kemp J, Ilett KF, Booth J, Hackett LP (1985) Excretion of doxepin and N-desmethyldoxepin in human milk. *Br. J. Clin. Pharmacol., 20:*, 497–499.
2. Matheson I, Pande H, Alertsen AR (1985) Respiratory depression caused by N-desmethyldoxepin in breast milk. *Lancet, ii,* 1124.

ETHOSUXIMIDE

GENERAL

Ethosuximide is an antiepileptic drug used mainly to treat simple absence seizures. It is absorbed from the adult gastrointestinal tract and is not significantly bound to plasma proteins. Ethosuximide is extensively metabolised but no active metabolites are known. The plasma half-life of ethosuximide is 55 h in adults and 32–38 h in newborn infants (4).

EVALUATION OF DATA

Passage of ethosuximide into human milk has been reported as follows:

Treatment conditions Dose × Frequency × Duration; Route; No. of patients; Lactation stage	Concentration (mg/l)		Milk/plasma ratio	Maximum observed milk conc. (mg/l)	Absolute dose to infant (mg/kg/day)		Ref.
	Milk	Plasma			Ave	Max	
500 mg × 2/d × LT; p.o.; 1; 3–5 d	60–70	60–75	0.94	–	–	–	(1)
? × LT; p.o.; 4; 3–32 d	21.3 (18–24)	29.3 (18–39)	0.79	24.0	3.2	3.6	(2)
250 mg × 2/d × LT; p.o.; 1; 1–5 months	44.7	55.9	0.8	54.9	6.7	8.2	(3)
3.5–23.6 mg/kg/d × LT; p.o.; 5; 3–28 d	49.5	57.4	0 86	77.0	7.4	11.5	(4)
250–500 mg × 2/d × LT; p.o.; 4; 3 d–5 months	35.5	37.4	0.94 (0.79–1.03)	54.9	5.3	8.2	(5)

LT, long term. Reference (1) reports numerous serum and 3 milk samples taken over 53 days after delivery. The milk concentrations are estimated from a graph. Average concentrations with the ranges in brackets are given in reference (2). Reference (3) presents average values for 6 paired milk and blood samples taken at intervals over 5 months after delivery, 3–5 h after the morning dose of ethosuximide. The milk to plasma ratio refers to mature milk. The maximum milk concentration is the highest value recorded by the patient. Reference (4) gives average values based on 12 paired samples from the mothers. The maximum milk concentration is the highest value recorded in an individual. Average milk and plasma concentrations are presented in reference (5) and the maximum milk concentration is the highest value noted in an individual. All studies were conducted under steady-state conditions of dosing.

RELATIVE DOSE IN MILK

The amount of ethosuximide that a suckling infant would ingest in a day is on average 63.5% (35.3 × 900/500)* (5) and at maximum 98.8% (54.9 × 900/500)* (5) of the weight-adjusted maternal daily dose.

* An explanation of the calculation (s) appears on pp. 71–72.

DATA ON THE INFANT

The plasma ethosuximide concentration in the breast-feeding infant reported in reference (3) was 29.6 mg/l and in those in reference (4) the concentrations were 15.0–40.0 mg/l; abnormal behaviour such as sedation, poor suckling and hyperexcitability was noted in 7 of the latter group. Three of the suckling infants reported in reference (4) had plasma ethosuximide concentrations in the range 16.9–23.0 mg/l (mean 20.4 mg/l) but no adverse effects were noted. The fourth baby was partially breast-fed and ethosuximide was not found in the plasma. The therapeutic plasma concentration of ethosuximide in adults is 40–100 mg/l.

ASSESSMENT AND RECOMMENDATIONS

The risk to the suckling infant of administering ethosuximide to its mother is significant because a substantial quantity of drug passes into milk and because adverse effects can be attributed to it. Breast-feeding should be regarded as unsafe.

REFERENCES

1. Koup JR, Rose JQ, Cohen ME (1978) Ethosuximide pharmacokinetics in a pregnant patient and her newborn. *Epilepsia, 19,* 535–539.
2. Kaneko S, Sato T, Suzuki J (1979) The levels of anticonvulsants in breast milk. *Br. J. Clin. Pharmacol., 7,* 624–626.
3. Rane A, Tunell R (1981) Ethosuximide in human milk and in plasma of a mother and her nursed infant. *Br. J. Clin. Pharmacol., 12,* 855–858.
4. Kuhnz W, Koch S, Jakob S, Hartmann A, Helge H, Nau H (1984) Ethosuximide in epileptic women during pregancy and lactation period. Placental transfer, serum concentrations in nursed infants and clinical status. *Br. J. Clin. Pharmacol., 18,* 671–677.
5. Soderman P, Rane A, Tunell, R (1986) *111 World Conference on Clinical Pharmacology and Therapeutics*, Stockholm, (Abstract)

FENTANYL

GENERAL

Fentanyl is a synthetic opioid that is used to provide anaesthesia before, during and after surgical procedures, and during labour and delivery. It readily causes respiratory depression in overdose. Fentanyl may be given by a variety of routes, has a large apparent distribution volume (4 l/kg) and is extensively metabolised by the liver to products that are thought to be inactive. The plasma half-life is 1–6 h and lengthens with repeated doses.

EVALUATION OF DATA

Passage of fentanyl into human milk has been reported as follows:

Treatment conditions: Dose × Frequency × Duration; Route; No. of patients; Lactation stage	Concentration (μg/l): Milk	Concentration (μg/l): Serum	Milk/serum ratio	Maximum observed milk conc. (μg/l)	Absolute dose to infant (μg/kg/day): Ave	Absolute dose to infant (μg/kg/day): Max	Ref.
2 μg/d × 1/d × 1 d; i.v.; 13; 1 d	0.40	0.19	2.1	0.97	–	0.06	(1)
50–400 μg × 1 d × 1 d; i.v.; 10; 1 d	(see below)	–	–	–	–	–	(2)

In (1) fentanyl was given for analgesia or anaesthesia during Caesarean section (n = 8) or tubal ligation (n = 5). Milk and serum samples were taken for 10 h after dosing; the concentration-time profiles were concurrent at 0.75 and 2 h but the serum concentration thereafter was negligible. The table gives the mean peak concentration in milk (at 0.75 h) and the maximum concentration is the highest value recorded in an individual. Milk fentanyl concentrations declined rapidly to reach 0.15 μg/l at 4 h and <0.1 μg/l at 6 h. In (2) fentanyl was given during labour. The milk concentration 4 h later was <0.5 μg/l in 6 mothers and 0.12–0.15 μg/l in 3 mothers, i.e. similar to the values in (1).

RELATIVE DOSE IN MILK

As fentanyl citrate (mol. wt. 529) was administered but the free base (mol. wt. 337) was assayed a factor of 1.57 (529/337) is included in the calculation. Assuming a maternal weight of 60 kg and (for the purpose of the calculation) suckling at peak concentration, an infant would ingest in a feed at maximum 0.9% (0.4 × 180 × 1.57/120)* of the weight-adjusted maternal single dose of fentanyl. More realistically, an infant suckling, say, 12 h after a single dose to the mother would ingest negligible amounts of the drug.

* An explanation of the calculation (s) appears on pp. 71–72.

DATA ON THE INFANT

No data are available from the quoted studies.

ASSESSMENT OF DATA

Single dose data indicate that the risk to the suckling infant of administering fentanyl to its mother is low on the basis that the quantity of drug that passes into milk is small. Breast-feeding after a single analgesic dose should be regarded as safe.

REFERENCES

1. Steer PL, Biddle CJ, Marley WS, Lantz RK, Sulik PL (1992) Concentration of fentanyl in colostrum after an analgesic dose. *Can. J. Anaesth. (Toronto), 39*, 231–235.
2. Leuschen MP, Wolf LJ, Rayburn WF (1990) Fentanyl excretion in breast milk. *Clin. Pharm., 9*, 336–337.

FLUNITRAZEPAM

GENERAL

Flunitrazepam is a benzodiazepine drug that is used in short courses principally as an hypnotic. It is rapidly absorbed from the adult gastrointestinal tract and is 78% bound to plasma proteins. Flunitrazepam is extensively metabolised in the liver; both major metabolites, desmethylflunitrazepam and the 7-amino derivative, are pharmacologically active. The plasma half-life of flunitrazepam is 29 h.

EVALUATION OF DATA

Passage of flunitrazepam into human milk has been reported as follows:

Treatment conditions: Dose × Frequency × Duration; Route; No. of patients; Lactation stage	Concentration (μg/l)		Milk/ plasma ratio	Maximum observed milk conc. (μg/l)	Absolute dose to infant (μg/kg/day)		Ref.
	Milk	Plasma			Ave	Max	
1–2 mg/d × 1/d; i.v.; 5 1 week	1.7	4.2	0.41	7.0	0.3	1.1	(1)
2 mg/d × 1 d; p.o.; 5; 1 d	2	3	0.67	–	0.3	–	(2)

Reference (1) reports on flunitrazepam given for i.v. anaesthesia. The milk and plasma concentration-time profiles were defined for 24 h after dosing and were concurrent; the table gives average values based on the areas under the respective curves. The maximum milk concentration was the highest value recorded in an individual. In reference (2) the concentrations quoted are average values measured 11 h after the single dose and are estimated from a graph. Neither study was conducted under steady-state conditions of dosing.

RELATIVE DOSE IN MILK

The amount of flunitrazepam that a suckling infant would ingest in a feed is at maximum 0.6% (7 × 180/2000)* of the weight-adjusted maternal single dose (1).

DATA ON THE INFANT

No effects were reported in the infants studied.

ASSESSMENT OF DATA

The data indicate that when a single dose of flunitrazepam is administered to a

* An explanation of the calculation (s) appears on pp. 71–72.

nursing mother, the quantity of drug ingested by her infant in milk is small. The evaluated studies do not, however, address the issue of accumulation to steady-state of flunitrazepam and its pharmacologically active metabolites. The risk to the infant suckling after a single dose to the mother would appear to be low, but may become significant if regularly repeated doses are given.

REFERENCES

1. Jensen OH, Bredesen JE, Lindbaek E (1981) Transfer of flunitrazepam to mothers' milk. *Tiddskr. Nor. Laegeforen, 101,* 504–505.
2. Kanto J, Aaltonen L, Langas L, Erkkola R, Pitkänen Y (1979) Placental transfer and breast milk levels of flunitrazepam. *Curr. Ther. Res., 26,* 539–546.

FLUOXETINE

GENERAL

Fluoxetine is an antidepressant that acts by inhibiting uptake of 5-hydroxytryptamine. It is well absorbed from the adult gastrointestinal tract, 90% bound to plasma proteins and it is extensively metabolised by processes that become non-linear at higher doses. The principal product, norfluoxetine, retains pharmacological activity. The plasma half-life of fluoxetine is 3.6 days and that of norfluoxetine is 6 days.

EVALUATION OF DATA

Passage of fluoxetine into human milk has been reported as follows:

Treatment conditions Dose × Frequency × Duration; Route; No. of patients; Lactation stage	Concentration (μg/l) Milk	 Plasma	Milk/ plasma ratio	Maximum observed milk conc. (μg/l)	Absolute dose to infant (μg/kg/day) Ave	 Max	Ref.
20 mg × 1/d × 2 months; p.o.; 1; 5 months	28.8 (41.6)	100.5 (194.5)	–	–	–	–	(1)
20 mg × 1/d × 53 d; p.o.; 1; 18 weeks	17* (13)	124* (141)	0.14 (0.09)	–	–	–	(2)
20 mg × 1/d × 53 d; p.o.; 1; 4 months	67** (52)	135** (149)	0.5 (0.35)	–	–	10.1 (7.8)	(2)

*8 h post-dose; **4 h post-dose. The figures in brackets refer to norfluoxetine.

RELATIVE DOSE IN MILK

The amount of fluoxetine and norfluoxetine that a suckling infant would ingest in a day is at maximum 5.5% (67 + 52 × 900/20000)* of the weight-adjusted maternal daily dose.

DATA ON THE INFANT

The infants in (1) and (2) continued to breast-feed while their mothers received fluoxetine and exhibited no drug-related effects.

* An explanation of the calculation (s) appears on pp. 71–72.

ASSESSMENT OF DATA

Data from 3 cases under conditions of steady-state dosing suggest that the risk to the suckling infant of administering fluoxetine to its mother is low on the basis that the quantity of drug that passes into milk is small. A decision about the advisability of breast-feeding is probably best determined by the factors pertinent to the individual case. When the maternal dose is high, exposure to the infant to the drug may be reduced by limiting the number of feeds per day.

REFERENCES

1. Isenberg KE (1990) Excretion of fluoxetine in human milk. *J. Clin. Psychiatyr, 51*, 169.
2. Burch KJ, Wells BG (1992) Fluoxetine/norfluoxetine concentrations in human milk. *Pediatrics, 89*, 676–677.

FLUPENTIXOL

GENERAL

Flupentixol (flupenthixol is a thioxanthene neuroleptic drug with little sedative effect. It is readily absorbed from the adult gastrointestinal tract but oral bioavailability is about 40% as flupentixol is subject to first pass metabolism. Flupentixol is also available as the decanoate which is given as a depot i.m. injection every 2–4 weeks. Binding to plasma proteins exceeds 95%. The plasma half-life of oral flupentixol is 35 h and that of the decanoate is 17 h.

EVALUATION OF DATA

Passage of flupentixol into human milk has been reported as follows:

Treatment conditions Dose × Frequency × Duration; Route; No. of patients; Lactation stage	Concentration (μg/l)		Milk/ plasma ratio	Maximum observed milk conc. (μg/l)	Absolute dose to infant (μg/kg/day)		Ref.
	Milk	Plasma			Ave	Max	
2 mg × 1/d × LT; p.o.; 1; 30 d	1.8	1.5	1.2	–	0.27	–	(1)
40 mg every 2 weeks × LT; depot i.m.; 1; 41 d	1.8	1.3	1.4	–	0.27	–	(1)
60 mg every 3 weeks × LT; depot i.m.; 1; 17 d	1.8	1.4	1.3	–	0.27	–	(1)
4 mg × 1/d × LT; p.o.; 1; 6–6 d	2.8	–	0.55–0.83	–	0.42	–	(2)

LT, long term. Paired milk and plasma samples were taken from patients under steady-state conditions of dosing, i.e. the concentration-time profile was not defined in (1). Reference (2) defined the concentration-time profiles which appeared to be concurrent. The milk concentration is the mean of 7 measurements.

RELATIVE DOSE IN MILK

The amount of flupentixol that an infant would ingest in a day is on average 0.6% (2.8 × 900/4000)* (2) of the weight-adjusted maternal daily dose.

DATA ON THE INFANT

The authors report that the infants, who were also exposed to flupentixol in utero,

* An explanation of the calculation (s) appears on pp. 71–72.

were normal on routine clinical examination and appeared to be growing normally (1). Infant serum on day 6 and 7 postpartum contained flupentixol <0.2 and 0.3 μg/l respectively, and reflect placental as well as breast milk transfer (2).

ASSESSMENT OF DATA

The data indicate that when flupentixol is administered to a nursing mother, the quantity of drug that is ingested by her infant in breast milk is small. A decision about the advisability of breast-feeding is probably best determined by the factors pertinent to the individual case. When the maternal dose is high, exposure of the infant to the drug may be reduced by limiting the number of feeds per day.

REFERENCES

1. Kirk L, Jorgensen A (1980) Concentrations of cis (Z)-flupentixol in maternal serum, amniotic fluid, umbilical cord serum and milk. *Psychopharmacology, 72*, 107–108.
2. Matheson I, Skjæraasen J (1988) Milk concentrations of flupenthixol, nortriptyline and zuclopenthixol and between-breast differnces in two patients. *Eur. J. Clin. Pharmacol., 35*, 217–220.

FLUVOXAMINE

GENERAL

Fluvoxamine is an antidepressant drug that acts by inhibiting neuronal uptake of 5-hydroxytryptamine. It is well absorbed from the adult gastrointestinal tract, is 77% bound to plasma proteins and is completely metabolised to products that are excreted in the urine. The plasma half-life is 15 h.

EVALUATION OF DATA

Passage of fluvoxamine into human milk has been reported as follows:

Treatment conditions Dose × Frequency × Duration; Route; No. of patients; Lactation stage	Concentration (mg/l) Milk	 Plasma	Milk/ plasma ratio	Maximum observed milk conc. (mg/l)	Absolute dose to infant (mg/kg/day) Ave	 Max	Ref.
100 mg × 2/d × 14 d; p.o..; 1; 12 weeks	90	310	0.29	–	–	–	(1)

Single milk and plasma samples were taken 4.75 h after a dose; steady-state conditions are assumed to have been reached.

RELATIVE DOSE IN MILK

The amount of fluvoxamine that a suckling infant would ingest in a day is 0.6% (90 × 900/146 300)* of the weight-adjusted maternal daily dose (1). The calculation takes account of the fact that fluvoxamine malate 200 mg contains 146.3 mg of fluvoxamine base.

DATA ON THE INFANT

The infant did not exhibit drug-related effects.

ASSESSMENT AND RECOMMENDATIONS

Limited data suggest that the risk to the suckling infant of administering fluvoxamine to its mother is low on the basis that the quantity of drug that passes into milk is small. A decision about the advisability of breast-feeding is probably best deter-

* An explanation of the calculation (s) appears on pp. 71–72.

mined by the factors pertinent to the individual case. When the maternal dose is high, exposure to the infant to the drug may be reduced by limiting the number of feeds per day.

REFERENCE

1. Wright S, Dawling S, Ashford JJ (1991). Excretion of fluvoxamine in breast milk. *Br. J. Clin. Pharmacol., 31*, 209.

GLUTETHIMIDE

GENERAL

Glutethimide is an hypnotic drug. It is irregularly absorbed from the adult gastrointestinal tract and 54% is bound to plasma proteins. Glutethimide is extensively metabolised in the liver and some of the products are pharmacologically active. The terminal plasma half-life is 5–22 h.

EVALUATION OF DATA

Passage of glutethimide into human milk has been reported as follows:

Treatment conditions	Concentration (mg/l)		Milk/ plasma ratio	Maximum observed milk conc. (mg/l)	Absolute dose to infant (mg/kg/day)		Ref.
Dose × Frequency × Duration; Route; No. of patients; Lactation stage	Milk	Plasma			Ave	Max	
500 mg × 1/d × 1 d; p.o.; 13; ?	0.27	2.0	0.15	0.27	0.04	–	(1)

The milk concentration quoted is the mean value in 90 samples collected 8 h after dosing. Concentrations 12, 16, 20 and 23 h after dosing were 0.27, 0.22, 0.12 and 0.04 mg/l respectively. In 32 of the samples, no drug was detected but the values from all 90 samples were included in calculating the means. All milk concentrations were measured in hind milk.

RELATIVE DOSE IN MILK

The amount of glutethimide that a suckling infant would ingest in a feed is at maximum 0.1 % (0.27 × 180/500)* of the weight-adjusted maternal single dose (1).

DATA ON THE INFANT

No data are available.

ASSESSMENT OF DATA

The risk to the suckling infant of administering a single dose of glutethimide to its mother is low on the basis that the quantity of drug that passes into milk is small. When glutethimide is taken as an occasional single dose, breast-feeding would ap-

* An explanation of the calculation (s) appears on pp. 71–72.

pear to be safe. There are no data on which to base a recommendation when glutethimide is taken in regularly repeated doses.

REFERENCES

1. Curry SH, Ridall D, Gordon JS, Simpson P, Binns T, Rondel RK, McMartin C (1971) Disposition of gluthetimide in man. *Clin. Pharmacol. Ther.*, *12*, 849–857.

HALOPERIDOL

GENERAL

Haloperidol is a neuroleptic drug with strong antipsychotic effects. It is readily absorbed from the adult gastrointestinal tract and 40% is metabolised in first-pass through the liver. Metabolites are excreted in the faeces and urine. There is wide intersubject variation in plasma concentration. It is 92% bound to plasma proteins and the plasma half-life is 18 h.

EVALUATION OF DATA

Passage of haloperidol into human milk has been reported as follows:

Treatment conditions: Dose × Frequency × Duration; Route; No. of patients; Lactation stage	Concentration (μg/l)		Milk/ plasma ratio	Maximum observed milk conc. (μg/l)	Absolute dose to infant (μg/kg/day)		Ref.
	Milk	Plasma			Ave	Max	
29.2 × 1/d × 6 d; p.o.; 1; 6 weeks	5	–	–	–	–	–	(1)
5 mg × 2/d × 7 d; p.o.; 1; 4 weeks	21	33	–	23.5	–	–	(2)
3–4 mg × 1/d × ?; p.o.; 2; ?	17–32	–	–	–	–	–	(3)

In reference (1) the mean daily dose is quoted; the milk concentration was measured taken 11 h after a dose. On the 12th day of treatment, 9 h after haloperidol 12 mg, the milk concentration was 2 μg/l. The milk and plasma values in reference (2) are the means from the 6th and 7th days of treatment. The maximum milk concentration was the highest value recorded in the patient.

RELATIVE DOSE IN MILK

The amount of haloperidol that a suckling infant would ingest in a day is 0.2–2.1% (5 × 900/29 200)–(23.5 × 900/10 000)* (1,2) of the weight-adjusted maternal daily dose. Data from reference (3) give a maximum relative daily dose of 9.6% (32 × 900/3000)*.

DATA ON THE INFANT

A sample of the infant's urine collected on the 21st day of treatment to the mother contained haloperidol 1.5 μ/l (2). The baby did not appear to be sedated, fed well and achieved her developmental milestones at 6 months and 1 year.

* An explanation of the calculation (s) appears on pp. 71–72.

ASSESSMENT OF DATA

The data suggest that when haloperidol is administered to a nursing mother, the quantity of drug ingested by her infant in milk is small to moderate. A decision about the advisability of breast-feeding is probably best determined by the factors pertinent to the individual case. When the maternal dose is high, exposure to the infant to the drug may be reduced by limiting the number of feeds per day.

REFERENCES

1. Stewart RB, Karas B, Spring PK (1980) Haloperidol excretion in human milk. *Am. J. Psychiatry., 137*, 849–850.
2. Whalley LJ, Blain PG, Prime JK (1981) Haloperidol secreted in breast milk. *Br. Med. J., 282*, 1746–1747.
3. Ohkubo T, Shimoyama R, Sugawara K (1992) Measurement of haloperidol in human breast milk by high-performance liquid chromatography. *J. Pharmacol. Sci., 81*, 947–949.

IMIPRAMINE

GENERAL

Imipramine is a tricyclic antidepressant with properties similar to amitriptyline, but with less sedative effect. It is well absorbed from the adult gastrointestinal tract and is extensively demethylated by first-pass metabolism in the liver to form desipramine which is pharmacologically active. Imipramine and desipramine are 80–95% bound to plasma proteins. The plasma half-life of imipramine is 6–20 h and of desipramine is 12–54 h.

EVALUATION OF DATA

Passage of imipramine and desipramine into human milk has been reported as follows:

Treatment conditions	Concentration (μg/l)		Milk/plasma ratio	Maximum observed milk conc. (μg/l)	Absolute dose to infant (μg/kg/day)		Ref.
Dose × Frequency × Duration; Route; No. of patients; Lactation stage	Milk	Plasma			Ave	Max	
200 mg × 1/d × LT; p.o.; 1; 2 months	17 (26)	21 (41)	–	29 (35)	–	–	(1)

LT, long term. The figures in brackets refer to desipramine. The milk concentrations quoted are the means of 6 samples taken 1–23 h after the dose of imipramine on the 16–18th days of treatment. The maximum milk concentrations are the highest individual values recorded in the patient. The plasma concentrations were estimated on the 22nd day after the start of therapy and were below the recommended therapeutic range (100–300 μg/l).

RELATIVE DOSE IN MILK

The amount of imipramine and desipramine that a suckling infant would ingest in a day is on average 0.2% (17 + 26 × 900/200 000)* and at maximum 0.3% (29 + 35 × 900/200 000)* of the weight-adjusted maternal daily dose (1). Note, however, that maternal plasma concentrations were unexpectedly low for the dose administered, by a factor of ×3–4.

DATA ON THE INFANT

No data are available.

* An explanation of the calculation (s) appears on pp. 71–72.

ASSESSMENT OF DATA

This case report suggest when imipramine is administered to a nursing mother, the quantity of imipramine and desipramine that is ingested by her infant in milk is small. A decision about the advisability of breast-feeding is probably best determined by the factors pertinent to the individual case. When the maternal dose is high, exposure to the infant to the drug may be reduced by limiting the number of feeds per day.

REFERENCES

1. Sovner R, Orsulak PJ (1979) Excretion of imipramine and desipramine in human breast milk. *Am. J. Psychiatry., 136,* 451–452.

LITHIUM

GENERAL

Lithium salts are used in the treatment of manic-depressive illness. Lithium is well absorbed from the adult gastrointestinal tract and is not bound to plasma proteins. It is excreted by the kidney. The plasma half-life is 8–45 h in adults but it is longer in neonates. It is customary to monitor the plasma concentration as the therapeutic range is narrow (0.8–1.5 mmol/l) and toxic effects are common when the concentration exceeds 2 mmol/l.

EVALUATION OF DATA

Passage of lithium into human milk has been reported as follows:

Treatment conditions: Dose × Frequency × Duration; Route; No. of patients; Lactation stage	Concentration (mmol/l) Milk	Concentration (mmol/l) Plasma	Milk/plasma ratio	Maximum observed milk conc. (mmol/l)	Absolute dose to infant (mmol/kg day) Ave	Absolute dose to infant (mmol/kg day) Max	Ref.
10–20 mmol/d × LT; p.o.; 1; 1 week	0.6	1.5	0.4	–	–	–	(1)
16.4 mmol/d × LT; p.o.; 1; 70 d	0.12	0.5	0.24	–	0.02	–	(2)
?; p.o.; 4; 1–10 weeks	0.38	0.69	0.6	0.56	–	0.08	(3)
9–15 mmol/d × 1–3 d; p.o.; 1; 2 weeks	0.51	0.55	0.91	0.8	0.08	0.12	(4)
20 mmol/d× 3 d; p.o.; 1; 3 weeks	1.54	1.10	1.32	–	0.23	–	(4)

LT, long term. 1 mmol = 61 mg lithium carbonate = 94 mg lithium citrate. References (1) and (2) report patients from whom single milk samples were taken under steady-state conditions of dosing. The interval between the dose and the samples was not stated. The data in reference (3) are mean values (and exclude those also quoted in this paper from other sources). Reference (4) is a case report of a patient in whom treatment was started with lithium carbonate 600 mg the first day, 800 mg on the second day, 1000 mg the third day, and 1200 mg the fourth day. Milk concentrations rose more rapidly than plasma concentrations; breast-feeding ceased on the 21st day post partum when the milk to plasma ratio was 1.65. A further report of serial concentrations of lithium in maternal serum and milk during breast-feeding is in accord with these findings (5).

RELATIVE DOSE IN MILK

A suckling infant would ingest on average 54.0% (0.6 × 900/10)* (1) and at maximum 80.0% (0.8 × 900/9)* (4) of the weight-adjusted maternal daily dose of lithium.

* An explanation of the calculation (s) appears on pp. 71–72.

DATA ON THE INFANT

Tremor and involuntary movements were reported in a 2 month old suckling infant who had higher lithium concentrations (1.4 mmol/l) than his mother (0.7 mmol/l) (6). Schou and Amdisen (2), who summarised eight cases, reported serum concentrations in breast-fed infants to be one half that of their mothers' serum during the first week of life, and one-third during the following weeks.

ASSESSMENT AND RECOMMENDATIONS

The risk to the suckling infant of administering lithium to its mother is significant on the basis of the quantity of drug that passes into milk and the observation of drug-related effects. Breast-feeding should be regarded as unsafe.

REFERENCES

1. Tunnessen WW, Hertz CG (1972) Toxic effects of lithium in newborn infants: a commentary. *J. Paediatr., 81*, 804–807.
2. Weinstein MR, Goldfield M (1972) Lithium carbonate treatment during pregnancy. *Dis. Nerv. Sys., 30,* 828–832.
3. Schou M, Amdisen A (1973) Lithium and pregancy. 1ll. Lithium ingestion by children breast-fed by women on lithium treatment. *Br. Med. J., 2,* 138.
4. Shimizu M, Matsuda H, Sakaue N, Ikeda R, Mimuro I (1981) A few findings on lithium levels in mother milk. *Seishin Shinkeigaku Zasshi, 83*, 399–405.
5. Sykes PA, Quarrie J, Alexander FW (1976) Lithium carbonate and breast-feeding. *Br. Med. J., 4*, 1299.
6. Skausig OB, Schou M (1977) Breast-feeding during lithium treatment. *Ugeskr. Laeg., 139*, 400–401.

LORAZEPAM

GENERAL

Lorazepam is a benzodiazepine drug that is used in short courses as an anxiolytic and hypnotic. It is almost completely absorbed from the adult gastrointestinal tract, 85% bound to plasma proteins and is metabolised to products that are not pharmacologically active. The plasma half-life is 15 h

EVALUATION OF DATA

Passage of lorazepam into human milk has been reported as follows:

Treatment conditions	Concentration (μg/l)		Milk/ plasma ratio	Maxi- mum observed milk conc. (μg/l)	Absolute dose to infant (μg/kg/day)		Ref.
Dose × Frequency × Duration; Route; No. of patients; Lactation stage	Milk	Plasma			Ave	Max	
2.5 mg × 2/d × 5 d; p.o.; 1; 5 d	12 (35)	–	–	–	–	–	(1)
3.5 mg/d × 1 d; p.o.; 4; 1 week	9	41	0.22	–	–	–	(2)

The mother quoted in reference (1) was probably under steady-state dosing conditions. The interval between the taking of the last dose and the single milk sample is not stated. The concentration of lorazepam glucuronide appears in brackets. In reference (2) lorazepam was given as premedication for postpartum sterilisation; the table gives average milk and plasma concentrations 4 h after dosing.

RELATIVE DOSE IN MILK

Breast milk has been shown to have considerable beta-glucuronidase activity (3) and for the purpose of the calculation it has been assumed that lormetazepam glucuronide (mol. wt. 514) is deconjugated and that lorazepam (mol. wt. 321) is absorbed by the infant. On this basis the suckling infant would ingest in a day 5.3% (12 + 35 × 900 × 321/5000 × 514)* of the weight-adjusted maternal daily dose of lorazepam and its glucuronide (1).

DATA ON THE INFANT

No sedative effects were noted in the neonate (1).

* An explanation of the calculation (s) appears on pp. 71–72.

ASSESSMENT OF DATA

Limited data suggest that the risk to the suckling infant of administering a short course of lorazepam to its mother is low on the basis that the amount of drug that passes into milk is small. Breast-feeding is probably safe if a mother takes lorazepam for a short period.

REFERENCES

1. Whitelaw AGL, Cummings AJ, McFadyen IR (1981) Effects of maternal lorazepam on the neonate. *Br. Med. J., 282,* 1106–1108.
2. Summerfield RJ, Nielsen MS (1985) Excretion of lorazepam into breast milk. *Br. J. Anaesth., 57,* 1042–1043.
3. Gourley GR, Arend RA (1986) Beta-glucuronidase and hyperbilirubinaemia in breast-fed babies. *Lancet, i,* 644–646.

LORMETAZEPAM

GENERAL

Lormetazepam is a benzodiazepine hypnotic drug that is used in short courses for insomnia. In adults its bioavailability after oral administration is about 80% and it is 88% bound to plasma proteins. Lormetazepam is conjugated with glucuronic acid which is excreted in the urine. Its plasma half-life is 10 h.

EVALUATION OF DATA

Passage of lormetazepam into human milk has been reported as follows:

Treatment conditions: Dose × Frequency × Duration; Route; No. of patients; Lactation stage	Concentration (μg/l)		Milk/ plasma ratio	Maximum observed milk conc. (μg/l)	Absolute dose to infant (μg/kg/day)		Ref.
	Milk	Plasma			Ave	Max	
2 mg × 1/d × 10 d; p.o.; 5; 2–13 d	<0.2 (1.0)	3.5 (29.5)	<0.06	–	–	–	(1)

The figures in parentheses refers to lormetazepam glucuronide. The study was undertaken under steady-state conditions of dosing and milk and plasma were sampled twice daily for 10 days. The table gives average concentrations 12 h after each daily dose. Unknown radioimmunoactive material was present in blank milk from 3 subjects but not in the remaining 2, in whom the milk concentration was generally <2 μg/l.

RELATIVE DOSE IN MILK

Breast milk has been shown to have considerable beta-glucuronidase activity (2) and for the purpose of the calculation it has been assumed that lormetazepam glucuronide (mol. wt. 528) is deconjugated and lormetazepam (mol. wt. 335) is absorbed by the infant. On this basis a suckling infant would ingest in a day on average less than 0.3% (0.2 + 1 × 900 × 335 /2000 × 528)* of the weight-adjusted maternal daily dose of lormetazepam and lormetazepam glucuronide (1).

DATA ON THE INFANT

Unconjugated lormetazepam did not exceed the detection limit of 0.09 μg/l in any infant. Inactive lormetazepam glucuronide was present in plasma of all 5 infants and the mean concentration declined from 0.6 on the 1st day to 0.3 μg/l on the 9th day, indicating that their elimination capacity may have increased during this pe-

* An explanation of the calculation (s) appears on pp. 71–72.

riod. The highest lormetazepam glucuronide concentration recorded in any infant was 1.35 μg/l. No drug effects were observed in the five babies during the period of observation.

ASSESSMENT OF DATA

The risk to the suckling infant of administering lormetazepam to its mother is low on the basis that the amount of drug that passes into milk is small. Breast-feeding may be regarded as safe provided the period of exposure to the drug is short.

REFERENCES

1. Humpel M, Stopelli I, Milia S, Rainer E (1982) Pharmacokinetics and biotransformation of the new benzodiazepine, lormetazepam, in man. III. Repeated administration and transfer to neonates via breast milk. *Eur. J. Clin. Pharmacol., 21*, 421–425.
2. Gourley GR, Arend RA (1986) Beta-glucuronidase and hyperbilirubinaemia in breast-fed babies. *Lancet, i,* 644–646.

MAPROTILINE

GENERAL

Maprotiline is a tetracyclic antidepressant drug. It is slowly but completely absorbed from the adult gastrointestinal tract and is 90% bound to plasma proteins. Maprotiline is extensively demethylated to its principal active metabolite, desmethylmaprotiline. The plasma half-life of maprotiline is 48 h.

EVALUATION OF DATA

Passage of maprotiline into human milk has been reported as follows:

Treatment conditions — Dose × Frequency × Duration; Route; No. of patients; Lactation stage	Concentration (mg/l)		Milk/ plasma ratio	Maximum observed milk conc. (mg/l)	Absolute dose to infant (mg/kg/day)		Ref.
	Milk	Plasma			Ave	Max	
100 mg × 1/d × 1 d; p.o.; ?; ?	0.03–0.11	0.02–0.07	1.4	0.11	–	–	(1)
50 mg × 3/d × LT; p.o.; ?; ?	0.26	0.22	1.4	–	–	–	(1)

LT, long term. Milk and plasma concentration-time profiles were defined for 48 h after the single dose and were concurrent; the peak concentration in milk occurred at 8 h. In the repeated dose study, milk and plasma samples were taken daily for the 5 days; the values quoted are the concentrations on the 5th day and appear not to represent steady-state conditions. The values quoted in the table are taken from figures in the paper.

RELATIVE DOSE IN MILK

The amount of maprotiline that a suckling infant would ingest in a feed is at maximum 0.2% (0.11 × 180/100)* of the weight-adjusted maternal single dose, and in a day is 1.6% (0.26 × 900/150)* of the weight-adjusted maternal daily dose. Note that this estimate does not include any active metabolites which may be present in milk.

DATA ON THE INFANT

No data are available.

ASSESSMENT OF DATA

Limited data suggest that the quantity of maprotiline that passes into milk is small,

* An explanation of the calculation (s) appears on pp. 71–72.

but the estimate does not include pharmacologically active metabolites that are known to be produced. A decision about the advisability of breast-feeding is probably best determined by the factors pertinent to the individual case.

REFERENCES

1. Lloyd AH (1977) Practical considerations in the use of maprotiline (Ludiomil) in general practice. *J. Int. Med. Res., 5 (Suppl. 4),* 122–129.

METACLAZEPAM

GENERAL

Metaclazepam is a benzodiazepine with properties similar to those of diazepam. It is rapidly absorbed from the adult gastrointestinal tract and is metabolised in the liver. The plasma half life of metaclazapam and also of its desmethyl metabolite is 11 h.

EVALUATION OF DATA

Passage of metaclazepam into human milk has been reported as follows:

Treatment conditions	Concentration (μg/l)		Milk/ plasma ratio	Maxi- mum observed milk conc. (μg/l)	Absolute dose to infant (μg/kg/day)		Ref.
Dose × Frequency × Duration; Route; No. of patients; Lactation stage	Milk	Plasma			Ave	Max	
20 mg × 1/d × 1 d; p.o.; 10; 3–5 d	7.2[a] (4.6)	17.4	0.22 (0.16)	40 (310	1.08	6.0	(1)
	16.2[b] (8.6)	–	0.4 (0.28)	85 (38)	–	–	(1)

Values for desmethylmetaclazepam appear in brackets. Blood and milk was sampled 0.5, 1, 1.5, 2, 3, 4, 6, 9, 12, 16, 20 and 24 h after a single dose on day 3[a] and 5[b] postpartum. The milk to plasma ratio was calculated from the areas under the milk and plasma concentration-time curves.

RELATIVE DOSE IN MILK

A suckling infant would ingest in a day on average 1.1% (16.2 + 8.6 × 900/20 000)* and at maximum 5.5% (85+38 × 900/20 000) of the weight-adjusted maternal daily dose of metaclazepam.

DATA ON THE INFANT

No data are available.

ASSESSMENT OF DATA

Limited data suggest that the risk to the suckling infant of administering metaclazepam to its mother is low on the basis that the amount of drug that passes into the milk is small. Breast-feeding is probably safe provided the period of exposure to the drug is short, e.g. a few days, as in the quoted study.

* An explanation of the calculation (s) appears on pp. 71–72.

REFERENCES

1. Schotter A, Müller R, Günther C, Hausleiter HJ, Achtert G. (1989) Transfer of metaclazepam and its metabolites into breast milk. *Arzneimittelforschung, 39,* 1468–1470.

METHADONE

GENERAL

Methadone is a synthetic opioid drug whose pharmacological actions are similar to those of morphine. Its principal uses are to control severe pain and to treat opioid dependence. Methadone is well absorbed from the adult gastrointestinal tract and about 85% is bound to plasma proteins. It undergoes extensive biotransformation in the liver and the major metabolites are excreted in the urine and the bile. The half-life after repeated dosing is 25 h.

EVALUATION OF DATA

Passage of methadone into human milk has been reported as follows:

Treatment conditions	Concentration (mg/l)		Milk/plasma ratio	Maximum observed milk conc. (mg/l)	Absolute dose to infant (mg/kg/day)		Ref.
Dose × Frequency × Duration; Route; No. of patients; Lactation stage	Milk	Plasma			Ave	Max	
10–80 mg/d (mean 52 mg) × LT; p.o.; 10; 3–10 d	0.27	0.47	0.83	0.57	0.04	0.09	(1)
50 mg/d × LT; p.o.; 1; 7 d	0.03 (2 h) 0.04 (6 h)	0.44 (2 h) 0.36 (6 h)	0.07–0.11	0.12 (d 6,4 h)	0.01–0.01	0.02 –	(2)
25–50 mg/d × LT; p.o.; 2; 7 d	–	–	0.05–1.2	–	–	–	(3)
28–36 mg × LT; p.o.; 2; 1–3 weeks	–	–	0.32, 0.61	0.07	–	0.01	(4)

LT, long term. Reference (1) reports on patients enrolled in a methadone maintenance programme. The milk and plasma concentrations are the average of single samples, i.e. the concentration-time profiles were not defined. The maximum milk concentration was the highest value recorded in an individual who took methadone 80 mg/d. The patient reported in reference (2) was receiving methadone maintenance treatment for narcotic addiction. The milk and blood samples were taken at the stated times after the last dose. Reference (3) defined the concentration-time profile in milk; the peak concentration occurred 2–4 h after dosing. Reference (4) reported that the concentration-time profiles were concurrent in 2 mothers whose milk to plasma ratios are given in the table. The maximum milk concentration was the highest value reported in one of the mothers and is taken from a graph. Steady-state dosing conditions are assumed to apply in all the studies.

RELATIVE DOSE IN MILK

The amount of methadone that a suckling infant would ingest in a day is on average 0.9–4.7% (0.05 × 900/50) - (0.27 × 900/52)* (1, 2) and at maximum 6.4% (0.57 × 900/80)* (1) of the weight-adjusted maternal daily dose.

* An explanation of the calculation (s) appears on pp. 71–72.

DATA ON THE INFANT

Infants who had been exposed to methadone in utero experienced withdrawal symptoms in the first days after delivery; no adverse effects were reported during the nursing period (1, 2, 4). Methadone ingested in breast milk may have contributed to the death of an infant (5).

ASSESSMENT AND RECOMMENDATIONS

The risk to the suckling infant of administering methadone to its mother would appear to be low on the basis that the quantity of drug that appears in milk is small. Breast-feeding is probably safe provided the maternal dose is low and the mother is warned to seek medical advice if her infant appears sedated.

REFERENCES

1. Blinick G. Inturrisi CE, Jerez E, Wallach R (1975) Methadone assays in pregnant women and progeny. *Am. J. Obstet. Gynecol., 121,* 617–621.
2. Kreek MJ, Schecter A, Gutjaln CL, Bowen D, Field F, Queenan J, Merkatz I (1974) Analyses of methadone and other drugs in maternal and neonatal body fluids: use in evaluation of symptoms in a neonate of mother maintained on methadone. *Am. J. Drug Alc. Abuse, 1,* 409–419.
3. Kreek MJ (1979) Methadone disposition during the perinatal period in humans. *Pharmacol. Biochem. Behav., 11 (Suppl.),* 7–13.
4. Pond SM, Kreek MJ, Tong TG, Raghunath J, Benowitz NL (1985) Altered methadone pharmacokinetics in methadone-maintained pregnant women. *J. Pharmacol. Exp. Ther., 233,* 1–6.
5. Smialek JE, Aronow R (1977) Methadone deaths in children. *J. Am. Med. Assoc., 238,* 2516–2517.

MIANSERIN

GENERAL

Mianserin is a tetracyclic antidepressant drug. It is rapidly absorbed from the adult gastrointestinal tract and 96% bound to plasma proteins. Mianserin is extensively metabolised and some of the products retain weak pharmacological activity. The plasma half-life is 16 h.

EVALUATION OF DATA

Passage of mianserin into human breast milk has been reported as follows:

Treatment conditions	Concentration (μg/l)		Milk/ plasma ratio	Maximum observed milk conc. (μg/l)	Absolute dose to infant (μg/kg/day)		Ref.
Dose × Frequency × Duration; Route; No. of patients; Lactation stage	Milk	Plasma			Ave	Max	
60 mg/d × 9 d; p.o.; 1; 3 months	80 (10)	22 (20)	–	–	–	–	(1)
40 mg/d × 14 d; p.o.; 1; 5 months	20 (20)	25 (<10)	–	–	–	–	(1)

The figures in parentheses refer to desmethylmianserin. Steady-state dosing conditions can be assumed to apply. A single pair of milk and plasma samples was collected 15 h after the dose of mianserin in each case.

RELATIVE DOSE IN MILK

In a day a suckling infant would ingest, as mianserin and desmethylmianserin, 0.9% (20 + 20 × 900/40 000)* to 1.4% (80 + 10 × 900/60 000)* of the weight-adjusted maternal daily dose of mianserin (1).

DATA ON THE INFANT

A urine sample from the infant of the mother who took 40 mg/d contained mianserin 12 μg/l and desmethylmianserin 14 μg/l. No drug-related effects were noted in the infants.

ASSESSMENT AND RECOMMENDATIONS

Limited data suggest that the risk to the suckling infant of administering mianserin

* An explanation of the calculation (s) appears on pp. 71–72.

to its mother is low on the basis that the quantity of drug that passes into milk is small. A decision about the advisability of breast-feeding is probably best determined by the factors pertinent to the individual case.

REFERENCES

1. Buist A, Norman TR, Dennerstein L (1993) Mianserin in breast milk. *Br. J Clin. Pharmacol., 36,* 133–134.

MIDAZOLAM

GENERAL

Midazolam is a benzodiazepine drug with an action that is rapid in onset and short in duration. It is used to provide sedation before surgery and during minor procedures for which it is administered parenterally. Midazolam is absorbed from the adult gastrointestinal tract but its systemic availability is 44% due to first-pass metabolism by the liver; it is 96% bound to plasma proteins. A metabolite, hydroxymidazolam, is also pharmacologically active. The plasma half-life of both substances is 2–5 h, and in milk is 0.9–1.3 h (1).

EVALUATION OF DATA

Passage of midazolam and hydroxymidazolam into human milk has been reported as follows:

Treatment conditions Dose × Frequency × Duration; Route; No. of patients; Lactation stage	Concentration (μg/l)		Milk/plasma ratio	Maximum observed milk conc. (μg/l)	Absolute dose to infant (μg/kg/day)		Ref.
	Milk	Plasma			Ave	Max	
15 mg × 1/d × 5 d;	<3.0	10.0	–	–	<0.5	–	(1)
p.o.; 10; 7 d	(<3.0)	(4.0)	–	–	(<0.5)	–	
15 mg × 1/d × 1 d;	3.3	2.2	0.15	9	–	1.4	(1)
p.o.; 2; 2 months	(3.4)	–	–	(3)	–	(0.5)	

The figures for hydroxymidazolam appear in parentheses. In the repeated dose study (upper line of the table), milk and plasma were collected 7 h after administration of midazolam and the table gives average values for the 5 days. Steady-state conditions of dosing were not attained. In the single dose study (lower line) the concentration-time profile was defined for 7 h and the maximum milk concentration is given.

RELATIVE DOSE IN MILK

A suckling infant would ingest in a feed at maximum 0.1% (9 + 3 × 180/15 000)* of the weight adjusted maternal single dose (1).

DATA ON THE INFANT

All the infants were breast-fed and no drug effects were observed (1).

* An explanation of the calculation (s) appears on pp. 71–72.

ASSESSMENT AND RECOMMENDATIONS

The risk to the suckling infant of administering midazolam to its mother is low on the basis that the quantity of drug that passes into milk is small. Breast-feeding after single doses or during a short course of midazolam may be regarded as safe.

REFERENCES

1. Matheson I, Lunde PKM, Bredesen JE (1990) Midazolam and nitrazepam in the maternity ward: milk concentrations and clinical effects. *Br. J. Clin. Pharmacol., 30,* 787–793.

MOCLOBEMIDE

GENERAL

Moclobemide is a reversible monoamine oxidase-A inhibitor used in the treatment of depression. It is absorbed from the adult gastrointestinal tract and is 50% bound to plasma proteins. The action of moclobemide is terminated by metabolism which exhibits non-linear kinetics, and one N-oxidation product retains pharmacological activity. The plasma half-life in lactating women who took moclobemide 300 mg was 2.3 h (1).

EVALUATION OF DATA

Passage of moclobemide into human breast milk has been reported as follows:

Treatment conditions: Dose × Frequency × Duration; Route; No. of patients; Lactation stage	Concentration (mg/l)		Milk/plasma ratio	Maximum observed milk conc. (mg/l)	Absolute dose to infant (mg/kg/day)		Ref.
	Milk	Plasma			Ave	Max	
300 mg × 1/d × 1 d; p.o.; 6; 3–5 d	2.0 (3 h) 0.7 (6 h)	2.0 (3 h) 0.9 (6 h)	0.72	–	–	0.3	(1)

The concentration-time profiles were defined and appeared concurrent. The figures in the table are average values and were estimated from graphs in (1). [For comparison, the minimum steady-state plasma concentration in healthy males who took moclobemide 100 mg × 3/d was 0.22 mg/l (2)]. The active metabolite was detected in plasma but not in milk. The milk to plasma ratio was based on the linear correlation of milk and plasma values.

RELATIVE DOSE IN MILK

The amount of moclobemide that a suckling infant would ingest in a feed after a single dose is at maximum 1.2 % (2 × 180/300)* of the weight adjusted maternal dose.

DATA ON THE INFANT

No data are available.

ASSESSMENT AND RECOMMENDATIONS

Single dose data indicate that the risk to the suckling infant of administering mo-

* An explanation of the calculation (s) appears on pp. 71–72.

clobemide to its mother is low on the basis that the quantity of drug that passes into milk is small. There must be caution in extrapolating from single-dose data for a drug that may be given for several weeks, and also exhibits non-linear kinetics. A decision about the advisability of breast-feeding is probably best determined by the factors pertinent to the individual case.

REFERENCES

1. Pons G, Schoerlin MP, Tam YK, Moran C, Pfefen JP, Francoual Ch, Pedarriosse AM, Chavinie J, Olive G (1990). Moclobemide excretion in hman brast milk. *Br. J. Clin. Pharmacol., 29,* 27–31.
2. Schoerlin MP, Mayersohn M, Korn A (1987). Disposition kinetics of moclobemide, a mono amine oxidase-A enzyme inhibitor: single and multiple dosing in normal subjects. *Clin. Pharmacol. Ther., 42*, 395–404.

MORPHINE

GENERAL

Morphine, the principal alkaloid of opium, is used for the control of moderate to severe pain. It is rapidly absorbed after oral, subcutaneous or intramuscular administration, but bioavailability after oral dosing is low due to high first-pass metabolism in the liver. One of its metabolites, morphine-3-glucuronide, is pharmacologically active. Protein binding is 35%. In plasma the half-life of morphine is 3 h and that of the active metabolite is 2–6 h. The half-life of morphine in neonates is 14 h.

EVALUATION OF DATA

Passage of morphine into human milk has been reported as follows:

Treatment conditions: Dose × Frequency × Duration; Route; No. of patients; Lactation stage	Concentration (μg/l): Milk	Concentration (μg/l): Plasma	Milk/plasma ratio	Maximum observed milk conc. (μg/l)	Absolute dose to infant (μg/kg/day): Ave	Absolute dose to infant (μg/kg/day): Max	Ref.
5–10 mg × 1–2 doses in 4 h; i.v. + i.m.; 4; colostrum	500	300	1.1–3.6	500	–	75	(1)
4 mg × 6 h × 2 doses; epidural; 1; colostrum	82	–	–	82	–	12.3	(1)
0.1 mg/kg + PCA × 1/d × 1 d; i.v.; 5; 96 h + 5–30 mg p.o. as required after 20–43 h	65 (22)	–	–	95 (25)	–	14.3 (3.75)	(2)
5 mg × 6 h × 10 d; p.o.; 1; 21 days	10–100	–	–	100	–	15	(3)
5 mg x 1/day × 2 d; epidural; 30; colostrum	0.39–0.66 (0.6–1.6)	–	–		–		(4)

PCA, patient controlled analgesia. Milk and plasma concentration-time profiles were defined in (1) and were concurrent; the profile in milk was higher than that in plasma. The concentrations quoted are the highest observed in an individual who received morphine 10 mg i.v. plus 5 mg i.m. (first line) or morphine 4 mg followed by 4 mg 6 h later epidurally (second line). In reference (2) mothers undergoing elective caesarean section received morphine i.v. initially 0.1 mg/kg and subsequently by PCA until 20–43 h postpartum. The concentrations of morphine and morphine-3-glucuronide (in brackets) at 24 h are estimated from a graph; a histogram indicates that the mean dose of morphine received by this time was 90 mg. Reference (4) gives data on unconjugated and conjugated (in brackets) morphine from 3 of 24 mothers from whom colostrum was collected 12–36 h after epidural administration; these low values reflect the time lapse between exposure to the drug and collection of the samples.

RELATIVE DOSE IN MILK

A suckling infant would receive at maximum 6.0% (500 × 180/15000)* of the weight-adjusted maternal single dose of morphine (1). The single dose for a child is morphine 150 μg/kg and an infant would receive in a feed at maximum 10% (500 × 3/150)* of this (1).

DATA ON THE INFANT

The mother in (3) had received morphine during the last trimester. Her infant was healthy at birth and during breast-feeding had a serum concentration of 4 μg /l 4 h after maternal dosing.

ASSESSMENT AND RECOMMENDATIONS

The risk to the suckling infant of administering morphine to its mother appears low on the basis of the quantity of drug that passes into milk, especially if the time of nursing avoids the period 2 h after dosing when drug concentrations are highest. Breast-feeding may be regarded as safe when exposure to morphine is brief, e.g. for analgesia following birth.

REFERENCES

1. Feilberg VL, Rosenborg D, Broen Christensen C, Viby Mogensen J (1989) Excretion of morphine in human breast milk. *Acta Anaesthesiol. Scand., 33*, 426–428.
2. Wittels B, Scott DT, Sinatra R (1990) Exogenous opiods in human breast milk and acute neonatal neurobehaviour: A preliminary study. *Anesthesiology, 73,* 864–869.
3. Robieux I, Koren G, Vandenbergh H, Schneiderman J (1990) Morphine excretion in breast milk and resultant exposure of a nursing infant. *Clin. Toxicol., 28*, 365–370.
4. Zarowski MI, Ramanathan S, Turndorf H (1993) A two-dose epidural morphine regimen in cesarean section patients: pharmacokinetic profile. *Acta Anaesthesiol. Scand., 37,* 584–589.

* An explanation of the calculation (s) appears on pp. 71–72.

NALBUPHINE

GENERAL

Nalbuphine is an opioid analgesic with mixed agonist-antagonist activity. High (90%) presystemic metabolism renders the oral route unsuitable and it is available only for parenteral use. Nalbuphine is negligibly bound to plasma proteins. The plasma half-life is 3 h.

EVALUATION OF DATA

Passage of nalbuphine into human milk has been reported as follows:

Treatment conditions: Dose × Frequency × Duration; Route; No. of patients; Lactation stage	Concentration (μg/l): Milk	Concentration (μg/l): Plasma	Milk/plasma ratio	Maximum observed milk conc. (μg/l)	Absolute dose to infant (μg/kg/day): Ave	Absolute dose to infant (μg/kg/day): Max	Ref.
20 mg × 1/d × 1 d; i.m.; 7; 1–2 d	25	40	1.2	25	–	3.8	(1)

Nalbuphine was administered for postoperative pain. The table gives the peak milk concentration for the mother with the highest values. The milk to plasma ratio is based on area measurements.

RELATIVE DOSE IN MILK

The amount of nalbuphine that a suckling infant would ingest in a feed is at maximum 0.2% (25 × 180/20 000)* of the weight-adjusted maternal single dose (1).

DATA ON THE INFANT

No data are available.

ASSESSMENT AND RECOMMENDATIONS

The risk to the suckling infant of administering single doses of nalbuphine to its mother is low on the basis that the quantity of drug that passes into milk is small. Breast-feeding following single doses may be regarded as safe.

REFERENCE

1. Wischnik A, Wetzelsberger N, Lücker PW (1988) Elimination von nalbuphin in die muttermilch. *Arzneim-Forsch./Drug Res., 38,* 1496–1498.

* An explanation of the calculation (s) appears on pp. 71–72.

NEFOPAM

GENERAL

Nefopam is used to relieve moderate severe pain; its mechanism of action is unclear but may involve inhibition at dopamine, noradrenaline and serotonin receptors in the CNS. It is well absorbed from the adult gastrointestinal tract, 70% bound to plasma proteins and is extensively metabolised to products that do not retain pharmacological activity. The plasma half-life of 4 h.

EVALUATION OF DATA

Passage of nefopam into human milk has been reported as follows:

Treatment conditions	Concentration (μg/l)		Milk/ plasma ratio	Maximum observed milk conc. (μg/l)	Absolute dose to infant (μg/kg/day)		Ref.
Dose × Frequency × Duration; Route; No. of patients; Lactation stage	Milk	Plasma			Ave	Max	
60 mg × 4 h × 48–85 h; p.o.; 5; 1–4 d	90.4	96.7	1.21	299.0	13.6	44.9	(1)

Nefopam was administered for post-episiotomy pain. Paired milk and plasma samples were taken daily for 5 d; the table gives mean values for all samples.

RELATIVE DOSE IN MILK

The amount of nefopam that a suckling infant would ingest in a day would be on average 0.2% (90.4 × 900/360 000)* and at maximum 0.75 % (299 × 900/360 000)* of the weight related maternal daily dose.

DATA ON THE INFANT

No data are available.

ASSESSMENT AND RECOMMENDATIONS

The risk to the suckling infant of administering nefopam to its mother is low on the basis that the quantity of drug that passes into milk is small. Breast-feeding may be regarded as safe.

* An explanation of the calculation (s) appears on pp. 71–72.

REFERENCE

1. Liu DTY, Savage JM, Donnell D (1987) Nefopam excretion in human milk. *Br. J. Clin. Pharmacol.*, *23*, 99–101.

NITRAZEPAM

GENERAL

Nitrazepam is a benzodiazepine drug that is used as an hypnotic. It is well absorbed from the adult gastrointestinal tract, 87% bound to plasma proteins and almost completely metabolised to inactive products. The plasma half-life is 25 h.

EVALUATION OF DATA

Passage of nitrazepam into human milk after repeated doses has been reported as follows:

Treatment conditions Dose × Frequency × Duration; Route; No. of patients; Lactation stage	Concentration (μg/l) Milk	 Plasma	Milk/ plasma ratio	Maximum observed milk conc. (μg/l)	Absolute dose to infant (μg/kg/day) Ave	 Max	Ref.
5 mg × 1/d × 5 d; p.o.; 9; 1 week	13	47	0.27	20	2	3	(1)

Milk and blood samples were taken 7 h after dosing from the 1st to the 5th day after delivery; the table gives the average concentrations on the 5th day when steady-state dosing conditions had probably been attained. In another study, milk and blood samples were taken 13 h after administration of ^{14}C-labelled nitrazepam 10 mg per day for 5 days (2). Assuming that unchanged nitrazepam in milk represented 65% of total nitrazepam equivalents, as in plasma, the average milk nitrazepam concentration may be estimated to be 50 μg/l on the 5th day.

RELATIVE DOSE IN MILK

A suckling infant would ingest in a day on average 2.3% (13 × 900/5000)* and maximum 3.6% (2 × 900/5000)* of the weight-adjusted maternal daily dose (1).

DATA ON THE INFANT

Nitrazepam in plasma was below the level of detection (3 μg/l) in a 6 day old suckling infant on the 5th day of drug administration to its mother (1). No drug-related effects were reported in breast-fed infants.

ASSESSMENT OF DATA

The risk to the suckling infant of administering nitrazepam to its mother is low on

* An explanation of the calculation (s) appears on pp. 71–72.

the basis that the quantity of drug that passes into milk is small. Breast-feeding during short-term use of nitrazepam would appear to be safe.

REFERENCES

1. Matheson I, Lunde PKM, Bredesen JE (1990) Midazolam and nitrazepam in the maternity ward: milk concentrations and clinical effects. *Br. J. Clin. Pharmacol., 30,* 787–793.
2. Rieder J, Wendt G (1973) Pharmacokinetics and metabolism of the hypnotic nitrazepam. In: Garattini S, Mussini E, Randall LO (Eds) *The Benzodiazepines*, pp 99–127. Raven Press, New York.

OXAZEPAM

GENERAL

Oxazepam is a benzodiazepine drug that is used short-term for its anxiolytic and hypnotic properties. It is completely absorbed from the adult gastrointestinal tract, 96% bound to plasma proteins and extensively metabolised to products that are pharmacologically inactive. The plasma half-life is 9 h in adults, and 20 h in newborns (2).

EVALUATION OF DATA

Passage of oxazepam into human milk has been reported as follows:

Treatment conditions Dose × Frequency × Duration; Route; No. of patients; Lactation stage	Concentration (μg/l)		Milk/ plasma ratio	Maximum observed milk conc. (μg/l)	Absolute dose to infant (μg/kg/day)		Ref.
	Milk	Plasma			Ave	Max	
10 mg × 3/d × 3 d; p.o.; 1; ?	30	200	0.15	–	–	–	(1)
15–30 mg/d × LT; p.o.; 1; 2 weeks	11–26	–	0.1	26	–	4	(2)
10 mg × 3/d × 3 d; p.o.; 1; 7 months	24–30	200	0.1–0.3	–	–	–	(3)

LT, long term. The mother reported in reference (1) gave blood samples each morning and the breasts were emptied each morning and evening for 5 d. The table gives milk and plasma concentrations estimated from a graph at apparent steady-state conditions of dosing. The milk and plasma concentration-time profiles were not concurrent. Reference (2) describes a mother who received oxazepam daily throughout the third trimester. The table shows the range of 12 milk samples that were taken immediately before and 4 h after drug administration during the first two weeks after delivery. Conjugated oxazepam in milk was <5 μg/l. Reference (3) describes a mother who took oxazepam at the time of weaning; she gave milk every morning and evening 4–7 h after a dose and the table gives the range of concentrations recorded.

RELATIVE DOSE IN MILK

A suckling infant would ingest in a day 0.9% (30 × 900/30 000)* of the weight-adjusted maternal daily dose of oxazepam (1).

DATA ON THE INFANT

The plasma concentration of oxazepam plus its conjugate in the infant was 20 μg/l

* An explanation of the calculation (s) appears on pp. 71–72.

on the 5th day after delivery. The concentration of conjugated oxazepam in the infant's urine was 94 μg/l on the 5th and 2.3 μg/l on the 7th postpartum day (1).

ASSESSMENT OF DATA

Limited data suggest that the risk to the suckling infant of administering oxazepam to its mother is low on the basis that the quantity of drug that passes into milk is small. Breast-feeding during short-term use is probably safe.

REFERENCES

1. Norrbrink L (1977) Oxazepam in modersmjölk. *Ronden, 2,* 26.
2. Rane A, Sundwall S, Tomson G (1979) Oxazepamabstinens i nyföddhetsperioden. *Lakartidningen, 76,* 4416–4417.
3. Wretlind M (1987) Excretion of oxazepam in breast milk. *Eur. J. Clin. Pharmacol., 33,* 209–210.

PARACETAMOL

GENERAL

Paracetamol (acetaminophen) is an antipyretic and analgesic drug. It is rapidly and completely absorbed from the adult gastrointestinal tract, <20% bound to plasma proteins and extensively metabolised by the liver. One product is an epoxide that is effectively scavenged by glutathione after therapeutic doses. The plasma half-life is 2 h.

EVALUATION OF DATA

Passage of paracetamol into human milk has been reported as follows:

Treatment conditions	Concentration (mg/l)		Milk/ plasma ratio	Maximum observed milk conc. (mg/l)	Absolute dose to infant (mg/kg/day)		Ref.
Dose × Frequency × Duration; Route; No. of patients; Lactation stage	Milk	Plasma			Ave	Max	
500 mg × 1/d × 1 d; p.o.; 3; ?	4.2 (2 h)	5.6 (2 h)	0.76	4.4 (2 h)	–	0.66	(1)
650 mg × 1/d × 1 d; p.o.; 11; 2–22 months	10–15 (1–2 h)	12	1.08	15 (1–2 h)	–	2.25	(2)
(phenacetin) 648 mg 1/d × 1 d; p.o.; 1; 7, 13 weeks	0.89	1.09	0.81 0.91 (1 h) 1.42 (12 h)	–	–	–	(3)
1000 mg × 1/d × 1 d; p.o.; 4; 2–8 months	6.1	4.9	1.24	10.3	0.92	1.55	(4)

Reference (1) quoted average peak concentrations of milk and plasma and the maximum milk concentration was the highest value reported in an individual. The absorption profile was not assessed but the half-life of decline of drug concentration was 2.64 h in milk and 2.74 h in plasma. The milk to plasma ratio is based on area measurements. Protein binding in milk was on average 2.5% and that in plasma was 19.8%. The concentration-time profiles were defined in reference (2) and were similar in milk, plasma and saliva. The table gives the range of peak milk concentrations. The milk to plasma ratio of 1.08 is the average for one patient. These workers estimated that an infant would ingest on average 0.88 mg of paracetamol assuming 90 ml of milk were ingested 3, 6 and 9 h after the dose to the mother (0.14% of the dose). In one patient, concurrent profiles with a similar half-life, with and without nursing, indicated rapid equilibration of drug between milk and plasma. Reference (3) reports two women 7 (subject 1) and 13 (subject 2) weeks post partum who received an oral dose of two tablets of a combination product containing phenacetin 324 mg/tab. Paracetamol produced by metabolism of phenacetin appeared in milk. Average milk and plasma concentrations and the milk to plasma ratios based on the respective areas under the concentration-time curves (0–12 h) are given for subject 1; the ratio at 1 and 12 h for subject 2 appears below. The authors calculated that the infant of subject 2 would ingest 0.44 mg of paracetamol in the 12 h after the dose. The data indicate that paracetamol formed from phenacetin gives similar milk and plasma profiles to those from dosing with paracetamol. Reference (4) defined milk and plasma concentration-time curves and these were not concurrent. While references (1), (2) and (4) include an adequate number of samples to define the single dose concentration-time profile for acetaminophen in milk, the profile after repeated doses remains unknown.

RELATIVE DOSE IN MILK

A suckling infant would ingest in a feed at maximum 4.2% (15 × 180/650)* of the weight-adjusted maternal single dose (2). The infant single dose of acetaminophen is 10 mg/kg and a breast-feeding baby would ingest in a feed at maximum 4.5% (15 × 3/10)* of this (2).

DATA ON THE INFANT

Reference (2) recorded no drug effects. Neonates excreted significantly greater proportions of unchanged paracetamol and lesser proportions of paracetamol sulphate than did healthy volunteers aged 11–80, compatible with deficient sulphate conjugation in that age-group (4). A 2-month old infant whose mother was receiving paracetamol developed a rash which disappeared when the drug was discontinued and returned when paracetamol was re-administered (5).

ASSESSMENT AND RECOMMENDATIONS

The risk to the suckling infant of administering paracetamol to its mother is low on the basis that the quantity of drug that passes into milk is small. Breast-feeding appears to be safe but there is a need for data in nursing mothers who are taking repeated doses of paracetamol.

REFERENCES

1. Bitzen P-O, Gustafsson B, Jostell KG, Melander A, Wahlin-Boll E (1981) Excretion of paracetamol in human breast milk. *Eur. J. Clin. Pharmacol., 20*, 123–125.
2. Berlin Jr CM, Yaffe SJ, Ragni M (1980) Disposition of acetaminophen in milk, saliva, and plasma of lactating women. *Pediatr. Pharmacol., 1*, 135–141.
3. Findlay JWA, deAngelis RL, Kearney MF, Welch RM, Findlay JM (1981) Analgesic drugs in breast milk and plasma. *Clin. Pharmacol. Ther., 29,* 625–633.
4. Notarianni LJ, Oldham HG, Bennett PN (1987) Passage of paracetamol into breast milk and its subsequent metabolism by the neonate. *Br. J. Clin. Pharmacol., 24*, 63–67.
5. Matheson I, Lunde PKM, Notarianni LJ (1985) Infant rash caused by paracetamol in breast milk? *Pediatrics, 76*, 651–652.

* An explanation of the calculation (s) appears on pp. 71–72.

PERPHENAZINE

GENERAL

Perphenazine is a phenothiazine drug that is used to manage psychotic disorders, and also to control severe nausea and vomiting. It is well absorbed from the adult gastrointestinal tract and is extensively metabolised in the liver (60–70% in first-pass after oral administration); some of the products of metabolism retain pharmacological activity. Protein binding is 92%. The plasma half-life is 10 h.

EVALUATION OF DATA

Passage of perphenazine into human milk has been reported as follows:

Treatment conditions	Concentration (μg/l)		Milk/ plasma ratio	Maximum observed milk conc. (μg/l)	Absolute dose to infant (μg/kg/day)		Ref.
Dose × Frequency × Duration; Route; No. of patients; Lactation stage	Milk	Plasma			Ave	Max	
24 mg/d × ?; p.o.; 1; 1 month	3.2	4.9	0.7–1.1	3.2	–	0.48	(1)
16 mg/d × ?; p.o.; 1; > 1 month	2.1 (1.8–3.1)	2.0 (2.0–3.4)	–	3.1	–	0.47	(1)

The mother first received 24 mg/d (upper line), then the dose was reduced to 16 mg/d (lower line) because of extrapyramidal effects. The milk concentration on the higher dose refers to a 24 h total collection; that on the lower dose refers to a 12 h total collection. The milk concentrations in brackets give the range from 3 consecutive 4 h total collections.

RELATIVE DOSE IN MILK

A suckling infant would ingest in a day at maximum 0.2 % (3.1 × 900/16 000)* of the weight-adjusted maternal single dose of perphenazine (1).

DATA ON THE INFANT

The infant showed no evidence of drug effects.

ASSESSMENT OF DATA

Limited data indicate that the risk to the suckling infant of administering per-

* An explanation of the calculation (s) appears on pp. 71–72.

phenazine to its mother is low on the basis that the quantity of drug that passes into milk is small. Short-term use, e.g. to control nausea and vomiting would appear to be safe. A decision about the advisability of breast-feeding during longer-term exposure is probably best determined by the factors pertinent to the individual case.

REFERENCES

1. Olesen OV, Bartels U, Poulsen JH (1990) Perphenazine in breast milk and serum. *Am. J. Psychiatr., 147,* 1378–1379.

PETHIDINE

GENERAL

Pethidine (meperidine) is a synthetic opioid drug that is frequently used for obstetric analgesia. It is absorbed from the adult gastrointestinal tract but systemic availability is only 50% because of first-pass metabolism in the liver. The metabolite norpethidine may provoke excitatory effects. Pethidine is 40% bound to plasma proteins. The plasma half-life of pethidine in adults is 2–4 h and of norpethidine is 14–21 h. In neonates the half-lives of pethidine and norpethidine are 13 h and 63 h respectively.

EVALUATION OF DATA

Passage of pethidine into human milk has been reported as follows:

Treatment conditions: Dose × Frequency × Duration; Route; No. of patients; Lactation stage	Concentration (μg/l): Milk	Concentration (μg/l): Plasma	Milk/ plasma ratio	Maximum observed milk conc. (μg/l)	Absolute dose to infant (μg/kg/day): Ave	Absolute dose to infant (μg/kg/day): Max	Ref.
50 mg × 1/d × 1 d; i.m.; 9; 3–8 d	82	73	1.12	207	12	31	(1)
?; ?; 3; 8–72 h	36 (225)	–	1.12	–	–	–	(2)
1.0 mg/kg + PCA × 1/d × 1 d; i.v.; 5; 96 h + 50–300 mg p.o. as required after 20–43 h	475 (400)	–	–	–	–	–	(3)

The figures in parentheses refer to norpethidine. PCA, patient controlled anaesthesia. Reference (1) defined the milk and serum concentration-time profiles over 2–25 h. The table gives average values and the milk to serum ratio is based on paired samples obtained at 5, 9 and 13 h after dosing. The maximum milk concentration occurred 2 h after dosing and the value in the table is the highest recorded in an individual. The milk concentration had fallen to 20 μg/l by 25 h after dosing. Reference (2) quotes average values for pethidine and norpethidine. In reference (3) mothers undergoing elective caesarean section received pethidine i.v. initially 1 mg/kg and subsequently by PCA until 20–43 h postpartum. The concentrations of pethidine and norpethidine at 24 h are estimated from a graph; a histogram indicates that the mean dose of pethidine received by this time was 600 mg.

RELATIVE DOSE IN MILK

The amount of pethidine and norpethidine that a suckling infant would ingest in a feed is at maximum 0.8% (207 × 180/50 000)* (1) of the weight-adjusted maternal

* An explanation of the calculation (s) appears on pp. 71–72.

single dose or in a day 1.3 % (475 + 400 × 900/600 000)* of the weight-adjusted maternal daily dose (3).

DATA ON THE INFANT

The salivary concentration of pethidine was higher in breast-fed than in bottle-fed babies whose mothers received the drug during labour (4). Reduced alertness to stimuli in neonates was significantly more pronounced with pethidine than with morphine (3).

ASSESSMENT AND RECOMMENDATIONS

The risk to the suckling infant of administering a single dose of pethidine to its mother is low on the basis that the quantity of drug that passes into milk is small. Breast-feeding after single doses would appear to be safe. If pethidine is given in repeated doses, breast-feeding may be unsafe as norpethidine may accumulate.

REFERENCES

1. von Peiker G, Müller B, Ihn W, Nöschel H. Ausscheidung von Pethidin durch die Muttermilch (1980) *Zentralbl. Gynakol., 102,* 537–541.
2. Quinn PG, Kuhnert BR, Kaine CJ, Syracuse CD (1986) Measurement of meperidine and normeperidine in human breast milk by selected ion monitoring. *Biomed. Environ. Mass Spectrom., 13*, 133–135.
3. Wittels B, Scott DT, Sinatra RS (1990) Exogenous opioids in human breast milk and acute neonatal neurobehaviour: a preliminary study. *Anesthesiology, 73*, 864–869.
4. Freeborn SF, Calvert RT, Black P, Macfarlane T, D'Souza SW (1980) Saliva and blood pethidine concentrations in the mother and the newborn baby. *Br. J. Obstet. Gynaecol., 87*, 966–969.

PHENOBARBITAL SODIUM

GENERAL

Phenobarbital sodium (phenobarbitone sodium) is a barbiturate that is used to control epilepsy. It is completely but slowly absorbed from the adult gastrointestinal tract and is 50% bound to plasma protein (less in neonates). Some 20–50% is excreted unchanged in the urine, the remainder as metabolites. The plasma half-life is 100 h in adults and in term neonates is 21–120 h (4). Phenobarbital sodium is an inducer of hepatic microsomal enzymes and can thus accelerate its own metabolism and that of other drugs. Prenatal exposure to phenobarbital sodium speeds its elimination from the new-born.

EVALUATION OF DATA

Passage of phenobarbital sodium into human milk has been reported as follows:

Treatment conditions: Dose × Frequency × Duration; Route; No. of patients; Lactation stage	Concentration (mg/l)		Milk/plasma ratio	Maximum observed milk conc. (mg/l)	Absolute dose to infant (mg/kg/day)		Ref.
	Milk	Plasma			Ave	Max	
? × LT; p.o.; ?; 3–32 d	10.4	19.3	0.45	33.0	1.56	4.95	(1)
? × LT; p.o.; ?; ?	4.8	11.5	0.36	33.0	0.72	4.95	(2)

LT, long term. Neither study defined the concentration-time profile. Reference (1) reports the mean of 6 paired serum and milk samples. Reference (2) gives the mean of 51 paired samples from an unknown number of mothers. The maximum milk concentrations are the highest values recorded in individuals in each study.

RELATIVE DOSE IN MILK

Doses are not given in the quoted reports but phenobarbital sodium 100 mg/day may be regarded as generally adequate for control of epilepsy. On this basis a suckling infant would ingest in a day on average 43.2–93.6% (4.8 × 900/100)-(10.4 × 900/100)* (2,1) and at maximum 297.0% (33.0 × 900/100)* (1, 2) of the weight-adjusted maternal daily dose.

DATA ON THE INFANT

Forty-two infants of 32 epileptic mothers were observed for harmful side effects of antiepilepsy drug therapy (2). Poor weight gain and a high incidence of vomiting

* An explanation of the calculation (s) appears on pp. 71–72.

and inadequate suckling in some of the infants may have been due to phenobarbital sodium and other antiepilepsy drugs received in milk. Sedation from phenobarbital sodium ingested in breast milk may have contributed to the death of a 13-day old infant whose blood concentration was 8.3 mg/l (3).

ASSESSMENT AND RECOMMENDATIONS

The risk to the suckling infant of administering phenobarbital sodium to its mother is significant because the quantity of drug that passes into milk is substantial, and adverse effects can be attributed to it. Breast-feeding should be regarded as unsafe.

REFERENCES

1. Kaneko S, Sato T, Suzuki K (1979) The levels of anticonvulsants in breast milk. *Br. J. Clin. Pharmacol., 7,* 624–626.
2. Kaneko S, Suzuki K, Sato T, Ogawa Y, Nomura Y (1982) The problems of antiepileptic medication in the neonatal period: is breast-feeding advisable? In: Janz D, Dam M, Richens A, Bossi L, Helge H, Schmidt D (Eds) *Epilepsy, Pregnancy and the Child*, pp 343–348. Raven Press, New York.
3. Juul S (1969) Fenemalforgiftning via modermaelken? *Ugeskr. Laeg., 131*, 2257–2258.
4. Rane A (1978) Clinical pharmacokinetics of antiepileptic drugs in children. *Pharmacol. Ther., 2,* 251–267.

PHENYTOIN

GENERAL

Phenytoin is used for the treatment of epilepsy. In the adult its systemic availability by the oral route is 97% and it is 90% bound to plasma proteins. Phenytoin is metabolised to products that are inactive. The formation of p-OH-phenytoin is subject to saturation kinetics so that the steady-state plasma concentrations of phenytoin increase disproportionately to the dose and the plasma half-life varies from 10–40 h in adults. In infants, the half-life is in the same range, provided they have been exposed prenatally to the drug via the mother (4).

EVALUATION OF DATA

Passage of phenytoin into human milk has been reported as follows:

Treatment conditions	Concentration (mg/l)		Milk/ plasma ratio	Maxi-mum observed milk conc. (mg/l)	Absolute dose to infant (mg/kg/day)		Ref.
Dose × Frequency × Duration; Route; No. of patients; Lactation stage	Milk	Plasma			Ave	Max	
200–400 mg/d × LT; p.o.; 6; 1–3 months	1.61	8.39	0.13	2.95	0.24	0.44	(1)
?; p.o.; 9; ?	0.8	4.5	0.2	1.4	0.12	0.21	(2)
?; p.o.; ?; 3–32 d	0.7	2.8	0.2	2.2	0.11	0.33	(3)
250 mg × 2/d × LT; p.o.; 1; 1 week	0.26	0.58	0.45	-	-	-	(4)
300 mg × 1–2/d × LT; p.o.; 2; 4–6 d	1.9	4.2		2.6	0.29	0.39	(5)

LT, long term. The concentration-time profile was defined in (1) and indicated little variation in milk or plasma concentration throughout the dose interval. The milk and plasma figures are average values and the maximum milk concentration is the highest value recorded in an individual. The data in (2) are the averages of paired samples from 9 mothers and those in (3) are the averages of 59 paired samples. The maximum milk concentration is the highest value recorded in an individual. The data in (5) are average values of 7 paired samples from 2 mothers. All studies were conducted under steady-state conditions of dosing.

RELATIVE DOSE IN MILK

The amount of phenytoin that a suckling infant would ingest in a day is on average 0.5–4.8% (0.26 × 900/500)-(1.61 × 900/300)* (1, 4) and at maximum 8.9% (2.95 × 900/300)* (1) of the weight-adjusted maternal daily dose.

* An explanation of the calculation (s) appears on pp. 71–72.

DATA ON THE INFANT

No adverse effects have been reported in infants.

ASSESSMENT AND RECOMMENDATIONS

The risk to the suckling infant of administering phenytoin to its mother is low on the basis that the quantity of drug that passes into milk is small. Breast-feeding may be regarded as safe.

REFERENCES

1. Steen B, Rane A, Lonnerholm G, Falk O, Elwin CE, Sjoqvist F (1982) Phenytoin excretion in human breast milk and plasma levels in nursed infants. *Ther. Drug Monit., 4,* 331–334.
2. Kaneko S, Sato T, Suzuki K (1979) The levels of anticonvulsants in breast milk. *Br. J. Clin. Pharmacol., 7,* 624–626.
3. Kaneko S, Suzuki K, Sato T, Ogawa Y, Nomura Y (1982) The problems of antiepileptic medication in the neonatal period: is breast-feeding advisable? In: Janz D, Dam M, Richens A, Bossi L, Helge H, Schmidt D (Eds) *Epilepsy, Pregnancy and the Child*, pp 343–348. Raven Press, New York.
4. Rane A, Garle M, Borga O, Sjoqvist F (1974) Plasma disappearance of transplacentally transferred phenytoin (diphenylhydantoin) in the newborn studied by mass fragmentography. *Clin. Pharmacol. Ther., 15,* 39–45.
5. Mirkin B (1971) Diphenylhydantoin: placental transport, fetal localisation, neonatal metabolism, and possible teratogenic effects. *J. Pediatr., 78*, 329–337.

PINAZEPAM

GENERAL

Pinazepam is a benzodiazepine that is used as for its sedative and anxiolytic properties. After administration by mouth to the adult, pinazepam is extensively extracted in its first pass through the liver, being metabolised by it to desmethyldiazepam (see diazepam, p. 421).

EVALUATION OF DATA

Passage of desmethyldiazepam into human milk after administration of pinazepam to women before delivery has been reported as follows:

Treatment conditions Dose × Frequency × Duration; Route; No. of patients; Lactation stage	Concentration (μg/l)		Milk/ plasma ratio	Maximum observed milk conc. (μg/l)	Absolute dose to infant (μg/kg/day)		Ref.
	Milk	Plasma			Ave	Max	
5 mg × 1/d × 3–8 d; p.o.; 9; 2 d	6	63	0.1	–	1	–	(1)
10 mg × 1/d × 1 d; p.o.; 4; 2–3 d	6	52	1	11	1	2	(2)

Administration of pinazepam ceased up to 24 h before delivery and the studies were conducted 2–3 days later. Neither study was conducted under steady-state dosing conditions and neither defined the concentration-time profile. Pinazepam was not detectable in milk in either study and the concentrations given are those of the metabolite, desmethyldiazepam. The milk and plasma concentrations are average values and the maximum concentration is the highest value recorded in an individual.

RELATIVE DOSE IN MILK

The calculation must be interpreted in the light of the fact that dosing was not continued until steady-state conditions were reached and that administration of pinazepam ceased 2–4 days before milk was assayed. With this qualification a suckling infant would ingest in a day on average 1.2 % (6 × 900 × 1.14/5000)* and at maximum 2.3% (11 × 900 × 1.14/5000)* of the weight-adjusted maternal daily dose (1). As pinazepam (mol. wt. 309) was administered but desmethyldiazepam (mol. wt. 271) was assayed in milk, a factor of 1.14 (309/271) was introduced into the calculation.

* An explanation of the calculation (s) appears on pp. 71–72.

DATA ON THE INFANT

There are no data in the quoted study (but see diazepam, p. 422).

ASSESSMENT OF DATA

The relative dose estimate would have been higher had the evaluated studies been carried out under steady-state conditions of dosing, e.g. after 2–3 weeks of drug administration. Under the conditions of the study, concentrations of desmethyldiazepam in milk were in general lower than those obtained following administration of diazepam to nursing mothers. Therefore it seems likely that the risk to the infant is low if its mother receives occasional small doses of pinazepam. If dosing with pinazepam is prolonged, if the baby is premature or if the mother in addition received the drug shortly before delivery, there would be greater risk of drug effects in the infant, notably poor suckling or somnolence.

REFERENCES

1. Pacifici GM, Cuoci L, Guarneri M, Fornaro P, Arcidacono G, Cappelli N, Moggi G, Placidi GF (1984) Placental transfer of pinazepam and its metabolite, N-desmethyldiazepam in women at term. *Eur. J. Clin. Pharmacol., 27,* 307–310.
2. Pacifici GM, Placidi GF (1977) Rapid and sensitive electron-capture gas chromatographic method for the determination of pinazepam and its metabolites in human plasma, urine and milk. *J. Chromatogr., 135,* 133–139.

PRAZEPAM

GENERAL

Prazepam is a precursor of, and indeed a prodrug for, desmethyldiazepam (see diazepam p. 421) which is used for its anxiolytic and sedative properties. The elimination half-life of desmethyldiazepam is 30–90 h.

EVALUATION OF DATA

Passage of desmethyldiazepam into human milk after administration of prazepam to mothers has been reported as follows:

Treatment conditions Dose × Frequency × Duration; Route; No. of patients; Lactation stage	Concentration (μg/l)		Milk/ plasma ratio	Maximum observed milk conc. (μg/l)	Absolute dose to infant (μg/kg/day)		Ref.
	Milk	Plasma			Ave	Max	
20 mg × 3/d × 3 d; p.o.; 5; ?	86	823	0.1	–	13	–	(1)

The women were not breast-feeding. Steady-state conditions of dosing were not attained. The milk and plasma concentrations quoted are average values and were taken 12 h after the last dose of prazepam. Analysis of samples for a further 48 h showed that desmethyldiazepam concentration declined at about the same rate in milk as in plasma.

RELATIVE DOSE IN MILK

The calculation must be interpereted in the light of the fact that steady-state conditions of dosing were not attained and the first estimate of drug in milk was made 12 h after the last dose of prazepam. With these qualifications a suckling infant would ingest in a day on average 1.5% (86 × 900 × 1.2/60 000)* of the weight-adjusted maternal daily dose of prazepam (1). Note that as prazepam (mol. wt. 325) was administered but desmethyldiazepam (mol. wt. 271) was assayed in milk, a factor of 1.2 (325/271) has been introduced into the calculation.

DATA ON THE INFANT

No data are available in the quoted study (but see diazepam, p. 422)

* An explanation of the calculation (s) appears on pp. 71–72.

ASSESSMENT OF DATA

The relative dose estimate would have been significantly higher had the evaluated study been carried out under steady-state conditions of dosing, e.g. after 2–3 weeks of drug administration. Under the conditions of the study the concentrations of desmethyldiazepam in milk are of the same order as those obtained following administration of diazepam to nursing mothers. Therefore it seems likely that the risk to the infant is low if its mother receives occasional small doses of prazepam. If dosing with prazepam is prolonged, if the baby is premature or if the mother in addition received the drug shortly before delivery, there would be greater risk of drug effects in the infant, notably poor suckling or somnolence.

REFERENCES

1. Brodie RR, Chasseaud LF, Taylor T (1981) Concentrations of N-descyclopropylmethylprazepam in whole-blood, plasma and milk after administration of prazepam to humans. *Biopharm. Drug Dispos.*, *2*, 56–68.

PRIMIDONE

GENERAL

Primidone is an antiepilepsy drug that is structurally related to phenobarbital. It is well absorbed from the adult gastrointestinal tract and is 19% bound to plasma proteins. The parent compound is metabolised to two active products, phenobarbital (see p. 479) and phenyl-ethyl-malon-amide (PEMA). The half-life of the generated phenobarbital is 100 h, that of PEMA is 40–60 h and that of the parent primidone is 6–12 h. About half the dose is excreted as the unchanged parent compound in the urine.

EVALUATION OF DATA

Passage of primidone and metabolites into human milk has been reported as follows:

Treatment conditions Dose × Frequency × Duration; Route; No. of patients; Lactation stage	Concentration (mg/l) Milk	 Plasma	Milk/ plasma ratio	Maximum observed milk conc. (mg/l)	Absolute dose to infant (mg/kg/day) Ave	 Max	Ref.
1000 mg × 1/d × LT; p.o.; 1; LT	9.1 (11.2)	18.8 (39.7)	0.48 (0.28)	–	1.37 (1.68)	–	(1)
? × LT; p.o.; ?; 3–32 d	2.3	2.8	0.81	6.7	0.35	1.01	(2)
? × LT; p.o.; ?; ?	2.1	3.4	0.7	8.3	0.32	1.25	(3)
7.3 mg/kg × 1/d × LT; p.o.; 4; 4–27 d	4.2 (2.8) 1.95[a]	6.1 (6.1) 2.7[a]	0.72 (0.41) 0.76[a]	8.2 (5.2) 2.8[a]	0.72 (0.42) 0.29[a]	1.23 (0.78) 0.42[a]	(4)
500 mg × 2/d × LT; p.o.; 2; 5 d–4 months	8.7 (5.9)	10.9 (15.3)	0.80 (0.39)	12.6 (15.9)	1.31 (0.89)	1.89 (2.39)	(5)
? x LT; p.o.; 35; ?	–	–	0.72 (0.36)	–	0.38–1.9	–	(6)

LT, long term. The figures in parentheses refer to phenobarbital; [a]refers to PEMA. The concentrations reported in reference (1) are estimated from the skim fraction in the milk; it appears that only one sample was taken. Reference (2) reports average data in 12, reference (3) in 51 and reference (4) in 8 paired milk and plasma samples, i.e. the concentration-time profiles were not defined. The mothers also received other anti-epilepsy drugs. In reference (5) blood and milk drug concentrations were monitored in the same patient during two consecutive pregnancies and for several months afterwards. The values quoted are means of both colostrum and mature milk. The maximum milk concentrations throughout the table are the highest values recorded in individuals.

RELATIVE DOSE IN MILK

A suckling infant would ingest in a day as primidone and phenobarbitone derived from it, on average 13.1–18.3% (8.7 + 5.9 × 900/1000)-(9.1 + 11.2 × 900/1000)* (5,1) and at maximum 25.7% (12.6 + 15.9 × 900/1000)* (5) of the weight-adjusted maternal daily dose of primidone.

DATA ON THE INFANT

No drug effects were reported in infants in reference (1). Poor weight gain, a high incidence of vomiting and inadequate suckling due to tiredness, were noted in reference (3) and may have been due to primidone or other antiepilepsy drugs. Of the 14 infants described in reference (4), 6 exhibited lethargy, hypotonia and poor suckling during the first 5 days after birth. Two infants developed marked withdrawal symptoms. In one of the fully breast-fed babies the steady-state plasma concentration during the second and third postnatal weeks were, for primidone 0.8–1.0 mg/l and for phenobarbitone 1.5–3.0 mg/l. Reference (5) reports that in 2 infants the mean plasma concentration of primidone was 1.3 mg/l and of phenobarbital was 5.1 mg/l. They did not exhibit drug effects and developed physically and gained weight normally. Neonatal steady-state serum concentration of phenobarbital varied between 1.9 and 12 mg/l.

ASSESSMENT AND RECOMMENDATIONS

The suckling infant is at risk of drug effects if primidone is administered to its mother because the quantity of primidone and its metabolites that pass into milk is significant, and because adverse effects have been observed in nursed infants. Breast-feeding should generally be regarded as unsafe but if there is a strong indication to suckle, the infant should be observed for the appearance of ascribable drug effects given above.

REFERENCES

1. Niebyl J, Blake D, Freeman J, Luff R (1979) Carbamazepine levels in pregnancy and lactation. *Obstet. Gynecol., 53,* 139–140.
2. Kaneko S, Sato T, Suzuki K (1979) The levels of anticonvulsants in breast milk. *Br. J. Clin. Pharmacol., 7,* 624–626.
3. Kaneko S, Suzuki K, Sato T, Ogawa Y, Nomura Y (1982) The problems of antiepileptic medication in the neonatal period: is breast-feeding advisable? In: Janz D, Dam M, Richens A, Bossi L, Helge H, Schmidt D (Eds) *Epilepsy, Pregnancy and the Child,* pp 343–348. Raven Press, New York.
4. Nau H, Rating D, Hauser I, Jager E, Koch S, Helge H (1980) Placental transfer and pharmacokinetics of primidone and its metabolites phenobarbital, PEMA and hydroxyphenobarbital in neonates and infants of epileptic mothers. *Eur. J. Clin. Pharmacol., 18,* 31–42.
5. Söderman P, Elwin C-E, Liden A. *Excretion in milk and blood levels of primidone and pheno-*

* An explanation of the calculation (s) appears on pp. 71–72.

barbital in mother and child during primidone treatment. 111 World Conference on Clinical Pharmacology and Therapeutics, Stockholm, 1986, (Abstract).

6. Kuhnz W, Koch S, Helge H, Nau H (1988) Primidone and phenobarbital during lactation period in epileptic women: total and free drug serum levels in the nursed infants and their effects on neonatal behavior. *Dev. Pharmacol. Ther., 11,* 147–154.

PROPOFOL

GENERAL

Propofol is a short-acting intravenous anaesthetic agent used for the induction and maintenance of general anaesthesia. It is 97% bound to plasma proteins and is rapidly and almost completely metabolised to products that appear not to be pharmacologically active. The half-life in plasma is 30–60 min.

EVALUATION OF DATA

Passage of propofol into human milk has been reported as follows:

Treatment conditions: Dose × Frequency × Duration; Route; No. of patients; Lactation stage	Concentration (mg/l): Milk	Concentration (mg/l): Plasma	Milk/plasma ratio	Maximum observed milk conc. (mg/l)	Absolute dose to infant (mg/kg/day): Ave	Absolute dose to infant (mg/kg/day): Max	Ref.
2.5 mg/kg × 1/d × 1 d; i.v.; 4; 1 d	0.14–0.24 (4 h) 0.09–0.16 (8 h)	–	–	–	–	–	(1)
5 mg/kg/h × 1/d × 1/d; i.v. 3; 1 d	0.74 (5 h) 0.048 (24 h)	2.1 (delivery)	–	–	–	–	(1)
305.5 × 1/d × 1 d; i.v.; 2; 1 d	0.47 (12 h)	0.52 (12 h)	0.9	–	–	–	(2)

Propofol was given to induce and then maintain anaesthesia in women undergoing cesaerean section. The table gives the range of concentrations noted during induction (mean dose used 149.5 mg) and the highest individual concentrations recorded during maintenance (mean dose used 5.05 mg/kg). Mean values are given in (2)

RELATIVE DOSE IN MILK

Assuming a maternal weight of 60 kg and suckling at 24 h, an infant would ingest in a feed at maximum 0.03% (0.048 × 180/300)* of the maternal maintenance dose of propofol (1). Alternatively, an infant suckling 12 h after delivery would ingest 0.28% (0.47 × 180/303.5) of the maternal single dose (2)

DATA ON THE INFANT

The mean propofol concentration in heel prick blood 2 h after delivery, i.e. transplacentally received, was 0.78 mg/l.

* An explanation of the calculation (s) appears on pp. 71–72.

ASSESSMENT AND RECOMMENDATIONS

The risk to the infant suckling 12–24 h after administration of propofol to its mother has ceased is negligible on the basis that the quantity of drug that passes into milk is very small. Breast-feeding at this time should be regarded as safe.

REFERENCES

1. Dailland P, Cockshott ID, Lirzin JD, Jacquinot P, Jorrot JC, Devery J, Harmey J-L, Conseiller C (1989) Intravenous profofol during cesarean section: placental transfer, concentrations in breast milk, and neonatal effects. *Anaesthesiology, 71*, 827–834.
2. Schmitt JP, Schwoerer D, Diemunsch P, Gauthier-Lafaye J (1987) Passage du propofol dans le colostrium. Données préliminaires. *Ann. Fr. Anesth. Réanim. (Paris), 6*, 267–268.

PYRIDOSTIGMINE

GENERAL

Pyridostigmine is a cholinesterase inhibitor that is used to treat myasthenia gravis. It is poorly absorbed from the adult gastrointestinal tract. Pyridostigmine is eliminated in the urine mainly in the unchanged form; the plasma half-life after oral administration is 4 h. Plasma concentrations between 50 and 100 μg/l are needed to restore neuromuscular transmission in myasthenic patients.

EVALUATION OF DATA

Passage of pyridostigmine into human milk has been reported as follows:

Treatment conditions — Dose × Frequency × Duration; Route; No. of patients; Lactation stage	Concentration (μg/l) Milk	Plasma	Milk/plasma ratio	Maximum observed milk conc. (μg/l)	Absolute dose to infant (μg/kg/day) Ave	Max	Ref.
60 mg × 3/d × LT; p.o.; 1; 35 d	15	25	0.6	17	2.3	2.6	(1)
60 mg × 5/d × LT; p.o.; 1; 60 d	24	80	0.3	25	3.6	3.8	(1)

LT, long term. The mothers received pyridostigmine under steady-state conditions of dosing. The milk and plasma concentrations are average values derived from the areas under the respective concentration-time curves.

RELATIVE DOSE IN MILK

A suckling infant would ingest in a day on average 0.08% (15 × 900/180 000)* and at maximum 0.09% (17 × 900/180 000)* of the weight-adjusted maternal daily dose of pyridostigmine.

DATA ON THE INFANT

There were no drug effects in the two infants. Pyridostigmine could not be identified in plasma from one infant (limit of detection 2 μg/l).

ASSESSMENT OF DATA

The risk to the suckling infant of administering pyridostigmine to its mother is low

* An explanation of the calculation (s) appears on pp. 71–72.

on the basis that the quantity of drug that passes into milk is small. Breast-feeding may be regarded as safe.

REFERENCES

1. Hardell LI, Lindstrom B, Lonnerholm G, Osterman PO (1982) Pyridostigmine in human breast milk. *Br. J. Clin. Pharmacol., 14,* 565–567.

QUAZEPAM

GENERAL

Quazepam is a benzodiazepine drug that is used as an hypnotic. It is extensively metabolised to 2-oxoquazepam (OQ) and N-desalkyl-2-oxoquazepam (DOQ); the latter is identical to N-desalkylflurazepam. Binding of quazepam and its major metabolites to plasma proteins exceeds 95%. Quazepam has a plasma half-life of 25 h, DOQ of 72 h and OQ of 40 h.

EVALUATION OF DATA

Passage of quazepam and its two major metabolites into human milk has been reported as follows:

Treatment conditions — Dose × Frequency × Duration; Route; No. of patients; Lactation stage	Concentration (μg/l)		Milk/ plasma ratio	Maxi- mum observed milk conc. (μg/l)	Absolute dose to infant (μg/kg/day)		Ref.
	Milk	Plasma			Ave	Max	
15 mg/d × 1 d; p.o.; 4; ?	18	3	6.0	216	2.7	32.4	(1)
2-oxoquazepam	4	2	2.0	44	0.6	6.6	
N-desalkyl-2-oxoquazepam	2	18	0.1	3	0.3	0.5	

The concentration-time profiles were defined in milk and plasma and were concurrent; the milk and plasma concentrations are derived from the respective area calculations. The maximum concentration quoted is the highest value recorded in an individual. The authors report that the total collection for 48 h in the 4 mothers contained on average the equivalent of 0.017 mg (0.1%) of the dose of quazepam. This is probably a large underestimate, since sucking empties the breast more efficiently.

RELATIVE DOSE IN MILK

A suckling infant would ingest in a feed at maximum 3.2% (216 + 44 + 3 × 180/15 000)* of the weight-adjusted maternal single dose of quazepam and its active metabolites (1).

DATA ON THE INFANT

The mothers agreed to cease breast-feeding; there are thus no data on the infant (but see diazepam, p. 422).

* An explanation of the calculation (s) appears on pp. 71–72.

ASSESSMENT OF DATA

The risk to the suckling infant of administering quazepam to its mother as a single dose is low on the basis that the quantity of drug that passes into milk is small. Breast-feeding after occasional such doses may be regarded as safe. There are no data on which to base a recommendation for repeated dosing but quazepam and its active metabolites are eliminated slowly and would accumulate in the infant.

REFERENCES

1. Hilbert JM, Gural RP, Symchowicz S, Zampaglione N (1984) Excretion of quazepam into human milk. *J. Clin. Pharmacol., 24,* 457–462.

SALICYLATES

GENERAL

Salicylates (in particular aspirin) have antipyretic, analgesic and anti-inflammatory properties and act by inhibiting prostaglandin synthesis. Salicylates are well absorbed from the adult gastrointestinal tract and bind extensively to plasma proteins. After therapeutic doses, 5–10% is eliminated unchanged by the kidney and the remainder is metabolised in the liver by a process that exhibts saturation kinetics such that unexpected accumulation can occur with repeated doses. Significant metabolic disturbance results from salicylate overdose. Use of aspirin in children has been discontinued in many countries because of its causal association with Reye's syndrome.

EVALUATION OF DATA

Passage of salicylates (aspirin) into human milk has been reported as follows:

Treatment conditions	Concentration (mg/l)		Milk/ plasma ratio	Maxi- mum observed milk conc. (mg/l)	Absolute dose to infant (mg/kg/day)		Ref.
Dose × Frequency × Duration; Route; No. of patients; Lactation stage	Milk	Plasma			Ave	Max	
500 mg × 1/d × 1 d; p.o.; 6; 2–8 months	5.8	–	–	7.8	0.87	1.17	(1)
1000 mg × 1/d × 1 d; p.o.; 6; 2–8 months	16.0	–	–	21.0	2.4	3.2	(1)
1500 mg × 1/d × 1 d; p.o.; 6; 2–8 months	39.0	–	–	48.0	5.85	7.2	(1)
1307 mg × 1/d × 1 d; p.o.; 4; 23–43 d	–	–	–	–	0.04⊕	0.07⊕	(2)
650–975 mg × 3–6/d × 7 weeks; p.o.; 1; 4 months	3.0 (3–10)	92.0 (72–108)	0.06 (0.04–0.08)	10.0	–	1.5	(3)
908 mg × 1/d × 1 d; p.o.; 2; 7, 13 weeks			0.03–0.05	1.12	0.17		(4)
1000 mg × 1/d × 1 d; p.o.; 8; ?	0.1–2.0	0.7–81.9	0.024–0.14	2.4 (6 h)		0.36	(5, 6)
2.4 g/d × 7 weeks; p.o.; 1; 7 weeks		1.63 mmol/l					(8)

⊕The dose (mg/kg) to the infants was based on salicylate recovered from their urine. Reference (1) describes mothers who received single doses of aspirin 500, 1000 and 1500 mg orally in a crossover design one hour after breakfast; milk samples were collected for 6 h thereafter. The peak concentration in milk occurred on average 2.6 h after a dose. The table gives average peak milk concentrations for each dose for all subjects; these showed a clear dose dependency and the data may be compared with the findings in references (5) and (6) below. The maximum milk concentrations are the highest values recorded in individual mothers. Reference (2) reports 4 nursing women who each received a single dose of sodium salicylate 20 mg/kg (equivalent to acetylsalicylic acid [aspirin] 1307 mg). Recovery of salicylate in infant urine was 0.18–0.36% of maternal dose and in some infants, elimination continued 15 h after that from the mother was complete. The mother reported in reference (3) gave milk and blood samples for 8 h after aspirin 975 mg. The table gives the range of concentrations recorded. Reference (4) reports on two mothers, 7 and 13 weeks post partum, who received a single oral dose of 2 tablets of a combination drug containing aspirin 454 mg per tablet. The concentration of salicylic acid declined more slowly in milk than plasma, suggesting accumulation and a potential for a higher milk to plasma ratio with repeated doses. Two other references (5,6) report results from the same study of 8 lactating women each of whom received a single oral dose of microencapsulated aspirin 1 g. The maximum milk to plasma ratio of 0.14 was seen at 24 h after the dose, but prior to this, the range was much less (0.024–0.041). All reports describing single dose studies establish a milk to plasma ratio of <1.

RELATIVE DOSE IN MILK

Where aspirin (mol. wt. 180) was given but salicylate (regarded as salicylic acid, mol. wt. 138) was assayed, a factor of 1.3 (180/138) is included in the calculation. On this basis a suckling infant would ingest in a feed at maximum 3.7–7.5% (7.8 × 180 × 1.3/500)-(48.0 × 180 × 1.3/1500)* of the weight-adjusted maternal single dose (1). The amount estimated by recovery of salicylate in infant urine was 0.18–0.36% of the dose taken by the mothers (2). Reference (4) found 0.46 mg (per 12 h) or an estimated 6.7 mg (per 48 h after 12 doses) of salicylate in two subjects given 908 mg dose(s) of aspirin in a combined drug preparation. The actual accumulation of salicylic acid to steady-state in milk or in infant plasma after repeated doses of aspirin to the breast-feeding woman has not been evaluated. Reference (3) describes a mother under conditions of long-term dosing. Using this data a suckling infant would ingest in a day on average 2.4% (6 × 900 × 1.3/2925)* and at maximum 4.0% (10 × 900 × 1.3/2925)* of the weight-adjusted maternal daily dose. A larger maternal dose is consistent with accumulation and toxicity reported in one infant (7).

DATA ON THE INFANT

No drug-related effects were specifically reported by references (1–4). One case report (7) suggests salicylate toxicity secondary to maternal aspirin ingestion (3.9 gm/day) in a 16 day old nursing infant who had a serum salicylate concentration of 240 mg/1. Reference (8) quotes a serum salicylate of 65 mg/l in a partially breast-fed infant whose mother took aspirin 2.4 g/d (maternal serum salicylate 225 mg/l).

ASSESSMENT AND RECOMMENDATIONS

The milk to plasma ratio for salicylic acid was consistently <1. Thus only a small

* An explanation of the calculation (s) appears on pp. 71–72.

amount of salicylate is delivered to the infant in milk following a single maternal dose. The data do not allow an assessment of accumulation of salicylate in milk and in infant plasma; such information is especially important for a drug whose elimination processes are saturable. Safety assessment requires such data and also those on metabolic effects, extent of displacement of endogenous substances (e.g. bilirubin) from plasma proteins by salicylic acid in the very young infant and the role of salicylate in the causation of Reye's syndrome. Until these issues are clarified, administration of salicylate or its derivatives to nursing women should be regarded as unsafe, particularly when administered on a long-term basis.

REFERENCES

1. Jamali F, Keshavarz E (1981) Salicylate in breast milk. *Int. J. Pharmacol., 8*, 285–290.
2. Levy, G (1975) Salicylate pharmacokinetics in the human neonate. In: Morselli PL, Garattini S, Sereni F (Eds) *Basic and Therapeutic Aspects of Perinatal Pharmacology*, pp 319–329. Raven Press, New York.
3. Bailey DN, Weibert RT, Naylor AJ, Shaw RF (1982) A study of salicylate and caffeine excretion in the breast milk of two nursing mothers. *J. Anal. Toxicol., 6*, 64–68.
4. Findlay JWA, DeAngelis RL, Kearney MF, Welch RM, Findlay JM (1981) Analgesic drugs break milk and plasma. *Clin. Pharmacol. Ther., 29*, 625–633.
5. Putter J (1976) Übersicht über die Pharmakokinetick der Acetylsalicylsäure. *Med. Welt., 27*, 1362–1365.
6. Putter J, Satravaha P, Stockhausen H (1974) Quantitative Bestimmung der Hauptmetaboliten der Acetylsalizylsäure. *Z. Geburtshilfe Perinatol., 178*, 135–138.
7. Clark JH, Wilson WG (1981) A 16-day old breast-fed infant with metabolic acidosis caused by salicylates. *Clin. Pediatr., 20*, 53–54.
8. Unsworth J, d'Assis-Fonseca A, Beswick DT, Blake DR (1987) Serum salicylate levels in a breast-fed infant. *Ann. Rheum. Dis., 46*, 638–639.

SERTRALINE

GENERAL

Sertraline is an antidepressant drug that acts by inhibiting the uptake of serotonin into presynaptic nerves. It is well absorbed from the adult gastrointestinal tract, undergoes extensive presystemic metabolism and is 98% bound to plasma proteins. The plasma half-life is 26 h.

EVALUATION OF DATA

Passage of sertraline into human milk has been reported as follows:

Treatment conditions — Dose × Frequency × Duration; Route; No. of patients; Lactation stage	Concentration (μg/l)		Milk/ plasma ratio	Maxi- mum observed milk conc. (μg/l)	Absolute dose to infant (μg/kg/day)		Ref.
	Milk	Plasma			Ave	Max	
100 mg/d × LT; p.o.; 1; 3, 7 weeks	30 (ave.)	48 (12 h)	0.65	43	4.5	6.45	(1)

LT, long term. The concentration-time profile was defined for milk. The maximum concentration was recorded at 5 h after the dose and the average concentration is based on the area measurement. The milk to plasma ratio is based on measurements 13 h (milk) and 13 h (plasma) after the dose.

RELATIVE DOSE IN MILK

A suckling infant would ingest in a day on average 0.27% (30 × 900/100 000)* and at maximum 0.39% (43 × 900/100 000)* of the weight-adjusted maternal daily dose of sertraline (1).

DATA ON THE INFANT

No sertraline was measured in the infant's plasma (assay limit 0.5 μg/l) and no drug effects were noted in the infant.

ASSESSMENT OF DATA

Data from a single mother suggest that the risk to the suckling infant of administering sertraline to its mother is low on the basis that the quantity of drug that passes

* An explanation of the calculation (s) appears on pp. 71–72.

into milk is small. Breast-feeding would appear to be safe but more information is required before a definite recommendation can be made.

REFERENCES

1. Altshuler LL, Burt VK, McMullen M, Hendrick V (1995) Breastfeeding and sertraline: a 24-hour analysis. *J. Clin. Psychiatry, 56,* 243–245..

SULPIRIDE

GENERAL

Sulpiride is a dopamine antagonist with antipsychotic actions similar to those of chlorpromazine; it is used to treat schizophrenia. Sulpiride is absorbed from the adult gastrointestinal tract and 80–90% is excreted unchanged in the urine. The plasma half-life is 7 h. Sulpiride stimulates prolactin secretion and enhances milk yield in mothers with insufficient breast milk (1).

EVALUATION OF DATA

Passage of sulpiride into human milk has been reported as follows:

Treatment conditions	Concentration (mg/l)		Milk/plasma ratio	Maximum observed milk conc. (mg/l)	Absolute dose to infant (mg/kg/day)		Ref.
Dose × Frequency × Duration; Route; No. of patients; Lactation stage	Milk	Plasma			Ave	Max	
50 mg × 2/d × 7 d; p.o.; 20; 3–7 d	0.97	–	–	1.97	0.145	0.300	(1)
50 mg × 2/d × 5 d; p.o.; 45; 5 d	0.83	–	–	1.46	0.125	0.220	(2)

Milk samples were taken 2 h (1) or 4 h (2) after a dose of sulpiride. The milk concentrations quoted in both studies are average values and the maximum concentrations are the highest values recorded in individuals. The mean milk yield in the first 5 postpartum days was significantly greater in these mothers who received sulpiride than in control groups of mothers who received no sulpiride (1, 2). No significant changes were observed in milk fat, protein or lactose.

RELATIVE DOSE IN MILK

A suckling infant would ingest in a day on average 8.7% (0.97 × 900/100)* and at maximum 17.7% (1.97 × 900/100)* of the weight-djusted maternal daily dose of sulpiride (1).

DATA ON THE INFANT

No data are reported.

ASSESSMENT OF DATA

The risk to the suckling infant of administering sulpiride to its mother is significant

* An explanation of the calculation (s) appears on pp. 71–72.

on the basis that the quantity of drug that passes into milk is high. Breast-feeding should be regarded as unsafe.

REFERENCES

1. Aano T, Shioji T, Aki T, Hirota K, Nomura A, Jurachi K (1979) Augmentation of puerperal lactation by oral administration of sulpiride. *J. Clin. Endocrinol. Metabol., 48*,478–482.
2. Pollati FK (1982) Sulpiride isomers and milk secretion in puerperium. *Clin. Exp. Obstet. Gynaecol., 9,* 144–147.

SUMATRIPTAN

GENERAL

Sumatriptan is an agonist of 5-hydroxytryptamine-like receptors that is used to treat migraine. It is administered subcutaneously or orally and is rapidly absorbed by these routes; there is high pre-systemic metabolism after administration by mouth. About 80% is metabolised and the remainder is excreted unchanged in the urine. The plasma half-life is 2 h.

EVALUATION OF DATA

Passage of sumatriptan into human milk has been reported as follows:

Treatment conditions Dose × Frequency × Duration; Route; No. of patients; Lactation stage	Concentration (μg/l)		Milk/ plasma ratio	Maximum observed milk conc. (μg/l)	Absolute dose to infant (μg/kg/day)		Ref.
	Milk	Plasma			Ave	Max	
6 mg × 1/d × 1 d; sc.; 5; 22 weeks	87	80	4.9	87	–	13.3	(1)

The milk and plasma concentration-time profiles were not concurrent, the peak value in milk occurring later than that in plasma. The table gives mean maximum values.

RELATIVE DOSE IN MILK

A suckling infant would ingest in a feed at maximum 2.6% (87 × 180/6000)* of the weight-adjusted maternal single dose of sumatriptan. This estimate would be lower if, as in the adult, sumatriptan undergoes pre-systemic metabolism.

DATA ON THE INFANT

No data are available.

ASSESSMENT AND RECOMMENDATIONS

The risk to the suckling infant of administering sumatriptan to its mother is low on the basis that the quantity of drug that passes into milk is small. Sumatriptan is normally administered only in occasional doses, and such use would appear to be safe.

* An explanation of the calculation (s) appears on pp. 71–72.

REFERENCES

1. Wojnar-Horton RE, Hackett LP, Yapp P, Dusci LJ, Paech M, Ilett KF (1996) Distribution and excretion of sumatriptan in human milk. *Br. J. Clin. Pharmacol., 41*, 217–221.

TEMAZEPAM

GENERAL

Temazepam is a short-acting benzodiazepine that is used to treat insomnia. It is well absorbed from the adult gastrointestinal tract and is about 80% bound to plasma proteins. Temazepam is extensively metabolised to products that are, in the main, pharmacologically inactive but include a small quantity of oxozepam which is active. The plasma half-life is 5–12 h.

EVALUATION OF DATA

Passage of temazepam into human milk has been reported as follows:

Treatment conditions Dose × Frequency × Duration; Route; No. of patients; Lactation stage	Concentration (μg/l) Milk	 Plasma	Milk/plasma ratio	Maximum observed milk conc. (μg/l)	Absolute dose to infant (μg/kg/day) Ave	 Max	Ref.
10–20 mg × 1/d × >2d; p.o.; 10; 2 weeks	28 (<5)	53 (8)	–	–	–	–	(1)

Plasma and milk were sampled 15 h after at least 2 doses. Steady-state trough concentrations were obtained. In 9 mothers temazepam was below the limit of detection (5 μg/l); the table gives the concentrations of temazepam in the 10th mother. Oxazepam was <5 μg/l in all milk samples.

RELATIVE DOSE IN MILK

A suckling infant would ingest in a feed 15 hours after dosing 0.3% (28 × 180/20 000)* of the weight-adjusted maternal dose of temazepam.

DATA ON THE INFANT

Neither temazepam nor its metabolite oxazepam could be detected (<5 μg/l) in the plasma of 2 infants. No drug-related adverse related were observed in any of the ten breast-fed infants (1).

ASSESSMENT OF DATA

The risk to the suckling infant of administering a single dose of temazepam to its mother is negligible on the basis that the quantity of drug that passes into milk is

* An explanation of the calculation (s) appears on pp. 71–72.

very small. Breast-feeding after a single dose may be regarded as safe but any effects after repeated doses to the mother are not known.

REFERENCES

1. Lebeders TH, Wojnar-Horton RE, Tapp P, Roberts MJ, Dusci LJ, Hacket LP, Ilett KF. (1992) Excretion of temazepam in breast milk. *Br. J. Clin. Pharmacol., 33*, 204–206.

THIOPENTAL SODIUM

GENERAL

Thiopental sodium (thiopentone) is a rapidly-acting barbiturate used for the induction of general anaesthesia. It is administered by i.v. injection and is 50–80% bound to plasma proteins. Thiopental distributes initially to highly perfused tissues and then redistributes to lean tissues and fat. The drug is completely metabolised by the liver. The half-life of the terminal phase of elimination from plasma is 9 h.

EVALUATION OF DATA

Passage of thiopental into human milk has been reported as follows:

Treatment conditions: Dose × Frequency × Duration; Route; No. of patients; Lactation stage	Concentration (μg/l)		Milk/plasma ratio	Maximum observed milk conc. (μg/l)	Absolute dose to infant (μg/kg/day)		Ref.
	Milk	Plasma			Ave	Max	
4.4–7.0 mg/kg × 1/d × 1 d; i.v.; 8; > 2 weeks	99	233	0.42	899	15	135	(1)
3.8–6.3 mg/kg × 1 × 1 d; i.v.; 8; colostrum	42	92	0.46	95	6	14	(1)

The upper line of the table refers to mothers who received thiopental sodium to induce anaesthesia for minor elective surgery; the first samples were collected 2 h after drug administration. The lower line refers to mothers who underwent caesarean section and the first samples were taken after 4 h and hence exhibit lower concentrations. Blood and milk concentrations were defined for 36 h. The table gives mean figures based on area measurements; the maximum concentration is the average for the groups at the first sampling, i.e. 2 h and 4 h respectively.

RELATIVE DOSE IN MILK

Assuming a maternal weight of 60 kg, a suckling infant would ingest in a feed on average 0.06% (99 × 180/326 250)* of the weight-adjusted maternal dose of thiopental sodium.

DATA ON THE INFANT

All the infants delivered by caesarean section obtained maximal Apgar scores.

ASSESSMENT OF DATA

The risk to the infant of suckling after its mother has received thiopental sodium is

* An explanation of the calculation (s) appears on pp. 71–72.

negligible on the basis that the quantity of drug that passes into milk is very small. Breast-feeding may be regarded as safe.

REFERENCES

1. Andersen LW, Qvist T, Hertz J, Morgensen F (1987) Concentrations of thiopentone in mature breast milk and colostrum following an induction dose. *Acta Anaesthesiol. Scand.*, *31*, 30–32.

TRAZODONE

GENERAL

Trazodone is a triazolpyridine drug that is used to treat depression. It may act by inhibiting serotonin reuptake by neurones. Trazodone is rapidly absorbed from the adult gastrointstinal tract and is 90% bound to plasma proteins. Trazodone is extensively metabolised and the plasma half-life is 1–4 h.

EVALUATION OF DATA

Passage of trazodone into human milk has been reported as follows:

Treatment conditions Dose × Frequency × Duration; Route; No. of patients; Lactation stage	Concentration (μg/l)		Milk/ plasma ratio	Maximum observed milk conc. (μg/l)	Absolute dose to infant (μg/kg/day)		Ref.
	Milk	Plasma			Ave	Max	
50 mg × 1/d × 1 d; p.o.; 5; 3–8 months	100	704	0.142	100	–	15	(1)

The concentration-time profiles were defined and were concurrent. The milk concentration is the maximum for the group and is taken from a graph. The milk to plasma ratio is based on area measurements.

RELATIVE DOSE IN MILK

A suckling infant would ingest in a feed at maximum 0.4% (100 × 180/50 000)* of the weight-adjusted single dose of trazodone. (1).

DATA ON THE INFANT

No data are available.

ASSESSMENT OF DATA

The data indicate that the risk to the suckling infant of administering a single dose of trazodone to its mother is negligible on the basis that the quantity of drug that passes into milk is small. The normal use of trazodone, however, requires repeated dosing and the consequences to the infant of such exposure are not known. A deci-

* An explanation of the calculation (s) appears on pp. 71–72.

sion about the advisability of breast-feeding is probably best determined by the factors pertinent to the individual case.

REFERENCES

1. Verbeek RK, Ross SG, McKenna EA (1987) Excretion of trazodone in breast milk. *Br. J. Clin. Pharmacol.*, 22, 367–370.

SODIUM VALPROATE

GENERAL

Sodium valproate is used to treat several forms of epilepsy. It is rapidly absorbed from the adult gastrointestinal tract and 90% is bound to plasma proteins. Sodium valproate and is extensively metabolised; some of the products appear to retain antiepilepsy activity. The plasma half-life is 13–21 h in adults but is 47 h in neonates (4).

EVALUATION OF DATA

Passage of sodium valproate into human milk has been reported as follows:

Treatment conditions — Dose × Frequency × Duration; Route; No. of patients; Lactation stage	Concentration (mg/l) Milk	Plasma	Milk/ plasma ratio	Maximum observed milk conc. (mg/l)	Absolute dose to infant (mg/kg/day) Ave	Max	Ref.
300–2400 mg/d × LT; p.o.; 11; 3–6 d	1.8	36.4	0.05	3.9	0.285	0.585	(1)
250 mg × 2/d × LT; p.o.; 1; 1–6 d	(0.18) (0.47) 0.32	(9.9) (34.3) 22.1	0.01–0.02	0.47	0.048	0.071	(2)
1600 mg/d × LT; p.o.; 1; 5, 29d	5.1	76.7	–	7.2	0.77	1.08	(3)
600–1800 mg/d × LT; p.o.; 6; 3–82 d	1.4	45.1	0.03	5.4	0.21	0.71	(4)

LT, long term. Reference (1) reports average milk and plasma concentrations in samples taken simultaneously. When measurements were repeated on different days in 4 mothers similar results were obtained The milk and serum concentrations quoted in parentheses in reference (2) were taken 62 h and 130 h after delivery, 16 h and 3 h after dosing respectively; the mean values appear on the line below. Average concentrations for the 5th and 29th days after delivery are given in reference (3). Reference (4) gives data on 16 paired milk and plasma samples and the means appear in the table. The maximum milk concentration is the highest value recorded in an individual. All studies were conducted under steady-state conditions of dosing.

RELATIVE DOSE IN MILK

The average dose of sodium valproate quoted in reference (4) was 1032 mg/d assuming a maternal weight of 60 kg. On this basis a suckling infant would ingest in a day on average 1.2% (1.4 ×900/1032)* and at maximum 4.7% (5.4 × 900/1032)* of the average weight-adjusted maternal daily dose of sodium valproate.

* An explanation of the calculation (s) appears on pp. 71–72.

DATA ON THE INFANT

No data are available.

ASSESSMENT AND RECOMMENDATIONS

The risk to the suckling infant of administering sodium valproate to its mother is low in the basis that the quantity of drug that passes into milk is small. Breast-feeding would appear to be safe.

REFERENCES

1. Von Unruh GE, Froescher W, Hoffman F, Nielsen M (1984) Valproic acid in breast milk. How much is really there? *Ther. Drug Monit., 6,* 272–276.
2. Dickinsson R, Harland R, Lynn R, Smith B, Gerber N. (1979) Transmission of valproic acid (Depakene) across the placenta: Half-life of the drug in mother and baby. *J. Pediatr., 94*, 832–835.
3. Alexander FW (1979) Sodium valproate and pregnancy. *Arch. Dis. Child., 54*, 240.
4. Nau H, Rating S, Koch S, Hanser I, Helge H (1981) Valproic acid and its metabolites: placental transfer, neonatal pharmacokinetics, transfer via the mother's milk and clinical status in neonates of epileptic mothers. *J. Pharmacol. Exp. Ther., 219*, 768–777.

ZOLPIDEM

GENERAL

Zolpidem is an imidazopyridine hypnotic which has sedative effects similar to the benzodiazepines. It is rapidly absorbed from the adult gastrointestinal tract, 92% bound to plasma proteins and metabolised in the liver to products that appear to be pharmacologically inactive. The plasma half life is 2 h.

EVALUATION OF DATA

Passage of zolpidem into human milk has been reported as follows:

Treatment conditions Dose × Frequency × Duration; Route; No. of patients; Lactation stage	Concentration (μg/l) Milk	 Plasma	Milk/plasma ratio	Maximum observed milk conc. (μg/l)	Absolute dose to infant (μg/kg/day) Ave	 Max	Ref.
20 mg × 1/d × 1 d; p.o.; 5; 3–4 d	(see below)	90–364	0.13	–	–	–	(1)

Milk and plasma were sampled before and 3, 13 and 16 h after dosing. The 3 h collection of milk was pooled and the amounts excreted were 0.004–0.019% of the dose given. The milk:plasma ratios figure is based on concentrations at 3 h. No zolpidem was detected 13 and 16 h after dosing.

RELATIVE DOSE IN MILK

The relative dose cannot be calculated as no milk concentrations are quoted in (1). Alternatively, the amount of zolpidem excreted in milk 3 h after dosing, when the plasma concentration was highest, was on average 0.08% of the administered dose.

DATA ON THE INFANT

No data are available.

ASSESSMENT OF DATA

The data indicate that the risk to the suckling infant of administering zolpidem to its mother is low on the basis that the quantity of drug that passes into milk is small. Zolpidem has a short half life, no accumulation was found during multiple dose kinetic studies, and it is metabolised to inactive metabolites (2). Breast-feeding would appear to be safe.

REFERENCES

1. Pons G, Francoual C, Guillet PH, Moran C, Herman P, Bianchetti G, Thierelin JF (1989) Zolpidem excretion in breast milk. *Eur. J. Clin. Pharmacol., 37*, 245–248.
2. Thenot JP, Hermann Ph, Durand A, Burke JT, Allen J, Garrigou D, Vajta S, Albin H, Thebault JJ, Olive G, Warrington SJ. (1988) Pharmacokinetics and metabolism of zolpidem in various animal species and in humans. In: Sauvanet JP, Langer SZ, Morselli PL (Eds) *Imidazopyridines in Sleep Disorders*, pp 139–153. Raven Press, New York.

ZOPICLONE

GENERAL

Zopiclone is a cyclopyrrolone hypnotic which has effects similar to the benzodiazepines. It is rapidly absorbed from the adult gastrointestinal tract, 45% is bound to plasma proteins and it is extensively metabolised. The plasma half-life is 5 h.

EVALUATION OF DATA

Passage of zopiclone into human milk has been reported as follows:

Treatment conditions Dose × Frequency × Duration; Route; No. of patients; Lactation stage	Concentration (μg/l) Milk	Plasma	Milk/plasma ratio	Maximum observed milk conc. (μg/l)	Absolute dose to infant (μg/kg/day) Ave	Max	Ref.
7.5 mg × 1/d × 1 d; p.o.; 3; ?	–	–	0.6	50	–	7.5	(1)
7.5 mg × 1/d × 1 d; p.o.; 12; 3–6 d	11	23	0.51	34	2	5	(2)

The concentration-time profiles were defined in both studies and were concurrent. The table gives average milk and plasma concentrations and milk to plasma ratios which were derived from the areas under the respective concentration-time curves. The maximum concentration in milk is an average values for the group. Zopiclone was not detectable in milk 22 h after dosing in 7 of the 12 women and varied between 2.8 and 4.4 μg/l in 5 (2).

RELATIVE DOSE IN MILK

A suckling infant would receive in a feed at maximum 0.8% (34 × 180/7500)* of the weight-adjusted maternal single dose of zopiclone (2). Alternatively, as zopiclone is given only once daily, a suckling infant would receive in a day 4.1% (34 × 900/7500)* of the weight-adjusted maternal daily dose (2).

DATA ON THE INFANT

The infants were monitored but no drug-related effects were observed (2).

ASSESSMENT OF DATA

The risk to the suckling infant of administering a single dose of zopiclone to its

* An explanation of the calculation (s) appears on pp. 71–72.

mother is low on the basis that the quantity of drug that passes into milk is small. Breast-feeding after occasional such doses may be regarded as safe. There are no data on which to base a recommendation for regularly repeated use.

REFERENCES

1. Gaillot J, Heusse D, Hougton GW, Marc Aurele J, Dreyfus JF (1983) Pharmacokinetics and metabolism of zopiclone. *Pharmacology, 27 (Suppl. 2),* 76–91.
2. Matheson I, Sande HA, Gaillot J, Vegdahl K (1990) Zopiclone excretion in breast milk. *Br. J. Clin. Pharmacol., 30,* 267–271.

ZUCLOPENTHIXOL

GENERAL

Zuclopenthixol is a thioxanthene drug that has strong antipsychotic activity; it may act through dopaminergic mechanisms. It is rapidly absorbed from the adult gastrointestinal tract, 98% is bound to plasma proteins and it is extensively metabolised to products that are pharmacologically inactive. The plasma half-life is 20 h.

EVALUATION OF DATA

Passage of zuclopenthixol into human milk has been reported as follows:

Treatment conditions: Dose × Frequency × Duration; Route; No. of patients; Lactation stage	Concentration (μg/l) Milk	Concentration (μg/l) Plasma	Milk/plasma ratio	Maximum observed milk conc. (μg/l)	Absolute dose to infant (μg/kg/day) Ave	Absolute dose to infant (μg/kg/day) Max	Ref.
4–50 mg /d × ?; p.o.; 5; 4 d–10 months	1.0–2.0	3.5–12.0	0.12–0.56	–	0.3	–	(1)
50 mg/2 weeks × ?; p.o.; 1; 3 d	9.0	66.0	0.14	–	1.35	–	(1)
24 mg/d × 2–4 d; p.o.; 1; 2 weeks	20.0	22.0	0.4–0.7 (1.1–2.2)[a]	–	3.0	–	(2)
14 mg/d × 5–8 d; p.o.; 1; 2 weeks	5.0	9.0	0.2–0.7	–	0.8	–	(2)

[a]Postfeed. The studies in (1) were carried out under apparent steady-state conditions of dosing. The 5 mothers who received zuclopenthixol by mouth gave milk samples prior to the morning dose, i.e. the concentration-time profiles were not defined. The table gives the range of values estimated from a figure in the report. One mother received zuclopenthixol (50 mg) by depot injection. In reference (2) milk was collected from one mother after 2, 3, 4, 6, 7 and 8 days treatment in the third week postpartum prior to the morning dose. After 24 mg from day 1–4 the dose was reduced to 14mg from day 5. Steady-state was reached after 5 days.

RELATIVE DOSE IN MILK

The amount of zuclopenthixol that a suckling infant would ingest in a day varies between 0.2% (9 × 900/50 000)* and 0.5% (2 × 900/4000)* of the weight-adjusted maternal dose (1).

DATA ON THE INFANT

No drug effects were observed in the infants (1).

* An explanation of the calculation (s) appears on pp. 71–72.

ASSESSMENT OF DATA

The data suggest that when zuclopenthixol is administered to a nursing mother, the quantity of drug that her infant ingests in milk is very small. A decision about the advisability of breast-feeding is probably best determined by the factors pertinent to the individual case.

REFERENCES

1. Aaes-Jørgensen T, Bjørndal F, Bartels U (1986) Zuclopenthixol levels in serum and breast milk. *Psychopharmacology, 90*, 417–418.
2. Matheson I, Skjæraasen J (1988) Milk concentration of flupenthixol, nortriptyline and zuclopenthixol and between-breast diffences in two patients. *Eur. J. Clin. Pharmacol., 35,* 217–220.

DIPROPHYLLINE

GENERAL

Diprophylline (dyphylline) though not a methylxanthine, is structurally related to theophylline and is used to treat asthma. It is incompletely absorbed from the adult gastrointestinal tract and in contrast to theophylline, diprophylline is eliminated mainly by the kidney. The plasma half-life is 4 h.

EVALUATION OF DATA

Passage of diprophylline into human milk has been reported as follows:

Treatment conditions — Dose × Frequency × Duration; Route; No. of patients; Lactation stage	Concentration (mg/l) Milk	Plasma	Milk/plasma ratio	Maximum observed milk conc. (mg/l)	Absolute dose to infant (mg/kg/day) Ave	Max	Ref.
5 mg/kg × 1/d × 1 d; i.m.; 20; ?	–	–	2.08	14.1	–	2.1	(1)

Samples were taken for 5 h after diprophylline and the authors report that rates of elimination from milk and serum were equivalent. The milk to serum ratio was calculated from the respective values assumed to be present at zero time by extrapolation from the concentration data points. The peak concentration was in fact attained by 2 h in most volunteers when the serum concentration is estimated to be 6.8 mg/l ($=Co.e^{-kt}$, where Co = conc. at zero time, k = 0.229 and t = 2 h): this corresponds to a milk concentration of 14.1 mg/l.

RELATIVE DOSE IN MILK

Assuming a maternal weight of 60 kg, the dose received was 300 mg. On this basis a suckling infant would ingest in a feed at maximum 8.5% (14.1 × 180/300)* of the weight-adjusted maternal single dose of diprophylline (1).

DATA ON THE INFANT

No data are reported. The authors calculated, however, that the maximum plasma concentration achieved in an infant would be 4.6 mg/l which is 68% of the estimated peak maternal concentration (6.8 mg/l) (1).

ASSESSMENT AND RECOMMENDATIONS

Only single dose data are available and diprophylline is commonly administered in

* An explanation of the calculation (s) appears on pp. 71–72.

multiple doses. The findings suggest a risk of drug effects under conditions of steady-state dosing because of the quantity of drug that passes into milk. Furthermore, xanthines, to which diprophylline is structurally related, are eliminated slowly by the neonate and may accumulate (see theophylline p. 529). If a decision is taken to breast-feed then the baby should be observed for signs of xanthine excess, e.g. irritability or disturbed sleep.

REFERENCES

1. Jarboe CH, Cook LN, Malesic J, Fleischaker J (1981) Dyphylline elimination kinetics in lactating women: blood to milk transfer. *J. Clin. Pharmacol.*, *21*, 405–410.

ENPROFYLLINE

GENERAL

Enprofylline, a xanthine, is used as a bronchodilator. It is absorbed from the adult gastrointestinal tract and it is eliminated mainly in the urine. The plasma half-life is 1.5 h.

EVALUATION OF DATA

Passage of enprofylline into human milk has been reported as follows:

Treatment conditions Dose × Frequency × Duration; Route; No. of patients; Lactation stage	Concentration (mg/l) Milk	 Plasma	Milk/ plasma ratio	Maximum observed milk conc. (mg/l)	Absolute dose to infant (mg/kg/day) Ave	 Max	Ref.
150 mg × 2/d × 5 d; p.o.; 6; 6–8 months	0.71	0.89	0.8	–	0.11	–	(1)

The table gives the overall average milk and plasma concentrations for the group (over 6 h on each of 3 days).

RELATIVE DOSE IN MILK

The quantity of enprofylline that an infant would ingest in a day is on average 2.1% (0.7 × 900/300)* of the weight-adjusted maternal daily dose.

DATA ON THE INFANT

No data are available.

ASSESSMENT AND RECOMMENDATIONS

The risk to the suckling infant of administering enprofylline to its mother is low on the basis that the quantity of drug that passes into milk is small. Xanthines are eliminated slowly by the neonate, however, and may accumulate (see theophylline p. 529). If a decision is taken to breast-feed then the baby should be observed for signs of xanthine excess, e.g. irritability or disturbed sleep.

REFERENCE

1. Laursen LC, Borgå O, Ljungholm K, Weeke B (1988) Transfer of enprofylline into breast milk. *Ther. Drug Monit., 10,* 150–152.

* An explanation of the calculation (s) appears on pp. 71–72.

PSEUDOEPHEDRINE

GENERAL

Pseudoephedrine is a sympathomimetic drug that is used principally as a decongestant of the upper respiratory tract, often in combination with a histamine H_1-receptor antagonist. It is a base. Pseudoephedrine is well absorbed from the adult gastrointestinal tract. Its rate of elimination in the urine is dependent on urine pH. The plasma half-life was 5.2–8.0 h at pH 5.6–6.0 and increased to 9.2–16.0 h at pH 8.0 (1)

EVALUATION OF DATA

Passage of pseudoephedrine into human milk has been reported as follows:

Treatment conditions	Concentration (mg/l)		Milk/ plasma ratio	Maximum observed milk conc. (mg/l)	Absolute dose to infant (mg/kg/day)		Ref.
Dose × Frequency × Duration; Route; No. of patients; Lactation stage	Milk	Plasma			Ave	Max	
60 mg × 1/d × 1 d; p.o.; 3; 14, 14, 72 weeks	0.264	0.134	1.97	1.0	0.04	0.15	(2)

The mothers took a tablet of an antihistamine-decongestant product which also contained triprolidine hydrochloride 2.5 mg. The concentration-time profiles were defined and were concurrent. The milk and plasma concentrations are average values calculated from the areas under the concentration-time curves. The maximum milk concentration is the highest value attained by an individual and was estimated from a graph.

RELATIVE DOSE IN MILK

A suckling infant would ingest in a feed at maximum 3.0% (1.0 × 180/60)* of the weight-adjusted maternal single dose (1).

DATA ON THE INFANT

No data are reported.

ASSESSMENT AND RECOMMENDATIONS

The risk to the suckling infant of administering a single dose of pseudoephedrine to

* An explanation of the calculation (s) appears on pp. 71–72.

its mother is low on the basis that the quantity of drug that passes into milk is small. Breast-feeding after occasional such doses would appear to be safe.

REFERENCES

1. Kuntzman RG, Tsai I, Brand L, Mark LC (1971) The influence of urinary pH on the plasma half-life of pseudoephedrine in man and dog and a sensitive assay for its determination in human plasma. *Clin. Pharmacol. Ther., 12,* 62–67.
2. Findley JWA, Butz RF, Sailstad JM, Warren JT, Welch RM (1984) Pseudoephedrine and triprolidine in plasma and breast milk of nursing mothers. *Br. J. Clin. Pharmacol., 18,* 901–906.

TERBUTALINE

GENERAL

Terbutaline is a selective beta$_2$-adrenoceptor stimulant drug that is used to treat asthma. Terbutaline can be administered by inhalation, orally or intravenously; availability by the oral route is about 15% due to pre-systemic elimination. It is 25% bound to plasma proteins. Metabolism inactivates for about half of the dose and the remainder is eliminated unchanged in the urine. The half-life in adults is 16 h.

EVALUATION OF DATA

Passage of terbutaline into human milk has been reported as follows:

Treatment conditions Dose × Frequency × Duration; Route; No. of patients; Lactation stage	Concentration (μg/l)		Milk/plasma ratio	Maximum observed milk conc. (μg/l)	Absolute dose to infant (μg/kg/day)		Ref.
	Milk	Plasma			Ave	Max	
2.5 mg × 3/d × LT; p.o.; 2; 3 weeks	3.4	1.8	1.9 (1.8–2.9)	4.6	0.5	0.7	(1)
5 mg × 3/d × LT; p.o.; 1; 8 weeks	3.5	2.0–4.8	–	–	0.5	–	(2)
?; ?; ?; 1; 6 weeks	2.5 (pre-dose)	1.9 (pre-dose)	1.3	–	–	–	(2)
	3.8 (4 h)	3.7 (4 h)	1.0				

Neither study fully defined the concentration-time profiles but the concentrations in milk appeared to fluctuate less than those in plasma. The milk and plasma concentrations quoted for reference (1) are average values during one (1) or two (2) dose intervals or are paired samples at the times stated (2). The maximum milk concentration is the highest value recorded in an individual. Both studies were conducted under steady-state conditions of dosing.

RELATIVE DOSE IN MILK

As terbutaline sulphate (mol. wt. 274) was administered but terbutaline base (mol. wt. 225) was assayed a factor of 1.22 (274/225) is included in the calculation. A suckling infant would ingest in a day on average 0.5% (3.4 × 900 × 1.22/7500)* and at maximum 0.7% (4.6 × 900 × 1.22/7500 × 225)* of the weight-adjusted maternal daily dose of terbutaline (1).

* An explanation of the calculation (s) appears on pp. 71–72.

DATA ON THE INFANT

Terbutaline was not detected in two plasma samples from one of the infants reported in reference (2) using a gas chromatography-mass spectrometry assay with a detection limit of 0.1 μg/l, and the infant showed no signs of beta-adrenergic stimulation.

ASSESSMENT AND RECOMMENDATIONS

The risk to the suckling infant of administering terbutaline orally to its mother appears to be low on the basis that the quantity of drug that passes into milk is small. Breast-feeding may be regarded as safe. There are no data in mothers taking terbutaline by inhalation, but exposure of the infant to the drug is likely to be even less by this route.

REFERENCES

1. Boréus LO, de Château P, Lindberg C, Nyberg L. Terbutaline in•breast milk (1982) *Br. J. Clin. Pharmacol., 13*, 731–732.
2. Lönnerholm G, Lindström B (1982) Terbutaline excretion into breast milk. *Br. J. Clin. Pharmacol., 13*, 729–730.

TERFENADINE

GENERAL

Terfenadine is a histamine H_1-receptor antagonist that is used to treat allergic conditions. It is non-sedative. Terfenadine is almost completely absorbed from the adult gastrointestinal tract and is 70% bound to plasma proteins. It is extensively metabolised such that only the major metabolite which is pharmacologically active, and no parent drug, was detected in plasma (1). The plasma half-life is 20 h.

EVALUATION OF DATA

Passage of terbutaline metabolite into human milk has been reported as follows:

Treatment conditions: Dose × Frequency × Duration; Route; No. of patients; Lactation stage	Concentration (μg/l) Milk	Plasma	Milk/plasma ratio	Maximum observed milk conc. (μg/l)	Absolute dose to infant (μg/kg/day) Ave	Max	Ref.
60 mg × 12 h × 48 h; p.o.; 4; 5–12 months	27 (ave) 41 (max)	133 (ave) 309 (max)	0.12–0.28	41	4.05	6.15	(1)

The milk and plasma concentration-time profiles were defined under conditions of steady-state dosing. The table gives average values for terfenadine metabolite.

RELATIVE DOSE IN MILK

A suckling infant would ingest in a day on average 0.2% (0.027 × 900/120)* and at maximum 0.3% (0.041 × 900/120)* of the weight-adjusted maternal daily dose.

DATA ON THE INFANT

No data are available.

ASSESSMENT AND RECOMMENDATIONS

The risk to the suckling infant of administering terfenadine to its mother appears to be low on the basis that the quantity of drug that passes into milk is small. Breast-feeding may be regarded as safe.

REFERENCES

1. Lucas BD, Purdy CY, Scarim SK, Benjamin S, Abel SR, Hilleman DE (1995) Terfenadine pharmacokinetics in breast milk in lactating women. *Clin. Pharmacol. Ther., 57,* 398–402.

* An explanation of the calculation (s) appears on pp. 71–72.

THEOBROMINE

GENERAL

Theobromine is a methylxanthine that has been used as a drug and is present in significant amounts in chocolate. It is well absorbed from the adult gastrointestinal tract and is extensively metabolised. The plasma half-life is 5.7 h (1).

EVALUATION OF DATA

Passage of theobromine into human milk has been reported as follows:

Treatment conditions — Dose × Frequency × Duration; Route; No. of patients; Lactation stage	Concentration (mg/l) Milk	Concentration (mg/l) Plasma	Milk/ plasma ratio	Maximum observed milk conc. (mg/l)	Absolute dose to infant (mg/kg/day) Ave	Absolute dose to infant (mg/kg/day) Max	Ref.
240 mg × 1/d × 1 d; p.o.; 3–37 weeks	3.7–7.5 (5.3 (ave.))	4.5–7.8 (5.7 (ave.))	0.6–1.06 0.82	7.5	0.80	1.13	(1)

The mothers refrained from tea, coffee, cola drinks and chocolate for 24 h then consumed 113 g of milk chocolate within 10 min. The milk and plasma concentration profiles were defined and were concurrent. The table gives the range and average of the values.

RELATIVE DOSE IN MILK

A suckling infant would ingest in a feed on average 3.5% (5.3 × 180/240)* and at maximum 5.6% (7.5 × 180/240)* of the weight-adjusted quantity of chocolate consumed by the mothers.

DATA ON THE INFANT

No data are available.

ASSESSMENT AND RECOMMENDATIONS

The risk to the suckling infant of theobromine from chocolate consumed by its mother is low on the basis that the quantity of theobromine that passes into milk is small. Xanthines are eliminated slowly by the neonate, however, and may accumulate (see theophylline p. 529). Breast-feeding following occasional such ingestion of chocolate appears safe.

* An explanation of the calculation (s) appears on pp. 71–72.

REFERENCES

1. Resman BH, Blumenthal P, Jusko WJ (1977) Breast milk distribution of theobromine from chocolate. *J. Pediatr.*, *93*, 477–480.

THEOPHYLLINE

GENERAL

Theophylline is a xanthine bronchodilator that is used to treat asthma. It is almost completely absorbed from the adult gastrointestinal tract. Some 60% is bound to plasma proteins and 36% in newborns (1). The action of theophylline is terminated principally by metabolism in the liver by both first order and capacity limited kinetic processes. The plasma half-life is age-dependent, being 6.7 h in adults but 30 h in premature infants (1, 2). The slower elimination in newborns is presumably due to a developmentally deficient hepatic oxidising activity; in this age group about 50% of theophylline is excreted unchanged.

EVALUATION OF DATA

Passage of theophylline into human milk has been reported as follows:

Treatment conditions	Concentration (mg/l)		Milk/ plasma ratio	Maximum observed milk conc. (mg/l)	Absolute dose to infant (mg/kg/day)		Ref.
Dose × Frequency × Duration; Route; No. of patients; Lactation stage	Milk	Plasma			Ave	Max	
300, then 200 mg 5 h later × 1/d × 1 d; p.o.; 12; ?	2.8	4.0	0.7 (0.6–0.89)	6.0	0.42	0.9	(3)
3.2–5.3 mg/kg × 1/d × 1 d (20 min); i.v.; 3; ?	–	–	0.67 (0.60–0.73)	–	–	–	(4)
4.25 mg/kg × 1/d × 1 d; p.o.; 3; ?	–	–	0.67 (0.61–0.73)	4.2	–	–	(5)
200 mg × 4/d × LT; p.o.; 2; ?	–	–	0.75 (0.63–0.87)	–	–	–	(5)

LT, long term. The milk and plasma concentration-time profiles were defined in references (3–5) over 4–14 h after single doses of theophylline and were concurrent. The concentrations quoted in reference (3) derive from the 300 mg dose and are average values; the maximum concentration is the highest value recorded in an individual. In reference (5) the maximum milk concentration was estimated from a graph. Steady-state dosing conditions are presumed to apply to the patients receiving long term theophylline.

RELATIVE DOSE IN MILK

A suckling infant would ingest in a feed at maximum 3.6% (6.0 x 180/300)* (3) of the weight-adjusted maternal single dose. The data in reference (5) gives a relative single dose estimate of 3.0% (4.2 x 180/255), assuming a maternal weight of 60 kg. The only available repeated dose report (5) does not quote milk concentrations and so does not allow a direct estimate of relative daily dose. The milk to plasma ratio of 0.75, however, is consistent with the findings from single dose studies. The work of others indicates that theophylline 8.2 mg/kg/12 h (16.4 mg/kg/day) would give a steady-state serum concentration of 15 mg/l (6, 7) which would produce, from reference (5), a milk concentration of 11.25 mg/l (15×0.75). On this basis a suckling infant would ingest in a day 10.3% ($11.25 \times 15/16.4$)* of the weight-adjusted child's daily dose.

DATA ON THE INFANT

Irritability and fretful sleeping were noted in one infant and was related in time to maternal use of aminophylline; 5 other nursing mothers did not observe irritability in their children after they had taken theophylline (5).

ASSESSMENT AND RECOMMENDATIONS

The data suggest a risk of drug effects in the suckling infant if theophylline is administered to its mother, because of the quantity of drug that passes into milk and its slow elimination rate in the very young. Adverse effects in a breast-feeding baby have been reported in the literature. Nevertheless theophylline is usually a safe drug when used in moderate doses to treat apnoea in premature infants. A decision to breast-feed is probably reasonable if the maternal dose is moderate but the baby should be observed for signs of xanthine excess, e.g. irritability or disturbed sleep.

REFERENCES

1. Aranda JV, Sitar DS, Parsons WD, Loughnan PM, Neims AH (1976) Pharmacokinetic aspects of theophylline in premature newborns. *N. Engl. J. Med., 295*, 413–416.
2. Dothey CI, Tserng K-Y, Kaw SK, King KC (1989) Maturation changes of theophylline pharmacokinetics in preterm infants. *Clin. Pharmacol. Ther., 45,* 461–468.
3. Reinhardt D, Richter O, Brandenburg G (1983) Pharmakokinetik des Arzneimittelübergangs von stillenden Muttern auf ihre Säuglinge am Beispiel des Theophyllins. *Monatsschr. Kinderheilkd., 131*, 66–70.
4. Stec GP, Greenberger P, Ruo TI, Henthorn T, Morita Y, Atkinson AJ, Paterson R (1980) Kinetics of theophylline transfer to breast milk. *Clin. Pharmacol. Ther., 28*, 404–408.
5. Yurchak AM, Jusko WJ. Theophylline secretion into breast milk (1976) *Pediatrics, 57*, 518–520.
6. Hendeles L, Weinberger M (1983) Improved efficacy and safety of theophylline in the control of airways hyperreactivity. *Pharmacol. Ther., 18*, 91–105.
7. Weinberger M, Hendeles L, Wong L, Vaughn L (1981) Relationship of formulation and dosing interval to fluctuation of serum theophylline concentration in children with chronic asthma. *J. Pediatr., 99,* 145–152.

TRIPROLIDINE

GENERAL

Triprolidine is a histamine H_1-receptor antagonist that is used for the symptomatic relief of allergic conditions such as urticaria and hay fever. It is well absorbed from the adult gastrointestinal tract and 90% is bound to plasma proteins. Triprolidine appears to be extensively metabolised. The plasma half-life is 3 h.

EVALUATION OF DATA

Passage of triprolidine into human milk has been reported as follows:

Treatment conditions Dose × Frequency × Duration; Route; No. of patients; Lactation stage	Concentration (μg/l) Milk	 Plasma	Milk/ plasma ratio	Maximum observed milk conc. (μg/l)	Absolute dose to infant (μg/kg/day) Ave	 Max	Ref.
2.5 mg × 1/d × 1 d; p.o.; 3; 14, 14, 72 weeks	2.4	6.0	0.50, 0.56	–	0.36	–	(1)

The mothers took a tablet of an antihistamine-decongestant product which also contained pseudoephedrine 60 mg. The concentration-time profiles were defined and were not concurrent; the peak milk concentration occurred 2 h after dosing. The table gives average concentrations calculated from the areas under the concentration-time curves for milk from 3 mothers and for plasma from 2 mothers; the milk to plasma ratios refer to these 2 mothers.

RELATIVE DOSE IN MILK

As triprolidine hydrochloride (mol. wt. 332) was administered but triprolidine (mol. wt. 278) was assayed a factor of 1.19 (332/278) is included in the calculation. A suckling infant would ingest in a feed on average 0.2% (2.4 × 180 × 1.19/2500)* of the weight-adjusted maternal single dose (1).

DATA ON THE INFANT

No data are reported.

ASSESSMENT AND RECOMMENDATIONS

The risk to the suckling infant of administering a single dose of triprolidine to its

* An explanation of the calculation (s) appears on pp. 71–72.

mother is low on the basis that the quantity of drug that passes into milk is small. Breast-feeding after occasional such doses may be regarded as safe.

REFERENCES

1. Findley JWA, Butz RF, Sailstad JM, Warren JT, Welch R (1984) Pseudoephedrine and triprolidine in plasma and breast milk of nursing mothers. *Br. J. Clin. Pharmacol., 18*, 901–906.

Drugs and Human Lactation
P.N. Bennett, editor

7. Vitamins, minerals and essential trace elements

C.J. Bates and A. Prentice

INTRODUCTION

The response of breast milk to maternal supplementation with vitamins and essential trace elements is a fundamentally different problem from that of the passage of drugs into milk after being given to the mother. By definition, milk must contain all the essential trace nutrients, because they are essential for the survival and development of the infant. Control mechanisms have arisen, in the course of evolution, which ensure that, in nearly all instances, the milk contains sufficient of these nutrients to meet the infants' minimum requirements. Nutrients are often transported into the milk at the expense of depleting maternal tissues, if maternal intakes are low and maternal nutrient status is consequently poor. Conversely, there have also arisen mechanisms, for at least some of the nutrients, which ensure that excessive amounts do not appear in the milk, when the maternal intake is very high. It is therefore important to define whether the purpose of maternal supplementation is to correct deficiency in her own tissues, or to improve the status of her suckling infant.

The effect of supplementation often depends on the status of the mother beforehand. If it is poor, and the milk nutrient level is lower than normal, a small increment in maternal intake will often correct it. If maternal status is already good, additional amounts of a nutrient given to the mother may have little effect on milk concentrations. For some nutrients, such as selenium, iodine, fluorine, vitamins D and K, very large doses to the mother can produce a substantial increase in breast-milk concentration.

In considering the effect of maternal supplementation on breast-milk nutrient concentrations, we may ask:

a. Are there any effects of supplementation?
b. If so, are they related to maternal status?
c. Are they dose-related, and if so, how? Are there differences between oral and other routes of administration to the mother?

d. Is a maternal dose transferred rapidly and transiently, or slowly via long-term stores? Is there any adaptation to high or low intakes within a population, over long periods of time?

e. Is there an important effect of stage of lactation? (For instance, vitamins A and E are present in very high levels in colostrum, and decline very rapidly over the first few days, a pattern which does not occur for most water-soluble vitamins). Progressive changes in secretory patterns during the course of lactation may confound the interpretation of supplementation studies if stage of lactation is not taken into account. The same may be true for variations during the course of a feed. Some nutrients show differing magnitudes of response to supplementation at different stages of lactation.

f. Are there any circumstances in which toxic amounts might be transferred to the milk?

Some of the differences between mean values in different studies are likely to be attributable to differences in assay techniques, and in particular the earlier assays may have been inaccurate because of inappropriate techniques.

VITAMINS

Table 1 provides some background information, namely: (a) some means of individual daily intakes of vitamins in Britain, from National Food Survey data (5–7), (b) estimates of minimum requirements by adults, (c) recommended or reference daily intakes of vitamins for adults and for infants, as set by three expert committees (3, 10, 11), and (d) a tentative estimate of the upper limit of safe intakes for some nutrients. Recommended vitamin intakes for young infants traditionally reflect those of breast milk of well-nourished mothers. Table 2 shows mean vitamin concentrations in breast milk of healthy women from a survey in the UK, conducted by the Department of Health and Social Security. Table 3 provides a 'quick reference' to the main conclusions from the sections on individual vitamins, to indicate where deficiency or toxicity effects might occur, and whether a response to maternal supplementation has been observed. One important conclusion is that although megadose vitamin toxicity has been reported for several vitamins, the transfer of toxic amounts to the breast milk has been recorded only for vitamin D.

The section on individual vitamins summarises the most relevant of the available studies, since ca. 1945, from a variety of communities, and the effects on them of maternal supplementation. There are, of course, difficulties with interpretation of some of the older studies, arising from uncertainties over the accuracy of the assay techniques. The early attempts to assay vitamins D, K and folate were clearly unreliable, and most have been omitted. For the other vitamins, a selection of the most important older studies have been included, especially if numbers of subjects were large, or if intercountry comparisons were interesting. A large study in Detroit during the 1940s was summarised by Macy (1), and another in the UK by Kon and

TABLE 1 *Mean daily contents of vitamins in British household diets, approximate minimum adult requirements upper limits and reference or recommended dietary amounts for adults and infants*

Vitamin	British household diets (Refs. 5–7)	Approximate minimum requirements (adults)	Advised upper limits for regular intakes (Refs. 8; 11)		Reference nutrient intakes or RDAs for adults[a]			Reference nutrient intakes or RDAs for 0–6 month old infants[a]		
			Adult	Infant	UK (Ref. 11)	USA (Ref. 10)	WHO (Ref. 3)	UK (Ref. 11)	USA (Ref. 10)	WHO (Ref. 3)
A[b] (mg)	1.59	0.25	9.0	0.9[f]	0.65	0.9	0.75	0.35	0.375	0.35
B1 (thiamine) (mg)	1.16	0.23	3000	–	0.9	1.1	1.1	0.2	0.3	0.3
B2 (riboflavin) (mg)	1.74	0.8	–	–	1.2	1.5	1.5	0.4	0.4	0.5
B6 (pyridoxine)(mg)	1.35	1.0	50?	–	1.3	2.1	1.8	0.2	0.3	–
Niacin +Try/60)(mg)[c]	14.9	4.4	3000?	–	15	15	17	3	6	5.4
Pantothenate (mg)	5.1	?	–	–	3–7[d]	4–7	–	1.7	2[d]	–
Biotin (μg)	33	?	–	–	10–200[d]	30–100	–	–	10	–
Folate (μg)	19.1	100	–	–	200	190	200	50	25	20[e]
B12 (μg)	6.6	1.0	–	–	1.5	2	2	0.3	0.3	0.1
C (mg)	57	10	–	–	40	60	30	25	30	20
D (μg)	3	?	?	50[f]	–	5	2.5	8.5	–	10
E (mg)	8.3	?	–	–	3.5[d]	9	–	[g]	3[d]	–
K (μg)	–	?	–	–	1 μg/kg	70	–	10 μg	5[d]	–

[a]Mean between males and females, if different for each.
[b]In retinol equivalents = μg retinol + (μg beta-carotene/6) + (μg other carotenoids/12).
[c]Try/60 = (mg dietary tryptophan/60) since tryptophan makes a significant contribution to niacin by conversion in vivo.
[d]'Safe and adequate' intakes or 'safe intakes' (UK), where the requirements are difficult to define.
[e]'Free' folate in the WHO recommendation, the fraction available to Lactobacillus casei before conjugase treatment.
[f]The toxicity of A and D is much more serious than the comparatively milk and transient effects produced by megadoses of other vitamins.
[g]0.4 mg/g polyunsaturated fatty acids.

TABLE 2 *UK breast-milk vitamin concentrations observed in a Department of Health and Social Security (DHSS) study*[a] *(Ref. 4)*

Vitamin	Mean breast-milk concentration
Water-soluble	
B1 (mg/l)	0.16
B2 (mg/l)	0.31
B6 (mg/l)	0.06
Niacin (mg/l)	2.30
Pantothenate (mg/l)	2.60
Biotin (μg/l)	7.6
Folate (μg/l)	52
C (mg/l)	0.1
	38
Fat-soluble	
A (mg/l)	0.60
Carotene	None found
D[b]	No valid data
E (mg/l)	3.5
K	Not measured

[a]Pooled sample of mature breast-milk from 96 mothers living in 5 towns in the UK during 1975.
[b]Values for vitamin D sulphate were reported, but the technique was subsequently found to be invalid.

TABLE 3 *Quick reference guide to vitamin deficiency and toxicity effects in breast milk*

Vitamin	Supplementation effect[a]	Stage of lactation effect	Deficiency in breast-fed infants	Toxicity in adults	Toxicity in breast-fed infants
A	+ (D)	H[d]	–	+	–
B1	(+) (D)	L[d]	+[c]	–	–
B2	+	*ι*	–	–	–
B6	+	L	–	+	–
Niacin	(+) (D)	L	–	(+)	–
Pantothenate	(+) (D)	(L)	–	–	–
Biotin	(+) (D)	L	–	–	–
Folate	(+) (D)	L	–	(+)	–
B12	+	H	+	–	–
C	+ (D)	(L)	–	(+)	–
D	+	Complex[b]	+	+	+
E	+	H	–	+	–
K	+	None	+	(+)	–

[a]Mature breast-milk response to maternal supplementation. (D) = effect of supplementation primarily in deficient subjects; otherwise minimal. The supplementation response may decrease (d) or increase (*ι*) as maturation occurs.
[b]Vitamin D decreases, but 25-hydroxycholecalciferol increases, as lactation progresses.
[c]Deficiency of thiamin has been reported in infants who are breast-fed, however those reports are old and poorly documented.

Mawson (2). Only studies of mature breast milk have been included in the tables, but comments have been added in the text to indicate whether levels in colostrum or early milk have been reported to be different. Likewise, the composition of milk from mothers of preterm babies (9) is not reviewed in detail here. The number of milk samples analysed in each study may be equal to, or greater than, the number of individual subjects studied, and in most cases the values given are the arithmetic mean of the individual sample values, except where a range seemed more appropriate. For complex studies with many variables, only part of the available data are portrayed.

REFERENCES AND SOME RECENT REVIEWS

1. Macy IG (1949) Composition of human colostrum and milk. *Am. J. Dis. Child., 78*, 589–603.
2. Kon SK, Mawson EH (1950) Human milk. Wartime studies of certain vitamins and other constituents. *Medical Research Council Special Report Series No. 269*, HMSO, London.
3. Passmore R, Nied BM, Rao MN, Beaton GH, DeMayer E (1974) *Handbook on Human Nutritional Requirements. FAO Nutritional Series No. 28*, FAO, Rome, or WHO Monograph Series No. 61, WHO, Geneva.
4. Department of Health and Social Security (1977) The composition of mature human milk. *Rep. Health Soc. Subj.*, 12. HMSO, London.
5. Spring JA, Robertson J, Buss DH (1979) Trace nutrients. III. Magnesium, copper, zinc, vitamin B_6, vitamin B_{12} and folic acid in the British household food supply. *Br. J. Nutr., 41*, 487–493.
6. Bull NL, Buss DH (1982) Biotin, pantothenic acid and vitamin E in the British household food supply. *Hum. Nutr. Appl. Nutr., 36A*, 190–196.
7. Ministry of Agriculture, Food and Fisheries (1982) *Household Food Composition and Expenditure, 1982 Annual Report of the National Food Survey Committee*, HMSO, London.
8. Miller DR, Hayes KC (1982) Vitamin excess and toxicity. *Nutr. Toxicol., 1*, 81–133.
9. Kirksey A, Rahmanifar A (1988) Vitamin and mineral composition of preterm human milk: Implications for the nutritional management of the preterm infant. In: Berger H (Ed) *Vitamins and minerals in pregnancy and lactation*, Nestlé Nutrition Workshop Series No. 16, pp 301–329. Raven Press, New York.
10. National Research Council (1989) Recommended Dietary Allowances, 10th revision. Subcommittee on the Tenth Edition of the RDA's. *Food and Nutrition Board, Committee on Life Sciences, National Research Council.* National Academy Press, Washington, DC.
11. Department of Health (1991) Dietary reference values for food energy and nutrients for the United Kingdom. *Rep. Health Soc. Subj., 41*. HMSO, London.

VITAMIN A

Country	No. of subjects[h] (or samples)	Weeks post-partum	Maternal intake (mg/day, RE)[a]	Breast milk vitamin A concentration (mg/l)	Breast milk carotenoid[e] concentration (mg/l)	Ref.
Batavia (Indonesia) (1936)	698	0–52	NS	0.12[g]	0.15	1
USA (1945)	189	0–52	NS	0.60		2
USA (1945)	37; 23		NS; 30 (S)[b]	0.66; 2.10		3
UK (1950)	1032–1390 (sa)[h]	17 (corr)	NS[c]	0.44	0.24	4
UK (1951)	3	4	NS	0.73	0.13	6
Germany (1958)	54	0–10	NS	0.45	0.9	7
India (1959	84	8–78	NS	0.21		8
India (1961)	50; 7		NS; 15 (S)	0.16; 0.88[d]		10
India (1962)	10	2.5	1.28 (NS)	0.48		11
Hungary (1963)	50; 3	3–10	NS; 16	0.30; 0.60[d]		12
Lebanon (1965)	10	4		0.36	0.16	13
Pakistan (1974)	9	6–26		0.48		15
Guatemala (1974)	17	16	NS	0.18	(0.37)	16 (see also 14)
Ethiopia (poor) (1976)	42		0.80 (NS)	0.30	0.26	17
Sweden (1976)	37		NS	0.47	0.18	17
India (1976)[f]				0.14		18
Ethiopia (1979)	52		NS	0.19		20
Indonesia (1979)	79	0–52	NS	0.13		21
Kenya (1981)	40–60	0–100	NS	0.34	0.3	23
Navajo Indian (1981)	23	3–9	0.75 (NS)	0.33	0.2	24
USA (1981)	10	5	1.38 (NS)	0.77	0.085	25
Canada (1985)	12	5	NS	0.62	0.23	27
Israel (1985)	7	4–5	NS	0.70		28
Egypt (1987)	35		NS	0.30	0.65	30
Gambia (1987)	18; 37	3–15	0.4 (NS); 1.0 (S)	0.71; 0.87		31
Netherlands (1987), pooled	4–34		NS	0.39		32
Indonesia (1988)			NS	0.17		33
USA (1990)	15	2–30	NS	0.49	0.078	34
Indonesia (1993)	76	4	NS	0.58[i]		36

[a]RE, retinol equivalents, calculated as wt of retinol (usually in retinyl esters), plus one-sixth of the wt of β-carotene plus one-twelfth of other biologically active carotenoids in food.

[B]NS, not supplemented, i.e. vitamin supplied from food alone; S = supplemented, i.e. vitamin supplied from food plus additional vitamin supplement)

[c]A daily supplement of 7.2 mg from birth to the 9th day in 9 women resulted in a slower decline in vitamin A levels than was seen in unsupplemented women, levels being about twice as high in the supplemented group on the 9th day.

[d]Transient peaks ca. 14 h after single oral doses.

[e]Most publications have not distinguished between the different varieties of carotenoids. For those which have (refs. 3, 18) the figure given is the sum of alpha- and beta-carotene concentrations. Absence of a figure in this column means that the analysis was not performed.

[f]These mothers had children who were marasmic and ill.

[g]Mean for native and Chinese subjects. European residents had higher values: mean 0.38.

[h](sa) after the number = no. of samples: otherwise number of subjects.

[i]Increased to 0.93 mg/l by a single 100 mg vitamin A supplement, at 2 weeks post-partum. 3 month post-partum values also recorded.

Vitamin A is required for vision, reproduction, and the maintenance of epithelial structures, via the equilibrium between normal and squamous (keratinized) epithelium. Apart from its role in the visual pigment cycle, the mode of action of vitamin A at the molecular level is poorly understood. In developed countries, dietary sources of vitamin A include a considerable proportion of preformed vitamin A from animal products, but in the diets of most developing countries, the major contributors to vitamin A are the carotenoid pigments, whose potency, on a weight basis, varies between about one-twelfth and half that of preformed vitamin A. Until recently the principal biological role of carotenoids in humans was assumed to be that of vitamin A precursors and supply. Now, carotenoids are thought to play additional, independent roles especially as antioxidants. The significance of breast milk carotenoids has, however, been little studied and it deserves attention. Like earlier workers (4, 27), Patton et al. (35) observed a steep fall in human milk carotenoids following parturition, and a ten-fold decrease in both carotenoids and retinoids during lactation. Carotenoids also changed with parity.

Vitamin A deficiency, leading most characteristically to eye lesions and blindness, but also probably to other types of morbidity, is most commonly encountered in preschool children, particularly in those parts of Asia and Africa where carotene-rich fruits and leafy vegetables do not form a normal part of the diet.

The extent to which infantile vitamin-A deficiency can arise, or be exacerbated, by inadequate breast-milk vitamin-A concentrations during suckling, is uncertain (29). Anecdotally, it is claimed that fully breast-fed infants never suffer from overt clinical deficiency, even in those communities where children after weaning commonly develop deficiency signs. There is, however, good evidence that the vitamin-A content of breast milk is influenced by maternal diet. Several studies of well-nourished western communities (2, 3, 4, 17) have indicated mean vitamin-A levels of mature milk to be in the range, 0.45–0.6 mg/1, whereas the level in poorly nourished communities was 0.15–0.4 mg/1 (1, 6, 12, 14, 17, 20). The concentration changes dramatically with stage of lactation, being many fold higher in colostrum and early milk than in mature milk. A bile salt-stimulated-lipase present in human milk may assist the liberation of retinol from its esters, a necessary prelude to its absorption by the infant (19). The contribution of milk precursor carotenoids (and β-carotene) to the vitamin-A potency of breast milk is normally much smaller than that of preformed vitamin A, but may be significant for populations who obtain most of their vitamin A from carotenoids (17, 24). The vitamin-A content in the liver is influenced by exposure to persistent pollutants such as dioxins (22). Whether these also affect breast-milk vitamin-A levels, is not known. Preformed vitamin A in milk is a mixture of retinol and retinyl-fatty acid esters (17).

Studies of the efficacy of maternal supplementation in increasing the concentration of vitamin A in breast milk are complicated by the fact that a large proportion of any single dose to the mother is stored in the liver. The major contributor to milk vitamin-A is the retinol attached to circulating retinol-binding protein, which reflects long-term body stores rather than recent intake. Relatively large single (or short-term) doses do have a measurable influence on breast-milk concentrations (3, 4, 5, 8, 10, 12, 36). Most recently, a group of Indonesian women who received 312 μmol (100 mg) vitamin A, in a placebo-controlled study at 2 weeks postpartum (36) exhibited a 65% enhancement of breast milk vitamin A concentration at 1 month, receding to 35% enhancement at 3 months, postpartum. These authors concluded that "milk vitamin A is an efficient indicator for monitoring the effects of vitamin A interventions in women", being better than serum vitamin A, for this purpose (36). It would perhaps be more informative to examine the effect of a long-term but moderate change in intake. In one study 9 Indian women were given 0.7–3.0 mg vitamin A daily (9); no effect on their milk vitamin-A concentrations was observed, but a small effect would probably have been lost in the background 'noise'. In another study (31), of 55 Gambian women, some of whom were given 0.65 mg vitamin A daily for periods of a few months up to 1.5 years, a significant 23% increase in breast-milk vitamin-A levels was observed.

Vitamin A (but not most naturally occurring carotenes) has important toxic effects in adults when regularly ingested in amounts around two orders of magnitude above the recommended dietary amount of 0.75–1.2 mg/day (26). No instances have yet been reported of breast-fed infants suffering any toxicity effects when the mother has been ingesting large doses of the vitamin, and indeed the characteristics of the transport processes between the maternal intestinal wall and mammary gland make it unlikely that such a situation could arise. In the event of a nursing mother being prescribed retinoids as therapy for example for skin diseases, monitoring of these vitamin A analogues in breast milk would be advisable. An even more serious danger would be towards a developing foetus in utero, since important teratogenic effects of high doses of vitamin A (or retinoids) to the mother are well documented (26).

REFERENCES

1. Meulemans O, de Haas JH (1936) The carotene and vitamin A contents of mothers milk at Batavia. *Ind. J. Pediatr.*, *3*, 133–145.
2. Lesher M, Brody JK, Williams HH, Macy IG (1945) Human milk studies. XXVI Vitamin A and carotenoid contents of colostrum and mature human milk. *Am. J. Dis. Child*, *70*, 182–192.
3. Hrubetz MC, Deuel HJ, Hanley BJ (1945) Studies on carotenoid metabolism. V. The effect of a high vitamin A intake on the composition of human milk. *J. Nutr*, *29*, 245–254.
4. Kon SK, Mawson EH (1950) Human milk; wartime studies of certain vitamins and other constituents. *Med. Res. Counc. Spec. Rep. Ser.*, *269*, 32–69, HMSO, London.
5. Sobel AE, Rosenberg A, Kramer B (1950) Enrichment of milk vitamin A in normal lactating women. *Am. J. Dis. Child.*, *80*, 932–943.
6. Chanda R, Owen EC, Cramond B (1951) The composition of human milk with special reference to the relation between phosphorus partition and phosphatase and to the partition of certain vitamins. *Br. J. Nutr.*, *5*, 228–242.

7. Lubke VF, Finkbeiner H (1958) Beitrag zum verhalten des Vitamin A und β-carotin-spiegles in der Graviditat, unter der Geburt und im Wochenbett. *Z. Vitaminforsch.*, *29*, 45–68.
8. Belavady B, Gopalan C (1959) Chemical composition of human milk in poor Indian women. *Ind. J. Med. Res.*, *45*, 234–245.
9. Belavady B, Gopalan C (1960) Effect of dietary supplementation on the composition of breast milk. *Ind. J. Med. Res.*, *48*, 518–523.
10. Venkatachalam PS, Belavady B, Gopalan C (1962) Studies on vitamin A nutritional status of mothers and infants in poor communities of India. *J. Pediatr.*, *61*, 262–268.
11. Ashdhir S, Puri B (1962) Chemical composition of human milk at three different stages. *Ind. J. Pediatr.*, *29*, 99–109.
12. Tarjan R, Kramer M, Szoke K, Lindner K (1963, 1965) The effect of different factors on the composition of human milk and its variations. 1. The effect of vitamin rich foods on the composition of human milk. II. The composition of human milk during lactation. *Nutr. Dieta*, *5*, 12–29; 7, 136–154.
13. Ajans ZA, Sarrif A, Husbands M (1965) Influence of vitamin A on human colostrum and early milk. *Am. J. Clin. Nutr.*, *17*, 139–142.
14. Contreras C, Arroyave G, Guzman MA (1969) Estudio comparitivo del contenido de proteinas, riboflavina, carotenos y vitamin A de la leche materna entre dos grupos de mujeres de bajo y alto nivel socio-economico. *Arch. Venez. Nutr.*, *12*, 69–91.
15. Lindblad BS, Rahimtoola RJ (1974) A pilot study of the quality of human milk in a lower socio-economic group in Karachi, Pakistan. *Acta Paediatr. Scand.*, *63*, 125–128.
16. Arroyave G, Beghin I, Flores M, DeGuido CS, Ticas JM (1974) Efectos del consumo de azucar fortificada con retinol, por la madre embarazada y lactante cuya dieta habituel es baja en vitamina A. Estudio de la madre y del nino. *Arch. Latinoam. Nutr.*, *24*, 485–512.
17. Gebre-Medhin M, Vahlquist A, Hofvander Y, Upsall L, Vahlquist B (1976) Breast milk composition in Ethiopian and Swedish mothers. 1. Vitamin A and β-carotene. *Am. J. Clin. Nutr.*, *29*, 441–451.
18. Pereira SM, Begum A (1976) Vitamin A deficiency in Indian children. *World Rev. Nutr. Diet.*, *24*, 192–216.
19. Fredrikzon B, Hernell O, Blackberg L, Olivecrona T (1978) Bile salt-stimulated lipase in human milk. Evidence of activity in vivo and of a role in the digestion of milk retinol esters. *Pediatr. Res.*, *12*, 1048–1052.
20. Thein M (1979) Study on milk vitamin A, serum vitamin A and serum protein levels of lactating mothers of Bochessa village, rural Ethiopia. *E. Afr. Med. J.* *56*, 542–547.
21. Boediman D, Ismail D, Iman S, Ismangoen, Ismadi SD (1979) Composition of breast milk after one year. *J. Trop. Pediatr. Environ. Child Health*, *25*, 107–110.
22. Thunberg T, Ahlborg VG, Hakansson H, Krantz C, Monier M (1980) Effect of 2,3,7,8-tetrachlorodibenzo-*p*-dioxin on the hepatic storage of retinol in rats with different dietary supplies of vitamin A (retinol). *Arch. Toxicol.*, *45*, 273–285.
23. van Steenbergen WM, Kusin JA, van Rens WM (1981) Lactational performance of Akamba mothers, Kenya. Breast feeding behaviour, breast milk yield and composition. *J. Trop. Pediatr.*, *27*, 155–161.
24. Butte NF, Calloway DH (1981) Evaluation of lactational performance of Navajo women. *Am. J. Clin. Nutr.*, *34*, 2210–2215.
25. Thomas MR, Pearsons MH, Demkowicz IM, Chan IM, Lewis CG (1981) Vitamin A and vitamin E concentration of the milk from mothers of preterm infants and milk of mothers of full-term infants. *Acta Vitaminol. Enzymol.*, *3*, 135–144.
26. Biesalski (1989) Comparative assessment of the toxicology of vitamin A and retinoids in man. *Toxicology*, *57*, 117–161.

27. Chappell JE, Francis T, Clandinin MT (1985) Vitamin A and E content of human milk at early stages of lactation. *Early Hum. Dev., 11*, 157–167.
28. Vaisman N, Mogilner BM, Sklan D (1985) Vitamin A and E content of preterm and term milk. *Nutr. Res., 5*, 931–935.
29. Wallingford JC, Underwood BA (1986) Vitamin A deficiency in pregnancy, lactation and the nursing child. In: Bauernfeind JC (Ed). *Vitamin A Deficiency and its Control*, pp 101–152. Academic Press, New York.
30. Hussein L, Drar A, Allam H, el Naggar B (1987) Lipid and retinol contents in the milk of Egyptian mothers with normal and sick infants. *Int. J. Vitam. Nutr. Res., 57*, 3–10.
31. Villard L, Bates CJ (1987) Effect of vitamin A supplementation on plasma and breast milk vitamin A levels in poorly nourished Gambian women. *Hum. Nutr. Clin. Nutr., 41C*, 47–58.
32. van Zoeren-Grobben D, Schrijver J, van den Berg H, Berger HM (1987) Human milk vitamin content after pasteurization, storage or tube feeding. *Arch. Dis. Child., 62*, 161–165.
33. Muhilal, Mirdiana A, Azis I, Saidin S, Jahari AB, Karyadi D (1988) Vitamin A-fortified monosodium glutamate and vitamin A status: a controlled field trial. *Am. J. Clin. Nutr., 48*, 1265–1270.
34. Kim Y, English C, Reich P, Gerber LE, Simpson KL (1990) Vitamin A and carotenoids in human milk. *J. Agric. Food Chem., 38*, 1930–1933.
35. Patton S, Canfield LM, Huston G, Ferris AM, Jensen RG (1990) Carotenoids of human colostrum. *Lipids, 25*, 159–165.
36. Stoltzfus RJ, Habicht J-P, Rasmussen KM, Hakimi M (1963) Evaluation of use in vitamin A intervention trials targeted at women. *Int. J. Epidemiol., 22*, 1111–1118.

THIAMINE (vitamin B_1)

Country	No. of subjects	Weeks postpartum	Maternal intake (mg/day)	Breast milk thiamine concentration (mg/l)	Ref.
USA (1945)			1.23 (NS)	0.15	2
UK (1950)	10	5–24	NS; > 9 (S)	0.17; 0.24	3
USA (1951)	1149 (sa); 37	8–40	1.31 (NS); 13 (S)	0.15; 0.22	4
UK (1951)	18; 18	4	NS	0.14	5
India (1959)	3	52–75	NS	0.17	6
India (1960)	31	12–16	0.21 NS); 1.23 (NS)	0.12; 0.16	7
India (1964)	14; 14	4–12	0.25 (NS); 5 (S); 20 (S)	0.11; 0.22; 0.27	9
Germany (1980)	10; 10; 10		NS	0.12	10
USA (1980)	?	6	1.3 (NS); 3.3 (S)	0.22; 0.24	11
USA (1980)	5; 7	26	1.5 (NS); 3.3 (S)	0.21; 0.23	12
Kenya (1981)	6; 6	0–100	NS	0.23	13
UK (1983)	28	10–35	NS	0.18	14
Gambia (1983)	26	0–26	NS; 1.4 (S)	0.16; 0.22	15
India (1987)	21; 2325	2–4	NS	0.08	16

NS, not supplemented; S, supplemented; (sa), no. of samples; otherwise no. of subjects.

Thiamine is the precursor of enzyme cofactors involved primarily in carbohydrate metabolism, of which cocarboxylase at the gateway between the glycolytic and tricarboxylic acid cycles is probably the most important site. Clinical deficiency (classical beriberi) is apparently much less common today than it was 100 years ago, but some concern about sporadic deficiency remains, especially in poor societies.

The thiamine content of breast milk rises sharply in the early stages of lactation (2, 3, 14), but the concentration in mature milk does not appear to be very responsive to moderate amounts of maternal supplementation (see Table) except early in lactation (3) or for malnourished women (7, 8). Although the existence of beriberi in breast-fed infants has been recorded (1, 17), there are no well-documented instances that are backed by breast milk analyses. There is no evidence that high-level supplementation to the mother could result in toxic amounts in the milk.

REFERENCES

1. Aykroyd WR, Krishnan BG (1941) Infantile mortality in the beriberi area of the Madras Presidency. *Ind. J. Med. Res., 29*, 703–708.
2. Roderuck CE, Williams HH, Macy IG (1945) Human milk studies. XXIII. Free and total thiamine contents of colostrum and mature human milk. *Am. J. Dis. Child., 70,* 162–170.
3. Kon SK, Mawson EH (1950) Human milk. Wartime studies of certain vitamins and other constituents. *Med. Res. Counc. Spec. Rep. Ser., 269*, 74–103.
4. Pratt JP, Hamil BM, Moyer EZ, Kaucher M, Roderuck C, Coryell MN, Miller S, Williams HH, Macy IG (1951) Metabolism of women during the reproductive cycle. XVIII The effect of multivitamin supplements on the secretion of B vitamins in human milk. *J. Nutr., 44,* 141–157.

5. Chanda R, Owen EC, Cramond B (1951) The composition of human milk with special reference to the relation between phosphorus partition and phosphatase and to the partition of certain vitamins. *Br. J. Nutr., 5*, 228–242.
6. Belavady B, Gopalan C (1959) Chemical composition of human milk in poor Indian women. *Ind. J. Med. Res., 47*, 234–245.
7. Deodhar AD, Ramakrishnan CV (1960) Studies on human lactation. Relation between the dietary intake of lactating women and the chemical composition of milk with regard to vitamin content. *J. Trop. Pediatr., 6,* 44–47.
8. Belavady B, Gopalan C (1960) Effect of dietary supplementation on the composition of breast milk. *Ind. J. Med. Res., 48,* 518–523.
9. Deodhar AD, Rajalakshmi R, Ramakrishnan CV (1964) Studies on human lactation. III Effect of dietary vitamin supplementation on vitamin contents of breast milk. *Acta Paediatr., 53,* 42–48.
10. Stolley H, Droese W (1980) Thiamine in breast feeding. In: Freier S, Bidelman AI (Eds) *Human Milk. Its Biological and Social Values.* Selected Papers from the International Symposium on Breast Feeding, Tel Aviv. Excerpta Medica, Amsterdam.
11. Nail PA, Thomas MR, Eakin R (1980) The effect of thiamin and riboflavin supplementation on the level of those vitamins in human breast milk and urine. *Am. J. Clin. Nutr., 33,* 198–204.
12. Thomas MR, Sneed SM, Wei C, Nail PA, Wilson M, Sprinkle EE (1980) The effects of vitamin C, vitamin B_6, vitamin B_{12}, folic acid, riboflavin and thiamin on the breast milk and maternal status of well-nourished women at 6 months postpartum. *Am. J. Clin. Nutr., 33,* 2151–2156.
13. van Steenbergen WM, Kusin JA, van Rens WM (1981) Lactational performance of Akamba mothers, Kenya. Breastfeeding behaviour, breast milk yield and composition. *J. Trop. Pediatr., 27,* 155–161.
14. Ford JE, Zechalko A, Murphy J, Brooke OG (1983) Comparison of the B vitamin composition of milk from mothers of preterm and term babies. *Arch. Dis. Child., 58*, 367–372.
15. Prentice AM, Roberts SB, Prentice A, Paul AA, Watkinson M, Watkinson AA, Whitehead RG (1983) Dietary supplementation of lactating Gambian women. I. Effect on breast-milk volume and quality. *Hum. Nutr. Clin. Nutr., 37C*, 53–64.
16. Bijur AM, Kumbhat MM (1987) Vitamin B composition of breast milk from mothers of pre-term and term babies. *Ind. Pediatr., 24,* 33–37.
17. Debuse PJ (1992) Shoshin beri-beri in an infant of a thiamine-deficient mother. *Acta Paediatr., 81,* 723–724.

RIBOFLAVIN (vitamin B_2)

Country	No. of subjects	Weeks post-partum	Maternal intake (mg/day)	Breast milk riboflavin concentration (mg/l)	Ref.
USA (1945)	187	4–24	NS	0.35	1
UK (1950)	752 (sa); 4	8–40	NS; 6 (S)	0.25; 1.5 (peak)	2
USA (1951)	17; 17	52–75	0.32 (NS); 18 (S)	0.41; 1.87	3
India (1959)	30	12–16	NS	0.17	4
India (1960)	15; 15	3–10	0.15 (NS); 0.41 (NS)	0.21; 0.31	5
Hungary (1963)	3; 3	4–12	NS; 4.5–6.7 (S)	0.18; 0.40	6
India (1964)	10; 10; 10		0.18 (NS); 3 (S); 10 (S)	0.20; 0.57; 0.74	7
UK (1979)	6; 9		1.3 (NS); 2.4 (NS)	0.31; 0.39	8
USA (1980)	6; 6	26	1.9 (NS); 5.3 (S)	0.24; 0.27	9
USA (1980)	5; 7	6	2.6 (NS); 5.0 (S)	0.48; 0.71	10
Kenya (1981)	28	0–100	NS	0.14	11
Gambia (1982)	30; 30	4–80	0.5 (NS0; 2.5 (S)	0.16; 0.22	12
UK (1983)	24	10–35	NS	0.30	14
Japan (1986)	22		NS	0.36	15
India (1986)	71		NS	0.23	16
India (1987)	25	2–4	NS	0.26	17
Netherlands (1987), pooled		4–34	NS	0.58	18
USA (1990)	5		11–29 (NS)	0.18–0.8	19
India (1991)	55	4–26	NS	0.22	20

NS, nt supplemented; S = supplemented; (sa), no. of samples; otherwise no. of subjects.

Riboflavin is the precursor of two cofactors (riboflavin phosphate, commonly known as flavin mononucleotide, and flavin adenine dinucleotide) in a wide variety of enzymes catalysing electron transfer redox reactions; it is an essential component of the mitochondrial electron transfer chain.

Human milk contains much less riboflavin than the milk of species such as the rat and the cow. Biochemical, but not clinical deficiency has been observed in breast-fed infants of deficient mothers (13). Maternal supplementation has an important and long-lasting effect on breast-milk riboflavin if the initial status of the mother is poor (5, 7–10, 12), but the effect diminishes and becomes more transient after dosing, as maternal status improves. Peak secretion into the milk occurs about 4 h after a riboflavin-rich meal or dietary supplement (2, 15). While milk-riboflavin levels seem not to change very markedly with stage of lactation (1, 2, 16), there is some evidence that maternal supplementation has the largest influence on milk levels at the later stages of lactation (2).

Here is little evidence of toxicity, even of very large doses of riboflavin in man, and no indication that riboflavin in breast milk of supplemented mothers could be toxic.

REFERENCES

1. Roderuck CE, Coryell MN, Williams HH, Macy IG (1945) Human milk studies. XXIV. Free and total riboflavin contents of colostrum and mature human milk. *Am. J. Dis. Child., 70,* 171–175.
2. Kon SK, Mawson EH (1950) Human milk. Wartime studies of certain vitamins and other constituents. *Med. Res. Counc. Spec. Rep. Ser., 269,* 104–120.
3. Pratt JP, Hamil BM, Moyer EZ, Kaucher M, Roderuck C, Coryell MN, Miller S, Williams HH, Macy IG (1951) Metabolism of women during the reproductive cycle. XVIII The effect of multivitamin supplements on the secretion of B vitamins in human milk. *J. Nutr., 44,* 141–157.
4. Belavady B, Gopalan C (1959) Chemical composition of human milk in poor Indian women. *Ind. J. Med. Res., 47,* 234–245.
5. Deodhar AD, Ramakrishnan CV (1960) Studies on human lactation. Relation between the dietary intake of lactating women and the chemical composition of milk with regard to vitamin content. *J. Trop. Pediatr., 6,* 44–47.
6. Tarjan R, Kramer M, Szoke K, Lindner K (1963) The effect of different factors on the composition of human milk and its variations. 1. The effect of vitamin-rich-foods on the composition of human milk. *Nutr. Diet., 5,* 12–29.
7. Deodhar AD, Rajalakshmi R, Ramakrishnan CV (1964) Studies on human lactation. III. Effect of dietary vitamin supplementation on vitamin contents of breast milk. *Acta Paediatr., 53,* 42–48.
8. Hughes J, Sanders TAB (1979) Riboflavin levels in the diet and breast milk of vegans and omnivores. *Proc. Nutr. Soc., 38,* 95A.
9. Thomas MR, Sneed SM, Wei C, Nail PA, Wilson M, Sprinkle EE (1980) The effects of vitamin C, vitamin B_6, vitamin B_{12}, folic acid, riboflavin and thiamin on the breast milk and maternal status of well-nourished women at 6 months postpartum. *Am. J. Clin. Nutr., 33,* 2151–2156.
10. Nail PA, Thomas MR, Eakin R (1980) The effect of thiamin and riboflavin supplementation on the level of those vitamins in human breast milk and urine. *Am. J. Clin. Nutr., 33,* 198–204.
11. van Steenbergen WM, Kusin JA, van Rens WM (1981) Lactational performance of Akamba mothers, Kenya. Breast feeding behaviour, breast milk yield and composition. *J. Trop. Pediatr., 27,* 155–161.
12. Bates CJ, Prentice AM, Watkinson M, Morrell P, Sutcliffe BA, Foord F, Whitehead RG (1982) Riboflavin requirements of lactating Gambian women: a controlled supplementation trial. *Am. J. Clin. Nutr., 35,* 701–709.
13. Bates CJ, Prentice AM, Paul AA, Prentice A, Sutcliffe BA, Whitehead RG (1982) Riboflavin status in infants born in rural Gambia, and the effect on a weaning food supplement. *Trans. R. Soc. Trop. Med. Hyg., 76,* 253–259.
14. Ford JE, Zechalko A, Murphy J, Brooke OG (1983) Comparison of the B vitamin composition of milk from mothers of preterm and term babies. *Arch. Dis. Child., 58,* 367–372.
15. Funai Y (1986) Studies on riboflavin in milk. 1. On riboflavin content in breast milk. *Tokushima J. Exp. Med., 3,* 194–200.
16. Bamji MS, Prema K, Jacob CM, Ramalakshmi BA, Madhavapeddi R (1986) Relationship between maternal vitamins B_2 and B_6 status and the levels of these vitamins in milk at different stages of lactation. A study in a low-income group of Indian women. *Hum. Nutr.: Clin. Nutr., 40C,* 119–124.
17. Bijur AM, Kumbhat MM (1987) Vitamin B composition of breast milk from mothers of pre-term and term babies. *Ind. Pediatr., 24,* 33–37.
18. van Zoeren-Grobben D, Schrijver J, van den Berg H, Berger HM (1987) Human milk vitamin content after pasteurization, storage or tube feeding. *Arch. Dis. Child., 62,* 161–165.
19. Roughead ZK, McCormick DB (1990) Flavin composition of human milk. *Am. J. Clin. Nutr., 52,* 854–857.
20. Bamji MS, Chowdhury N, Ramalakshmi BA, Jacob CM (1991) Enzymatic evaluation of riboflavin status of infants. *Eur. J. Clin. Nutr., 45,* 309–313.

NIACIN (nicotinic acid)

Country	No. of subjects	Weeks postpartum	Maternal intake (mg/day)	Breast milk niacin concentration (mg/l)	Ref.
USA (1945)	268 (sa)	4–52	NS	1.8	1
USA (1951)	17; 17	8–40	NS (19); S (140)	2.0; 3.9	2
India (1960)	18; 13	12–16	2.1 (NS); 7.3 (NS)	1.0; 1.5	3
India (1964)	10; 10; 10	4–12	2.4 (NS); 20 (S); 60 (S)	1.0; 2.5; 2.7	4
UK (1983)	24	10–35	NS	1.8	5
Gambia (1983)	21; 23	0–26	NS; 19 (S)	1.1; 1.6	6
India (1987)	25	2–4	NS	1.7	7

NS, not supplemented; S, supplemented; (sa), described as number of samples but apparently all from different subjects.
[a]Not including the contribution from tryptophan.

Niacin is a component of the pyridine nucleotide coenzymes (NAD and NADP) involved in electron transport and is thus central to energy metabolism, among other processes. There are several factors which complicate the link between dietary niacin intake and the appearance of 'clinical' deficiency signs (pellagra), of which one is the contribution to niacin by dietary tryptophan, and another is the poor availability of bound forms of niacin in cereals.

Data on the response of breast milk niacin to maternal supplementation are very limited. One early study in the USA (2) and two studies from developing countries: India (4) and The Gambia (6), observed a moderate response of breast milk niacin to maternal supplementation. The amounts of niacin in colostrum are smaller than those in mature milk (5). There is no evidence that a serious deficiency or an overload problem could occur in breast-fed children.

REFERENCES

1. Coryell MN, Harris ME, Miller S, Williams HH, Macy IG (1945) Human milk studies. XXII. Nicotinic acid, pantothenic acid and biotin contents of colostrum and mature human milk. *Am. J. Dis. Child., 70,* 150–161.
2. Pratt JP, Hamil BM, Moyer EZ, Kaucher M, Roderuck C, Coryell MN, Miller S, Williams HH, Macy IG (1951) Metabolism of women during the reproductive cycle. XVIII The effect of multivitamin supplements on the secretion of B vitamins in human milk. *J. Nutr., 44,* 141–157.
3. Deodhar AD, Ramakrishnan CV (1960) Studies on human lactation. Relation between the dietary intake of lactating women and the chemical composition of milk with regard to vitamin content. *J. Trop. Pediatr., 6,* 44–47.
4. Deodhar AD, Rajalakshmi R, Ramakrishnan CV (1964) Studies on human lactation. III. Effect of dietary vitamin supplementation on vitamin contents of breast milk. *Acta Paediatr., 53,* 42–48.
5. Ford JE, Zechalko A, Murphy J, Brooke OG (1983) Comparison of the B vitamin composition of milk from others of preterm and term babies. *Arch. Dis. Child., 58,* 367–372.
6. Prentice AM, Roberts SB, Prentice A, Paul AA, Watkinson M, Watkinson AA, Whitehead RG

(1983) Dietary supplementation of lactating Gambian women. I. Effect on breast-milk volume and quality. *Hum. Nutr: Clin. Nutr., 37C,* 53–64.

7. Bijur AM, Kumbhat MM (1987) Vitamin B composition of breast milk from mothers of pre-term and term babies. *Ind. Pediatr., 24,* 33–37.

PANTOTHENATE

Country	No. of subjects	Weeks post-partum	Maternal intake (mg/day)	Breast milk pantothenate concentration (mg/l)	Maternal blood (mg/l)	Infants blood (mg/l)	Ref.
USA (1945)	269 (sa)	4–52	NS	2.5			1
USA (1951)	17	8–40	NS (8)	2.5			2
India (1960)	15;12	12–16	1.8 (NS); 8.6 (NS)	1.0; 1.8			3
India (1964)	10; 10; 10	4–12	2.2 (NS); 20 (S); 50 (S)	1.0; 2.7; 3.0			4
India (1976)	24		NS	2.3	0.66	0.95	5
USA (1981)	22		7.6 (NS)	6.7			6
USA (1981)	17		NS	2.6			7
UK (1983)	26	10–35	S	2.6			8
Gambia (1983)	21	0–26	NS	2.0			9
India (1987)	25	2–4	NS	1.8			10

NS, not supplemented; S, supplemented; (sa), described as number of samples but apparently all from different subjects.

Pantothenic acid is part of the coenzyme A molecule, and is thus an essential part of the mechanism for utilisation of fatty acids. It is very widely distributed in foods, and all known natural diets appear to provide sufficient, at least to prevent gross deficiency symptoms. For this reason it has received less attention than most of the other vitamins in human nutrition. The data in the Table indicate that mean values for concentrations found in human milk have ranged between 1.0 and 6.7 mg/l in 6 different studies, but part of this variation could be methodological (5). There is an increase between early and mature milk (1, 4, 6), but little work has been done on the effects of supplementation. In view of the generally low toxicity of pantothenic acid, it is extremely unlikely that toxic amounts could be transferred to breast milk.

REFERENCES

1. Coryell MN, Harris ME, Miller S, Williams HH, Macy IG (1945) Human milk studies. XXII. Nicotinic acid, pantothenic acid and biotin contents of colostrum and mature human milk. *Am. J. Dis. Child., 70,* 150–161.
2. Pratt JP, Hamil BM, Moyer EZ, Kaucher M, Roderuck C, Coryell MN, Miller S, Williams HH, Macy IG (1951) Metabolism of women during the reproductive cycle. XVIII The effect of multivitamin supplements on the secretion of B vitamins in human milk. *J. Nutr., 44,* 141–157.
3. Deodhar AD, Ramakrishnan CV (1960) Studies on human lactation. Relation between the dietary intake of lactating women and the chemical composition of milk with regard to vitamin content. *J. Trop. Pediatr., 6,* 44–47.
4. Deodhar AD, Rajalakshmi R, Ramakrishnan CV (1964) Studies on human lactation. III. Effect of dietary vitamin supplementation on vitamin contents of breast milk. *Acta Paediatr., 53,* 42–48.
5. Srinivasan V, Belavady B (1976) Nutritional status of pantothenic acid in Indian pregnant and nursing women. *Int. J. Vitam. Nutr. Res., 46,* 433–438.

6. Johnston L, Vaughan L, Fox HM (1981) Pantothenic acid content of human milk. *Am. J. Clin. Nutr., 34,* 2205–2209.
7. Song WO, Chan GM, Wyse BW, Hansen RG (1981) Effect of pantothenic acid status on the content of the vitamin in human milk. *Am. J. Clin. Nutr., 40,* 317–324.
8. Ford JE, Zechalko A, Murphy J, Brooke OG (1983) Comparison of the B vitamin composition of milk from mothers of preterm and term babies. *Arch. Dis. Child., 58,* 367–372.
9. Prentice AM, Roberts SB, Prentice A, Paul AA, Watkinson M, Watkinson AA, Whitehead RG (1983) Dietary supplementation of lactating Gambian women. I. Effect on breast milk volume and quality. *Hum. Nutr. Clin. Nutr., 37C,* 53–64.
10. Bijur AM, Kumbhat MM (1987) Vitamin B composition of breast milk from mothers of pre-term and term babies. *Ind. Pediat., 24,* 33–37.

BIOTIN

Country	No. of subjects	Weeks postpartum	Maternal intake (μg/day)	Breast milk biotin concentration (μg/l)	Ref.
USA (1945)	266 (sa)	4–52	NS	8.1	1
USA (1951)	17	8–40	76 (NS)	8.4	2
India (1964)	10; 10; 10	4–12	30 (NS); 150 (S); 250 (S)	1.6; 4.2; 5.0	3
UK (1973)	27	10–13	NS	5.3	4
Gambia (1983)	19	0–26	NS	9.0	5
Finland (1985)	140	17	NS	0–27	6
USA (1992)	6	>8	NS	11.0	7
Japan (1992)	35	2–3	NS	5.2	9

NS, n supplemented; S, supplemented. (sa), described as number of samples but apparently all from different subjects.

Biotin is involved as a cofactor in carboxylation reactions of lipid metabolism. Deficiency has only rarely been encountered in human subjects: usually as a result of inborn errors of metabolism or use of 'raw egg white' diets. Very few studies have been carried out on concentrations in, or effect of supplementation on, human milk. A recent study (7, 8) has shown that nearly all the biotin in human milk was in the 'skim' (water-soluble) fraction, and it did not exhibit any consistent pattern of changes, or constancy, during the course of lactation, in contrast to one earlier study's conclusions (1). It is generally considered that neither biotin deficiency nor biotin toxicity pose any serious threat to normal babies. Rare instances of infants with greatly increased requirements, described as 'dependency syndromes' need to be detected and treated before serious damage can occur, however.

REFERENCES

1. Coryell MN, Harris ME, Miller S, Williams HH, Macy IG (1945) Human milk studies. XXII. Nicotinic acid, pantothenic acid and biotin contents of colostrum and mature human milk. *Am. J. Dis. Child., 70,* 150–161.
2. Pratt JP, Hamil BM, Moyer EZ, Kaucher M, Roderuck C, Coryell MN, Miller S, Williams HH, Macy IG (1951) Metabolism of women during the reproductive cycle. XVIII The effect of multivitamin supplements on the secretion of B vitamins in human milk. *J. Nutr., 44,* 141–157.
3. Deodhar AD, Rajalakshmi R, Ramakrishnan CV (1964) Studies on human lactation. III. Effect of dietary vitamin supplementation on vitamin contents of breast milk. *Acta Paediatr., 53,* 42–48.
4. Ford JE, Zechalko A, Murphy J, Brooke OG (1983) Comparison of the B vitamin composition of milk from mothers of preterm and term babies. *Arch. Dis. Child., 58,* 367–372.
5. Prentice AM, Roberts SB, Prentice A, Paul AA, Watkinson M, Watkinson AA, Whitehead RG (1983) Dietary supplementation of lactating Gambian women. I. Effect on breast-milk volume and quality. *Hum. Nutr. Clin. Nutr., 37C,* 53–64.
6. Salmenpera L, Perheentupa J, Pispa JP, Siimes MA (1985) Biotin concentrations in maternal plasma and milk during prolonged lactation. *Int. J. Vit. Nutr. Res., 55,* 281–285.

7. Mock DM, Mock NI, Langbehn SE (1992) Biotin in human milk: methods, location and chemical form. *J. Nutr., 122,* 535–545.
8. Mock DM, Mock NI, Dankle JA (1992) Secretory patterns of biotin in human milk. *J. Nutr., 122,* 546–552.
9. Hirano M, Honma K, Daimatsu T, Hayakawa K, Oizumi J, Zaima K, Kanke Y (1992) Longitudinal variations of biotin content in human milk. *Int. J. Vit. Nutr. Res., 62,* 281–282.

PYRIDOXINE (vitamin B6)

Country	No. of subjects	Weeks postpartum	Maternal intake	Breast milk pyridoxine concentrations (mg/l)	Ref.
India (1964)	10;10;10		0.35 (NS); 10 (S); 40 (S)	0.08; 0.14; 0.16	1
USA (1979)	7; 10	6	0.84 (NS; 5.11 (S)	0.20; 0.24	2
USA (1976)	6; 5		<2.5 (NS); >5.0 (NS)	0.13; 0.13	4
USA (1979)	21	2	NS	0.065	6
USA (1980)	6; 6	26	1.1 (NS); 5.3 (S)	0.21; 0.23	8
USA (1981)	7; 9	6	1.41 (NS); 5.12 (S)	0.12; 0.24	10
Gambia (1983)	21	0–26	NS	0.12	13
UK (1983)	25	0–35	NS	0.11	14
USA (1983)	7		>4 (S)	0.31	15
USA (1985)	24	8–12	2.0/4.4/11.3/21.1 (S)	0.09/0.19/0.25/0.41	17
USA (1985)	7; 14	14	1.5 (NS); 11.2 (S)	0.07; 0.18	18
USA (1985	9	8–26	2.5 (S)	0.2	19
USA (1985)	20	13–39	0.5/4.0 (S)	0.13/0.26	20
USA (1986)	40	30–100	NS	0.1	21
India (1986)	73		NS	0.07	22
USA (1986)	17		2.5/15 (S)	0.18/0.45	23
Netherlands (1987), pooled		4–34	NS	0.015	24
India (1987)	25	2–4	NS	0.095	25
USA (1990)	47	0–26	2.5/4.0/7.5/10.0 (S)	0.22/0.31/0.39/0.41	26
Egypt (1990)	66	8–26	NS	0.07	27
USA (1990)	40	5–36	0.5/4.0 (S)	0.15/0.3	29
USA (1992)	20	1–4	2/27 (S)	0.08/0.4	32
USA (1992)	10		NS	0.13	33

NS, not supplemented (basal intake may or may not be given); S, supplemented.

The main naturally occurring forms of B_6 are pyridoxal phosphate and pyridoxamine phosphate, with smaller amounts of pyridoxal and pyridoxine also present in tissues and body fluids including milk (15, 18, 28). B_6 coenzymes are essential cofactors for a very wide variety of enzymes, many of which catalyse group transfer reactions, e.g. transaminases and decarboxylases.

The minimum human requirement is poorly defined, and is closely linked to protein intake. The current recommended dietary amount for adult women is 1.6 mg/day in the USA (30), rising to 2.1 mg/day during lactation, and for 0–6 month old infants, 0.3 mg/day. The latter may prove to be unrealistically high, however, since recent evidence suggests that even well-nourished and supplemented mothers cannot provide a sufficiently high concentration in breast milk to meet this recommendation (11, 16, 17). In one study (20) the mean B_6 intake of breast-fed infants was found to vary between 0.06 mg/day when mothers were unsupplemented (maternal intake 2 mg/day) and 0.28 mg/day when the mothers received a 20 mg daily supplement of B_6. In the UK (31), the reference intake is

1.2 mg/day for adult women (including those who are pregnant or lactating), and 0.2 mg/day for 0–6-month-old infants.

With some exceptions (2, 8), studies of breast milk concentrations of B_6 during maternal supplementation do indicate a response to variations in maternal intake. The evidence concerning this relationship is summarized in the Table. Concentrations are generally lower in early milk than in mature milk (7, 9, 10, 11, 16, 17, 21), but the opposite may be true if the mothers have been supplemented during gestation but not postpartum (20). Very low concentrations in breast milk during the first 2 weeks of life may be a cause for concern (16), but further studies are required. Following oral supplements, peak breast-milk concentrations occur after about 4 h (17). There is little information on the relation of maternal or infant blood B_6 concentrations to milk concentrations.

No deleterious effects on the breast-fed infant have been documented as a result of very high maternal intakes during lactation, although intakes of the order of 100 times the recommended daily amount (RDA) are antilactogenic, and have been used therapeutically to treat cases of galactorrhoea-amenorrhoea (3, 5). No antilactogenic action was detectable after supplementation with doses moderately above the RDA (9, 17).

Vitamin B_6 is sometimes prescribed as therapy for postnatal depression, but its efficacy in this respect remains controversial, and there are well-documented cases of neurotoxic effects of long-term high dose therapy which should be taken into account before prescribing large doses of this vitamin (12).

REFERENCES

1. Deodhar AD, Rajalakshmi R, Ramakrishnan CV (1964) Studies on human lactation. III. Effect of dietary vitamin supplementation on vitamin contents of breast milk. *Acta Paediatr., 53,* 42–48.
2. Thomas MR, Kawamoto J, Sneed SM, Eakin R (1979) The effects of vitamin C, vitamin B_6 and vitamin B_{12} supplementation on the breast milk and maternal status of well-nourished women. *Am. J. Clin. Nutr., 32,* 1679–1685.
3. Foukas MD (1973) An antilactogenic effect of pyridoxine. *J. Obstet. Gynaecol. Br. Commonw., 80,* 718–720.
4. West KD, Kirksey A (1976) Influence of vitamin B_6 intake on the content of the vitamin in human milk. *Am. J. Clin. Nutr., 29,* 961–969.
5. McIntosh EN (1976) Treatment of women with the galactorrhoea-amenorrhoea syndrome with pyridoxine (vitamin B_6). *J. Clin. Endocrinol. Metab., 42,* 1192–1195.
6. Roepke JLB, Kirksey A (1979) Vitamin B_6 nutriture during pregnancy and lactation. II. The effect of long-term use of oral contraceptives. *Am. J. Clin. Nutr., 32,* 2257–2264.
7. Roepke LB, Kirksey A (1979) Vitamin B_6 nutriture during pregnancy and lactation. Vitamin B_6 intake, levels of the vitamin in biological fluids, and condition of the infant at birth. *Am. J. Clin. Nutr., 32,* 2249–2256.
8. Thomas MR, Sneed SM, Wei C, Nail PA, Wilson M, Sprinkle EE (1980) The effects of vitamin C, vitamin B_6 and vitamin B_{12}, folic acid, riboflavin and thiamin on the breast milk and maternal status of well-nourished women at 6 months postpartum. *Am. J. Clin. Nutr., 33,* 2151–2156.
9. Ejderhamn J, Hamfelt A (1980) Pyridoxal phosphate concentration in blood in newborn infants

and their mothers compared with the amount of extra pyridoxol taken during pregnancy and breast feeding. *Acta Paediatr. Scand., 69,* 327–330.

10. Sneed SM, Zane C, Thomas MR (1981) The effects of ascorbic acid, vitamin B_6, B_{12} and folic acid supplementation on the breast milk and maternal status of low socio-economic lactating women. *Am. J. Clin. Nutr., 34,* 1338–1346.
11. Reynolds RD (1982) Inability of breast milk to provide the RDA of vitamin B_6. *J. Am. Coll. Nutr., 1,* 125–126.
12. Miller DR, Hayes KC (1982) Vitamin excess and toxicity. *Nutr. Toxicol., 1,* 81–133.
13. Prentice AM, Roberts SB, Prentice A, Paul AA, Watkinson M, Watkinson AA, Whitehead RG (1983) Dietary supplementation of lactating Gambian women. 1. Effect on breast-milk volume and quality. *Hum. Nutr. Clin. Nutr., 37C,* 53–64.
14. Ford JE, Zechalko A, Murphy J, Brooke OG (1983) Comparison of the B-vitamin composition of milk from mothers of preterm and term babies. *Arch. Dis. Child., 58,* 367–372.
15. Vanderslice JT, Brownlee SG, Maire CE, Reynolds RD, Polansky M (1983). Forms of vitamin B_6 in human milk. *Am. J. Clin. Nutr., 37,* 867–871.
16. Wilson RG, Davis RE (1984) Vitamin B_6 intake and plasma pyridoxol phosphate concentrations in the first two weeks of life. *Acta Paediatr. Scand., 73,* 218–224.
17. Styslinger L, Kirksey A (1985) Effects of different levels of vitamin B_6 supplementation on vitamin B_6 concentrations in human milk and vitamin B_6 intakes of breast fed infants. *Am. J. Clin. Nutr., 41,* 21–31.
18. Morrison LA, Driskell JA (1985) Quantities of B_6 vitamins in human milk by HPLC. Influence of maternal vitamin B_6 status. *J. Chromatogr., 337,* 249–258.
19. Andon MB, Howard MP, Moser PB, Reynolds RD (1985) Nutritionally relevant supplementation of vitamin B_6 in lactating women: effect on plasma prolactin. *Pediatrics, 76,* 769–773.
20. Reinken L, Dockx F (1985) Vitamin B_6 and protein concentrations in breast milk from mothers of preterm and term infants. *Klin. Paediatr., 197,* 40–43.
21. Karra MV, Udipi SA, Kirksey A, Roepke JLB (1986) Changes in specific nutrients in breast milk during extended lactation. *Am. J. Clin. Nutr., 43,* 495–503.
22. Bamji MS, Prema K, Jacob CM, Ramalakshmi BA, Madhavapeddi R (1986) Relationship between maternal vitamins B_2 and B_6 status and the levels of these vitamins in milk at different stages of lactation. A study in low-income group of Indian women. *Hum. Nutr. Clin. Nutr., 40C,* 119–124.
23. Borschel MW, Kirksey A, Hannemann RE (1986) Effects of vitamin B_6 intake on nutriture and growth of young infants. *Am. J. Clin. Nutr., 43,* 7–15.
24. van Zoeren-Grobben D, Schrijver J, van den Berg H, Berger HM (1987) Human milk vitamin content after pasteurization, storage or tube feeding. *Arch. Dis. Child., 62,* 161–165.
25. Bijur MS, Kumbhat MM (1987) Vitamin B composition of breast milk from mothers of pre-term and term babies. *Ind. Pediatr., 24,* 33–37.
26. Chang SJ, Kirksey A (1990) Pyridoxine supplementation of lactating mothers: relation to maternal nutrition status and vitamin B_6 concentrations in milk. *Am. J. Clin. Nutr., 51,* 826–831.
27. McCullough AL, Kirksey A, Wachs TD, McCabe GP, Bassily NS, Bishry Z, Galal OM, Harrison GG, Jerome NW (1990) Vitamin B_6 status of Egyptian mothers: relation to infant behaviour and maternal-infant interactions. *Am. J. Clin. Nutr., 51,* 1067–1074.
28. Hamaker BR, Kirksey A, Borschel MW (1990) Distribution of B_6 vitamers in human milk during a 24 hour period after oral supplementation with different amounts of pyridoxine. *Am. J. Clin. Nutr., 51,* 1062–1066.
29. Moser-Veillon PB, Reynolds RD (1990) A longitudinal study of pyridoxine and zinc supplementation of lactating women. *Am. J. Clin. Nutr., 52,* 135–141.
30. National Research Council (1989) *Recommended Dietary Allowances.* Subcommittee on the

Tenth Edition of the RDA's Food and Nutrition Board Committee on Life Sciences, The National Academy of Sciences.

31. Department of Health (1991) *Report on Health and Social Subjects No. 41*. Dietary Reference Values for Food Energy and Nutrients for the United Kingdom. HMSO, London.
32. Kang-Yoon SA, Kirksey A, Giacola G, West K (1992) Vitamin B-6 status of breast-fed neonates: influence of pyridoxine supplementation on mothers and neonates. *Am. J. Clin. Nutr., 56,* 548–558.
33. Coburn SP, Mahuren JD, Pauley TA, Ericson KL, Townsend DW (1992) Alkaline phosphatase activity and pyridoxal phosphate concentrations in the milk of various species. *J. Nutr., 122,* 2348–2353.

FOLATE

Country	No. of subjects	Weeks postpartum	Maternal intake	Breast milk folate concentrations (μg/l)	Ref.
India (1964)	10; 10;10	4–12	NS; 300 (S); 10000 (S)	2; 4; 5.6[a]	1
India (1965)	10	>2	NS	16[a]	2
USA (1980)	19	26	194 (NS); 960 (S)	50; 55	3
Japan (1980)	6; 6	3–25	NS; 1000 (S)	130; 137[a]	4
Navajo Indian (1981)	16; 16	3–9	NS	56	5
USA (1981)	10	6	340 (NS); 1010 (S)	43; 49	6
Japan (1981)	7; 9		NS	45	7
USA (1982)	15	>2	NS	33	8
USA (1982)	80		NS (clinically deficient)	10[b]	8
UK (1983)	1	10–35	NS	42	9
Norway (1983)	26	4–40	NS	53	10
Gambia (1983)	30	0–26	NS	38	11
USA (1983)	21	6, 12	NS	79	12
USA (1984	132	5–7	NS	49	13
India (!985)	65		NS	11[c]	14
USA (1986)	18	30–100	NS	40	15
USA (1986)	29	6	NS	85	16
India (1987)	16	2–4	NS	14	17
Netherlands (1987), pooled	25	4–34	NS	32	18
USA (1987)	27	4		53[d]	19
Brazil (1988)	9	1–5	NS	25	20
Brazil (1989)	11	4–40	NS	47[e]	21
Brazil (1990)	113	4–12	NS	38	22
USA (1991)	8		NS	110	24

NS, not supplemented; S, supplemented.
[a]See text for comments on methodology.
[b]A 5000 μg daily supplement increased the milk folate content to around 50 μg/l.
[c]Figure given for 'frequent meat-eaters'; other groups had lower values.
[d]Includes changes between 4 and 40 weeks post partum, of the 27 subjects 21 were taking 400–1000 μg supplemental folate/day.
[e]Includes changes between 1 and 40 weeks post-partum.

The folates arc a family of compounds which are involved as coenzymes in the transfer of C-1 units between molecules; a central role is in the synthesis of DNA and hence cell division, but there are many other functions also involving the various folate coenzymes. Several studies have reported reduced growth rates and haematological abnormalities attributable to folate deficiency in premature infants who have received damaged or unsuitable milk formulae, and naturally occurring folates are known to be labile in the presence of heat and oxygen. Infants who are fully or mainly breast-fed appear to be protected. Although there is little well-documented quantitative information on the relationship between natural folate intake and the concentration of folate compounds in breast milk (partly because the measurement of the folate content of diets is difficult and time-consuming), it is clear from several studies that breast-milk folate concentrations are not very sensitive to moderate variations in intake, and that maternal folate deficiency is unlikely to affect the milk folate concentrations, until fairly severe depletion of maternal tissues has occurred. Most recent studies have found about 50 μg folate per litre in mature milk (see Table); those earlier studies which reported much lower or much higher values probably used inappropriate assay conditions. Milk folate assays, which are usually based on the stimulation of growth of *Lactobacillus casei*, are critically dependent on factors such as preservation by an antioxidant, the correct conditions of conjugase treatment to release monoglutamate forms completely, and the correct choice of pH during the assay. Folate concentrations rise considerably as lactation progresses from colostrum to mature milk (7–10, 13). Recent studies (12, 19, 23, 24) found that human milk contains a mixture of mono and polyglutamate folates, notably 5-methyl tetrahydropteroylglutamate; the polyglutamates needing conjugase treatment before assay (24). There is controversy over the proportion of polyglutamates in human milk folates (24, 25). There has been some interest in trying to elucidate the role of the folate-binding proteins which are present in milk, since they may aid intestinal absorption and limit the removal of milk folate by the intestinal flora. There is no evidence to suggest that large doses of folate given to the mother could raise folate concentrations in the milk to the extent of harming the infant, and many infants who receive supplements of much larger amounts of folate than could ever occur in breast milk appear to thrive quite satisfactorily.

REFERENCES

1. Deodhar AD, Rajalakshmi R, Ramakrishnan CV (1964) Studies on human lactation. III. Effect of dietary vitamin supplementation on vitamin contents of breast milk. *Acta Paediatr., 53,* 42–48.
2. Ramasastri BV (1965) Folate activity in human milk. *Br. J. Nutr., 19,* 581–586.
3. Thomas MR, Sneed SM, Wei C, Nail PA, Wilson M, Sprinkle EE (1980) The effects of vitamin C, vitamin B_6, vitamin B_{12}, folic acid riboflavin and thiamin on the breast milk and maternal status of well-nourished women at 6 months postpartum. *Am. J. Clin. Nutr., 33,* 2151–2156.
4. Tamura T, Yoshimura Y, Arakawa T (1980) Human milk folate and folate status in lactating mothers and their infants. *Am. J. Clin. Nutr., 33,* 193–197.
5. Butte NF, Calloway DH (1981) Evaluation of lactational performance of Navajo women. *Am. J. Clin. Nutr., 34,* 2210–2215.
6. Sneed SM, Zane C, Thomas MR (1981) The effects of ascorbic acid, vitamin B_6, vitamin B_{12} and folic acid supplementation on the breast milk and maternal nutritional status of low socio-economic lactating women. *Am. J. Clin. Nutr., 34,* 1338–1346.
7. Imamura A (1981) Iron, folate and vitamin B_{12} in maternal blood and breast milk. *Acta Obstet. Gynaecol. Jpn., 33,* 1053–1061.
8. Cooperman JM, Dweck HS, Newman LJ, Garbarino C, Lopez R (1982) The folate in human milk. *Am. J. Clin. Nutr., 36,* 576–580.
9. Ford JE, Zechalko A, Murphy J, Brooke OG (1983) Comparison of the B vitamin composition of milk from mothers of preterm and term babies. *Arch. Dis. Child., 58,* 367–372.

10. Ek J (1983) Plasma, red cell and breast milk folacin concentrations inlactating women. *Am. J. Clin. Nutr., 38,* 929–935.
11. Prentice AM, Roberts SB, Prentice A, Paul AA, Watkinson M, Watkinson AA, Whitehead RG (1983) Dietary supplementation of lactating Gambian women. I. Effect on breast-milk volume and quality. *Hum. Nutr. Clin. Nutr., 37C,* 53–64.
12. Smith AM, Picciano MF, Deering RH (1983) Folate supplementation during lactation: maternal folate status, human milk folate content, and their relationship to infant folate states. *J. Pediatr. Gastroenterol., 2,* 622–628.
13. Eitenmiller RR, Bryan WD, Khalsa IK, Feeley RM, Barnhart HM (1984) Folate content of human milk during early lactational stages. *Nutr. Res., 4,* 391–397.
14. Bijur AM, Desai AG (1985) Composition of breast milk with reference to vitamin B_{12} and folic acid in Indian mothers. *Ind. J. Pediatr., 52,* 147–150.
15. Karra MV, Udipi SA, Kirksey A, Roepke JLB (1986) Changes in specific nutrients in breast milk during extended lactation. *Am. J. Clin. Nutr., 43,* 495–503.
16. Brown CM, Smith AM, Picciano MF (1986) Forms of human milk folacin and variation patterns. *J. Pediatr. Gastroenterol Nutr., 5,* 278–282.
17. Bijur AM, Kumbhat MM (1987) Vitamin B composition of breast milk from mothers of pre-term and term babies. *Ind. Pediatr., 24,* 33–37.
18. van Zoeren-Grobben D, Schrijver J, van den Berg H, Berger HM (1987) Human milk vitamin content after pasteurisation, storage, or tube-feeding. *Arch. Dis. Child., 62,* 161–165.
19. Udipi SA, Kirksey A, Roepke JLB (1987) Diurnal variations in folacin levels in human milk: use of a single sample to represent folacin concentration in milk during a 24-h period. *Am. J. Clin. Nutr., 45,* 770–779.
20. Trugo NMF, Donangelo CM, Koury J, Barretosilva MI, Freitas LA (1988) Concentration and distribution pattern of selected micronutrients in pre-term and term milk from urban Brazilian mothers during early lactation. *Eur. J. Clin. Nutr., 42,* 497–507.
21. Donangelo CM, Trugo NMF, Koury JC, Barretosilva MI, Freitas LA, Feldheim W, Barth C (1989) Iron, zinc, folate and vitamin B_{12} nutritional status and milk composition of low-income Brazilian mothers. *Eur. J. Clin. Nutr., 43,* 253–266.
22. Lehti KK (1990) Breast milk folic acid and zinc concentrations of lactation, low socio-economic, Amazonian women and the effect of age and parity on the same two nutrients. *Eur. J. Clin. Nutr., 44,* 675–680.
23. Selhub J (1989) Determination of tissue folate composition by affinity chromatography followed by high-pressure ion pair liquid chromatography. *Anal. Biochem., 182,* 84–93.
24. O'Connor DL, Tamura T, Picciano MF (1991) Pteroylpolyglutamates in human milk. *Am. J. Clin. Nutr., 53,* 761–762; 930–934.
25. Cooperman JM, Lopez R (1991) Pteroylglutamates in human milk. *Am. J. Clin. Nutr., 54,* 760–761.

VITAMIN B12

Country	No. of subjects	Weeks postpartum	Maternal intake (μg/day)	Breast milk vitamin B12 concentration (ng/l)	Maternal serum or plasma (ng/l)	Infants plasma (ng/l)	Ref.
India (1964)	10; 10; 10	4–12	NS; 50 (S); 200 (S)	78; 88; 100			2
UK (1971)	10	1	NS	605	490		3
UK (1971)	1	1	1 mg i.m. (S)	4000	2500		3
USA (1978)	1		NS	75	160	20[a]	4
USA (1979)	6; 7	6	2.1 (NS); 11.9 (S)	610; 1100	540; 560		5
USA (1980)	6; 6	26	2.9 (NS); 11(S)	640; 870	690; 710		6
UK (1980)	16	2–26	NS	260			7
USA (1981)	19	8–150	NS	970			8
USA (1981)	7; 9	6	5.2 (NS); 11.8 (S)	550; 790	660; 640		9
Japan (1981)	15		NS	320			10
USA (1982)	1		NS	51	99	23[b]	11
UK (1983)	23	10–35	NS	230			13
Gambia (1983)	16	0–26	NS	160			14
India (1985)	17		NS	110[d]			15
Netherlands (1987), pooled		4–34	NS	410			16
Brazil (1988)	9	1–5	NS	1030			17
Brazil (1989)	10	4–40	NS	910	450		18
USA (1990)	6		NS	500[e]	475		20
Netherlands (1992)	10	8–14	NS	440[c]			21
Brazil (1994)	9	0–12	NS	330[f]			23
Denmark (1994)	6	1	NS	270	298		24

NS, not supplemented (basal intake may be given); S, supplemented.
[a]Normal range quoted: 150–1000 ng/l.
[b]Normal range quoted: 215–800 ng/l.
[c]Figures given for omnivores; subjects consuming macrobiotic diets had 360 ng/l.
[d]Figures given for 'frequent meat-eaters'; other groups had lower values.
[e]Figures given for omnivores: vegetarians had lower values.
[f]Range 10–1100: lower during 3rd month than during first 2 months postpartum.

Vitamin B_{12} is involved in molecular rearrangements requiring adenosyl cobalamin as cofactor and in C_1 transfer processes requiring methyl cobalamin and folic acid. Deficiency interferes with normal folate utilisation, especially for DNA synthesis, which accounts for the fact that both B_{12} and folate deficiencies result in megaloblastic anaemia. B_{12} deficiency also has irreversible neurological effects, and this makes untreated B_{12} deficiency especially dangerous. In addition, the nature of pernicious anaemia, in which B_{12} absorption is impaired by lack of intrinsic factor, makes it frequently mandatory to treat the condition with injections of B_{12}, and this fact places the medical problems associated with B_{12} in a somewhat different category from those of most other vitamins.

Until recently, dietary B_{12} deficiency in subjects with normal intestinal function was considered rare, but cases of pure dietary deficiency are now being brought to light, and can apparently affect breast-fed infants of mothers consuming vegan or strict vegetarian diets, whose contents of B_{12} are extremely low (1, 4, 19, 22). There are also at least 2 recorded cases of deficiency in infants whose mothers had untreated pernicious anaemia (11, 12).

Since some subjects requiring parenteral B_{12} for pernicious anaemia may breastfeed their infants, the effects of large parenteral doses of B_{12} on maternal breast milk B_{12} concentration need to be considered. It is clear that parenteral doses can increase the B_{12} milk level very considerably over the baseline amount (3). B_{12} given by mouth, on the other hand, seems to have a relatively small effect (5, 6). It is unclear whether infants who receive breast milk in which the B_{12} concentration has been raised grossly above the natural levels by maternal parenteral dosage are in danger of toxicity effects. There are no recorded instances of its causing any overt clinical problems, and B_{12} is generally considered non-toxic even in very large doses, in adults. A recent study (24) has shown that biologically inactive vitamin B_{12} analogues do not appear in human milk, even when they do appear in human plasma. Human milk contains more ado-cobalamin and relatively less methyl-cobalamin, than does plasma (24).

Most recent studies of normal mature breast milk from unsupplemented mothers have found B_{12} concentrations around 200–1000 ng/l. A study of 2 severely deficient infants and their mothers (4, 22) revealed milk concentrations at least an order of magnitude lower. An early study from India (2) reported very low levels, but it is uncertain whether these genuinely reflected poor status in the low-income malnourished subjects studied, or inadequate assay methodology (8).

Specker et al. (20) have recently reported that low levels of milk B_{12} in vegetarian women are associated with methylmalonic aciduria in their infants.

As in the case of folate, B_{12}-binding proteins occur in breast milk. There are at least two types (R-type or cobalophilin), and transcobalamin II (8); these may have an important role in protecting the vitamin from intestinal micro-organisms and in facilitating absorption by the infant. In early studies, B_{12} levels appeared to be considerably more concentrated in colostrum than in mature milk (7, 10, 12). In a recent study from Brazil, however, the concentration remained almost constant from colostrum, through transitional milk to the second month, but then fell significantly by the third month post-partum (23). Unsaturated B_{12} binding capacity rose significantly by the third month post-partum (23), and there was a strong inter-subject correlation between milk cobalamin levels and the unsaturated B_{12}-binding capacity in milk.

REFERENCES

1. Jadhav M, Webb JKG, Vaishnava S, Baker SJ (1962) Vitamin B_{12} deficiency in Indian infants. A clinical syndrome. *Lancet, ii,* 903–907.
2. Deodhar AD, Rajalakshmi R, Ramakrishnan CV (1964) Studies on human lactation. III. Effect of dietary vitamin supplementation on vitamin contents of breast milk. *Acta Paediatr., 53,* 42–48.

3. Craft IL, Matthews DM, Linnell JC (1971) Cobalamins in human pregnancy and lactation. *J. Clin. Pathol., 24,* 449–455.
4. Higginbottom MC, Sweetman L, Nyhan WL (1978) A syndrome of methyl malonic aciduria, homocystinuria, megaloblastic anaemia and neurologic abnormalities of a vitamin B_{12}-deficient breast-fed infant of a strict vegetarian. *N. Engl. J. Med., 299,* 317–323.
5. Thomas MR, Kawamoto J, Sneed SM, Eakin R (1979) The effects of vitamin C, vitamin B_6 and vitamin B_{12} supplementation on the breast milk and maternal status of well-nourished women. *Am. J. Clin. Nutr., 32,* 1679–1685.
6. Thomas MR, Sneed SM, Wei C, Neil PA, Wilson M, Sprinkle EE (1980) The effects of vitamin C, vitamin B_6, vitamin B_{12}, folic acid, riboflavin and thiamin on the breast milk and maternal status of well-nourished women at 6 months postpartum. *Am. J. Clin. Nutr., 33,* 2151–2156.
7. Samson RR, McClelland DBL (1980) Vitamin B_{12} in human colostrum and milk. *Acta Paediatr. Scand., 69,* 93–99.
8. Sandberg DP, Begley JA, Hall CA (1981) The content, binding and forms of vitamin B_{12} in milk. *Am. J. Clin. Nutr., 34,* 1717–1724.
9. Sneed SM, Zane C, Thomas MR (1981) The effects of ascorbic acid, vitamin B_6, vitamin B_{12}, and folic acid supplementation on the breast milk and maternal status of low socio-economic lactating women. *Am. J. Clin. Nutr., 34,* 1338–1346.
10. Imamura A (1981) Iron, folate and vitamin B_{12} in maternal blood and breastmilk. *Acta Obstet. Gynaecol. Jpn., 33,* 1053–1061.
11. Johnson PR, Roloff JS (1982) Vitamin B_{12} deficiency in an infant strictly breast-fed by a mother with latent pernicious anaemia. *J. Pediatr., 100,* 917–919.
12. Hoey H, Linnell JC, Oberholzer VG, Laurance BM (1982) Vitamin B_{12} deficiency in a breast-fed infant of a mother with pernicious anaemia. *J. R. Soc. Med., 75,* 656–658.
13. Ford JE, Zechalko A, Murphy J, Brooke OG (1983) Comparison of the B vitamin composition of milk from mothers of preterm and term babies. *Arch. Dis. Child., 58,* 367–372.
14. Prentice AM, Robert SB, Prentice A, Paul AA, Watkinson M, Watkinson A, Whitehead RG (1983) Dietary supplementation of lactating Gambian women. I. Effect on breast-milk volume and quality. *Hum. Clin. Nutr., 37C,* 53–64.
15. Bijur AM, Desai AG (1985) Composition of breast milk with reference to vitamin B_{12} and folic acid in Indian mothers. *Ind. J. Pediatr., 52,* 147–150.
16. van Zoeren-Grobben D, Schrijver J, van den Berg H, Berger HM (1987) Human milk vitamin content after pasteurisation, storage, or tube feeding. *Arch. Dis. Child., 62,* 161–165.
17. Trugo NMF, Donangelo CM, Koury J, Barretosilva MI, Freitas LA (1988) Concentration and distribution pattern of selected micronutrients in preterm and term milk from urban Brazilian mothers during early lactation. *Eur. J. Clin. Nutr., 42,* 497–507.
18. Donangelo CM, Trugo NMF, Koury JC, Barretosilva MI, Freitas LA, Feldheim W, Barth C (1989) Iron, zinc folate and vitamin B_{12} nutritional status and milk composition of low-income Brazilian mothers. *Eur. J. Clin. Nutr., 43,* 253–266.
19. Doyle JJ, Langevin AM, Zipursky A (1989) Nutritional vitamin B_{12} deficiency in infancy. *Ped. Hematol. Oncol., 6,* 161–172.
20. Specker BL, Black A, Allen L, Morrow F (1990) Vitamin B_{12}: low milk concentrations are related to low serum concentrations in vegetarian women and to methylmalonic aciduria in their infants. *Am. J. Clin. Nutr., 52,* 1073–1076.
21. Dagnelie PC, van Staveren WA, Roos AH, Tuinstra LGMTh, Burema J (1992) Nutrients and contaminants in human milk from mothers on macrobiotic and omnivorous diets. *Eur. J. Clin. Nutr., 46,* 355–366.
22. Kühne T, Bubl R, Baumgartner R (1991) Maternal vegan diet causing a serious infantile neurological disorder due to vitamin B_{12} deficiency. *Eur. J. Pediatr., 150,* 205–208.

23. Trugo NMF, Sardinha F (1994) Cobalamin and cobalamin-binding capacity in human milk. *Nutr. Res., 14,* 23–33.
24. Adjalla C, Mabert D, Benhayoun S, Berthelsen J G, Nicolas JP, Guéant JL, Nexo E (1994) Forms of cobalamin and vitamin B_{12} analogs in maternal plasma, milk, and cord plasma. *J. Nutr. Biochem., 5,* 406–410.

VITAMIN C (ascorbic acid)

Country	No. of subjects	Weeks post-partum	Maternal intake (mg/day)	Breast milk vitamin C concentration (mg/l)	Maternal or serum plasma (mg/l)	Infants plasma (mg/l)	Ref.
Poland (1937)	6	0–70	400–500 (S)	58			2
USA (1945)	233	0–52	NS	52			4
Australia (1946)	258	>1.5		37			5
USA (1947)	6; 6		100–230 (NS); 850–1000 (S)	64; 87	4.7; 13.1	107; 10	6
UK (1950)	1116 (sa)	3–24	NS	33			7
Botswana (1952)	84		NS	24			8
S. African Bantu (1954)	266	4–100	NS	29			9
India (1959)	37	52–75	NS	32			10
India (1960)	13; 14	12–16	0.6; 8.5	24; 45			11
India (1962)	10	2.5	80–208 (NS)	40			12
India (1964)	10; 10; 10	4–12	1.5 (NS); 100 (S); 200 (S)	61			13
India (1965)	10	4–30	NS (4)	25	3.5		14
Thailand (1978)	204			58			15
USA (1979)	6; 7	6	174 (NS); 215 (S)	61; 87	38.6; 21.4		16
USA (1980)	12	26	130 (NS)	35	5.5		17
USA (1981)	7; 9	6	152 (NS); 193 (S)	61; 72	8.7; 11.7		18
Kenya (1981)	61	0–100	NS	60			19
Gambia (1982–3)	100; 80; 80	6–100	<10 (NS); 34 (S); 100 (S)	20; 34; 55	2; 2.5; 7.2		20,21
Finland (1984)	200	12–50	138 (NS)	45	10	13	22
USA (1985)	7; 8	7–13	NS; > 1000 (S)	85; 110			23
USA (1985)	1		1500 (S)	105			24
USA (1986)	39	30–100	NS	75			25
Austria (1987)	200	4–5	NS	58	7.9		26

NS, not supplemented (basal intake may or may not be given); S, supplemented. (sa), no. of samples; otherwise no. of subjects.

The biological role of vitamin C is poorly understood. As a powerful water-soluble reducing agent and metal chelator it modulates the absorption and function of certain metal ions, particularly iron and copper, and it has a fairly specific role in maintaining the activity of certain mixed function oxidases which have iron at the active site. Its role in the prolyl and lysyl hydroxylases of collagen synthesis account for a least some of the lesions of classical scurvy, and avoidance of these lesions requires a daily intake in adults of only 6–10 mg. The question, whether other biological functions of vitamin C may require a higher intake to achieve maximum competence, has not yet been fully resolved, and the criteria upon which recommended intakes of vitamin C are based, vary with different authorities. The intake needed to saturate turnover processes within the body, and approach tissue saturation for the majority of normal people is about 100 mg/day. The extra requirement in lactating women to provide the vitamin C secreted in breast milk is thought to be in the region of 30–80 mg/day.

Normal breast milk vitamin C concentrations range between 40 and 90 mg/l; these decline to a moderate extent as lactation progresses (4, 17). In situations where maternal intake is very low (<10 mg/day) and the concentration in maternal plasma is practically undetectable, breast milk concentrations may fall as low as 20 mg/l or less (8–11, 14). The ceiling level, at high maternal intakes, is probably around 70–110 mg/l (1, 3, 4, 18, 22). Supplementation of poorly nourished women with the vitamin increases their breast milk vitamin C concentration (13, 21), but supplementation of well-nourished women does not (16, 18, 23). It appears that the upper limit in milk is probably well regulated: partly by limitations on maternal intestinal absorption capacity, and partly by the mechanisms of transferral to the milk. Apart from minor symptoms of intestinal intolerance, there are no well-established toxic effects of large doses of vitamin C given orally to adults in amounts up to 10–40 g/day, but many authorities would, nevertheless, advise caution over regular ingestion of daily amounts greater than 500 mg to 1 g, since adverse effects may occur in minority groups with unusual genetic characteristics or medical conditions. With regard to effects on lactation and the composition of breast milk, however, there are no indications that very high maternal intakes are likely to result in undesirable concentrations in breast milk. Likewise, there are no well established instances of clinical deficiency occurring in breast-fed infants of malnourished mothers, and it appears likely that the maintenance of minimally adequate concentrations of vitamin C in breast milk probably takes precedence over the maintenance of maternal stores. Further studies are needed on the quantitative aspects of these observations.

REFERENCES

1. Selleg I, King CG (1936) The vitamin C content of human milk and its variation with diet. *J. Nutr., 11,* 599–606.
2. Widenbauer von F, Kuhner A (1937) Ascorbinsäurestudien an stillenden Frauen. *Z. Vitaminforsch., 6,* 50–75.
3. Toverud KV (1939) The vitamin C requirements of pregnant and lactating women. *Z. Vitaminforsch., 8,* 237–247.
4. Munks B, Robinson A, Williams HH, Macy IG (1945) Human milk studies. XXV. Ascorbic acid and dehydroascorbic acid in colostrum and mature human milk. *Am. J. Dis. Child., 70,* 176–181.
5. Winikoff D (1946) Ascorbic acid in the milk of Melbourne women. *Med. J. Australia, 1,* 205–210.
6. Munks B, Kaucher M, Myer EZ, Harris ME, Macy IG (1947) Metabolism of women during the reproductive cycle. XI. Vitamin C in diets, breast milk, blood and urine of nursing mothers. *J. Nutr., 33,* 601–619.
7. Kon SK, Mawson EH (1950 Human Milk. Wartime studies of certain vitamins and other constituents. *Med. Res. Counc. Spec. Rep. Ser., 269,* 232–240.
8. Squires BT (1952) Ascorbic acid content of the milk of Tswana women. *Trans. R. Soc. Trop. Med. Hyg., 46,* 95–98.

9. Walker ARP, Arvidsson UB, Draper WL (1954) The composition of breast milk of South African Bantu mothers. *Trans. R. Soc. Trop. Med. Hyg., 48,* 395–399.
10. Belavady B, Gopalan C (1959) Chemical composition of human milk in poor Indian women. *Ind. J. Med. Res., 47,* 234–245.
11. Deodhar AD, Ramakrishnan CV (1960) Studies on human lactation. Relation between the dietary intake of lactating women and the chemical composition of milk with regard to the vitamin content. *J. Trop. Pediatr., 6,* 44–47.
12. Ashdhir S, Puri B (1962) Chemical composition of human milk at three different stages. *Ind. J. Pediatr., 29,* 99–109.
13. Deodhar AD, Rajalakshmi R, Ramakrishnan CV (1964) Studies on human lactation. III. Effect of dietary vitamin supplementation on vitamin contents of breast milk. *Acta Paediatr., 53,* 42–48.
14. Rajalaksmi R, Deodhar AD, Ramakrishnan CV (1965) Vitamin C secretion during lactation. *Acta Paediatr. Scand., 54,* 375–382.
15. Chatranon W, Siddhikol C, Chavalittamrong B (1978) Ascorbic acid and dehydroascorbic acid in breast milk of Thai mothers. *J. Med. Assoc. Thai., 62,* 315–317.
16. Thomas MR, Kawamoto J, Sneed SM, Eakin R (1979) The effects of vitamin C, vitamin B_6, and vitamin B_{12} supplementation on the breast milk and maternal status of well nourished women. *Am. J. Clin. Nutr., 32,* 1679–1685.
17. Thomas MR, Sneed SM, Wei C, Nail PA, Wilson M, Sprinkle II (1980) The effects of vitamin C, vitamin B_6, vitamin B_{12}, folic acid, riboflavin and thiamine on the breast milk and maternal status of well-nourished women at 6 months postpartum. *Am. J. Clin. Nutr., 33,* 2151–2156.
18. Sneed SM, Zane C, Thomas MR (1981) The effects of ascorbic acid, vitamin B_6, vitamin B_{12}, folic acid supplementation on the breast milk and maternal status of low socioeconomic lactating women. *Am. J. Nutr., 34,* 1338–1346.
19. van Steenbergen WM, Kusin JA, van Rens WM (1981) Lactational performance of Akamba mothers, Kenya, Breast-feeding behaviour, breast milk yield and composition. *J. Trop. Pediatr., 27,* 155–161.
20. Bates CJ, Prentice AM, Prentice A, Paul AA, Whitehead RG (1982) Seasonal variations in ascorbic acid status and breast milk ascorbic acid levels in rural Gambian women in relation to dietary intake. *Trans. R. Soc. Trop. Med. Hyg., 76,* 341–347.
21. Bates CJ, Prentice AM, Prentice A, Lamb WH, Whitehead RG (1983) The effect of vitamin C supplementation on lactating women in Keneba, a West African rural community. *Int. J. Vit. Nutr. Res., 53,* 68–76.
22. Salmenpera L (1984) Vitamin C nutrition during prolonged lactation: optimal in infants while marginal in some mothers. *Am. J. Clin. Nutr., 40,* 1050–1056.
23. Byerley LO, Kirksey A (1985) Effects of different levels of vitamin C intake on the vitamin C concentration in human milk and the vitamin C intakes of breast-fed infants. *Am. J. Clin. Nutr., 41,* 665–671.
24. Anderson DM, Pittard WB (1985) Vitamin E and C concentrations in human milk with maternal megadosing. A case report. *J. Am. Diet. Assoc., 85,* 715–717.
25. Karra MV, Udipi SA, Kirksey A, Roepke JLB (1986) Changes in specific nutrients in breast milk during extended lactation. *Am. J. Clin. Nutr., 43,* 495–503.
26. Heinz-Erian P, Achmüller M, Berger H, Brabec W, Nirk S, Rufer R (1987) Vitamin C konzentration in maternalem plasma, fruchtwasser, nabel- schnurblut, im plasma des neugeborenen und in kolostrum, transitarischer und reifer frauenmilch. *Pediatr. Padol., 22,* 163–178.

VITAMIN D

Country	No. of subjects	Weeks postpartum	Maternal intake (μg/day)	Breast milk vitamin D concentration (μg/l)[a]	Ref.
Denmark (1980)	?	1	NS	0.37	2
USA (1981)	3		10–20 (NS)	0.43	3
Israel (1982)	36	1–3	NS	0.4[b]	4
USA (1982)	3	Mid-lactation	NS	0.5	5
USA (1982)	3; 3		NS; 62 (S)	<0.5; 3.5	6
USA (1984)	1	2	2500 (S)	180	9
Finland (1984)	4; 4		NS; 25 (S)	0.2; 0.29	10
Germany (1984)	14	1–20	NS	0.9	11
USA (1985)	15; (10)		13; (9)[d]	0.76; (0.24)[c,d]	15
Japan (1985)	10	1	NS	0.79	16
USA (1986)	51	2–13	.ca 10	0.71	17
France (1986)	11; (1)	2	NS; (+30)[e]	0.69; (1.02)[c,e]	18
Spain (1987)	14		NS	2.1	19
USA (1987)	9	4	NS	0.58	20
Netherlands (1987), pooled		4–34	NS	0.06[f]	21
Finland (1988)	80	8, 20	NS (+25)	1.47 (2.05)	22
Japan (1988)	10		NS	0.07	23
Japan (1988)	23	1–17	NS	0.78[c]	24
Netherlands (1989)	39	1–3	NS	0.13[f]	25

NS, not supplemented; S, supplemented.

[a]Where the original data were in international units, they have been divided by 40 to give a μg vitamin D equivalent, regardless of the forms actually present.

[b]Hydroxylated metabolites only.

[c]Sum of vitamin D and hydroxylated metabolites, quoted separately in original publication.

[d]Results for dark-skinned mothers in parentheses following those for light-skinned mothers.

[e]Results for one supplemented subject given in parentheses after the results for 11 unsupplemented subjects.

[f]Hydroxylated forms only.

[g]Mean of 4 seasonal values, 2 lactation stages, and fore and hind milk. Half were supplemented (25 μg/day). Sum of vitamin D + 25(OH)D.

Vitamin D3 (cholecalciferol) is synthesised in the skin in the presence of UV light, as well as being present naturally in a small number of foods. It is required as part of the complex regulatory system for transport and control of calcium, being converted via the 25-hydroxy to the 1,25-dihydroxy derivative, which is the main active form in vivo. Early studies used a rat (line test) bioassay for vitamin D. During the past decade, there have arisen conflicting reports about the vitamin D potency of milk, with the suggestion that water-soluble forms might be of major importance. Recent reinvestigations of human and cows' milk by HPLC-based procedures, combined with competitive binding assays, have shown, however, that only fat-soluble forms are present (3, 5, 7, 11) of which 25-hydroxy vitamin D is probably the most important, at least in terms of biological potency (5, 7, 11). It represents 30–75% of the vitamin D by weight, and increases in concentration during lactation, unlike vitamin D per se, which decreases (11). The 25-hydroxy derivative may be of particular value to newborn infants, whose enzyme system for conversion of vitamin D to the 25-hydroxy form is poorly developed (1). Milk, like plasma and some other body components, contains a binding protein for vitamin D and its hydroxylated metabolites (27).

As can be seen from the Table, the milk vitamin D from unsupplemented human subjects in several recent studies was found to be very low in comparison with the infants' recommended daily amount of around 10 μg cholecalciferol/day and there have been several recent reports of rickets (or biochemical deficiency) developing in breast-fed infants (8, 12, 13). Milk from dark-skinned mothers (in the USA) had a lower level of vitamin D than that from white mothers (15). Vitamin D in milk from a vitamin D-deficient subject was undetectable (26). Although adequate exposure to sunlight seems to constitute the safest, and most natural way of acquiring an adequate vitamin D status in infancy, some infants undoubtedly require dietary supplementation. This is particularly true in the winter, when breast milk vitamin D levels decline markedly in northern countries (12). Vitamin D is toxic in large doses and the safety margin between currently accepted safe and adequate intakes and those suspected of causing toxicity effects (such as hypercalcaemia) is smaller than that found for most other vitamins.

An increase in maternal vitamin D intake usually results in some increase in breast-milk concentrations (6, 18, 22). Supplements of 25 or 50 μg of vitamin D to Finnish mothers (22) significantly increased their breast milk vitamin D levels in February and April when a seasonal low-point was encountered. Exposure of the mother to ultraviolet light can also increase breast-milk vitamin D concentrations, but not to toxic levels (6, 14, 17).

The considerably raised vitamin D concentration in the breast milk of a woman treated with vitamin D 2500 μg per day for hypoparathyroidism (9) resulted in a high serum calcium concentration in her breast-fed infant, and this vitamin D concentration was similar to that known to have caused hypercalcaemia in previous instances of accidental vitamin D overdosage from formula feeds. Although the evidence is clearly very limited, it does appear that therapeutic amounts of vitamin D given to nursing mothers for certain medical conditions may result in greatly increased breast-milk concentrations, which could in turn result in toxicity to the infant. The authors of this study (9) recommended that in such cases, the infant's serum calcium concentrations and possible symptoms of vitamin D toxicity should be closely monitored throughout breast-feeding. Likewise, Ala-Houhala et al. (22) warned that "the responses (to supplementation with 25 or 50 μg/day) were highly variable and the safety of such a dose of vitamin D over prolonged periods should be examined." Clearly this subject requires some further study.

REFERENCES

1. Hoff N, Haddad J, Teitelbaum S, McAlister W, Hillman LS (1979) Serum concentrations of 25-hydroxyvitamin-D in rickets of extremely premature infants. *J. Pediatr., 94,* 460–466.

2. Leerbeck E, Sondergaard H (1980) The total content of vitamin D in human milk and cow's milk. *Br. J. Nutr., 44,* 7–12.
3. Hollis BW, Roos BA, Draper HH, Lambert PW (1981) Vitamin D and its metabolites in human and bovine milk. *J. Nutr., 111,* 1240–1248.
4. Weisman Y, Bawnik JD, Eisenberg Z, Spirer Z (1982) Vitamin D metabolites in human milk. *J Pediatr., 100,* 745–748.
5. Reeve LE, Chesney RW, DeLuca HF (1982) Vitamin D of human milk: identification of biologically active forms. *Am. J. Clin. Nutr., 36,* 122–126.
6. Hollis BW, Greer FR, Tsang RC (1982) The effects of oral vitamin D supplementation and ultraviolet phototherapy on the antirachitic sterol content of human milk. *Calcif. Tissue Int., 34 Suppl. 1),* 552.
7. Hollis B W (1983) Improved quantitation of vitamin D_2, vitamin D_3, 25-hydroxyvitamin D_2 and 25-hydroxyvitamin D_3 in human milk. *Anal. Biochem., 131,* 211–219.
8. Markestad T (1983) Plasma concentrations of vitamin D metabolites in unsupplemented breast-fed infants. *Eur. J. Pediatr., 141,* 77–80.
9. Greer FR, Hollis BW, Napoli JL (1984) High concentrations of vitamin D_2 in human milk associated with pharmacological doses of vitamin D_2. *J. Pediatr., 105,* 61–64.
10. Parviainen MT, Koskinen T, Ala-Houhala M, Visakorpi JK (1984) A method for routine estimation of vitamin D activity in human and bovine milk. *Acta Vitaminol. Enzymol., 6,* 211.
11. Kunz C, Niesen M, Lileenfeld-Toal HV, Burmeister W (1984) Vitamin D, 25-hydroxy-vitamin D and 1,25 dihydroxy-vitamin D in cows' milk, infant formulas and breast milk during different stages of lactation. *Int. J. Vitam. Nutr. Res., 54,* 141–148.
12. Markestad T, Kolmannskog S, Arntzen E, Toftegaard L, Haneberg B, Aksnes L (1984) Serum concentrations of vitamin D metabolites in exclusively breast-fed infants at 70° north. *Acta Paediatr. Scand., 73,* 29–32.
13. Anonymous (1984) Rickets in a breast-fed infant. *Nutr. Rev., 42,* 380–382.
14. Greer FR, Hollis BW, Cripps DJ, Tsang RC (1984) Effects of maternal ultraviolet B irradiation on vitamin D content of human milk. *J. Pediatr., 105,* 431–433.
15. Specker BL, Tsang RC, Hollis BW (1985) Effect of race and diet on human-milk vitamin D and 25-hydroxyvitamin D. *Am. J. Dis. Child., 139,* 1134–1137.
16. Yamaoka K, Seino Y, Yabuchi H, Tanaka Y, Nishimura K (1985) 25-hydroxyvitamin D and 1,25 hydroxyvitamin D in human breast milk in Japan. *J. Bone Min. Metab., 3,* 127–132.
17. Hollis BW, Pittard WB, Reinhardt TA (1986) Relationships among vitamin D, 25-hydroxyvitamin D, and vitamin D-binding protein concentrations in the plasma and milk of human subjects. *J. Clin. Endocrinol. Metab., 62,* 41–44.
18. Cancela L, Le Boulch N, Miravet L (1986) Relationships between the vitamin D content of maternal milk and the vitamin D status of nursing women and breast-fed infants. *J. Endocrinol., 110,* 43–50.
19. Ballester I, Cortes E, Moya M, Campello MJ (1987) Improved method for quantifying vitamin D in proprietory infants formulas and in breast milk. *Clin. Chem., 33,* 796–799.
20. Atkinson SA, Reinhardt TA, Hollis BW (1987) Vitamin D activity in maternal plasma and milk in relation to gestational stage at delivery. *7,* 1005–1011.
21. van Zoeren-Grobben D, Schrijver J, van den Berg H, Berger HM (1987) Human milk vitamin content after pasteurisation, storage, or tube-feeding. *Arch. Dis. Child., 62,* 161–165.
22. Ala-Houhala M, Koskinen T, Parvainen MT, Visakorpi JK (1988) 25-hydroxyvitamin D and vitamin D in human milk: effects of supplementation and season. *Am. J. Clin. Nutr., 48,* 1057–1060.
23. Nakao H (1988) Nutritional significance of human milk vitamin D in neonatal period. *Kobe J. Med. Sci., 34,* 121–128.

24. Takeuchi A, Okano T, Tsugawa N, Katayama M, Mimura Y, Kobayashi T (1988) Determination of vitamin D and its metabolites in human and cow's milk. *J. Micronutr. Anal., 4,* 193–208.
25. Hoogenboezem T, Degenhart HJ, Keizer-Schrama SMPF de M, Bouillon R, Grose WFA, Hackeng WHL, Visser HKA (1989) Vitamin D metabolism in breast-fed infants and their mothers. *Ped. Res., 25,* 623–628.
26. Jensen RG (1989) Lipids in human milk composition and fat-soluble vitamins. In: Lebenthal E (Ed) *Textbook of Gastroenterology and Nutrition,* (2nd edn.). pp 157–208. Raven Press, New York.
27. Ena JM, Pérez MD, Aranda P, Sanchez L, Calvo M (1992) Presence and changes in the concentration of vitamin D-binding protein throughout early lactation in human and bovine colostrum and milk. *J. Nutr. Biochem., 3,* 498–502.

VITAMIN E

Country	No. of subjects	Weeks post-partum	Maternal intake (mg/day)	Breast milk vitamin E concentration[a] (mg/l)	Ref.
USA (1947)	4	4–34	NS	1.4	1
USA (1952)	10	3–36	NS	2.4	2
USA (1964)	20	6	NS	1.75	3
Germany (1965)	200	20	NS	8.5	5
Japan (1966)	49		NS	5	6
Japan (1975)	3		NS	1.8	7
Sweden (1981)	24	2–20	NS	3.2	8
USA (1981)	10	5	17 (NS)	8.4	9
India (1981)	30	4–12	NS	4.3	10
USA (1985)	1		1100 (S)	11	12
Israel (1985)	23	5	NS	1.1	13
Finland	62	>2	NS	4.9	14
Canada (1985)	24	5	21 (NS)	3	15
USA (1985)	7	12–16	NS	3.7	16
Canada (1986)	12	2	NS	5.8	17
Germany (1986)		5	NS	3	18
Netherlands (1987), pooled		4–34	NS	3.2	19
Germany (1987)	63[b]	5	NS	2.8	20
USA (1987)	5	4	NS	3.7[c]	21
USA (1989)	–	–	NS	3.4	23
International (1991)	99	1–4	NS	4.6–8.0	25
China (1993)	72	0–2	NS	4.6–7.8[d]	26

NS, not supplemented; S, supplemented.
[a]Alpha-tocopherol equivalent.
[b]From 13 subjects.
[c]Of which 3.05 mg/l is the alpha-form and the remainder gamma.
[d]No consistent difference between term and pre-term milk.

Although the role of vitamin E as a lipid-soluble antioxidant, protecting polyunsaturated fatty acids in particular, is well recognised, there is still much to be learned about its biological significance, and in particular its significance in human nutrition. Simple dietary deficiency is unlikely to occur in normal human subjects, but there are recorded instances of favourable responses to vitamin E supplementation in subjects with certain genetic abnormalities or in those subjected to oxidative stress: one example being the protection of preterm infants who are exposed to high oxygen tensions, from damage to their sensitive ocular tissues (retrolental fibroplasia). The vitamin E content of milk from mothers of preterm infants appears to be similar to that of mothers of term infants (20). The risk-benefit ratio of giving supplemental vitamin E to newborn infants needs to be assessed further.

The concentration of vitamin E (mainly α-tocopherol) in human milk is higher than that in cows' milk, and is generally found to be much higher in colostrum and transitional milk than in mature milk (18, 20, 26), which parallels the situation for vitamin A. Some early studies on colostrum, omitted from the Table, are summarised in Ref. (7), and there are two detailed reviews of vitamin E in human milk (11, 22). Very little is known about the effects of maternal deprivation or supplementation with vitamin E, on breast-milk concentrations. A moderate increase in milk vitamin E was observed after substituting sunflower oil for lard in the maternal diet (4). One mother, who had been taken 100–140 times the US recommended daily amount since pregnancy had milk vitamin E concentrations 'above the normal range' (12), but the increment was undoubtedly much smaller than the increment in maternal intake, and in view of the relatively low toxicity of vitamin E, unlikely to have been harmful. Another mother who received a similar amount (1.1 mg) as a single dose in the 11th week of lactation exhibited a 6.6 fold increase in breast milk vitamin E by the third day after the dose, falling to baseline by the fifth day (24). However, the peak concentration of 4.1 mg/l was well within the ranges recorded without supplements by other workers.

REFERENCES

1. Quaife ML (1947) Tocopherols (vitamin E) in milk: Their chemical determination and occurrence in human milk. *J. biol. Chem., 169,* 513–514.
2. Harris PL, Quaife ML, O'Grady P (1952) Tocopherol content of human milk and of cows' milk products used for infant feeding. *J. Nutr., 46,* 459–466.
3. Woodruff CW, Bailey MC, Davis JT, Rogers N, Coniglio GL (1964) Serum lipids in breast-fed infants and in infants fed evaporated milk. *Am. J. Clin. Nutr., 14,* 83–90.
4. Kramer M, Szoke K, Lindner K, Tarjan R (1965) The effect of different factors on the composition of human milk and its variations. III. Effect of dietary fats on the lipid composition of human milk. *Nutr. Diet., 7,* 71–79.
5. Herre HD (1965) Variations in the vitamin E content of human milk as affected by season, duration of lactation and degree of heating. *Monatsschr. Kinderheilkd., 113,* 95–97.
6. Kuratani H (1966) Vitamin E content of milk and serum in children. *Acta Paediatr. Jpn., 8,* 55.
7. Kobayashi H, Kanno C, Yamauchi K, Tsugo T (1975) Identification of alpha-, beta-, gamma- and delta-tocopherols and their contents in human milk. *Biochim. Biophys. Acta, 380,* 282–290.
8. Jansson L, Akesson B, Holmberg L (1981) Vitamin E and fatty acid composition of human milk. *Am. J. Clin. Nutr., 34,* 8–13.
9. Thomas MR, Pearsons MH, Demkowicz IM, Chan IM, Lewis CG (1981) Vitamin A and vitamin E concentration of the milk from mothers of pre-term infants and milk of mothers of full term infants. *Acta Vitaminol. Enzymol., 3,* 135–144.
10. Jagadeesan V, Prema K (1981) Lactation and vitamin E status: Relationship between plasma and milk levels at different lactational periods. *Nutr. Rep. Int., 23,* 135–141.
11. Lammi-Keefe CJ, Jensen RG (1984) Lipids in human milk: a review. II. Composition and fat-soluble vitamins. *J. Paediatr. Gastroenterol., 3,* 172–198.
12. Anderson DM, Pittard WB (1985) Vitamin E and C concentrations in human milk with maternal megadosing: a case report. *J. Am. Diet. Assoc., 85,* 715–717.
13. Vaisman N, Mogilner BM, Sklan D (1985) Vitamin A and E content of preterm and term milk. *Nutr. Res., 5,* 931–935.
14. Syvaoja EL, Piironen V, Varo P, Koivistoinen P, Salminenen K (1985) Tocopherols and tocotrienols in Finnish foods, human milk and infant formulas. *Int. J. Vitam. Nutr. Res., 55,* 159–166.
15. Chappell JE, Francis T, Clandinin MT (1985) Vitamin A and E content of human milk at early stages of lactation. *Early Hum. Dev., 11,* 157–167.

16. Lammi-Keefe CJ, Jensen RG, Clark RM, Ferris AM (1985) Tocopherol, total lipid and linoleic acid contents of human milk. In: Schaub J (Ed) *Composition and Physiological Properties of Human Milk*, pp 241–245. Elsevier, New York.
17. Chappell JE, Francis T, Clandinin MT (1986) Simultaneous high performance liquid chromatography analysis of retinol esters and tocopherol isomers in human milk. *Nutr. Res., 6,* 849–852.
18. Harzer G, Haug M, Bindels JG (1986) Biochemistry of maternal milk in early lactation. *Hum. Nutr.: Clin. Nutr., 40A,* 11–18.
19. van Zoeren-Grobben D, Schrijver J, van den Berg H, Berger HM (1987) Human milk vitamin content after pasteurisation, storage, or tube feeding. *Arch. Dis. Child., 62,* 161–165.
20. Haug M, Laubach C, Burke M, Harzer GI (1987) Vitamin E in human milk from mothers of preterm and term infants. *J. Pediatr. Gastroenterol. Nutr., 6,* 605–609.
21. Moffatt PA, Lammi-Keefe CJ, Ferris AM, Jensen RG (1987) Alpha and gamma tocopherols in pooled mature human milk after storage. *J. Pediatr. Gastroenterol. Nutr., 6,* 225–227.
22. Jensen RG (1989) Lipids in human milk - composition and fat-soluble vitamins. In: Lebenthal E (Ed) *Textbook of Gastroenterology and Nutrition in Infancy,* 2nd edn., pp 157–208. Raven Press, New York.
23. Collins SE, Jackson MB, Lammi-Keefe CJ, Jensen RG (1989) The simultaneous separation and quantitation of human milk lipids. *Lipids, 24,* 746–749.
24. Kanno C, Kobayashi H, Yamauchi K (1989) Transfer of orally-administered α-tocopherol into human milk. *J. Nutr. Sci. Vitaminol., 35,* 649–653.
25. Boersma ER, Offringa PJ, Muskiet FAJ, Chase VM, Simmons IJ (1991) Vitamin E, lipid fractions, and fatty acid composition of colostrum, transitional milk and mature milk: an international comparative study. *Am. J. Clin. Nutr., 53,* 1197–1204.
26. Zheng M-C, Zhou LS, Zhang GF (1993) Alpha-tocopherol content of breast milk in China. *J. Nutr. Sci. Vitaminol., 39,* 517–520.

VITAMIN K

Country	No. of subjects	Weeks postpartum	Maternal intake	Breast milk vitamin K concentration (μg/l)	Forms detected	Ref.
Japan (1981)	19		NS	4.7		3
UK (1982)	20; 1		NS; 20 (S)	2.1; 140 (after 12 h)	K1	4
Japan (1982)	43		NS	9.2	K1	6
Indonesia (1983)	13		NS	8.9		7
Japan (1984)	337	4–7	NS	4.5	K1 + K2	10
Germany (1987)	9	3–5	NS	1.2	K1	12
France (1987)	10	3	NS	9.2	K1	13
Japan (1988)	23		NS	2.1	K1 + K2	14
USA (1991)	15	4–26	NS	2.9	K1	16
USA (1991)	23; 11	6–26	NS; 20,000 (S)	1; 130	K1	17
Austria (1993)	36	1–12	NS; 88 (S)	1.6; 1.6	K1	18

NS, not supplemented; S, supplemented.

Vitamin K is an essential component of the blood-clotting cascade, and a small proportion (ca. 1:5000) of otherwise normal infants suffer from persistent bleeding, which responds to vitamin K therapy (1, 2, 5, 8–11). In some of these, intracranial bleeding can be life-threatening. Several studies (8, 10, 11) have reported an association between persistent or delayed onset of bleeding and breast-feeding, which is consistent with the detection of only very small amounts of vitamin K in breast milk or colostrum (4, 10). The amount in breast milk of mothers whose infants suffered from intracranial bleeding was low (10). A single oral dose of vitamin K (20 mg) to the mother substantially increased her breast-milk vitamin K_1 (4). Doses of 0.5–3 mg of vitamin K_1 to the mother produced fairly substantial vitamin K increments to 25–30 μg/l, 12 to 24 h later (12). A much smaller dose of around 88 μg, given for up to 12 weeks, had no detectable effect on breast milk vitamin K levels (18). The efficacy of maternal supplementation in preventing infantile haemorrhage, and the possible toxicity of large doses via the breast-milk, have not been studied. Neonatal vitamin K deficiency is controlled, in many countries, by a single prophylactic i.m. injection of vitamin K (ca. 0.5–1.0 mg) to all babies soon after birth (8); there is some recent evidence, albeit controversial, that oral doses may be safer (19). The water-soluble form (menadione) has significant toxicity when given directly to the neonate, and the naturally occurring, fat-soluble forms (e.g. phytomenadione) are therefore preferred. The vitamin K content of human milk has recently been reviewed (15), and it was concluded that menaquinones (K_2) probably do not occur there.

REFERENCES

1. Sutherland JM, Glueck HI, Gleser G (1967) Hemorrhagic disease of the newborn. Breast feeding as a necessary factor in the pathogenesis. *Am. J. Dis. Child., 113,* 524–533.

2. Keenan WJ, Jewett T, Glueck HI (1971) Role of feeding and vitamin K in hypoprothrombinemia of the newborn. *Am. J. Dis. Child., 122,* 271–277.
3. Shirahata A, Nojiri T, Miyaji Y et al. (1981) Vitamin K contents of infant formula products and breast milk. *Igaku No Ayumi, 118,* 857–859.
4. Haroon Y, Shearer MJ, Rahim S, Gunn WG, McEnery G, Barkhan P (1982) The content of phylloquinone (vitamin K_1) in human milk, cows' milk and infant formula foods determined by high-performance liquid chromatography. *J. Nutr., 112,* 1105–1117.
5. Jiminez R, Navarrette M, Jiminez E, Mora LA, Robles G (1982) Vitamin K-dependent clotting factors in normal breast-fed infants. *J. Pediatr., 100,* 424–426.
6. Miyagi Y (1982) Study on the idiopathic vitamin K in breast milk and formula milk. *Acta Paediatr. Jpn., 86,* 1320–1326.
7. Isarangkura PB, Mahadandana C, Panstienkul B et al. (1983) Vitamin K levelin maternal breast milk of infants with acquired prothrombin complex deficiency syndrome. *SE Asian J. Trop. Med. Publ. Health, 14,* 275–76.
8. O'Connor ME, Livingstone DS, Hannah J, Wilkins D (1983) Vitamin K deficiency and breast-feeding. *Am. J. Dis. Child., 40,* 601–602.
9. American Academy of Pediatrics (1971) Vitamin K supplementation for infants receiving milk substitute infant formulas and for those with rate malabsorption. *Pediatrics, 137,* 483–487.
10. Motohara K, Matsukura M, Matsuda I, Iribe K, Ikeda T, Kondo Y, Yonekubo A, Yamamoto Y, Tsuchiya F (1984) Severe vitamin K deficiency in breast-fed infants. *J. Pediatr., 105,* 943–945.
11. Von Kries R, Wahn V, Kolefzko B, Gobel U (1984) Late manifestations of vitamin K deficiency in breast-fed infants. *Monatsschr. Kinderheilkd., 132,* 293–295.
12. Von Kries R, Shearer M, McCarthy PT, Haug M, Harzer G, Gobel U (1987) Vitamin K_1 content of maternal milk: influence of the stage of lactation, lipid composition and vitamin K_1 supplements given to the mother. *Ped. Res., 22,* 513–517.
13. Fournier B, Sann L, Guillaumont M, Leclerq M (1987) Variations of phylloquinone concentration in human milk at various stages of lactation and in cow's milk at various seasons. *Am. J. Clin. Nutr., 45,* 551–558.
14. Isshiki H, Suzuki Y, Yonekubo A, Hasegawa H, Yamamoto Y (1988) Determination of phylloquinone and menaquinone in human milk using high performance liquid chromatography. *J. Dairy Sci., 71,* 627–632.
15. Canfield LM, Hopkinson JM (1989) State of the art vitamin K in human milk. *J. Pediatr. Gastroenterol. Nutr., 8,* 430–441.
16. Canfield LM, Hopkinson JM, Lima AF, Silva B, Garza C (1991) Vitamin K in colostrum and mature human milk over the lactation period - a cross-sectional study. *Am. J. Clin. Nutr., 53,* 730–735.
17. Greer FR, Marshall S, Cherry J, Suttic JW (1991) Vitamin K status of lactating mothers, human milk, and breast-feeding infants. *Pediatrics, 88,* 751–756.
18. Pietschnig B, Haschke F, Vanura H, Shearer M, Veitl V, Kellner S, Schuster E (1993) Vitamin K in breast milk: no influence of maternal dietary intake. *Eur. J. Clin. Nutr., 47,* 209–215.
19. Golding J, Greenwood R, Birmingham K, Mott M (1992) Childhood cancer, intramuscular vitamin K, and pethidine given during labour. *Br. Med. J., 305,* 341–346.

MINERALS AND TRACE ELEMENTS

EFFECTS OF DIETARY SUPPLEMENTATION ON THE ESSENTIAL MINERALS AND TRACE ELEMENTS IN HUMAN MILK

There is only limited information about the effects of maternal deficiency and supplementation on the secretion of minerals and trace elements in human milk. For the most part, studies have been confined to mothers with no indication of poor mineral or trace element status and to the early stages of lactation. Maternal diet appears to have relatively little influence on the concentration of most of the nutritionally-relevant trace elements in breast milk (13). It is possible that marginal maternal deficiency has an influence on breast-milk concentrations only after prolonged lactation, so that a response to supplementation is restricted to the later stages of lactation. This has been shown to be the case for zinc (9), but it has not been investigated in detail for other elements.

All essential minerals and trace elements are found in breast milk. At the present time, data are available only on the effects of maternal dietary intake and supplementation on the breast-milk concentrations of the metals calcium, chromium, copper, iron, magnesium, manganese, sodium and zinc, and of the non-metals fluorine, iodine and selenium. The data for these 11 elements are discussed in this chapter together with relevant background information. The studies reviewed have been restricted to those performed on man, as many animal models have proved inappropriate for establishing dietary influences on human lactation. For example, in rats supplementation of the diet with iron results in increased milk iron concentration (4, 6) and iron deficiency produces low milk iron concentrations (4). There is no evidence that lactating humans with haematological signs of iron deficiency have reduced breast-milk iron secretion or that supplementation increases breast-milk iron concentration (1–3, 28).

The measurement of breast-milk minerals and trace elements has proved technically difficult. New techniques are being developed (7, 10, 11, 19, 22–24) which may help to extend the repertoire and the accuracy of analytical values. Differences in methodology between studies have often made direct comparisons between mothers living in different communities very difficult. In recent years some attempt at standardisation has been made and it appears that there are substantial differences in the trace element and mineral concentrations of breast-milk in different parts of the world (7, 8, 25). The reasons for these differences are not clear. In some cases it is unlikely to be directly related to dietary intake. In Malaysia, for example, mothers of different ethnic origins were shown to produce milk of different iron content but this was not related to maternal iron status (1). For clarity, this review has considered only those studies which have investigated the influence of maternal dietary intake and supplementation within the same mothers, within mothers of the same community or measured by the same workers. In addition, no values have been given in the text for the 'normal' concentration of each element in breast milk. A full discussion of the problems in determining the elemental composition of human milk and a comprehensive review of reported values has been published by the International Atomic Energy Agency (7).

The secretion of many of the minerals and trace elements in breast milk varies, sometimes very considerably, with stage of lactation (12, 16, 26). These changes in composition are likely to be under the control of mechanisms which are independent of substrate availability, e.g. hormonal, and are not generally correlated with maternal dietary intake. Relationships between maternal intake of an element and breast-milk element concentrations must therefore be studied in mothers at the same stage of lactation. Details of study design are included in the tables of this review.

The effects of deficient and excessive intakes of many essential minerals and trace elements are largely unknown, especially for infants. For a few elements there have been sufficient data for reference nutrient intakes or recommended dietary allowances to be made or for safe-and-adequate levels to be calculated (5). Where appropriate, the effects of deficiency and toxicity are discussed in the sections on the individual elements. The definition of deficient and excessive intakes is further complicated by the wide variations in bioavailability observed between different dietary forms of the elements, and the effects of interactions with other dietary constituents. The bioavailability of breast-milk elements to the human infant is generally far greater than the same element in cow's milk or formula milks. A comparison of the absolute concentrations of the essential minerals and trace elements between human milk and other milks can therefore be misleading in terms of its biological efficacy, and is not discussed here.

This review summarises the evidence whether supplementation of the maternal diet is advisable for lactating mothers, whether it constitutes a convenient route for the supplementation of breast-fed infants, and whether there is any risk of toxicity for the breast-fed child. Maternal dietary intake has been shown to influence the breast-milk concentration of fluorine, iodine and selenium and possibly manganese and zinc. Supplementation of lactating mothers with some of these elements may be associated with a risk of toxicity in the infant and should be approached with caution. The fluorine content of breast milk, however, is much lower than drinking water, so that maternal supplementation is unlikely to lead to adverse reactions in the breast-fed child. Breast-milk secretions of iron, chromium, copper, sodium and magnesium seem relatively unresponsive to maternal dietary supplementation. Calcium may or may not be responsive, and studies to test this are in progress. The likelihood of toxicity in infants as a result of maternal supplementation with these elements is small.

Studies carried out since the last period of review (up to 1985) are documented in references (10–28) below, and in the reference lists of sections dealing with individual elements. These have added detail to the picture in various ways, but have not altered the broad conclusions, stated above.

REFERENCES

1. Loh TT, Sinnathury TA (1971) Haematological data and milk iron in Malaysian women. *Aust. N. Z. J. Obstet. Gynaecol., 11,* 254–258.
2. Picciano MF, Guthrie HA (1976) Copper, iron and zinc contents of mature human milk. *Am. J. Clin. Nutr., 29,* 242–254.
3. Murray MJ, Murray AB, Murray NJ, Murray MB (1978) The effect of iron status of Nigerian mothers on that of their infants at birth and 6 months and on the concentration of Fe in breast-milk. *Br. J. Nutr., 39,* 627–630.
4. Keen CL, Lonnerdal B, Sloan MV, Hurley LS (1980) Effect of dietary iron, copper and zinc chelates or nitrilotriacetic acid (NTA) on trace metal concentrations in rat milk and maternal and pup tissues. *J. Nutr., 110,* 897–906.
5. National Academy of Sciences (1980) *Recommended Dietary Allowances,* 9th edn. National Academy of Sciences, Washington, DC.
6. Anaokar SG, Garry PS (1981) Effect of maternal iron nutrition during lactation on milk iron and rat neonatal iron status. *Am. J. Clin. Nutr., 34,* 1505–1512.
7. Iyengar GV (1982) Elemental composition of human and animal milk, a review. *IAEA-Tecdoc.*, Vol. 269, IAEA, Vienna.
8. Iyengar GV, Parr RM (1985) Trace elements in human milk from several global regions. In: Schaub J (Ed) *Composition and Physiological Properties of Human Milk,* pp. 17–44. Elsevier, Amsterdam.
9. Krebs NF, Hambidge KM, Jacobs MA, Rasbach JO (1985) The effects of a dietary zinc supplement during lactation on longitudinal changes in maternal zinc status and milk zinc concentrations. *Am. J. Clin. Nutr., 41,* 560–570.
10. Casey CE, Howell RR, Lonnerdal B, Moser PB, Picciano MF, Rumball SV (1985) Principles of trace element analysis and notes on some important elements. In: Jensen RG, Neville MC (Eds) *Human Lactation. Milk Components and Methodologies,* pp 223–236. Plenum Press, New York.
11. Neville MC, Keller RP, Lonnerdal B, Atkinson S, Wade CL, Butte N, Moser PB (1985) Measurement of electrolyte and macromineral concentrations in human milk. In: Jensen RG, Neville MC (Eds) *Human Lactation. Milk Components and Methodologies,* pp 129–140. Plenum Press, New York.
12. Finley DA, Lonnerdal B, Dewey KG, Grivetti LE (1985) Inorganic constituents of breast milk from vegetarian and non-vegetarian women: relationships with each other and with organic constituents. *J. Nutr., 115,* 772–781.
13. Lonnerdal B (1986) Effects of maternal dietary intake on human milk composition. *J. Nutr., 116,* 499–513.
14. Howell RR, Palma PA, West MS, Caprioli RM, Seifert WE (1986) Trace elements in human milk: differences over time and between population groups. In: Howell RR, Morriss FH Jr, Pickering LK (Eds) *Human Milk in Infant Nutrition and Health,* pp 28–50. Charles C. Thomas, Illinois.
15. Adcock EW III, Brewer ED, Caprioli RM, West MS (1986) Macronutrients, electrolytes and minerals in human milk: differences over time and between population groups. In: Howell RR, Morriss FH Jr, Pickering LK (Eds) *Human Milk in Infant Nutrition and Health,* pp 3–27. Charles C. Thomas, Illinois.
16. Karra MV, Udipi SA, Kirksey A, Roepke JL (1986) Changes in specific nutrients in breast milk during extended lactation. *Am. J. Clin. Nutr., 43,* 495–503.
17. Lonnerdal B (1987) Trace element binding ligands in human milk: function in trace element utilization. In: Goldman AS, Atkinson SA, Hanson LA (Eds) *Human Lactation 3. The Effects of Human Milk on the Recipient Infant,* pp 61–70. Plenum Press, New York.

18. Butte NF, Garza C, O'Brian Smith E, Wills C, Nichols BL (1987) Macro- and trace-mineral intakes of exclusively breast-fed infants. *Am. J. Clin. Nutr., 45,* 42–48.
19. Schramel P, Lill G, Hasse S, Kloze BJ (1988) Mineral- and trace element concentrations in human breast milk, placenta, maternal blood and the blood of the newborn. *Biol. Trace Elements Res., 16,* 67–75.
20. George DE, Franceska BA (1989) Human milk in comparison to cow milk. In: Lebenthal E (Ed) *Textbook of Gastroenterology and Nutrition in Infancy*, 2nd edn., pp 239–261. Raven Press, New York.
21. Harzer G, Haschke F (1989) Micronutrients in human milk. In: Renner E (Ed) *Micronutrients in Milk and Milk-Based Food Products,* pp 125–237. Elsevier, London.
22. Nagra SA (1989) Longitudinal study in biochemical composition of human milk during the first year of lactation. *J. Trop. Paediatr., 35,* 126–128.
23. Li JZ, Yoshinaga J, Suzuki T, Abe M, Morita M (1990) Mineral and trace element content of human transitory milk identified with inductively coupled plasma atomic emission spectrometry. *J. Nutr. Sci. Vitaminol., 36,* 65–74.
24. Coni E, Stacchini A, Caroli S, Falconieri P (1990) Analytical approach to obtaining reference values for minor and trace elements in human milk. *J. Anal. Atomic Spectrom., 5,* 581–586.
25. Parr RM, DeMaeyer EM, Iyengar VG, Byrne AR, Kirkbright GF, Schoch G, Niinisto L, Pineda O, Vis HL, Hofvander Y, Omololu A (1991) Minor and trace elements in human milk from Guatemala, Hungary, Nigeria, Philippines, Sweden and Zaire - Results from a WHO/IAEA Joint Project. *Biol. Trace Elements Res., 29,* 51–75.
26. Yoshinaga J, Li JZ, Suzuki T, Karita K, Abe M, Fuju H, Mishina J, Morita M (1992) Trace elements in human transitory milk-variation caused by biological attributes of mother and infant. *Biol. Trace Elements Res., 31,* 159–170.
27. Anderson RR (1993) Longitudinal changes of trace elements in human milk during the first 5 months of lactation. *Nutr. Res., 13,* 499–510.
28. Zapata CV, Donangelo CM, Trugo NMF (1994) Effect of iron supplementation during lactation on human milk composition. *J. Nutr. Biochem., 5,* 331–337.

CALCIUM

Country	No. of mothers		Maternal status	Study design	Age of child (months)	Normal diet (mg/day)	Supplementation			Effect	Ref.
	NS	S					Amount (mg/day)	Route	Time		
India (1960)	59	–	G	Y	1–3	170, 330, 440, 1144	–	–	–	0	1
USA (1978)	11	–	G	N	1–32	1100	–	–	–	0	3
USA (1979)	12	21	G	Y	<0.5	900	300	MM	C	0	2
USA (1983)	14	88	G	Y	0–1.5	-	200–300	MM	C	0	6
Gambia (1994)	30	30	L	Y	0–18	300	700	MC	C	0	19

0, No effect on breast-milk calcium concentration; C, chronic ingestion; G, good mineral status, no evidence of maternal deficiency; L, dietary intake regarded as low; MC, by mouth, calcium as carbonate; MM, by mouth, multivitamin and mineral mixture; N, no allowance made for stage of lactation; NS, non-supplemented mothers; S, supplemented mothers; Y, allowance made for stage of lactation.

An adult human contains approximately 1.2 kg of calcium, primarily in the bones. The calcium in the skeleton is in dynamic equilibrium; about 700 mg of calcium enter and leave the bones each day. In addition calcium is involved in blood coagulation, muscle contraction, myocardial function and maintaining the integrity of membranes (13). Homeostatic mechanisms exist to control plasma calcium concentrations within narrow limits. Different populations around the world consume widely different amounts of calcium with no apparent detriment to health. There is, however, some evidence from studies of infantile tetany through the use of non-human milk formulae with different calcium and phosphorus contents and ratios from those of human milk, that young infants may be sensitive to moderate variations in intakes of these nutrients, and that human milk can be considered as a 'gold standard' (14).

A significant proportion of breast-milk calcium (16%) is associated with the lipid fraction (5, 8) although this may be a function of milk storage; little calcium appears to be associated with the lipid layer in freshly-expressed breast-milk (19). In the aqueous layer the calcium is distributed between whey proteins and low molecular weight compounds and very little is associated with casein. This is in contrast to cow's milk where 40% of milk calcium is casein-bound (5). The concentration of calcium in breast milk changes little during early lactation (2), rises slightly until 6 weeks (4) and gradually declines there-after (3, 4, 9–11, 15, 17). Breast milk calcium can vary at least two-fold between mothers, but it appears independent of maternal age, parity, and milk output (15, 17).

There is little evidence that breast-milk calcium concentrations are greatly influenced by maternal dietary intake (1–3, 6, 11, 12). Few studies, however, have investigated the effects of calcium supplements in mothers lactating for more than 6 months or those on potentially sub-optimal calcium intakes. In general, breast-milk calcium concentrations in different populations are similar (11, 12) although one report observed high calcium contents in the milks of Ethiopian mothers consuming diets low in calcium (7). The reason for this finding is unknown. In contrast to this, breast-milk calcium levels in The Gambia and Zaire, where maternal intakes are low, were significantly lower at an equivalent stage of lactation than in the UK, where maternal intakes are much higher (15–17). The Gambian mothers also exhibited a low ratio of calcium to phosphorus (16). It is not yet known whether diet, or other factors, are responsible for these differences.

A recent study in The Gambia in which mothers were supplemented with 700 mg Ca/day for 1 year showed no effect on breast-milk calcium concentrations (19).

SUMMARY

a. The effect of maternal dietary deficiency of calcium during prolonged lactation on the secretion of breast-milk calcium is poorly understood, and is currently being assessed.

b. Calcium supplementation of mothers with apparently adequate calcium status does not affect breast-milk calcium concentrations.

REFERENCES

1. Karmarkar MG, Ramakrishnan CV (1960) Studies on human lactation. Relation between the dietary intake of lactating women and the chemical composition of milk with regard to principal and certain inorganic constituents. *Acta Paediatr., 49,* 599–604.
2. Kirksey A, Ernst JA, Roepke JL, Tsai T-L (1979) Influence of mineral intake and use of oral contraceptives before pregnancy on the mineral content of human colostrum and of more mature milk. *Am. J. Clin. Nutr., 32,* 30–39.
3. Vaughan LA, Weber CW, Kemberling SR (1979) Longitudinal changes in the mineral content of human milk. *Am. J. Clin. Nutr., 32,* 2301–2306.
4. Greer FR, Tsang RC, Levin RS, Searcy JE, Wu R, Steichen JJ (1982) Increasing serum calcium and magnesium concentrations in breast-fed infants: longitudinal studies of minerals in human milk and in sera of nursing mothers and their infants. *J. Pediatr., 100,* 59–64.
5. Fransson G-B, Lonnerdal B (1983) Distribution of trace elements and minerals in human and cow's milk. *Pediatr. Res., 17,* 912–915.
6. Feeley RM, Eitenmiller RR, Jones JB, Barnhart H (1983) Calcium, phosphorus and magnesium contents of human milk during early lactation. *J. Pediatr. Gastroenterol. Nutr., 2,* 262–267.
7. Fransson G-B, Gebre-Medhin M, Hambraeus L (1984) The human milk contents of iron, copper, zinc, calcium and magnesium in a population with a habitually high intake of iron. *Am. J. Clin. Nutr., 73,* 471–476.
8. Fransson GB, Lonnerdal B (1984) Iron, copper, zinc, calcium and magnesium in human milk fat. *Am. J. Clin. Nutr., 39,* 185–189.

9. Karra MV, Udipi SA, Kirksey A, Roepke JLB (1986) Changes in specific nutrients in breast milk during extended lactation. *Am. J. Clin. Nutr., 40,* 635–646.
10. Karra MV, Kirksey A (1988) Variation in zinc, calcium and magnesium concentrations of human milk within a 24 hour period from 1 to 6 months of lactation. *J. Pediatr. Gastroenterol. Nutr., 7,* 100–106.
11. Karra MV, Kirksey A, Galal O, Bassily NS, Harrison GG, Jerome NW (1988) Zinc, calcium and magnesium concentrations in human milk from American and Egyptian women throughout the first 6 months of lactation. *Am. J. Clin. Nutr., 47,* 642–648.
12. Moser PB, Reynolds RD, Acharya S, Howard P, Andon MB (1988) Calcium and magnesium dietary intakes and plasma and milk concentrations of Nepalese lactating women. *Am. J. Clin. Nutr., 47,* 735–739.
13. National Academy of Sciences (1989) *Recommended Dietary Allowances*, 10th edn., pp 174–184. National Academy of Sciences, Washington, DC.
14. Greer FR (1989) Calcium, phosphorus and magnesium: how much is too much for infant formulas? *J. Nutr., 119,* 1846–1851.
15. Laskey MA, Prentice A, Shaw J, Zachou T, Ceesay SM, Vasquez-Velasquez L, Fraser DR (1990) Breast-milk calcium concentrations during prolonged lactation in British and rural Gambian mothers. *Acta Paediatr. Scand., 79,* 507–512.
16. Laskey MA, Dibba B, Prentice A (1991) Low ratios of calcium to phosphorus in the breast-milk of rural Gambian mothers. *Acta Paediatr. Scand., 80,* 250–251.
17. Prentice A, Barclay DV (1991) Breast milk calcium and phosphorus concentrations of mothers in rural Zaire. *Eur. J. Clin. Nutr., 45,* 611–617.
18. Neville MC, Keller RP, Casey C, Allen JC (1994) Calcium partitioning in human and bovine milk. *J. Dairy Sci., 77,* 1964–1975.
19. Prentice A, Jarjou LMA, Dibba B, Sawo Y, Cole TJ, Stirling DM, Fairweather-Tait S Calcium requirements of lactating women: effects of a calcium supplement on the breast-milk calcium concentration of rural Gambian women. *Proc. Nutr. Soc., 53*, 258A.

CHROMIUM

Country	No. of mothers		Maternal status	Study design	Age of child (months)	Normal diet (μg/day)	Supplementation			Effect	Ref.
	NS	S					Amount (μg)	Route	Time		
Finland (1980)	10	–	L	Y	2.5	30	–	–	–	0	1
USA (1990)	6	–	G	Y	2.3	–	600	Oral	Bolus	+	8
USA (1993)	17	–	G	Y	2	41	–	–	–	0	7

0, no effect on breast-milk chromium concentration; +, breast-milk concentration related to intake; L, dietary intake regarded as low, no signs of deficiency; NS, non-supplemented mothers; S, supplemented mothers; Y, allowance made for stage of lactation.

Marginal chromium deficiency has been associated with disturbances of glucose and lipid metabolism (1, 5). In vitro, chromium concentrations of 10^{-3} M are cytotoxic and concentrations as low as 10^{-7} M inhibit RNA synthesis (3). Toxicity by ingested chromium has not been reported in humans, and long-term supplementation trials have shown that intakes of chromium 2–3 times higher than normal are safe in adults (5).

Studies of chromium concentrations in breast milk have been hampered by methodological problems. A progressive improvement in the sensitivity and precision of techniques has occurred over the years with the result that normal breast-milk concentrations obtained in recent studies are much lower than those values reported earlier (6, 7).

The concentration of chromium in breast milk is not influenced by stage of lactation either during the initial onset of lactation or in mature milk (2, 4). The distribution of chromium between the different fractions of breast milk is unknown.

There have been no studies of the effect of maternal chromium supplementation or chromium deficiency on breast-milk chromium concentrations. An increase in breast-milk chromium was observed 24–48 h after an oral bolus of 600 μg chromium was given as chromium chloride to 6 mothers, 2–3 months postpartum (8). In two investigations of the relationship between maternal dietary intake and breast-milk chromium concentrations, however, no relationship could be detected (1, 7). The mothers in one of these studies (1) were consuming diets with exceptionally low levels of chromium. Likewise, no correlation could be detected between breast milk chromium, and serum or urinary chromium levels (7).

SUMMARY

Until more knowledge is gained about chromium secretion into breast milk it is not possible to speculate on the influence of chromium deficiency or supplementation in lactating mothers.

REFERENCES

1. Kumpulainen J, Vuori E, Makinen S, Kara R (1980) Dietary chromium intake of lactating Finnish mothers: effect on the chromium content of their breast-milk. *Br. J. Nutr., 44,* 257–263.
2. Kumpulainen J, Vuori E (1980) Longitudinal study of chromium in human milk. *Am. J. Clin. Nutr., 33,* 2299–2302.
3. Beisel WR (1982) Single nutrients and immunity. *Am. J. Clin. Nutr., 35 (Suppl.),* 417–468.
4. Casey CE, Hambidge KM, Neville MC (1985) Studies in human lactation: zinc, copper, manganese and chromium in human milk in the first month of lactation. *Am. J. Clin. Nutr., 41,* 1193–1200.
5. National Academy of Sciences (1989) *Recommended Dietary Allowances*, 10th edn., pp 241–243. National Academy of Sciences, Washington, DC.
6. Cocho JA, Cervilla JR, Reygoldar ML, Fdezlorenzo JR, Fraga JM (1992) Chromium content in human milk, cows milk and infant formulas. *Biol. Trace Elements Res., 32,* 105–107.
7. Anderson RA, Bryden NA, Patterson KY, Veillon C, Andon MB, Moser-Veillon PB (1993) Breast milk chromium and its association with chromium intake, chromium excretion and serum chromium. *Am. J. Clin. Nutr., 57,* 519–523.
8. Engelhardt S, Moser-Veillon PB, Mangels AR, Patterson KY, Veillan C 1990 Appearance of an oral dose of chromium (^{53}Cr) in breast milk? In: Atkinson SA, Hansen LA, Chandra RK (Eds) *Breastfeeding, Nutrition, Infection and Infant Growth in Developed and Emerging Countries,* pp 485–487. ARTS Biomedical, St John's Newfoundland, Canada.

COPPER

Country	No. of mothers		Maternal status	Study design	Age of child (months)	Normal diet (mg/day)	Supplementation			Effect	Ref.
	NS	S					Amount (mg/day)	Route	Time		
Denmark (1950)	10	7	G	Y	<0.5	–	200	i.v.	–	0	1
USA (1979)	12	21	D	Y	<0.5	–	2	MM	C	0	4
USA (1979)	38	–	G	N	1–32	3.4	–	–	–	0	5
Finland (1980)	15	–	G	Y	2, 5	1.8	–	–	–	0	7
USA (1983)	63	39	G	Y	0–1.5	–	2	MM	C	0	12
Nigeria (1986)	226	–	G	Y	0.2–6	1.6	–	–	–	0	17

0, no effect on breast-milk copper concentration; C, chronic ingestion of supplement; D, deficient mineral status, low serum copper concentration responsive to supplementation; G, good mineral status, no signs of deficiency reported; i.v., intravenous administration; MM, by mouth, multivitamin and mineral mixture self-administered; N, no allowance made for stage of lactation; NS, non-supplemented mothers; S, supplemented mothers; Y, allowance made for stage of lactation.

Severe copper deficiency in man is rarely related to dietary intake. Certain instances, however, have been recorded in children, notably either in those who were born prematurely and fed on cow's milk formula or in those who were malnourished. Dietary copper deficiency in these cases was associated with bone disease, anaemia and neutropenia (20). Marginal copper deficiency in adults, particularly in the presence of high zinc intakes, has been implicated in cardiovascular disease (2).

Although copper is very toxic to certain animals, it has low toxicity for man (23). Little is known, however, about its toxic effect in early infancy. In addition the toxicity may vary with chemical form.

Copper occurs predominantly in the aqueous fraction of breast milk (85%), part of which is associated with low molecular weight compounds and casein. Fifteen percent of breast-milk copper is found in the lipid layer (10, 11, 13). In one study, the milk of mothers delivering prematurely contained higher concentrations of copper than that of mothers delivering at term (9), but in another (21) this was not observed. The concentration of copper is highest in colostrum and decreases steadily with increasing stage of lactation (6, 14, 15, 17–19, 22).

Breast-milk copper secretion seems unresponsive to maternal copper supplementation (7, 18). No study, however, has investigated long-term copper supplementation and its effects on the cumulative ingestion of copper by infants breast-fed for 6 months or more (see the section on zinc). Intravenous administration of copper to mothers, which raised the serum concentrations considerably, did not influence breast-milk copper concentrations when measured at several time points during the day following the dose (1). The dietary intakes of copper within populations of healthy lactating mothers were not correlated with breast-milk copper concentrations (5, 7, 17). These studies were all based on mothers without signs of copper deficiency. One study (16) observed that malnourished Indian infants received breast-milk containing less copper, zinc and manganese than those who were better nourished of the same age group, but this is difficult to interpret. A single study has investigated a group of mothers with low serum copper concentrations due to long-term use of oral contraceptives. The breast milk of these mothers had copper concentrations indistinguishable from mothers with normal copper status (4). Relatively low copper concentrations were observed in the milk from Finnish (18) and Bangladeshi (23) mothers, but the reasons for this are not known.

High intakes of zinc are known to affect copper status adversely (8). There is no evidence that supplementation of lactating mothers with zinc or iron influences breast-milk copper concentrations (3, 8).

SUMMARY

From the limited evidence available breast-milk copper concentrations are unlikely to be affected by copper supplementation or by marginal copper deficiency. In addition, ingestion of other minerals by lactating mothers which adversely affect their own copper status are unlikely to influence breast-milk copper secretion.

REFERENCES

1. Munch Petersen S (1950) On the copper content in mother's milk before and after intravenous copper administration. *Acta Paediatr., 39,* 378–388.
2. Klevay LM (1975) The ratio of zinc to copper of diets in the United States. *Nutr. Rep. Int., 11,* 237–242.
3. Picciano MF, Guthrie HA (1976) Copper, iron and zinc contents of mature human milk. *Am. J. Clin. Nutr., 29,* 242–254.
4. Kirksey A, Ernst JA, Roepke JL, Tsai J-L (1979) Influence of mineral intake and use of oral contraceptives before pregnancy on the mineral content of human colostrum and of more mature milk. *Am. J. Clin. Nutr., 32,* 30–39.
5. Vaughan LA, Weber CW, Kemberling SR (1979) Longitudinal changes in the mineral content of human milk. *Am. J. Clin. Nutr., 32,* 2301–2306.
6. Vuori E, Kuitenen P (1979) The concentrations of copper and zinc in human milk: a longitudinal study. *Acta Paediatr. Scand., 68,* 33–37.
7. Vuori E, Makinen SM, Kara R, Kuitenen P (1980) The effects of dietary intakes of copper, iron, manganese and zinc on the trace element content of human milk. *Am. J. Clin. Nutr., 33,* 227–231.
8. Fischer PWF, Giroux A, Abbe MRL (1980) Effect of zinc supplementation on copper status in adult man. *Am. J. Clin. Nutr., 40,* 743–766.
9. Mendelson RA, Anderson GH, Bryan MH (1982) Zinc, copper and iron content of milk from mothers of preterm and full-term infants. *Early Hum. Dev., 6,* 145–151.
10. Fransson GB, Lonnerdal B (1982) Zinc, copper, calcium and magnesium in human milk. *J. Pediatr., 101,* 504–508.
11. Fransson GB, Lonnerdal B (1983) Distribution of trace elements and minerals in human and cows milk. *Pediatr. Res., 17,* 912–915.
12. Feeley RM, Eitenmiller RR, Jones JB, Barnhart H (1983) Copper, iron and zinc contents of human milk at early stages of lactation. *Am. J. Clin. Nutr., 37,* 443–448.

13. Fransson GB, Lonnerdal (1984) Iron, copper, zinc, calcium and magnesium in human milk fat. *Am. J. Clin. Nutr., 39,* 185–189.
14. Casey CE, Hambidge KM, Neville MC (1985) Studies in human lactation: zinc, copper, manganese and chromium in human milk in the first month of lactation. *Am. J. Clin. Nutr., 41,* 1193–1200.
15. Dorea JG, Horner MR, Campanate ML (1985) Lacteal zinc and copper in relation to volume, total ash and energy during the first three months of lactation of Brazilian women. *Acta Paediatr. Scand., 74,* 891–896.
16. Dang HS, Jaiswal DD, Wadhwani CN, Somesandaram S, Dacosta H (1985) Breast feeding: Mo, As, Mn, Zn and Cu concentrations in milk of economically poor Indian tribal and urban women. *Sci. Total Environ., 44,* 177–182.
17. Mbofung CMF, Atinmo T (1986) Relationship between breast milk content and intake of zinc, copper and iron of Nigerian women. *Ecol. Food Nutr., 18,* 91–98.
18. Salmenpera L, Perheentupa J, Pakarinen P, Siimes M (1986) Copper nutrition in infants during prolonged exclusive breast feeding: low intake but rising concentrations of copper and ceruloplasmin. *Am. J. Clin. Nutr., 43,* 251–257.
19. Burguera M, Burguera JL, Garaboto AM, Alarcon OM (1988) Iron and copper content of human milk at early stage of lactation in Venezuelan women. *Trace Elements Med., 5,* 60–63.
20. National Academy of Sciences (1989) *Recommended Dietary Allowances*, 10th edn., pp 224–230. National Academy of Sciences, Washington, DC.
21. Saner G, Garibagaoglu M (1988) Zinc, copper, iron and manganese levels in milk from mothers of preterm and term infants. *Nutr. Rep. Int., 37,* 211–217.
22. Casey CE, Neville MC, Hambidge KM (1989) Studies in human lactation: secretion of zinc, copper and manganese in human milk. *Am. J. Clin. Nutr., 49,* 773–785.
23. Simmer K, Ahmed S, Carlsson L, Thompson RPH (1990) Breast milk zinc and copper concentrations in Bangladesh. *Br. J. Nutr., 63,* 91–96.

IRON

Country	No. of mothers NS	S	Maternal status	Study design	Age of child (months)	Normal diet (mg/day)	Supplementation Amount (mg/day)	Route	Time	Effect	Ref.
India (1960)	32	–	G	Y	3.5	11, 19,	–	–	–	0	1
USA (1976)	13	37	G	Y	1.5–3	24, 33	>30	MM	C	0	4
India (1977)	11	–	G	YL	1–6	–	200	i.m.	–	0	5
Nigeria (1978)	63	–	G,D,X	YA	0.5, 6	–	–	–	–	0	6
USA (1978)	11	–	G	N	1–32	–	–	–	–	0	7
Finland (1980)	15	–	G	Y	2, 5	40	–	–	–	0	10
Nigeria (1986)	226	–	G	Y	0.2–6	16	–	–	–	+	18
Brazil (1994)	14	14	G	Y	0–3	27–	40	M	90–100 days	0	24

0, no effect on breast-milk iron concentration; +, breast-milk concentration related to intake; A, only aqueous breast-milk iron measured; C, chronic ingestion of supplement; D, iron deficient (haemoglobin <100 g/l + other signs); G, good mineral status, no signs of deficiency reported; i.m. intramuscular administration; L, only total lactoferrin and saturation percentage of lactoferrin measured; M, by mouth; MM, by mouth, multivitamin and mineral mixture self-administered; N, no allowance made for stage of lactation; NS, non-supplemented mothers; S, supplemented mothers; X, iron overload (haemoglobin >120 g/l + other signs); Y, allowance made for stage of lactation.

The primary function of iron is that of a constituent of haemoglobin. Anaemia occurs in iron deficiency, although it may only become apparent after depletion of body stores of the element. Unlike many of the other essential trace elements, dietary iron intake is often inadequate, especially in women due to menstrual losses or during pregnancy, and iron deficiency states are common. Daily supplements of iron are usually recommended for pregnant and lactating mothers in the range 30–60 mg/day (21).

Although the toxicity of dietary iron is regarded as low, many cases of iron poisoning of children have been reported. The lethal dose for a 2-year-old child is 3 g ferrous sulfate (21). In addition, iron excess has been associated with an increased susceptibility to infection (12). The toxicity of iron depends on its oxidation state and chemical form.

The distribution of iron in breast milk is still a matter of confusion. Recent studies have shown that a significant proportion of iron is associated with the lipid layer (33%), possibly bound to xanthine oxidase in the fat globule membrane (11, 15). Lactoferrin, the predominant whey protein in human milk, has a high affinity for iron with a greater binding constant than transferrin (3). Until recently it had been assumed that all breast-milk iron was associated with lactoferrin. It now seems likely that lactoferrin in breast milk is largely unsaturated and that some of the iron in the aqueous fraction is combined with low molecular weight compounds (8). A number of studies have concentrated on measuring only aqueous iron or lactoferrin-bound iron in breast milk. Such studies must now be regarded as incomplete.

The concentrations of iron and of lactoferrin in breast milk decrease moderately as lactation progresses (9, 18, 20, 22) and are highest in colostrum. The milk of mothers who deliver prematurely has a similar iron concentration to that of mothers who deliver at term (13, 19).

Apart from one study (18), breast-milk iron secretion was found to be unaffected by, and unrelated to, dietary intake or to short-term supplementation (1, 4–7, 10, 16, 24). In addition, breast-milk iron concentrations were not correlated with maternal haemoglobin or serum ferritin levels, plasma total-iron binding capacity or transferrin saturation (2, 6, 14). A recent study (24) recorded higher levels of iron ligands and of lactoferrin in human milk following 90–100 days of iron supplementation, 40 mg/day, as a controlled experiment. A report on a small number of subjects has suggested that extremely low maternal haemoglobin levels (20–80 g/l) may be associated with raised milk iron concentrations (17). However, breast-milk iron concentrations of mothers habituated to a diet containing very high amounts of iron were similar to those of mothers in other communities (16). Maternal iron supplementation does not appear to affect the secretion of other trace elements in breast milk (4, 23).

SUMMARY

a. Breast-milk iron secretion appears to be unresponsive to maternal iron status, to iron dietary intake and to maternal supplementation.

b. It is unlikely, therefore, that ingestion of iron supplements by lactating mothers will be associated with a risk of iron toxicity in their infants, that it will correct infantile iron deficiency or that it will lead to low breast-milk concentrations of other trace elements.

REFERENCES

1. Karmarker MG, Ramakrishnan CV (1960) Studies on human lactation. Relation between the dietary intake of lactating women and the chemical composition of milk with regard to principal and certain inorganic constituents. *Acta Paediatr., 49,* 599–604.
2. Loh TT, Sinnathury TA (1971) Haematological data and milk iron in Malaysian women. *Aust. N. Z. J. Obstet. Gynaecol., 11,* 254–258.
3. Aisen P, Leibman A (1972) Lactoferrin and transferrin: a comparative study. *Biochim. Biophys. Acta., 257,* 314–323.
4. Picciano MF, Guthrie HA (1976) Copper, iron and zinc contents of mature human milk. *Am. J. Clin. Nutr., 29,* 242–254.
5. Reddy V, Bhaskaram C, Raghuramulu N, Jagadeesan V (1977) Anti-microbial factors in human milk. *Acta Paediatr. Scand., 66,* 229–232.
6. Murray MJ, Murray AB, Murray NJ, Murray MB (1978) The effect of iron status of Nigerian mothers on that of their infants at birth and 6 months and on the concentration of Fe in breast-milk. *Br. J. Nutr., 39,* 627–630.

7. Vaughan LA, Weber CW, Kemberling SR (1979) Longitudinal changes in the mineral content of human milk. *Am. J. Clin. Nutr., 32,* 2301–2306.
8. Fransson G-B, Lonnerdal B (1979) Iron in human milk. *J. Pediatr., 96,* 380–384.
9. Siimes MA, Vuori E, Kuitenen P (1979) Breast-milk iron: a declining concentration during the course of lactation. *Acta Paediatr. Scand., 68,* 29–31.
10. Vuori E, Makinen SM, Kara R, Kuitenen P (1980) The effects of the dietary intakes of copper, iron, manganese and zinc on the trace element content of human milk. *Am. J. Clin. Nutr., 33,* 227–231.
11. Lonnerdal B, Keen CL, Hurley LS (1981) Iron, copper, zinc and manganese in milk. *Ann. Rev. Nutr., 1,* 149–174.
12. Beisel WR (1982) Single nutrients and immunity. *Am. J. Clin. Nutr., 35 (Suppl.),* 417–468.
13. Mendelson RA, Anderson GH, Bryan MH (1982) Zinc, copper and iron content of milk from mothers of preterm and full-term infants. *Early Hum. Dev., 6,* 145–151.
14. Celada A, Busset R, Gutierrex J, Herrera V (1982) No correlation between iron concentration in breast milk and maternal iron stores. *Helv. Paediatr. Acta., 37,* 11–16.
15. Fransson G-B, Lonnerdal B (1983) Distribution of trace elements and minerals in human and cow's milk. *Pediatr. Res., 17,* 912–916.
16. Fransson G-B, Gebre-Medhin M. Hambraeus L (1984) The human milk contents of iron, copper, zinc, calcium and magnesium in a population with a habitually high intake of iron. *Acta Paediatr. Scand., 73,* 471–476.
17. Fransson G-B, Agarwal KN, Gebre-Medhin M, Hambraeus L (1985) Increased breast-milk iron in severe maternal anaemia: physiological 'trapping' or leakage? *Acta Paediatr. Scand., 74,* 290–291.
18. Mbofung CMF, Atinmo T (1986) Relationship between breast milk content and intake of zinc, copper and iron of Nigerian women. *Ecol. Fd. Nutr., 18,* 91–98.
19. Trugo NMF, Donangelo CM, Koury JC, Barretosilva MI, Freitas LA (1988) Concentrations and distribution pattern of selected micronutrients in preterm and term milk from urban Brazilian mothers during early lactation. *Eur. J. Clin. Nutr., 42,* 497–507.
20. Donangelo CM, Trugo NMF, Koury JC, Barretosilva MI, Freitas LA, Feldheim W, Barth C (1988) Iron, zinc, folate and vitamin B_{12} nutritional status and milk composition of low-income Brazilian mothers. *Eur. J. Clin. Nutr., 43,* 253–266.
21. National Academy of Sciences (1989) *Recommended Dietary Allowances,* 10th edn., pp 195–205. National Academy of Sciences, Washington, DC.
22. Hirai Y, Kawakata N, Satoh K, Ikeda Y, Hibayasu S, Orimo H, Yoshino Y (1990) Concentrations of lactoferrin and iron in human milk at different stages of lactation. *J. Nutr. Sci. Vitaminol., 36,* 531–544.
23. Arnaud J, Prual A, Preziosi P, Cherouvrier F, Favier A, Galan P, Hercberg S (1993) Effect of iron supplementation during pregnancy on trace element (Cu, Se, Zn) concentrations in serum and breast milk from Nigerien women. *Ann. Nutr. Metab., 37,* 262–271.
24. Zapata CV, Donangelo CM, Trugo NMF (1994) Effect of iron supplementation during lactation on human milk composition. *J. Nutr. Biochem., 5,* 331–337.

MAGNESIUM

Country	No. of mothers		Mater-nal status	Study design	Age of child (months)	Normal diet (mg/day)	Supplementation			Effect	Ref.
	NS	S					Amount (mg/day)	Route	Time		
USA (1978)	38	–	G	N	1–32	365	–	–	–	0	3
USA (1979)	12	23	G	Y	<0.5	–	104	MM	C	0	2
USA (1982)	18	–	G	N	1–6	220	–	–	–	0	6
USA (1983)	29	73	G	Y	0–1.5	–	100	MM	C	0	7

0, no effect on breast-milk magnesium concentration; C, chronic ingestion of supplement; G, no signs of maternal magnesium deficiency; MM, by mouth, multivitamin and mineral mixture self-administered; N, no allowance made for stage of lactation; NS, non-supplemented mothers; S, supplemented mothers; Y, allowance made for stage of lactation.

Magnesium deficiency due to inadequate dietary intake is rare and is generally confined to pathological conditions. Its chief manifestations are neuromuscular dysfunction and behavioural disturbances (10). Hypomagnesaemia has been associated with infantile convulsions and tremors (1).

Large oral intakes of magnesium are well tolerated by adults although doses of magnesium salts greater than 3 g have a cathartic effect (10).

Magnesium occurs in the aqueous fraction of human milk, only 2% being associated with the lipid layer (4). In one study, the concentration of magnesium varied little with stage of lactation (3) after an initial small decrease during the first week postpartum (7), but in a more recent one (8, 9), there was a moderate increase between the first and sixth month of lactation in two dissimilar communities, and also a marked diurnal variation (8). A third study (12) recorded no differences in magnesium between the first and the twelfth month of lactation in Pakistani mothers. Clearly there is controversy about changes with stage of lactation.

Magnesium secretion into breast milk does not appear to be influenced by maternal magnesium supplementation or dietary intake (2, 3, 6, 7). The supplementation data, however, are confined to the early lactation of mothers with good mineral status. Perinatal infusion of magnesium sulfate, a treatment of pre-eclampsia, was reported to raise colostral levels of magnesium transiently by a small amount (5). This study, however, compared the concentration of magnesium in the secretions of non-lactating patients with breast-feeding controls which could well account for the differences observed. Cow's milk formulae, with a considerably higher magnesium content than human milk, do not, apparently, result in magnesium toxicity or other adverse effects (11).

SUMMARY

It seems unlikely, on the very limited information available, that magnesium supplementation of lactating mothers will influence breast-milk magnesium concentrations. There is no information on the effect of maternal magnesium deficiency on breast-milk magnesium secretion.

REFERENCES

1. Wong HB, Teh YF (1968) An association between serum-magnesium and convulsions in infants and children. *Lancet*, *ii*, 18–81.
2. Kirksey A, Ernst JA, Roepke JL, Tsai T-L (1979) Influence of mineral intake and use of oral contraceptives before pregnancy on the mineral content of human colostrum and of more mature milk. *Am. J. Clin. Nutr.*, *32*, 30–39.
3. Vaughan LA, Weber CW, Kemberling SR (1979) Longitudinal changes in the mineral content of human milk. *Am. J. Clin. Nutr.*, *32*, 2301–2306.
4. Fransson G-B, Lonnerdal B (1982) Zinc, copper, calcium and magnesium in human milk. *J. Pediatr.*, *101*, 504–508.
5. Cruikshank DP, Varner MW, Pitkin RM (1982) Breast milk magnesium and calcium concentrations following magnesium sulphate treatment. *Am. J. Obstet. Gynecol.*, *143*, 685–688.
6. Greer FR, Tsang RC, Levin RS, Searcy JE, Wu R, Steichen JJ (1982) Increasing serum calcium and magnesium concentrations in breast-fed infants: longitudinal studies of minerals in human milk and in sera of nursing mothers and their infants. *J. Pediatr.*, *100*, 59–64.
7. Feeley RM, Eitenmiller RR, Jones JB, Barnhart H (1983) Calcium, phosphorus and magnesium contents of human milk during early lactation. *J. Pediatr. Gastroenterol. Nutr.*, *2*, 262–267.
8. Karra MV, Kirksey A (1988) Variation in zinc, calcium and magnesium concentrations of human milk within a 24 hr period from 1 to 6 months of lactation. *J. Ped. Gastroenterol. Nutr.*, *7*, 100–106.
9. Karra MV, Kirksey A, Galal O, Bassily NS, Harrison GG, Jerome NW (1988) Zinc, calcium and magnesium concentrations in milk from American and Egyptian women throughout the first 6 months of lactation. *Am. J. Clin. Nutr.*, *47*, 642–648.
10. National Academy of Sciences (1980) *Recommended Dietary Allowances*, 9th edn., pp 125–133. National Academy of Sciences, Washington, DC.
11. Greer FR (1989) Calcium, phosphorus and magnesium: how much is too much for infant formulas? *J. Nutr.*, *119*, 1846–1851.
12. Nagra SA (1989) Longitudinal study in biochemical composition of human milk during first year of lactation. *J. Trop. Paediatr.*, *35*, 126–128.

MANGANESE

Country	No. of mothers		Mater-nal status	Study design	Age of child (months)	Normal diet (mg/day)	Supplementation			Effect	Ref.
	NS	S					Amount (mg/day)	Route	Time		
Finland (1980)	15	–	G	Y	2, 5	5	–	–	–	+	3

+, breast-milk concentration related to intake; G, good mineral status, no signs of deficiency reported; NS, non-supplemented mothers; S, supplemented mothers; Y, allowance made for stage of lactation.

Manganese is an essential component of several enzyme systems and signs of manganese deficiency can be readily induced in animals. These include growth retardation, poor reproductive performance and impaired glucose tolerance (11). Evidence of manganese deficiency in man is lacking, although there is some suggestion that it may be responsible for certain convulsive disorders (5).

Large amounts of manganese, at concentrations above 1000 μg/g diet, are required to produce toxic effects in animals. Adverse effects of dietary manganese in adult humans have not been reported, although the element is highly toxic to the central nervous system if inhaled or injected (11). Young infants, however, may be more susceptible to manganese toxicity because of poor biliary excretion (4).

Manganese occurs predominantly in the whey fraction of human milk (71%), most of which is associated with lactoferrin. Eighteen percent is found in the lipid layer and 11% is associated with casein (7). The concentration of manganese in breast milk has been reported to remain steady during lactation after an initial decrease in the first week postpartum (1, 8). Other authors report a progressive decrease in concentration as lactation proceeds (6, 9, 10) with an increase at the end of lactation (2, 10), possibly associated with weaning (10).

There have been no studies on the effects of manganese supplements or manganese deficiency on breast-milk manganese secretion. There has been a single study which reported a positive correlation between maternal dietary intake and breast-milk concentrations of manganese (3). It therefore seems possible that manganese supplementation could lead to increased manganese secretion in breast milk.

SUMMARY

a. The limited evidence available suggests that maternal dietary intake of manganese may influence breast-milk concentrations of manganese.

b. The effect of marginal manganese deficiency on manganese secretion by lactating mothers is unknown.

c. Although dietary manganese has low toxicity for adults, little is known about its toxic effects on the growing and developing infant.

d. Supplementation of lactating mothers with manganese should be approached with caution.

REFERENCES

1. Vaughan LA, Weber CW, Kemberling SR (1979) Longitudinal changes in the mineral content of human milk. *Am. J. Clin. Nutr., 32,* 2301–2306.
2. Vuori E (1979) A longitudinal study of manganese in human milk. *Acta Paediatr. Scand., 68,* 571–573.
3. Vuori E, Makinen SM, Kara R, Kuitenen P (1980) The effects of the dietary intakes of copper, iron, manganese and zinc on the trace element content of human milk. *Am. J. Clin. Nutr., 33,* 227–231.
4. Watkins JB (1981) Nutritional considerations in treatment of disease in children. In: Suskind RM (Ed) *Textbook of Pediatric Nutrition*, pp 493–500. Raven Press, New York.
5. Tanaka Y (1982) Manganese: its possible significance in childhood nutrition in relation to convulsive disorders. *J. Am. Coll. Nutr., 1,* 113–114.
6. Stastny D, Wogel RS, Picciano MF (1984) Manganese intake and serum concentrations of human milk-fed and formula-fed infants. *Am. J. Clin. Nutr., 39,* 872–878.
7. Lonnerdal B, Keen CL, Hurley LS (1985) Manganese binding proteins in human and cows milk. *Am. J. Clin. Nutr., 41,* 550–559.
8. Casey CE, Hambidge KM, Neville MC (1985) Studies in human lactation: zinc, copper, manganese and chromium in human milk in the first month of lactation. *Am. J. Clin. Nutr., 41,* 1193–1200.
9. Saner G, Garibagaoglu M (1988) Zinc, copper, iron and manganese levels in milk from mothers of preterm and term infants. *Nutr. Rep. Int., 37,* 211–217.
10. Casey CE, Neville MC, Hambidge KM (1989) Studies in human lactation: secretion of zinc, copper and manganese in human milk. *Am. J. Clin. Nutr., 49,* 773–785.
11. National Academy of Sciences (1989) *Recommended Dietary Allowances*, 10th ed., pp 230–235. National Academy of Sciences, Washington, DC.

SODIUM

Country	No. of mothers		Mater-nal status	Study design	Age of child (months)	Normal diet (mg/day)	Supplementation		Effect	Ref.
	NR	R					Amount	Time (day)		
Netherlands (1981)	22	13	G	Y	0.5	UN	UR	5	0	3

0, no effect of breast-milk sodium concentration; G, good sodium status, no sodium-related disease; NR, non-sodium-restricted mothers; R, sodium-restricted mothers; UN, urinary output on normal diet was 132 mmol Na/day; UR, urinary output on restricted diet was 74 mmol Na/day; Y, allowance made for stage of lactation.

There is epidemiological evidence that chronic excessive sodium intake is one of several factors associated with hypertension (8). Fears have been expressed that excessive sodium intake in early life may predispose an individual to hypertension (1). Practically all ingested sodium is absorbed and the kidney is responsible for maintaining sodium homeostasis.

The electrolyte composition of breast milk closely resembles intracellular fluid, and therefore has a high potassium/sodium ratio. In normal milk all sodium enters via the secretory cell, the concentration being controlled by a sodium-potassium pump on the cell membrane and by hormonal action (2, 4). Under certain circumstances, such as mastitis, the junctions between secretory cells open allowing sodium to flow directly into the milk from extracellular fluid down a paracellular pathway (5). When this occurs sodium concentrations up to 25 times higher than normal can be observed, sometimes in the milk of only one breast. During normal mature lactation, however, the sodium (and potassium) concentrations of milk change little (7).

We have found only two studies which investigated the effect of maternal dietary sodium intake on breast-milk sodium concentrations (3, 6). In the first (3), mothers consumed a diet with low levels of sodium, sufficient to reduce their urinary sodium excretion by almost a half, and no change in breast-milk sodium concentration was noted. In the second (6), breast milk sodium levels were measured at 15 min intervals for 2 h following lunch with either low or high sodium content: no effects of meal type or of postprandial duration were observed. Considering the tight control of sodium secretion in normal mature breast milk and of sodium concentrations in plasma in order to maintain osmotic pressure, it is very unlikely that dietary sodium intake would influence breast-milk sodium secretion in the absence of maternal dehydration.

SUMMARY

It is unlikely that maternal dietary sodium intake can influence breast-milk sodium secretion.

REFERENCES

1. Guthrie HA (1968) Infant feeding practices: a predisposing factor in hypertension? *Am. J. Clin. Nutr., 21,* 863–867.
2. Peaker M (1978) Iron and water transport in the mammary gland. In: Larson BL (Ed) *Lactation: a Comprehensive Treatise*, pp 437–462. Academic Press, New York.
3. De Filippi JP, Kaanders H, Hofman A (1981) Sodium in diet and milk of breast feeding women. *Acta Paediatr. Scand., 70,* 417–418.
4. Keenan BS, Buzek SW, Garza C (1983) Cortisol and its possible role in regulation of sodium and potassium in human milk. *Am. J. Physiol., 244,* E253–E261.
5. Prentice A, Prentice AM, Lamb WH (1985) Mastitis in rural Gambian mothers and the protection of the breast by milk antimicrobial factors. *Trans. R. Soc. Trop. Med. Hyg., 79,* 90–95.
6. Ereman RR, Lonnerdal B, Dewey KG (1987) Maternal sodium intake does not affect postprandial sodium concentrations in human milk. *J. Nutr., 117,* 1154–1157.
7. Nagra SA (1989) Longitudinal study in biochemical composition of human milk during first year of lactation. *J. Trop. Paediatr., 35,* 126–128.
8. National Academy of Sciences (1989) *Recommended Dietary Allowances,* 10th edn., pp 247–255. National Academy of Sciences, Washington, DC.

ZINC

Country	No. of mothers		Maternal status	Study design	Age of child (months)	Normal diet (mg/day)	Supplementation			Effect	Ref
	NS	S					Amount (mg/day)	Route	Time (days)		
USA (1978)	11	–	G	N	1–32	15	–	–	–	0	2
USA (1979)	14	19	G	Y	<1	11	17	MM	C	0	1
Finland (1980)	15	–	G	Y	2, 5	13	–	–	–	0	3
Australia (1981)	–	2	L	Y	3P	–	150	M	7	0	6
USA (1982)	–	2	L	Y	1–5, 4–6P	–	50–150	M	120, 70	0	10
USA (1983)	63	39	G	Y	1.5	–	15	M	C	0	11
USA (1983)	23	–	G	N	1–6	11	–	–	–	0	14
USA (1984)	–	11	G	Y	<3P	–	60, 50, 100, 150	M	7–14	0	15
USA (1985)	39	14	G	Y	0–12	11	15	M	C	+	16
Brazil (1985)	28	37	E	Y	1, 4	–	15	M	C	0	17
Nigeria (1986)	226	–	D	Y	0.2–6	8	–	–	–	+	23
USA (1990)	20	20	G	Y	1–8	12	25	MM	C	0	34

0, no effect on breast-milk zinc concentration; +, breast-milk concentration related to intake; C, chronic ingestion of supplement; D, dietary intakes low compared with RDA; E, endemic zinc deficiency, 25% of adults with serum zinc levels < 11.5 μmol/l; G, good mineral status, no signs of deficiency reported; L, low breast-milk concentrations, suckling infants were zinc deficient; M, taken by mouth; MM, by mouth, multivitamin and mineral mixture self-administered; N, no allowance made for stage of lactation; NS, non-supplemented mothers; P, premature infants; S, supplemented mothers; Y, allowance made for stage of lactation.

Marginal zinc deficiency is associated with loss of appetite, decreased taste acuity, skin changes, poor wound healing and failure to grow. Severe zinc deficiency leads to hypogonadism, dwarfism and acrodermatitis enteropathica. A few cases of severe zinc deficiency in breast-fed infants born prematurely have been reported and some instances have been associated with exceptionally low breast-milk zinc concentrations or daily zinc secretion (4, 6, 7, 10, 15, 18, 31). Attempts to improve the zinc status of these children by prescribing large doses of oral zinc sulfate to the mother failed to alter the secretion of zinc in breast milk (6, 10, 15).

Zinc toxicity produces gastrointestinal irritation and vomiting and occurs with the ingestion of 2 g zinc sulfate or more. In addition, zinc supplements above 15 mg/day taken over prolonged periods may exacerbate marginal copper deficiency (32). The distribution of zinc in breast milk is not fully elucidated (24, 33, 36). Earlier studies suggested that over 70% is present in the whey fraction associated with lactoferrin, serum albumin, citrate and possibly picolinate (5, 8) that only a small amount is bound to casein, while 18% is found in the fat layer (8, 12). More recent studies suggest that zinc may be distributed relatively evenly between whey, casein and fat compartments (33, 38) and compartmentation may vary with stage of lactation (33). In normal mothers the concentration of zinc in breast milk declines with increasing stage of lactation, being the highest in colostrum and early milk (2, 19, 20, 25, 28–30, 33, 35, 37). In one study, there was no evidence of diurnal variation (21), but in another diurnal variations did occur, depending on duration of lactation and presence of supplements (19). The milk of mothers who deliver prematurely contains similar quantities of zinc to the breast milk of mothers delivering at term (9, 13, 26), although the variability between mothers is higher (13). In a South African study (22), milk from thin mothers had the same zinc content as that from mothers of normal weight. There is little evidence that short-term maternal supplementation with physiological or pharmacological doses of oral zinc has any major effect on breast-milk zinc concentrations (1, 6, 10, 11, 15, 16, 34). Similarly, self-medication with multivitamin–mineral mixtures containing zinc appears to have little short-term effect on zinc secretion in milk (16). In one study, daily supplementation of mothers with zinc 15 mg (zinc sulfate) during the whole of lactation reduced the decrease in breast-milk zinc concentrations with stage and thereby increased the cumulative ingestion of zinc by their infants. This effect, however, was not apparent until after 6 months of lactation (16). In all these studies the mothers were healthy and had no signs of zinc deficiency. In two later studies (27, 29), a 25 or 50 mg daily zinc supplement to American women throughout lactation produced a small but significant increase in their breast milk zinc levels, over those of the control groups at equivalent stages of lactation. Three dietary surveys (2, 3, 14) have shown that, within populations of healthy mothers, the intake of zinc from the normal diet does not influence breast-milk zinc concentrations. An association between zinc intakes and breast-milk concentrations was observed in Nigerian mothers with low intakes compared to the RDA (23). Ingestion of 15 mg zinc per day (zinc sulfate) throughout pregnancy and 4 months of lactation by poor Amazonian mothers living in a population where low serum zinc concentrations were common did not alter breast-milk zinc concentrations (17) and a 25 mg zinc supplement failed to influence breast milk zinc levels in another recent study of American mothers (34). There have been no studies of mothers with severe zinc deficiency and it is not possible speculate whether maternal zinc deficiency is reflected in a decrease in breast-milk zinc secretion which might be responsive to zinc supplementation.

SUMMARY

a. There is little evidence of any major effect of maternal zinc supplementation on breast-milk zinc secretion in mothers of adequate zinc status during the first 6 months of lactation. Physiological or pharmacological doses of oral zinc to these mothers are unlikely to be toxic to the breast-fed infant or to correct infantile zinc deficiency.

b. The influence of maternal zinc deficiency on breast-milk zinc concentrations is unknown.

REFERENCES

1. Kirksey A, Ernst J, Roepke J, Tsai T-L (1979) Influence of mineral intake and use of oral contraceptives before pregnancy on the mineral content of human colostrum and of more mature milk. *Am. J. Clin. Nutr., 32,* 30–39.
2. Vaughan LA, Weber CW, Kemberling SR (1979) Longitudinal changes in the mineral content of human milk. *Am. J. Clin. Nutr., 32,* 2301–2306.
3. Vuori E, Makinen SM, Kara R, Kuitenen P (1980) The effects of the dietary intakes of copper, iron, manganese and zinc on the trace element content of human milk. *Am. J. Clin. Nutr., 33,* 227–231.
4. Aggett PJ, Atherton DJ, More J, Davey J, Delves HT, Harries TJ (1980) Symptomatic zinc deficiency in a breast-fed, preterm infant. *Arch. Dis. Child., 55,* 547–550.
5. Ainscough EW, Brodie AM, Plowman JE (1980) Zinc transport by lactoferrin in human milk. *Am. J. Clin. Nutr., 33,* 1314–1315.
6. Weymouth RD, Czarnecki D (1981) Symptomatic zinc deficiency in premature, breast-fed infants associated with defective mammary gland zinc secretion. *Aust. Pediatr. J., 17,* 131.
7. Ahmed S, Blair AW (1981) Symptomatic zinc deficiency in a breast-fed infant. *Arch. Dis. Child., 56,* 315–318.
8. Lonnerdal B, Keen CL, Hurley LS (1981) Iron, copper, zinc and manganese in milk. *Annu. Rev. Nutr., 1,* 149–174.
9. Mendelson RA, Anderson GH, Bryan MH (1982) Zinc, copper and iron content of milk from mothers of pre-term and full-term infants. *Early Hum. Dev., 6,* 145–151.
10. Zimmerman AW, Hambidge KM, Lepow ML, Greenberg RD, Stover ML, Casey CE (1982) Acrodermatitis in breast-fed premature infants: evidence for a defect of mammary zinc secretion. *Pediatrics, 69,* 176–183.
11. Feeley RM, Eitenmiller RR, Benton Jones J, Barnhart H (1983) Copper, iron and zinc contents of human milk at early stages of lactation. *Am. J. Clin. Nutr., 37,* 443–448.
12. Fransson G-B, Lonnerdal B (1983) Distribution of trace elements and minerals in human and cows milk. *Pediatr. Res., 17,* 912–915.
13. Moran JR, Vaughan R, Stroop S, Coy S, Johnston H, Greene HL (1983) Concentrations and daily total output of micronutrients in breast milk of mothers delivering preterm: a longitudinal study. *J. Pediatr. Gastroenterol. Nutr., 2,* 629–634.
14. Moser PB, Reynolds RD (1983) Dietary zinc intake and zinc concentrations of plasma, erythrocytes and breast-milk in antepartum and postpartum lactating and non-lactating women: a longitudinal study. *Am. J. Clin. Nutr., 38,* 101–108.
15. Moore CME, Moran JR, Greene HL (1984) Zinc supplementation in lactating women: evidence for mammary control of zinc secretion. *J. Pediatr., 105,* 600–602.
16. Krebs NF, Hambidge KM, Jacobs MA, Rasbach JO (1985) The effects of a dietary zinc supplement during lactation on longitudinal change in maternal zinc status and milk zinc concentrations. *Am. J. Clin. Nutr., 41,* 560–570.
17. Shrimpton R, Alencar FH, Vasconcelos JC, Rocha YR (1985) Effect of maternal zinc supplementation on the growth and diarrhoeal status of breast fed infants. *Nutr. Res., Suppl. 1,* 338–342.
18. Murphy JF, Gray OP, Rendall JR, Hann S (1985) Zinc deficiency: a problem with preterm breast-milk. *Early Hum. Dev., 10,* 303–307.
19. Casey CE, Hambidge KM, Neville MC (1985) Studies in human lactation: zinc, copper, manganese and chromium in human milk in the first month of lactation. *Am. J. Clin. Nutr., 41,* 1193–1200.
20. Dorea JG, Horner MR, Campanate ML (1985) Lacteal zinc and copper in relation to volume,

total ash and energy during the first three months of lactation of Brazilian women. *Acta Paediatr. Scand., 74,* 891–896.

21. Krebs NF, Hambidge KM, Jacobs MA, Mylet S (1985) Zinc in human milk: diurnal and within-feed patterns. *J. Pediatr. Gastroenterol. Nutr., 4,* 227–229.
22. Van der Elst CW, Dempster WS, Woods DL, Heese H de V (1986) Serum zinc and copper in thin mothers, their breast milk and their infants. *J. Trop. Paediatr., 32,* 111–114.
23. Mbofung CMF, Atinmo T (1986) Relationship between breast milk content and intake of zinc, copper and iron of Nigerian women. *Ecol. Fd. Nutr., 18,* 91–98.
24. Blakeborough P, Gurr MI, Salter DN (1986) Digestion of the zinc in human milk, cow's milk and a commercial baby food: some implications for human infant nutrition. *Br. J. Nutr., 55,* 209–217.
25. Harzer G, Haug M, Bindels JG (1986) Biochemistry of maternal milk in early lactation. *Hum. Nutr: Appl. Nutr., 40A (Suppl. 1),* 11–18.
26. Trugo NMF, Donangelo CM, Koury JC, Barretosilva ML, Freitas LA (1988) Concentration and distribution pattern of selected micronutrients in preterm and term milk from urban Brazilian mothers during early lactation. *Eur. J. Clin. Nutr., 42,* 497–507.
27. Karra MV, Kirksey A, Galal O, Bassily NS, Harrison GG, Jerome NW (1988) Zinc, calcium and magnesium concentrations in milk from American and Egyptian women throughout the first 6 months of lactation. *Am. J. Clin. Nutr., 47,* 642–648.
28. Lamounier JA, Danelluzzi JC, Vannucchi H (1989) Zinc concentrations in human milk during lactation: a 6 month longitudinal study in Southern Brazil. *J. Trop. Pediatr., 35,* 31–34.
29. Karra MV, Kirksey A, Galal O, Bassily NS, Harrison GG, Jerome NW (1989) Effect of short-term oral zinc supplementation on the concentration of zinc in milk from American and Egyptian women. *Nutr. Res., 9,* 471–478.
30. Casey CE, Neville MC, Hambidge KM (1989) Studies in human lactation: secretion of zinc, copper and manganese in human milk. *Am. J. Clin. Nutr., 49,* 773–785.
31. Atkinson SA, Whelan D, Whyte RK, Lonnerdal B (1989) Abnormal zinc content in human milk. Risk for development of nutritional zinc deficiency in infants. *Am. J. Dis. Child., 143,* 608–611
32. National Academy of Sciences (19890) *Recommended Dietary Allowances*, 10th edn., pp 144–147. National Academy of Sciences, Washington, DC.
33. Bates CJ, Tsuchiya H (1990) Zinc in breast milk during prolonged lactation: comparison between the UK and The Gambia. *Eur. J. Clin. Nutr., 44,* 61–69.
34. Moser-Veillon PB, Reynolds RD (1990) A longitudinal study of pyridoxine and zinc supplementation of lactating women. *Am. J. Clin. Nutr., 52,* 135–141.
35. Simmer K, Ahmed S, Carlsson L, Thompson RPH (1990) Breast milk zinc and copper concentrations in Bangladesh. *Br. J. Nutr., 63,* 91–96.
36. Michalke B, Munch DC, Schramel P (1991) Contribution to Zn-speciation in human breast milk: fractionation of organic compounds by HPLC and subsequent Zn-determination by DCP-AES. *J. Trace Elements Electrolytes Health Dis., 5,* 251–258.
37. Dorea JG, Costa THM, Marques AO (1993) Effects of contraceptives on mothers' serum and milk zinc. *J. Nutr. Biochem., 4,* 86–91.
38. Neville MC, Keller RP, Casey C, Allen JC (1994) Calcium partitioning in human and bovine milk. *J. Dairy Sci., 77,* 1964–1975.

FLUORINE

Country	No. of mothers		Maternal status	Study design	Age of child (months)	Normal diet (W)	Supplementation			Effect	Ref
	NS	S					Amount (mg/day)	Route	Time (days)		
Canada (1968)	164	–	G	N	–	0.25; 1.0	–	–	–	+	2
Netherlands (1974)	19	–	G	Y	0.2	0.1; 1.0	–	–	–	+	3
Sweden (1981)	–	5	G	Y	0.1	–	1.5	M	1	0	4
Finland (1982)	24	–	G	N	–	0.2; 1.7	–	–	–	+	5
Sweden (1983)	106	–	G	Y	<0.1	0.2; 1.0	–	–	–	+	6
Sweden (1984)	–	1	Os	Y	7	–	11.25	M	30	++	7

0, no effect on breast-milk concentration; +, breast-milk concentration (or sub-fraction) related to intake; ++, elevation in milk concentration peaking 2h after dose; G, good fluorine status, no signs of deficiency; M, by mouth; N, no allowance made for stage of lactation; NS, non-supplemented mothers; Os, mother suffering from osteoporosis; S, supplemented mothers; W, concentration in drinking water (mg/l); Y, allowance made for stage of lactation.

Fluorine, in its ionic form, is deposited in bones and teeth in a manner proportional to the dietary intake, while blood concentrations are controlled within narrow limits. Increasing incorporation of fluorine into tooth enamel provides increasing resistance to dental caries. It is also thought that fluorine may help to protect against periodontal disease and osteoporosis (12).

High fluorine intakes, in areas where the drinking water contains more than 2 mg/l, are associated with mottling of teeth. Chronic fluorine toxicity, fluorosis, occurs in people regularly consuming in excess of 20 mg/day (5).

Little is known about the compartmentation of fluorine in breast milk. Free ionic fluoride has been detected at levels of 4–11 μg/l (5). The remaining fluorine is present as a bound fraction and constitutes between 20 and 92% of the total (5). There is no evidence of diurnal variation, or differences in levels with stage of lactation (6). Levels in breast milk are generally 150–200 times lower than in fluoridated tapwater (11).

The concentration of breast-milk fluorine is influenced by maternal dietary intake but the effect is small (2–8). When high doses of sodium fluoride were given to a lactating mother as a treatment for osteoporosis, only 0.2% of the maternal dose reached the infant (7). Small differences in breast-milk concentrations are observed between mothers living in areas where drinking water contain different levels of fluorine (9–11, 13). The changes in breast-milk fluorine secretion caused by variations in maternal dietary intake even when the mother is consuming relatively high doses of fluorine, are well within the normal limits. The intake of fluorine by breast-fed children is much less than that of bottle-fed or mixed-fed infants. Occupational exposure of mothers to fluorine, however, has been reported to result in dental fluorosis of suckling infants (1).

SUMMARY

Breast-milk fluorine concentrations do reflect maternal dietary intake of fluorine. The effect, however, is small and is unlikely to cause excessive fluorine intakes by the breast-fed infant. Problems may arise for mothers on long-term fluoride therapy or who are occupationally exposed.

REFERENCES

1. Brinch VO, Roholm K (1934) Zwei Falle von 'mottled Enamel' nach chronischer Fluorvergiftung der Mutter. *Paradentium, 6,* 148–150.
2. Simpson WJ, Tuba J (1968) An investigation of fluoride concentrations in the milk of nursing mothers. *J. Oral Med., 23,* 104–106.
3. Dirks OB, Jongeling-Eijndhoven JMPA, Flissebaalje TD, Gedalia I (1974) Total and free ionic fluoride in human and cows milk as determined by gas-liquid chromatography and the fluoride electrode. *Caries Res., 8,* 181–186.
4. Ekstrand J, Boreus LO, De Chateau P (1981) No evidence of transfer of fluoride from plasma to breast milk. *Br. Med. J., 283,* 761–762.
5. Esala S, Vuori E, Helle A (1982) Effect of maternal fluorine intake on breast milk fluorine content. *Br. J. Nutr., 48,* 201–204.
6. Spak C-J, Hardell LI, Chateau PDE (1983) Fluoride in human milk. *Acta Paediatr. Scand., 72,* 699–701.
7. Ekstrand J, Spak C-J, Falch J, Afseth J, Ulvestad H (1984) Distribution of fluoride to human breast-milk following intake of high doses of fluoride. *Caries Res., 18,* 93–94.
8. Ekstrand J, Hardell LI, Spak CI (1984) Fluoride balance studies on infants in a l-ppm-water-fluoride area. *Caries Res., 18,* 87–92.
9. Machari KR (1984) Trace elements in breast milk in endemic fluorosis areas and normal areas. *Trace Elements Anal. Chem. Med. Biol., 3,* 323–329.
10. Dabeka RW, Karpinski KF, McKenzie AD, Bajdik CD (1986) Survey of lead, cadmium and fluoride in human milk and correlation of levels with environmental and food factors. *Fd. Chem. Toxicol., 24,* 913–921.
11. Ekstrand J (1989) Fluoride intake in early infancy. *J. Nutr.*, 1856–1860.
12. National Academy of Sciences (1989) *Recommended Dietary Allowances*, 10th edn., pp 235–240. National Academy of Sciences, Washington, DC.
13. Opinya GN, Bwibo N, Valderhang J, Birkeland JM, Lokken P (1991) Intake of fluoride and excretion in mothers' milk in a high fluoride (9 ppm) area in Kenya. *Eur. J. Clin. Nutr., 45,* 37–41.

IODINE

Country	No. of mothers		Maternal status	Study design	Age of child (months)	Normal diet (μg/day)	Supplementation			Effect	Ref.
	NS	S					Amount (mg/day)	Route	Time (days)		
USA (1934)	20	–	G,D	Y	1–11	–	–	–	–	+	1
USA (1982)	–	1	G	Y	7.5	–	50	V	6	++	2
USA (1984)	37	–	G	N	0.5–4.2	–	–	–	–	(+)	3

(+), breast-milk iodine concentration related to maternal consumption of iodised salt and cows milk; +, breast-milk concentration related to intake; ++, breast-milk iodine 4–5 times normal 3d after discontinuing medication, infant showed signs of iodine poisoning; D, poor iodine status, high risk of goitre; G, good iodine status, no signs of deficiency; N, no allowance made for stage of lactation; NS, non-supplemented mothers; S, supplemented mothers; V, vaginal gel (providone-iodine); Y, allowance made for stage of lactation.

Dietary iodine deficiency is a common problem in many areas of the world. Iodine supplements, e.g. iodised table salt, are often used to increase iodine intakes in such communities. The iodine requirement of adults is approximately 1 μg/kg body weight, while for breast-fed infants 30 μg/day is regarded as adequate (6). Intakes of dietary iodine appear to be safe for adults in amounts up to 1 mg. Chronic intakes above 300 μg/day, however, are associated with an increased risk of thyrotoxicosis (6). Little is known about the compartmentation of iodine in breast milk. Free ionic iodide was shown to constitute over 80% total breast-milk iodine in one study (3). The nature of the bound iodine fraction is not completely understood although iodine containing thyroid hormones have been detected. There are conflicting reports about the influence of stage of lactation on iodine concentrations. The early study suggested that the iodine concentration increased up to 3–5 months postpartum and declined thereafter (1). Another observed no relationship with age of child between 14 days and 42 months (3), while a third (4) recorded a progressive increase from colostrum to transitional and mature milk, and a fourth (7) recorded lower values beyond 60 days of lactation. Breast-milk iodine concentrations are influenced by maternal dietary intake (3–7). A wide range of concentrations (greater than 10-fold) was noted in one study of American mothers and this variation was associated with differing maternal consumption of iodised table salt and cow's milk (3). A recent study, however, (8) found only small non-significant differences in breast milk iodine levels between an endemic goiter region and a control region of Sicily, suggesting compensatory concentrations in the goiter region. Absorption of iodine from topical preparations can also lead to an increase in breast-milk iodine secretion. A case report observed iodine toxicity in an infant receiving breast milk from a mother who had used an iodine-containing vaginal gel (2), and another (5) reported hyperthyroidism in a 6-week-old girl whose mother had used topical iodine in pregnancy and lactation.

SUMMARY

a. Although the evidence is limited, breast-milk iodine secretion appears to be influenced by maternal dietary intake. It is likely that maternal iodine deficiency will result in decreased breast-milk iodine concentrations.

b. Excessive iodine intakes for children may be toxic. Iodine supplementation of lactating mothers is not advisable unless careful monitoring of the breast-milk concentration is undertaken.

c. Iodine supplementation of a lactating mother may correct infantile iodine deficiency but caution must be exercised.

d. Topical preparations of iodine should not be recommended to mothers during lactation.

REFERENCES

1. Turner RG (1934) Iodine and thyroid hyperplasia. I. The iodine content of human skimmed milk from goitrous and nongoitrous regions. *Am. J. Dis. Child., 48,* 1209–1227.
2. Postellon DC, Aronow R (1982) Iodine in mother's milk. *J. Am. Med. Assoc., 247,* 463.
3. Gushurst CA, Mueller JA, Green JA, Seodr F (1984) Breast-milk iodide: reassessment in the 1980s. *Pediatrics, 73,* 354–357.
4. Etling N, Padovani E, Fouque F, Tato L (1986) First-month variations in total iodine content of human breast milk. *Early Hum. Dev., 13,* 81–85.
5. Danziger Y, Pertzelan A, Mimouni M (1987) Transient congenital hypo-thyroidism after topical iodine in pregnancy and lactation. *Arch. Dis. Child., 62,* 295–296.
6. National Academy of Sciences (1989) *Recommended Dietary Allowances*, 10th edn, pp 213–217. National Academy of Sciences, Washington, DC.
7. Johnson LA, Ford HC, Doran J, Richardson VF (1990) A survey of the iodide concentration of human milk. *N. Z. Med. J., 103,* 393–394.
8. Vermiglio F, Lopresti VP, Finocchiaro MD, Battiato S, Grasso L, Ardita FV, Mancuso A, Trimarchi F (1992) Enhanced iodine concentrating capacity by the mammary gland in iodine-deficient lactating women of an endemic goiter region in Sicily. *J. Endocrinol. Invest., 15,* 137–142

SELENIUM

Country	No. of mothers		Maternal status	Study design	Age of child (months)	Normal diet (μg/day)	Supplementation			Effect	Ref.
	NS	S					Amount (μg/day)	Route	Time (months)		
Finland (1984)	18	46	G	Y	1–3	30	20	MF	–	+	2
Finland (1985)	–	1	MS	–	6–10	–	MS	M	–	+	4
Finland (1985)	67	134	G	Y	0.2–6	50–75	0, 100	M	6	+	7
USA (1987)	10	–	G	Y	1–6	80	–	–	–	0	14
USA (1993)	14	17	G	Y	1–5	–	200	M	1	+	24

+, breast-milk concentration related to dietary intake; G, dietary intake regarded as adequate; M, by mouth in food, supplement due to importation of selenium-rich USA grain; MS, mother had multiple sclerosis (daily dose of 0.02–0.04 mg selenium per kg body weight during study period); NS, non-supplemented mothers; S, supplemented mothers; Y, allowance made for stage of lactation.

Selenium is a constituent of glutathione peroxidase, an enzyme which protects cells from oxidative damage and it has other roles, including a role in thyroid hormone production. Primary selenium deficiency is uncommon in man, but can be precipitated in animals (17). Epidemiological studies have suggested an association between low selenium intakes and an increased incidence of cancer and coronary artery disease (5). Sodium selenite has been used to treat multiple sclerosis (4).

Selenium toxicity is observed in animals with dietary intakes higher than 3 μg per g diet (17). Toxicity has not been described in man but intakes above 200 μg/day in adults are regarded as unsafe (17). An increased frequency of dental caries has been associated with high selenium intakes during tooth formation (1).

Breast milk selenium is correlated positively with protein content and negatively with fat content (9). It correlates with glutathione peroxidase in the aqueous fraction (8, 12, 13). Selenium is also thought to be bound to several other proteins and low molecular weight compounds (8, 12, 13, 15). Milk produced at the end of a feed is richer in selenium than at the beginning (8). The concentration of selenium is highest in colostrum and decreases during the first month of lactation (6, 10, 14, 20). In some communities no further change in selenium concentration is observed as lactation progresses (6). In an area of low maternal selenium intakes, however, milk selenium concentrations continued to fall with duration of lactation, possibly due to maternal depletion (2). In West African (Gambian) women, both season (nutritional status) and parity influenced breast milk selenium levels (19).

Several studies have suggested that maternal selenium intake or selenium status strongly influence breast-milk selenium concentration (2, 3, 4, 7, 11, 14, 16). Mothers in Finland who were habituated to a low selenium intake had raised breast-milk selenium concentrations after the importation of selenium-rich grain (2), after the provision of yeast-selenium (7) and after selenium fertilisation of crops (21).

Yeast-selenium 100 μg/day was judged to be both safe and effective (7). Selenomethionine was more effective, as a supplement, than inorganic selenite (18) and, moreover, either selenomethionine or selenium-enriched yeast reduced the rate of decline of milk selenium levels as lactation progressed beyond 8 weeks (24). No direct correlations between breast-milk selenium concentrations and intake were seen in a group of American women consuming a wide range of selenium intakes (14). However, enormous (100-fold) differences in breast milk selenium concentrations have been recorded between selenium-deficient and endemic selenosis region of China (3, 16).

SUMMARY

a. The limited evidence suggests that breast-milk selenium secretion is influenced by maternal dietary intake.
b. It is possible, therefore, that infantile selenium deficiency may be corrected by supplementation of the mother. There are, however, no guidelines for safe limits of selenium intake by infants.
c. Supplementation of lactating mothers with infants of normal selenium status may lead to toxicity in the child. Caution should therefore be exercised.

REFERENCES

1. Hadjimarkos DM (1973) Selenium in relation to dental caries. *Food Cosmet. Toxicol., 11,* 1083–1095.
2. Kumpulainen J, Vuori E, Siimes MA (1984) Effect of maternal dietary selenium intake on selenium levels in breast-milk. *Int. J. Vitam. Nutr. Res., 54,* 251–255.
3. Picciano MF (1985) Form and distribution of selenium in human milk: factors exerting an influence. In: Schaub J (Ed) *Composition and Physiological Properties of Human Milk*, pp 77–85. Elsevier, Amsterdam.
4. Westermarck T, Salmi A, Lakoma E-L, Pohja P (1985) Selenium level in milk during long-term supplementation with sodium selenite to a patient with multiple sclerosis. *Nutr. Res., Suppl. 1,* 232–234.
5. Luo X, Wei H, Yang C, Xing J, Qiao C, Feng Y, Liu J, Wu Q, Liu Y, Stoecker BJ, Spallholz JE, Yang SP (1985) Selenium intake and metabolic balance of 10 men from a low selenium area of China. *Am. J. Clin. Nutr., 42,* 31–37.
6. Robberecht H, Roekens E, Van Caillie-Bertrand M, Deelstra H, Clara R (1985) Longitudinal study of the selenium content in human breast milk in Belgium. *Acta Paediatr. Scand., 74,* 254–258.
7. Kumpulainen J, Salmenpera L, Siimes MA, Koivistoinen P, Perheentupa J (1985) Selenium status of exclusively breast-fed infants as influenced by maternal organic or inorganic selenium supplementation. *Am. J. Clin. Nutr., 42,* 829–835.
8. Picciano MF, Mannan S (1986) Effect of maternal selenium nutrition on human milk content and form. In: Hamosh M, Goldman AS (Eds) *Human Lactation, Vol 2, Maternal and Environmental Factors*, pp 371–380. Plenum Press, New York.
9. Hojo Y (1986) Sequential study on glutathione peroxidase and selenium contents of human milk.

Sci. Total Environ., *52*, 83–91.
10. Walivaara R, Jansson L, Akesson B (1986) Selenium content of breast milk sampled in 1978 and 1983 in Sweden. *Acta Paediatr. Scand.*, *75*, 236–239.
11. Mannan S, Picciano MF (1987) Influence of maternal selenium status on human milk selenium concentration and glutathione peroxidase activity. *Am. J. Clin. Nutr.*, *46*, 95–100.
12. Debski B, Picciano MF, Milner JA (1987) Selenium content and distribution of human, cow and goat milk. *J. Nutr.*, *117*, 1091–1097.
13. Milner JA, Sherman L, Picciano MF (1987) Distribution of selenium in human milk. *Am. J. Clin. Nutr.*, *45*, 617–624.
14. Levander OA, Moser PB, Morris VC (1987) Dietary selenium intake and selenium concentrations of plasma, erythrocytes and breast-milk in pregnant and postpartum lactating and non-lactating women. *Am. J. Clin. Nutr.*, 46, 694–698.
15. Van Dael P, Deelstra H, Vlaemynck G, Vanrenterghem R (1988) Distribution of selenium in cow's and human milk. *J. Trace Elements Electr. Health Dis.*, *2*, 121 (Abstract).
16. Levander OA (1989) Upper limit of selenium in infant formulas. *J. Nutr.*, 119, 1869–1873.
17. National Academy of Sciences (1989) *Recommended Dietary Allowances*, 10th edn., pp 217–223. National Academy of Sciences, Washington, DC.
18. Mangels AR, Moser-Veillon PB, Patterson KY, Veillon C (1990) Selenium utilization during human lactation by use of stable-isotope tracers. *Am. J. Clin. Nutr.*, *52*, 621–627.
19. Funk MA, Hamlin L, Picciano MF, Prentice A, Milner JA (1990) Milk selenium of rural African women: influence of maternal nutrition, parity and length of lactation. *Am. J. Clin. Nutr.*, *51*, 220–224.
20. Ellis L, Picciano MF, Smith AM, Hamosh M, Mehta NR (1990) The impact of gestational length on human-milk selenium concentration and glutathione peroxidase activity. *Pediatr. Res.*, *27*, 32–35.
21. Kantola M, Vartiainen T (1991) Selenium content of breast milk in Finland after fertilization of soil with selenium. *J. Trace Elements Electr. Health. Dis.*, *5*, 283–284.
22. McGuire MK, Burgert SL, Milner JA, Glass L, Kummer R, Deering R, Boucek R, Picciano MF (1993) Selenium status of lactating women is affected by the form of selenium consumed. *Am. J. Clin. Nutr.*, *58*, 649–652.

Drugs and Human Lactation
P.N. Bennett, editor

8. Radiopharmaceuticals

Peter J. Mountford, Colin R. Lazarus and Susan Edwards

INTRODUCTION

Administration of a radiopharmaceutical to a breast-feeding mother will result in the passage of radioactivity into her milk. Her infant will then be exposed to the radiation emitted by the ingested radioactivity. To determine the risk to her infant, the radiation exposure can be quantified in terms of the corresponding value of effective dose which allows a direct comparison to be made between the detrimental risks from different types of exposure (e.g. administration of different types of radiopharmaceutical, diagnostic X-ray examinations, background radiation) (1). If the effective dose to her breast-fed infant is considered to be too high, then it can be reduced by instructing the mother to interrupt feeding. However beyond a certain length of interruption, it is impractical for a mother to maintain her milk supply, and there is no alternative but to advise her that feeding will have to cease altogether.

Before deciding whether to request a particular nuclear medicine procedure, the referring clinician and the mother will have to be advised of the appropriate instructions in order to make an informed decision. Therefore prior knowledge is required of the effective dose to the infant when feeding is resumed and of the appropriate period of interruption. To estimate the effective dose requires not only a prior knowledge of the temporal variation of the concentration of radioactivity in milk, but also the chemical form of the radioactivity since it determines the fractional absorption of the radioactivity in the infant's gut and its subsequent anatomical distribution and rate of clearance. If an interruption period is necessary, then it can only be determined from a prior knowledge of the effective half-life of the radioactivity in milk.

The passage of radioactivity into human milk and the potential hazard to a breast-fed infant were identified soon after the first radiopharmaceuticals were adopted for routine clinical use (2–6) and during the period of atmospheric nuclear weapons testing (7–9). Subsequently there has been a continual growth both in the number of the different types of radiopharmaceuticals and in their clinical applications, particularly during the last couple of decades. However until recently, data describing the magnitude and chemical form of the radioactivity secreted in human milk following radiopharmaceutical administration remained scarce. Moreover, various methods and assumptions had been used to analyse and interpret the data, with different criteria employed to decide the safe resumption of feeding.

Two appeals published by the British Nuclear Medicine Society have resulted in the collation of further data (10, 11). Further stimulation may have come from a growing realisation that for many radiopharmaceuticals an interruption was not necessary, resulting perhaps in a greater willingness to administer them to this group of patients. Coincident with this increase in available data has been the use of the same analytical method by the authors of recent large studies (12–14), and the classification of radiopharmaceuticals into different groups according to the appropriate recommendation for interrupting breast-feeding (13–15). However despite this recent growth in relevant information, secretion data on most radiopharmaceuticals are still limited to a few case reports, and for some, there are no data at all. Hence there remains a continuing need for nuclear medicine practitioners to grasp every opportunity to acquire such data.

GLOSSARY

Radionuclides

Radionuclide	Symbol
Phosphorus-32	^{32}P
Chromium-51	^{51}Cr
Gallium-67	^{67}Ga
Selenium-75	^{75}Se
Molybdenum-99	^{99}Mo
Technetium-99m	^{99m}Tc
Indium-111	^{111}In
Indium-113m	^{113m}In
Iodine-123	^{123}I
Iodine-125	^{125}I
Iodine-131	^{131}I
Thallium-201	^{201}Tl

Terminology

Electron capture	A mode of radioactive decay of a radionuclide in which an orbital electron is captured by the nucleus, with the emission of a neutrino and X-ray.
Isomeric transition	Decay of an excited state (i.e. an isomer) of a radionuclide to its ground state.

Abundance	The number of emissions (β-particle, X or γ-ray) produced per radioactive decay, with the value usually expressed as a percentage (i.e. the number of emissions per 100 decays) (16).
Physical half-life	The time for the initial administered radioactivity to be reduced to one half by physical decay (16).
Biological half-life	The time for the initial administered radioactivity to be reduced to one half by biological elimination.
Effective half-life	The time for the initial administered radioactivity to be reduced to one half by both physical decay and biological elimination.
Decay constant	An alternative parameter for describing the rate of decay or elimination which is mathematically convenient to use in an exponential decay equation. It is equal to ln(2) divided by the physical, biological or effective half-life depending on which decay constant is required.
Absorbed dose	The energy absorbed per unit mass of tissue by the absorption of ionising radiation.
Effective dose	The risk of stochastic effects following the absorption in tissue of ionising radiation. It is derived from the absorbed dose to each irradiated tissue weighted by a factor which accounts for the quality of the radiation (ionisation density) and by a factor which represents the proportion of the stochastic risk provided by that tissue to the total risk when the whole body is irradiated uniformly (1).
Bremsstrahlung radiation	Ionising radiation emitted by a charged particle (e.g. a β-particle or an electron) as it slows down in a medium and loses kinetic energy.

Units

Bq	The SI unit of radioactivity is the Becquerel (Bq) where 1 Bq = 1 disintegration per second.
eV	An electron gains a kinetic energy of 1 electron volt (eV) when it is accelerated through a potential difference of 1 volt.
Gy	The SI unit of radiation dose absorbed in tissue is the Gray (Gy) where 1 Gy = 1 joule per kilogram.
Sv	The SI unit of effective dose is the Sievert (Sv).

REFERENCES

1. International Commission on Radiological Protection (1991) *1990 Recommendations of the International Commission on Radiological Protection* (ICRP Publication 60). Pergamon Press, Oxford.

2. Honour AJ, Myant NB. Rowlands EN (1952) Secretion of radioiodine in digestive juices and milk in man. *Clin. Sci., 11,* 447–462.
3. Nurnberger CE, Lipscomb A (1952) Transmission of radioiodine (I^{131}) to infants through human maternal milk. *J. Am. Med. Assoc., 150,* 1398–1400.
4. Karjalainen P, Penttila IM, Pystynen P (1971) The amount and form of radioactivity in human milk after lung scanning, renography and placental localization by ^{131}I-labelled tracers. *Acta Obstet. Gynecol. Scand., 50,* 357–361.
5. Vagenakis AG, Abreau CM, Braverman LE (1971) Duration of radioactivity in the milk of a nursing mother following ^{99m}Tc administration. *J. Nucl. Med., 12,* 188.
6. Wyburn JR (1973) Human breast milk excretion of radionuclides following administration of radiopharmaceuticals. *J. Nucl. Med., 14,* 115–117.
7. Jarvis AA, Brown JR, Tiefenbach B (1963) Strontium-89 and strontium-90 levels in breast milk and in mineral supplement preparations. *Can. Med. Assoc. J., 88,* 136–139.
8. Straub CP, Murthy GK (1965) A comparison of Sr-90 component of human and cow's milk. *Pediatrics, 36,* 732–735.
9. Aarkrog A (1963) Caesium-137 from fall-out in human milk. *Nature, 197,* 667–668.
10. Harding LK (1987) Breast milk - more data required. *Nucl. Med. Commun., 10,* 125–126.
11. Mountford PJ, Harding LK (1989) Breast milk – still more data required. *Nucl. Med. Commun., 10,* 777–778.
12. Ahlgren L, Ivarsson S, Johansson L, Mattson S, Nosslin B (1985) Excretion of radionuclides in human breast milk after the administration of radiopharmaceuticals. *J. Nucl. Med., 26,* 1085–1090.
13. Mountford PJ, Coakley AJ (1989) A review of the secretion of radioactivity in human breast milk: data, quantitative analysis and recommendations. *Nucl. Med. Commun., 10,* 15–27.
14. Rubow S, Klopper J, Wasserman H, Baard B, van Niekerk M (1994) The excretion of radiopharmaceuticals in human breast milk: additional data and dosimetry. *Eur. J. Nucl. Med., 21,* 144–153.
15. Administration of Radioactive Substances Advisory Committee (1993) *Notes for Guidance on the Administration of Radioactive Substances to Persons for Purposes of Diagnosis, Treatment or Research.* Department of Health, London.
16. International Commission on Radiological Protection (1983) *Radionuclide Transformations. Energy and Intensity of Emissions.* (ICRP Publication 38). Pergamon Press, Oxford.

ASSESSMENT AND CONTROL OF RISK

The general method and assumptions described below for estimating the effective dose to a breast-fed infant have been applied to all known published data and to further data supplied by nuclear medicine practitioners following the appeals by the British Nuclear Medicine Society (1). Recommendations derived from this analysis have been based on the goal of reducing the effective dose to a young infant to 1 mSv. This value of effective dose is the single annual limit suggested in the UK by the National Radiological Protection Board (2) for members of the public following the recommendations recently issued by the International Commission on Radiological Protection (ICRP) (3). It is appropriate to treat the infant as a member of the public rather than under the less restricted conditions associated with the definition of medical exposure, because the infant will not benefit directly from the radiopharmaceutical administration (3). By comparison, a patient will receive an effective dose of about 1 mSv from a conventional X-ray examination of the pelvis or thoracic spine (2), and this level of effective dose corresponds to just less than one half of the average natural background radiation dose in the UK of 2.2 mSv (4).

The adverse effects of low level radiation exposure are: cancer which will not appear for many years, and genetic damage which will only manifest itself in subsequent generations. The risk of fatal and non-fatal cancers for the whole population is given by ICRP as $5 \times 10^{-2}\,Sv^{-1}$ and $1 \times 10^{-2}\,Sv^{-1}$, respectively, and the risk of severe hereditary effects is given as $1.3 \times 10^{-2}\,Sv^{-1}$ (3). Hence a dose of 1 mSv represents an increase in fatal cancer risk of 1 in 20 000 and an increased genetic risk of 1 in 77 000. These increases in risk compare with a natural cumulative risk of 1 in 1300 for fatal childhood cancer up to age 15 years, and an estimated natural frequency in the range 1–3 in 100 for genetic disease manifesting at birth (5).

The radioactivity retained by the mother will emit a beam of photon radiation external to the mother's body. Not only will this occur for γ-ray and X-ray emitting radionuclides, but external bremsstrahlung radiation will also be produced by β-particle radiation. The intensity of this radiation, and hence the corresponding dose will increase with decrease in distance from the mother's body, and hence it will only present a potential hazard to an infant when held in close contact to the mother. This close contact radiation risk to the infant has been evaluated in a few studies (6–10), but is not considered in this chapter.

Ingested activity

The more complete sets of secretion data have shown that the concentration in milk decreased exponentially with time of expression after a peak value which was reached at varying times after administration. Therefore if the volume of milk per feed V and the time between feeds τ are assumed constant, the total activity ingested for all feeds taken beyond the peak concentration, expressed as a fraction of the administered activity A, is given by

$$F = \sum_{j=1}^{m} c_j V / \{A[1 - \exp(-\lambda_j \tau)]\} \qquad (1)$$

where m is the number of exponential components for each of which c_j is the concentration of activity ingested in the first feed and λ_j is the effective decay constant.

It was assumed that the infant ingested 850 ml of milk per day (11) with an interval of 4 h between feeds (i.e. 6 feeds per day each of 142 ml). Assuming that the mother followed the advice given below and fed her infant at 1 h before radiopharmaceutical administration (i.e. at the last practical opportunity), then the first feed would be at 3 h after administration. Where the data showed a peak activity concentration before 3 h, the value of c_j and λ_j were derived from exponential curves fitted by least squares to the measurements. If the peak was reached after 3 h, then the fraction ingested in each feed taken between 3 h and the peak was calculated from the term aV/A where a is the activity concentration in that feed, and the total fractional activity was determined by adding these contributions to the value given by equation (1). If only graphical data were available, then the fractional ingested activity was calculated from the concentration at 3 h taken from the published graph and the reported value of the effective half-life.

If it can be assumed that the activity decays monoexponentially with time after administration, with a known decay constant λ, and there is a constant time between feeds, then by making just one measurement of the concentration of radioactivity c in milk, the actual activity which would be ingested if feeding was resumed at the next occasion can be predicted simply from (12)

$$I = cK \tag{2}$$

where K is a constant given by

$$K = V\exp(-\lambda\tau)/[1 - \exp(-\lambda\tau)] \tag{3}$$

and can be considered as the total 'effective ingestion volume' which accounts for the progressively decreasing importance of each feed with time after administration because of the corresponding decrease in activity concentration. Although suggested values of K have been published (12), they can be calculated for any of the radiopharmaceuticals described in this chapter using the tabulated half-life, and using whatever values of (constant) volume per feed and (constant) time between feeds may be considered appropriate.

Dosimetry

The effective dose D to a young infant was estimated from

$$D = AFe \tag{4}$$

by substituting the maximum usual administered activity permitted in the UK for A in the above equation (12). Because the variation with age of e, the effective dose to an infant per unit activity ingested, is not available, the effective dose to the infant was calculated from ICRP published values of the effective dose to an adult per unit activity ingested, increased by the ratio of the adult 'standard man' total body weight (70 kg) to the infant's body weight (13, 14). The value of e increases as the age of the infant decreases, and therefore to err on the side of caution, the infant's body weight was assumed to be 4 kg. Values of e for a 4 kg infant are given below for the radionuclides included in this chapter.

Radionuclide	e (mSv MBq^{-1})
^{51}Cr	0.17
^{67}Ga	4.4
^{111}In	7.0
^{123}I	3.9
^{125}I	350
^{131}I	438
^{99m}Tc	0.35
^{201}Tl	1.2

Interruption periods

If the radioactivity concentration expressed in milk decays monoexponentially with time after administration, then the period P (h) to interrupt feeding in order to reduce the infant's effective dose D to x (mSv) is given by

$$P = t_{1/2}[\ln(D/x)/\ln(2)] + 3 \qquad (5)$$

where $t_{1/2}$ (h) is the effective half-life of the activity in milk. If the radioactivity concentration in milk decayed with more than one exponential component, then for simplicity, the interruption period was calculated from the effective half-life of the longest decay component. In the following tables, the interruption time has been calculated for a value for x of 1 mSv.

Recommendations

Before a radiopharmaceutical is administered to a breast-feeding mother, the following questions should be answered which follow the principle of ensuring the radiation exposure of her infant will be as low as reasonably practicable:

a. Is an investigation essential?
b. Is there an alternative procedure which does not involve the administration of a radiopharmaceutical?
c. Is there an alternative radiopharmaceutical which yields a lower effective dose to the infant?
d. Can a diagnostic result be obtained from the procedure with less than the usual administered activity?
e. What is the possibility of a repeat investigation? If the study is to be repeated, the total effective dose to the infant from both investigations should not exceed 1 mSv even if the second procedure is carried out up to 1 year after the first.

The interruption period to give a lower effective dose than 1 mSv can be estimated from equation (5).

The mother can be reassured that if she follows the advice issued to her, then the effective dose to her infant will be no more than 1 mSv, and in most cases it will be a lot less than this value. She should be advised to express some milk and store it in a refrigerator, and to breast-feed her infant immediately before attending the nuclear medicine department. The stored milk can be used to feed her infant during the subsequent period of interruption. The advice for interrupting feeding will depend on which of the following four categories applies to the radiopharmaceutical to be administered.

I. *Interruption not essential:* breast-feeding need not be interrupted because the activity concentrations in milk are so small that the effective dose to the infant is equal to or less than 1 mSv. In practice, a mother can be reassured by advising a short *interruption* (e.g. 4 h), at the end of which milk should be expressed and discarded.

II. *Interruption for a definite period*: breast-feeding should be interrupted for the period given, starting from the time the radiopharmaceutical was administered to the mother. During this period of interruption, breast milk should be expressed at normal feeding times and discarded. Apart from the effective dose to the infant and the effective half-life of the radioactivity in milk, the other main criteria for including a radiopharmaceutical in this category is the quantity of available data.

III. *Interruption with measurement*: although the available data indicate that breast-feeding can be resumed after a period of interruption, they are too limited for a definite period to be recommended. Instead, the concentration of radioactivity in expressed milk should be measured, and feeding interrupted for the period (derived by the method described above) which will reduce the infant's effective dose to 1 mSv.

IV. *Cessation*: the period of interrruption calculated from the available data is so long that the mother will have to be advised to discontinue feeding altogether.

Colostrum

These four categories of recommendation apply to when the mother is producing mature milk. The sparse data available to describe the passage of radioactivity in the early stages of lactation, when she may still be producing colostrum, indicate that the pattern of secretion is different to mature milk (15). However because this data is sparse and the pattern is likely to vary between patients, then unless the radiopharmaceutical falls into category IV, mothers likely to be producing colostrum should be advised to follow the recommendations in category III for all other radiopharmaceuticals.

Radiopharmaceutical and radionuclide quality control

Animal and human studies have shown that the concentration of free pertechnetate ($^{99m}TcO_4^-$) and free iodide (I^-) in milk is higher than in plasma (16–18), and a review of the available human data has shown that higher concentrations of radioactivity are secreted in milk when a radiopharmaceutical has been administered which results in the circulating plasma containing free radioiodide or free pertechnetate (1). However, the advice contained in the chapter assumes that the radiopharmaceutical administered to the mother is purely in the chemical form stated, and contains no other radiochemical species. Therefore it is imperative to ensure that a negligible quantity of the unbound form of the radionuclide is administered with any radioiodinated or ^{99m}Tc-labelled radiopharmaceutical. Moreover radiopharmaceuticals labelled with ^{123}I may also contain ^{124}I and ^{125}I as contaminants, with the levels of contamination varying with the manufacturer. The data given below for ^{123}I-labelled radiopharmaceuticals refer only to the ^{123}I activity, and these contamination levels will need to be determined before a recommendation for resuming breast-feeding can be given.

High concentrations of radioactivity are also secreted when the circulating plasma contains radioactivity bound to breast milk protein. In the case of ^{67}Ga-citrate and ^{75}Se-methionine, protein-bound activity cannot be avoided, but for ^{111}In-leucocytes, protein-bound activity can be avoided by ensuring that a negligible quantity of non-cell bound activity is administered with the labelled leucocytes.

REFERENCES

1. Mountford PJ, Coakley AJ (1989) A review of the secretion of radioactivity in human breast milk: data, quantitative analysis and recommendations. *Nucl. Med. Commun., 10,* 15–27.
2. National Radiological Protection Board (1993) *Occupational, Public and Medical Exposure.* (Documents of the NRPB Vol 4 No 2) HMSO, London.
3. International Commission on Radiological Protection (1991) *1990 Recommendations of the International Commission on Radiological Protection* (ICRP Publication 60). Pergamon Press, Oxford.
4. Hughes JS, O'Riordan MC (1993) *Radiation Exposure of the UK Population 1993 Review* (NRPB-R263) HMSO, London.
5. National Radiological Protection Board (1993) *Board Statement on Diagnostic Medical Exposures to Ionising Radiation During Pregnancy.* (Documents of the NRPB Vol 4 No 4) HMSO, London.
6. Mountford PJ (1987) Estimation of close contact doses to young infants from surface dose rates on radioactive adults. *Nucl. Med. Commun., 8,* 857–863.
7. Mountford PJ, O'Doherty MJ, Forge NI, Jefferies A, Coakley AJ (1991) Radiation dose rates from adult patients undergoing nuclear medicine investigations. *Nucl. Med. Commun., 12,* 767–777.
8. Rubow S, Klopper J, Wasserman H, Baard B, van Niekerk M (1994) The excretion of radiopharmaceuticals in human breast milk: additional data and dosimetry. *Eur. J. Nucl. Med., 21,* 144–153.

9. O'Doherty MJ, Kettle AG, Eustance CP, Mountford PJ, Coakley AJ (1993) Radiation dose rates from adult patients receiving ^{131}I therapy for thyrotoxicosis. *Nucl. Med. Commun., 14,* 160–168.
10. Barrington SF, Kettle AG, O'Doherty MJ, Wells CP, Somer EJR, Coakley AJ (1996) Radiation dose rates from patients receiving iodine-131 therapy for carcinoma of the thyroid. *Eur. J. Nucl. Med., 23,* 123–130.
11. International Commission on Radiological Protection (1977) *Report of the Task Group on Reference Man* (ICRP Publication 23). Pergamon Press, Oxford.
12. Administration of Radioactive Substances Advisory Committee (1993) *Notes for Guidance on the Administration of Radioactive Substances to Persons for Purposes of Diagnosis, Treatment or Research.* Department of Health, London.
13. International Commission on Radiological Protection (1980) *Limits for Intakes of Radionuclides by Workers* (ICRP Publication 30). Pergamon Press, Oxford.
14. International Commission on Radiological Protection (1991) *Annual Limits on Intake of Radionuclides by Workers Based on the 1990 Recommendations* (ICRP Publication 61). Pergamon Press, Oxford.
15. Heaton B (1979) The build up of technetium in breast milk following the administration of $^{99}Tc^{m}O_4$ labelled macroaggregated albumin. *Br. J. Radiol., 52,* 149–150.
16. Mountford PJ, Heap RB, Hamon M, Fleet IR, Coakley AJ (1987) Suppression of technetium-99m and iodine-123 secretion in milk of lactating goats. *J. Nucl. Med., 28,* 1187–1191.
17. Ennis ME, Johnson JE, Ward GM, Boamah KN (1989) Technetium metabolism by lactating goats. *Health Phys., 57,* 321–330.
18. Honour AJ, Myant NB. Rowlands EN (1952) Secretion of radioiodine in digestive juices and milk in man. *Clin. Sci., 11,* 447–462.

NOTES ON THE TABLES

a. The radiopharmaceuticals are tabulated according to the alphabetical order of the radionuclide. Where the same radionuclide is used to label more than one radiopharmaceutical, then they are subgrouped according to the alphabetical order of the name of the unlabelled compound.

b. The abundance of β-particle and γ-ray emission is given as a percentage value in parentheses after the energy of the emission.

c. The radiopharmaceutical was administered once to each patient in every case analysed.

d. For a case to qualify for the above analysis, it had to include a measurement of the activity concentration in breast milk expressed on three different occasions after radiopharmaceutical administration.

e. The time to reach 1 mSv is the period for which feeding should be interrupted after the radiopharmaceutical was administered in order for the effective dose to the infant to reduce to this value.

f. The metabolic and dosimetric models used to derive the effective dose per unit activity ingested (e) were not designed specifically for young infants. These models should account for the following factors specific to young infants: the fractional absorption from the gut, anatomical distribution and metabolism of the different chemical forms of the radionuclides secreted in milk, and organ weighting factors for this age group. Moreover, information on the chemical form of the radioactivity secreted in milk following radiopharmaceutical administration remains limited. Hence the recommendations are based on 'worst case' assumptions (see note **g** below).

g. The 'worst case' assumptions include:- the maximum calculated value of fractional activity ingested, the maximum usual administered activity permitted in the UK (see reference (12) above), the maximum measured value of effective half-life, and values of effective dose to the infant per unit activity ingested (e) which were derived by increasing the adult values by body weight ratio. Effective dose probably increases with decrease in weight at a slower rate than given by this method and infants may excrete the radioactivity at a faster rate than adults.

h. The values of weight-corrected effective dose per unit activity ingested used in the dosimetry estimations apply to a specific chemical form of the radionuclide which is given in each table, together with a summary of the limited evidence describing the chemical form of the radioactivity in milk.

i. Although the effective dose per unit activity ingested to an infant weighing less than 4 kg will be greater than the values tabulated, this increase in effective dose will be countered by a lighter infant being more likely to ingest less than 850 ml per day .

j. The tabulated data and the recommendations apply to the secretion of mature milk only. If the mother is likely to be producing colostrum, then the recommendation given above should be followed.

k. Radionuclide purity is assumed in each case; in other words, the estimated effective dose to the infant and the corresponding recommendation is based on the assumption that no other contaminating radionuclide was administered.

FURTHER READING

1. Beasley TM, Palmer HE, Nelp WB (1966) Distribution and excretion of technetium in humans. *Health. Phys., 12,* 1425–1435.
2. Crawford-Brown KJ (1983) An age-dependent model for the kinetics of uptake and removal of radionuclides from the G.I.tract. *Health Phys., 44,* 609–622.
3. Taylor DM, Gerber GB, Stather JW (editors) (1992) Age-dependent factors in the biokinetics and dosimetry of radionuclides. Proceedings of a Workshop held in Schloss Elmau, Germany, November 5–8, 1991. *Radiat. Prot. Dosim., 41 (2–4).*
4. International Commission on Radiological Protection (1993) *Radiation Dose to Patients from Radiopharmaceuticals (Including Addendum 1)* (ICRP Publication 53, 2nd edn.). Pergamon Press, Oxford.
5. Coakley AJ, Mountford PJ (1985) Nuclear medicine and the nursing mother. *Br. Med. J., 291,* 159–160.
6. Romney BM, Nickoloff EL, Esser PD, Alderson PO (1986) Radionuclide administration to nursing mothers: mathematically derived guidelines. *Radiology, 160,* 549–554.

7. Fulton B, Moore L (1990) The galactopharmacopedia. Radiopharmaceuticals and lactation. *J. Human Lact., 6,* 181–184.
8. International Commission on Radiological Protection (1987) *Protection of the Patient in Nuclear Medicine* (ICRP Publication 52). Pergamon Press, Oxford.
9. Mountford PJ (1991) Radiation protection for the parent and child in diagnostic nuclear medicine. *Eur. J. Nucl. Med., 18,* 940–943.
10. Goldstone KE, Jackson PC, Myers MJ, Simpson AE (editors) (1991) *Radiation Protection in Nuclear Medicine and Pathology* (IPSM Report 63). Institute of Physical Sciences in Medicine, York.

RADIOACTIVE CHROMIUM

The radionuclide ^{51}Cr decays to stable vanadium by 100% electron capture, emitting γ-rays with an energy of 320 keV (9%). The physical half-life is 27.7 days.

The ICRP dosimetry data for ingested activity assumes a fractional absorption of 1% for chromium in its trivalent form (1, 2).

REFERENCES

1. International Commission on Radiological Protection (1980) *Limits for Intakes of Radionuclides by Workers* (ICRP Publication 30). Pergamon Press, Oxford.
2. International Commission on Radiological Protection (1991) *Annual Limits on Intake of Radionuclides by Workers Based on the 1990 Recommendations* (ICRP Publication 61). Pergamon Press, Oxford.

^{51}Cr-ETHYLENEDIAMINETETRAACETIC ACID

GENERAL

^{51}Cr-Ethylenediaminetetraacetic acid (^{51}Cr-EDTA) is used for determination of glomerular filtration rate. After intravenous injection the radiopharmaceutical is not bound by plasma proteins. Approximately 98% of the dose is normally excreted in urine within 24 h.

EVALUATION OF DATA

Analysis of the available data describing the passage of ^{51}Cr into milk gives the following results.

No. of cases; route	Fractional ingested activity (%)			Effective half-life (h)			Administered activity (MBq)	Effective dose to infant (mSv)	Time to reach 1 mSv (h)	Ref
	Max.	Min.	Mean	Max.	Min.	Mean				
3; i.v.	0.06	0.01	0.03	11	5	7.7	3	0.001	–	1,2

RADIOACTIVITY IN MILK

The fractional activity concentration was at a maximum value in the first milk sample which was measured at about 2 h after administration in one case (1) (7×10^{-5} % ml^{-1}) and at 10 h in both the other cases (1, 2) (1.8×10^{-4} and 1.2×10^{-5} % ml^{-1} respectively). It then decreased monoexponentially with a very minor proportion showing a much longer effective half-life.

ASSESSMENT

If any of the radioactivity in milk was bound to EDTA, then its rapid renal excretion would tend to reduce the infant's dose. After a single intravenous administration of 3 MBq of ^{51}Cr-EDTA, the maximum effective dose is estimated to be about 1 μSv for uninterrupted breast-feeding with the first feed taken at 3 h after radiopharmaceutical administration.

RECOMMENDATION

Category I. Interruption not essential

Breast-feeding need not be interrupted because the activity concentrations in milk and the estimated effective dose to the infant are small. In practice, a mother can be reassured by advising a short interruption (e.g. 4 h), at the end of which milk should be expressed and discarded.

REFERENCES

1. Ahlgren L, Ivarsson S, Johansson L, Mattson S, Nosslin B (1985) Excretion of radionuclides in human breast milk after the administration of radiopharmaceuticals. *J. Nucl. Med., 26,* 1085–1090.
2. Mattson S, Johansson L, Nosslin B, Ahlgren L (1981) Excretion of radionuclides in human breast milk following administration of ^{125}I-fibrinogen, ^{99}Tc^{m}-MAA, and ^{51}Cr-EDTA. In Watson EE, Schlafke AT, Coffey JL, Cloutier RJ (Eds) *Proc. 3rd Int. Radiopharmaceut. Dosimetry Symp.,* HHS Publications FDA 81–8166, pp 102–110. US Department of Health and Human Services, Rockville, MD.

RADIOACTIVE GALLIUM

The radionuclide ^{67}Ga has a physical half-life of 78.3 h and decays to stable zinc by electron capture with the following γ-ray emissions: 93 keV (38%), 185 keV (21%), 300 keV (17%) and 394 keV (5%).

The ICRP dosimetry data for ingested activity assumes a fractional absorption of 0.1% for all forms of gallium ingested (1, 2).

REFERENCES

1. International Commission on Radiological Protection (1980) *Limits for Intakes of Radionuclides by Workers* (ICRP Publication 30). Pergamon Press, Oxford.
2. International Commission on Radiological Protection (1991) *Annual Limits on Intake of Radionuclides by Workers Based on the 1990 Recommendations* (ICRP Publication 61). Pergamon Press, Oxford.

^{67}Ga-GALLIUM CITRATE

GENERAL

^{67}Ga-Gallium citrate is used for the localisation of some soft-tissue tumours, staging of Hodgkin's disease and lymphomas, localising areas of infection and inflammation, and following tumour response to therapy. Normal uptake is predominantly to bone, liver, red marrow, spleen, adrenals, kidney and gastrointestinal tract. After intravenous injection about 30% of the dose in the blood is bound to plasma protein, mainly transferrin. Plasma clearance is slow with about 20% of the dose in plasma at 24 h, and about 25% excreted in the kidneys at this time. A further 10% of the dose is excreted in the faeces over about 7 days. The blood clearance curve is biexponential with biological half-life components of about 6 h and 7 days.

EVALUATION OF DATA

Analysis of the available data describing the passage of ^{67}Ga into milk gives the following results.

No. of cases; route	Fractional ingested activity (%)			Effective half-life (h)			Administered activity (MBq)	Effective dose to infant (mSv)	Time to reach 1 mSv (h)	Ref
	Max.	Min.	Mean	Max.	Min.	Mean				
5; i.v.	16[a]	3.2	[b]	68	16	[b]	150	105	460	1–3

[a] From 72 h after administration (1).
[b] The combined mean value of all 5 cases could not be estimated because separate data was not published for the 4 cases in reference (3), but the above method of analysis was used in that reference which reported a mean fractional ingested activity for these 4 cases alone of 7.2%, and a mean effective half-life of 51 h

RADIOACTIVITY IN MILK

After intravenous administration of ^{67}Ga citrate, high concentrations of radioactivity have been found in human milk, and this radioactivity has been shown to be contained in the lactoferrin-rich protein fraction (4). Where the activity in milk had been measured at less than 2 days after administration (two cases), the maximum fractional activity concentration of 3.2×10^{-3} % ml^{-1} occurred in the first sample taken at 12 h in one case, but in the other patient, the peak fractional activity concentration of 1.9×10^{-3} % ml^{-1} was delayed until the third sample taken at 38 h (2). Thereafter, the activity concentration decreased monoexponentially with time after administration. Because of this possibility of a delayed peak in the activity concentration, in the case where the first breast milk sample was not expressed until 72 h after administration (fractional activity concentration of 5×10^{-3} % ml^{-1}), the fractional ingested activity was estimated for feeding being resumed at that later time, yet it produced the maximum value of fractional ingested activity (1). The data in other published cases were insufficient for analysis, but were consistent with that used in the above table (4–6).

EFFECT ON THE INFANT

In one case, a 9-month-old infant was breast-fed for 48 h after administration of 185 MBq of ^{67}Ga citrate (2). At the end of that period, the radioactivity retained by the infant was found to be 6.5 MBq (3.5% of the administered activity) and was restricted to the intestines. Breast-feeding was stopped, and the infant was treated with laxatives. By 96 h after administration, the retained activity had decreased to 0.6 MBq (0.3%). No adverse effects in the infant were reported.

ASSESSMENT

After a single intravenous administration of 150 MBq of ^{67}Ga citrate, the maximum effective dose is estimated to be 105 mSv for uninterrupted breast-feeding with the first feed taken at 3 h after radiopharmaceutical administration, requiring an interruption period of 460 h (19.2 days) to reduce it to 1 mSv. This effective dose estimate is based on the ICRP assumption of a fractional absorption of only 0.1%, and this assumption is consistent with the report describing an apparent absence of absorption of ^{67}Ga by the breast-fed infant with the activity being restricted to the intestines.

RECOMMENDATION

Category IV. Cessation

The period of interrruption calculated from the available data is so long that the mother will have to be advised to discontinue feeding altogether.

REFERENCES

1. Tobin RE, Schneider PB (1976) Uptake of ^{67}Ga in the lactating breast and its persistence in milk: case report. *J. Nucl. Med., 17,* 1055–1056.
2. Rubow S, Klopper J, Scholtz P (1991) Excretion of gallium 67 in human breast milk and its inadvertent ingestion by a 9-month-old child. *Eur. J. Nucl. Med., 18,* 829–833.
3. Rubow S, Klopper J, Wasserman H, Baard B, van Niekerk M (1994) The excretion of radiopharmaceuticals in human breast milk: additional data and dosimetry. *Eur. J. Nucl. Med., 21,* 144–153.
4. Hoffer PB, Huberty J, Khayam-Bashi H (1977) The association of Ga-67 and lactoferrin. *J. Nucl. Med., 18,* 713–717.
5. Greener AW, Conte PJ, Steidley KD (1970) Update on gallium-67 concentration in human breast milk. *J. Nucl. Med., 11,* 171–172.
6. Larson SM, Schall GL (1971) Gallium 67 concentration in human milk. *J. Am. Med. Assoc., 218,* 257.

RADIOACTIVE INDIUM

The radionuclide ^{111}In decays by electron capture to stable cadmium with a physical half-life of 67.9 h. Two γ-rays of energy 171 keV (91%) and 245 keV (94%) are emitted together with cadmium X-rays of energy 23–27 keV.

The ICRP dosimetry data for ingested activity assumes a fractional absorption of 2% for all compounds of indium (1, 2).

REFERENCES

1. International Commission on Radiological Protection (1980) *Limits for Intakes of Radionuclides by Workers* (ICRP Publication 30). Pergamon Press, Oxford.
2. International Commission on Radiological Protection (1991) *Annual Limits on Intake of Radionuclides by Workers Based on the 1990 Recommendations* (ICRP Publication 61). Pergamon Press, Oxford.

^{111}In-LEUCOCYTES

GENERAL

Autologous ^{111}In-leucocytes are used for localising sites of infection and inflammation. There is negligible release of ^{111}In from labelled leucocytes in plasma, but simultaneous administration of unbound ^{111}In will lead ultimately to some radioactivity bound to breast milk protein. The most commonly used labelling procedure relies on ^{111}In oxine as the radiopharmaceutical and results in a mixed cell preparation with most of the radioactivity bound to granulocytes, and the remainder bound to other types of leucocytes, platelets and erythrocytes. The normal uptake is to the liver, spleen and red bone marrow. After intravenous reinjection, about half of the radioactivity is taken up more or less immediately to these organs, and the remainder is cleared again to these organs from the blood with a half-life of about 7.5 h.

EVALUATION OF DATA

Analysis of the available data describing the passage of ^{111}In into milk gives the following results.

No. of cases; route	Fractional ingested activity (%)			Effective half-life (h)			Administered activity (MBq)	Effective dose to infant (mSv)	Time to reach 1 mSv (h)	Ref
	Max.	Min.	Mean	Max.	Min.	Mean				
3; i.v.	0.45	0.12	0.27	134	49	88	20	0.6	–	1–3

RADIOACTIVITY IN MILK

Administration of an excessive quantity of unbound ^{111}In will lead to greater concentrations of radioactivity in milk, and therefore care must be taken to minimise this quantity in the labelled cell suspension before reinjection. In each case, the fractional activity concentration showed a delayed peak with a maximum value in the samples measured at 13 h (1), 16 h (2) and 19 h (3) after administration followed by a monoexponential decrease. These maximum values were 3.1×10^{-5} % ml^{-1} (1), 6.2×10^{-5} % ml^{-1} (2) and 8.1×10^{-5} % ml^{-1} (3). In two cases, cell bound radioactivity in milk was considered unlikely, and a significant proportion of the activity in milk was associated with the protein precipitate (1, 2). The data in one other case were insufficient for analysis, but were consistent with that used in the above table (4).

ASSESSMENT

After a single intravenous administration of 20 MBq of ^{111}In-leucocytes, the maximum effective dose is estimated to be 0.6 mSv for uninterrupted breast-feeding with the first feed taken at 3 h after radiopharmaceutical administration.

RECOMMENDATION

Category I. Interruption not essential

Breast-feeding need not be interrupted because the activity concentrations in milk and the estimated EDE to the infant are small. In practice, a mother can be reassured by advising a short interruption (e.g. 4 h), at the end of which milk should be expressed and discarded.

REFERENCES

1. Mountford PJ, Coakley AJ (1985) Excretion of radioactivity in breast milk after an Indium-111 leukocyte scan. *J. Nucl. Med., 26,* 1096–1097.
2. Hesslewood SR, Thornback JR, Brameld JM (1988) Indium-111 in breast milk following administration of In-111 labelled leukocytes. *J. Nucl. Med., 29,* 1301–1302.
3. Hesslewood SR (1988) Unpublished data.
4. Butt D, Szaz KF (1986) Indium-111 radioactivity in breast milk. *Br. J. Radiol., 59,* 80.

RADIOACTIVE IODINE

Three radionuclides of iodine are routinely used in nuclear medicine: ^{123}I, ^{125}I and ^{131}I.

The radionuclide ^{123}I decays by electron capture to stable tellerium with a physical half-life of 13.2 h, and with the emission of a 159 keV (83%) γ-ray and a 28 keV tellerium X-ray. Radiopharmaceuticals labelled with ^{123}I may also contain ^{124}I and ^{125}I as contaminants, with the levels of contamination varying with the manufacturer. The data given below for ^{123}I-labelled radiopharmaceuticals refer only to the ^{123}I activity, and these contamination levels will need to be determined before a recommendation for resuming breast-feeding can be resumed.

The radionuclide ^{125}I decays by electron capture to stable tellerium with a physical half-life of 60.1 days, and with the emission of a 35 keV (7%) γ-ray and 25 keV tellerium X-rays.

The radionuclide ^{131}I decays by β-particle emission to stable xenon with a physical half-life of 8.04 days, and with the emission of a 192 keV (89%) β-particle, and a 365 keV (81%) γ-ray. In addition four other β-particles and eight other γ-rays are associated with its decay.

Radioiodine-labelled radiopharmaceuticals tend to produce high concentrations of radioactivity in milk, because some are prone to de-iodination in vivo and animal studies have shown that radioioidide is concentrated by the mammary gland. The concentration in milk will be affected by the degree of thyroid trapping of circulating radioiodide which in turn will depend on thyroid function as well as on the simultaneous administration of a thyroid-blocking agent such as potassium perchlorate. The concentration in milk will also be directly affected by the thyroid-blocking agent because the latter has been shown in animal studies to suppress the secretion of radioiodide in milk (1).

For each radioiodine-labelled radiopharmaceutical, it was assumed that only free radioiodide was secreted for which the ICRP dosimetry data assumes complete fractional absorption of ingested activity (2, 3).

REFERENCES

1. Mountford PJ, Heap RB, Hamon M, Fleet IR, Coakley AJ (1987) Suppression of technetium-99m and iodine-123 secretion in milk of lactating goats. *J. Nucl. Med., 28,* 1187–1191.
2. International Commission on Radiological Protection (1980) *Limits for Intakes of Radionuclides by Workers* (ICRP Publication 30). Pergamon Press, Oxford.
3. International Commission on Radiological Protection (1991) *Annual Limits on Intake of Radionuclides by Workers Based on the 1990 Recommendations* (ICRP Publication 61). Pergamon Press, Oxford.

^{123}I-METAIODOBENZYLGUANIDINE

GENERAL

Metaiodobenzylguanidine (MIBG) is an analogue of the adrenergic blocking agent guanethidine, and has an affinity for tissues endowed with sympathetic nerves such as adrenal medulla and myocardium. When radiolabelled with ^{123}I, it is used for the diagnosis and localisation of benign and malignant phaeochromocytomas, adrenal medulla hyperplasias, paragangliomas and neuroblastoma in children. After intravenous administration, there is initial rapid uptake by the liver, and with some accumulation in the lungs, heart, spleen, salivary glands and adrenal medulla. It is largely excreted unaltered by the kidneys although four major metabolic breakdown products have been isolated.

EVALUATION OF DATA

Analysis of the available data describing the passage of ^{123}I into milk gives the following results.

No. of cases; route	Fractional ingested activity (%)			Effective half-life (h)			Administered activity (MBq)	Effective dose to infant (mSv)	Time to reach 1 mSv (h)	Ref
	Max.	Min.	Mean	Max.	Min.	Mean				
2; i.v.	0.36	0.013	0.19	7.3	6.8	7.1	400	5.6	21	1,2

RADIOACTIVITY IN MILK

Speciation analysis indicated that the radioactivity in milk was not bound to MIBG, but was more likely to be in the form of free iodide (1). In the first case, the maximum fractional activity concentration of 5.6×10^{-4} % ml^{-1} occurred in the first sample expressed at 4.5 h after administration (1). In the second case, the fractional activity concentration showed a delayed peak with a maximum value of 2.7×10^{-5} % ml^{-1} at 5.3 h (2). Thereafter in both cases, the activity concentration decreased monoexponentially with time after administration.

ASSESSMENT

After a single intravenous administration of 400 MBq of ^{123}I-MIBG, the maximum effective dose from the ingested ^{123}I activity is estimated to be 5.6 mSv for uninterrupted breast-feeding with the first feed taken at 3 h after radiopharmaceutical administration, requiring an interruption period of 21 h to reduce it to 1 mSv.

RECOMMENDATION

Category III. Interruption with measurement

Although the available data indicate that breast-feeding can be resumed after a period of interruption, they are too limited for a definite period to be recommended. Instead, the concentration of radioactivity in expressed milk should be measured, and feeding interrupted for a period (derived by the method described in the first part of this chapter) which will reduce the infant's effective dose to 1 mSv. The effective dose from any ^{125}I activity in expressed milk must also be estimated before a recommendation that breast-feeding can be resumed, since this contamination could be the limiting factor for determining the appropriate period of interruption.

REFERENCES

1. Kettle AG, O'Doherty MJ, Blower PJ (1994) Secretion of [^{123}I] iodide in breast milk following administration of [^{123}I] *meta*-iodobenzylguanidine. *Eur. J. Nucl. Med., 21,* 181–182.
2. Hill JC, Waller ML (1996) Unpublished data.

^{123}I-ORTHOIODOHIPPURIC ACID

GENERAL

^{123}I-Orthoiodohippuric acid is used for functional imaging of the renal tract. It is excreted entirely by the kidneys, primarily (80%) by the proximal tubular cells with the remainder (20%) by glomerular filtration, and is therefore used to measure effective renal plasma flow. It is carried in the blood, weakly bound to protein.

EVALUATION OF DATA

Analysis of the available data describing the passage of ^{123}I into milk gives the following results.

No. of cases; route	Fractional ingested activity (%)			Effective half-life (h)			Administered activity (MBq)	Effective dose to infant (mSv)	Time to reach 1 mSv (h)	Ref
	Max.	Min.	Mean	Max.	Min.	Mean				
3; i.v.	3.9	1.1	2.1	5.8	3.5	4.7	20	3	11	1–3

RADIOACTIVITY IN MILK

The first sample measured in each case was expressed at 3.7 h (1), 5.0 h (2) and 2.9 h (3) and contained the maximum fractional activity concentrations of $1.2 \times 10^{-2}\%\ ml^{-1}$, $2.1 \times 10^{-2}\ \%\ ml^{-1}$ and $5.2 \times 10^{-3}\ \%\ ml^{-1}$ respectively. Thereafter, the activity concentration decreased monoexponentially with time after administration. Only a minor proportion (3–7%) of the radioactivity was associated with the protein precipitate (3).

ASSESSMENT

After a single intravenous administration of 20 MBq of ^{123}I-orthoiodohippuric acid, the maximum effective dose from the ingested ^{123}I activity is estimated to be 3 mSv for uninterrupted breast-feeding with the first feed taken at 3 h after radiopharmaceutical administration, requiring an interruption period of 11 h to reduce it to 1 mSv.

RECOMMENDATION

Category III. Interruption with measurement

Although the available data indicate that breast-feeding can be resumed after a period of interruption, they are too limited for a definite period to be recommended. Instead, the concentration of radioactivity in expressed milk should be measured, and feeding interrupted for a period (derived by the method described in the first part of this chapter) which will reduce the infant's effective dose to 1 mSv. The effective dose from any ^{125}I activity in expressed milk must also be estimated before a recommendation that breast-feeding can be resumed, since this contamination could be the limiting factor for determining the appropriate period of interruption.

REFERENCES

1. Rose MR, Prescott MC, Herman KJ (1990) Excretion of iodine-123-hippuran, technetium-99m-red blood cells, and technetium-99m-macroaggregated albumin into breast milk. *J. Nucl. Med., 31,* 978–984.
2. Rose MR, Prescott MC, Prince JR (1996) Unpublished data.
3. Mountford PJ, Coakley AJ (1989) Secretion of radioactivity in breast milk following administration of ^{123}I hippuran. *Br. J. Radiol., 62,* 388–389.

SODIUM ^{123}I-IODIDE

GENERAL

Sodium ^{123}I-iodide is usually administered orally for thyroid function imaging and for localisation of parathyroid adenoma as a dual radiopharmaceutical procedure with ^{201}Tl-chloride or ^{99m}Tc-hexakismethoxyisobutylisonitrile. After oral administration, absorption is rapid and complete, with normal uptake to the thyroid, stomach and intestines. The thyroid gland selectively traps iodide and radioiodide which are incorporated into the peptide-linked residues in thyroglobulin to form monoiodotyrosine and diiodotyrosine, some of which then forms thyroxine and small quantities of triiodothyronine. The latter two are then released into the blood when about 90% of thyroxine is protein-bound. Thyroid pathology can lead to a wide variation in radioiodide trapping over the range 0–55% of the administered activity. Excretion is predominantly by the renal tract, with some gastric and salivary secretion, and also into sweat.

EVALUATION OF DATA

Analysis of the available data describing the passage of ^{123}I into milk gives the following results.

No. of cases; route	Fractional ingested activity (%)			Effective half-life (h)			Administered activity (MBq)	Effective dose to infant (mSv)	Time to reach 1 mSv (h)	Ref
	Max.	Min.	Mean	Max.	Min.	Mean				
2; i.v.	16.3	2.6	9.5	6.6	5.8	6.2	20	13	27	1,2

RADIOACTIVITY IN MILK

One case showed a delayed peak in the fractional activity concentration with the second sample measured at 6 h after administration having a greater value (5×10^{-3} % ml^{-1}) than the first sample taken at 2 h (1). In the other case, the fractional activity concentration was at a maximum value of 2.9×10^{-2} % ml^{-1} in the first sample measured at 6.2 h after administration (2). Thereafter, the activity concentration decreased monoexponentially with time after administration in both cases. Only a minor proportion (8 ± 2%) of the radioactivity was associated with the protein precipitate (1).

The ^{125}I contamination activity concentrations were also measured in the second case with a maximum value of 0.054 kBq ml^{-1} at 6.2 h (2). Assuming a monoexponential decay over the period of the measurements (6.2–88.7 h), the effective half-life was calculated to be 13.3 h. The administered ^{125}I activity was not recorded, but the manufacturer specified it to be <0.6%. Using the method outlined in the first part of this chapter, the total activity ingested for uninterrupted feeding resumed 3 h after administration of 15 MBq of sodium ^{123}I-iodide was calculated to be 46 kBq.

ASSESSMENT

After a single intravenous administration of 20 MBq of ^{123}I-iodide, the maximum effective dose from the ingested ^{123}I activity is estimated to be 13 mSv for uninterrupted breast-feeding with the first feed taken at 3 h after radiopharmaceutical administration, requiring an interruption period of 27 h to reduce it to 1 mSv.

The effective dose from ^{125}I contamination is estimated from the second case (2) to be 21 mSv for an administration of 20 MBq of ^{123}I-iodide, requiring an interruption period of 61 h to reduce it to 1 mSv.

RECOMMENDATION

Category III. Interruption with measurement

Although the available data indicate that breast-feeding can be resumed after a period of interruption, they are too limited for a definite period to be recommended. Instead, the concentration of radioactivity in expressed milk should be measured, and feeding interrupted for a period (derived by the method described in the first part of this chapter) which will reduce the infant's effective dose to 1 mSv. The effective dose from any ^{125}I activity in expressed milk must also be estimated before a recommendation that breast-feeding can be resumed, since this contamination could be the limiting factor for determining the appropriate period of interruption.

REFERENCES

1. Hedrick WR, Di Simone RN, Keen RL (1986) Radiation dosimetry from breast milk excretion of radioiodine and pertechnetate. *J. Nucl. Med., 27,* 1569–1571.
2. Lawes SC (1992) ^{123}I excretion in breast milk - additional data. *Nucl. Med. Commun., 13,* 570–572.

^{125}I-HUMAN SERUM ALBUMIN

GENERAL

^{125}I-Human serum albumin (^{125}I-HSA) is used for the measurement of red cell mass and plasma volume. After intravenous injection, approximately 60–65% of the administered radioactivity is retained in the vascular system at 2 h after injection.

EVALUATION OF DATA

There is one publication describing two cases, but only one of these has sufficient data describing the passage of ^{125}I into milk for analysis giving the following results.

No. of cases; route	Fractional ingested activity (%)			Effective half-life (h)			Administered activity (MBq)	Effective dose to infant (mSv)	Time to reach 1 mSv (h)	Ref
	Max.	Min.	Mean	Max.	Min.	Mean				
1; i.v.	20			72			0.2	14	277	1

RADIOACTIVITY IN MILK

The fractional activity concentration reached a maximum value of 6×10^{-3} % ml^{-1} at 24 h after administration and then decreased monoexponentially thereafter (1). In one milk sample, 70% of the radioactive iodine was reported as being in an organic form.

EFFECT ON INFANT

In both cases the infants were fed with contaminated milk. The authors (1) calculated that the total intake by the infants was 10% and 12% of the administered activity respectively. No adverse effects were reported in the infants.

ASSESSMENT

After a single intravenous administration of 0.2 MBq of ^{125}I-HSA, the maximum effective dose is estimated to be 14 mSv for uninterrupted breast-feeding with the first feed taken at 3 h after radiopharmaceutical administration, requiring an interruption period of 277 h (11.5 days) to reduce it to 1 mSv.

RECOMMENDATION

Category IV. Cessation

The period of interrruption calculated from the available data is so long that the mother will have to be advised to discontinue feeding altogether.

REFERENCES

1. Bland EP, Crawford JS, Docker MF, Farr RF (1969) Radioactive iodine uptake by thyroid of breast-fed infants after maternal blood volume measurements. *Lancet, ii,* 1039–1041.

^{131}I-ORTHOIODOHIPPURIC ACID

GENERAL

^{131}I-Orthoiodohippuric acid is used for investigations of renal function using serial measurements of uptake with probe detectors. It is excreted entirely by the kidneys, primarily by the tubules, and is therefore used to measure effective renal plasma flow. Approximately 80% of the material is excreted by the proximal tubular cells and 20% is eliminated by glomerular filtration. It is carried in the blood, weakly bound to protein.

EVALUATION OF DATA

Analysis of the available data describing the passage of ^{131}I into milk gives the following results.

No. of cases; route	Fractional ingested activity (%)			Effective half-life (h)			Administered activity (MBq)	Effective dose to infant (mSv)	Time to reach 1 mSv (h)	Ref
	Max.	Min.	Mean	Max.	Min.	Mean				
6; i.v.	4.9	1.8	2.8	5.8	2.2	4.5	2	43	34	1

RADIOACTIVITY IN MILK

The peak activity concentration occurred in the first sample expressed at 2–3 h after administration in 4 cases, and in the other 2 cases, it was delayed to the second sample expressed at about 5–7 h after administration. The maximum fractional activity concentration of 1.3×10^{-2} % ml^{-1} was recorded at 3 h after administration. After the maximum value in each case, the activity concentration decayed monexponentially with time after administration. Other published data were insufficient for analysis, but were consistent with that used in the above table (2).

ASSESSMENT

After a single intravenous administration of 2 MBq of ^{131}I-orthoiodohippuric acid, the maximum effective dose is estimated to be 43 mSv for uninterrupted breast-feeding with the first feed taken at 3 h after radiopharmaceutical administration, requiring an interruption period of 34 h to reduce it to 1 mSv.

RECOMMENDATION

Category III. Interruption with measurement

Although the available data indicate that breast-feeding can be resumed after a period of interruption, they are too limited for a definite period to be recommended. Instead, the concentration of radioactivity in expressed milk should be measured, and feeding interrupted for a period (derived by the method described in the first part of this chapter) which will reduce the infant's effective dose to 1 mSv.

REFERENCES

1. Ahlgren L, Ivarsson S, Johansson L, Mattson S, Nosslin B (1985) Excretion of radionuclides in human breast milk after the administration of radiopharmaceuticals. *J. Nucl. Med., 26,* 1085–1090.
2. Karjalainen P, Penttila IM, Pystynen P (1971) The amount and form of radioactivity in human milk after lung scanning, renography and placental localization by ^{131}I-labelled tracers. *Acta Obstet. Gynecol. Scand., 50,* 357–361.

SODIUM ^{131}I-IODIDE

GENERAL

Sodium ^{131}I-iodide is usually administered orally (otherwise intravenously) for treatment of thyrotoxicosis, for treatment of thyroid cancer, or for localisation of thyroid metastases by γ camera imaging following surgical or radioiodide ablative treatment. After oral administration, absorption is rapid and complete, with normal uptake to the thyroid, stomach and intestines. The thyroid gland selectively traps iodide and radioiodide which are incorporated into the peptide-linked residues in thyroglobulin to form monoiodotyrosine and diiodotyrosine, some of which then forms thyroxine and small quantities of triiodothyronine. The latter two are then released into the blood when about 90% of thyroxine is protein-bound. Excretion is predominantly by the renal tract, with some gastric and salivary secretion, and also into sweat.

EVALUATION OF DATA

Analysis of the available data describing the passage of ^{131}I into milk gives the following results.

No. of cases; route	Fractional ingested activity (%)				Effective half-life			Administered activity (MBq)	Effective dose to infant (mSv)	Time to reach 1 mSv	Ref
	Max.	Min.	Mean		Max.	Min.	Mean				
7; oral[a]	46.4	10.8	26.8	(i)	14.8	5.0	9.7 h	400	81292	96.4 days	1–8
				[b](ii)	5.9	5.7	5.8 days				

[a] The route of administration is given as oral in 4 cases (1,3,4,8) and is not stated in the others.
[b] Biexponential decay was observed in only 2 cases.

RADIOACTIVITY IN MILK

In three cases where more than one sample was expressed during the first day after administration, the activity concentration showed a delayed peak with the second sample at 6 h (1, 3) and at 18 h (6, 7) having a greater activity concentration than the first sample taken at 2–3 h (1, 3) and at 12 h (6, 7) respectively. The maximum fractional activity concentration recorded from the 6 cases was 6.7×10^{-2} % ml^{-1} at 6 h after administration (1). Three cases showed a small increase in activity concentration just after the fourth (1, 5) and seventh (4, 5) day after administration. These increases remain unexplained but they may be related to the effects on the thyroid and circulating plasma radioiodide levels of the patient restarting thyroid drug treatment.

The concentration of radioactivity in milk decayed monoexponentially in 5 cases where the measurements had been recorded up to 5 days (1), 48 h (2, 3), 1 week (6, 7) and 100 h (8) after administration. In the 2 other cases, a biexponential decrease in the fractional activity concentration f_t (days) was recorded where measurements were made up to 38 days after administration (4):

$$f_t = 6.61 \times 10^{-4} \exp(-1.49t) + 1.56 \times 10^{-5} \exp(-0.12t)$$

and up to 13.3 days after administration (5):

$$f_t = 3.46 \times 10^{-5} \exp(-3.34t) + 1.43 \times 10^{-5} \exp(-0.12t)$$

The radioiodine was administered in four cases for treatment of thyrotoxicosis (1, 2, 4, 5), in one case for thyroid cancer (6, 7), in 1 case for a whole body scan of a hypothyroid patient (8), and in one case to a normal (3). The monoexponential decay for the thyroid cancer case measured over 1 week (6, 7) had an effective half-life of 11.0 h which was just within the range (monoexponential and first phase of biexponential decay) found for the thyrotoxic cases (5.0–11.1 h). The monoexponential decay measured over 100 h for the hypothyroid patient had an effective half-life of 14.8 h.

The data in other published cases were insufficient for analysis, but were consistent with that used in the above table (1, 3, 9, 10). In particular, the activity concentration produced by a thyroid cancer patient up to 32 days after radioiodine administration showed a biexponential decay with effective half lives reported to be 10.6 h and 4.4 days (10).

EFFECT ON INFANT

In only one report was an infant breast-fed after maternal administration of sodium ^{131}I-iodide (1). Uptake measurements of ^{131}I showed 34% of the administered activity in the mother's thyroid at 24 h after administration, falling to 10% at 10 days with a biological half-life of 9 days, compared with 3% of the administered activity in the infant's thyroid falling irregularly to 2% at 10 days. Although no effects on the infant were reported in the study, serious depression or ablation of thyroidal function is possible.

ASSESSMENT

After a single oral administration of 400 MBq of sodium ^{131}I-iodide, the maximum effective dose is estimated to be 81 292 mSv for uninterrupted breast-feeding with the first feed taken at 3 h after radiopharmaceutical administration, requiring an interruption period of 96.4 days to reduce it to 1 mSv.

RECOMMENDATION

Category IV. Cessation

The period of interrruption calculated from the available data is so long that the mother will have to be advised to discontinue feeding altogether.

REFERENCES

1. Nurnberger CE, Lipscomb A (1952) Transmission of radioiodine (I^{131}) to infants through human maternal milk. *J. Am. Med. Assoc., 150,* 1398–1400.
2. Miller H, Weetch RS (1955) The excretion of radioactive iodine in human milk. *Lancet, 269,* 1013.
3. Weaver JC, Kamm ML, Dobson RL (1960) Excretion of radioiodine in milk. *J. Am. Med. Assoc., 173,* 872–875.
4. Dydek GJ, Blue PW (1988) Human breast milk excretion of iodine-131 following diagnostic and therapeutic administration to a lactating patient with Grave's disease. *J. Nucl. Med., 29,* 407–410.
5. Hesslewood SR (1990) Unpublished data.
6. Rubow S, Klopper J (1988) Excretion of radioiodine in human milk following a therapeutic dose of I-131. *Eur. J. Nucl. Med., 14,* 632–633.
7. Rubow S, Klopper J, Wasserman H, Baard B, van Niekerk M (1994) The excretion of radiopharmaceuticals in human breast milk: additional data and dosimetry. *Eur. J. Nucl. Med., 21,* 144–153.
8. Spencer RP, Spitznagle LA, Karimeddini MK, Hosain F (1986) Breast milk of ^{131}I in a hypothyroid patient. *Nucl. Med. Biol. Int. J. Radiat. Appl. Instrum. Part B., 13,* 585.
9. Honour AJ, Myant NB, Rowlands EN (1952) Secretion of radioiodine in digestive juices and milk in man. *Clin. Sci., 11,* 447–462.
10. Robinson PS, Barker P, Campbell A, Henson P, Surveyor I, Young PR (1994) Iodine-131 in breast milk following therapy for thyroid carcinoma. *J. Nucl. Med., 35,* 1797–1801.

RADIOACTIVE TECHNETIUM

The decay of the radionuclide ^{99m}Tc to its ground state ^{99}Tc by isomeric transition yields a 140.5 keV γ-ray (89%) and some low energy X-rays. It has a physical half-life of 6.02 h, and is produced by the radioactive decay of the longer-lived parent radionuclide ^{99}Mo which is manufactured commercially as a column in a generator. By eluting the column with physiological saline, the ^{99m}Tc can be easily separated from its parent and produced in solution as sodium ^{99m}Tc-pertechnetate. Weekly delivery of the generator allows a hospital to have a continuous supply of this short-lived radionuclide on site as the radiolabel for local production of radiopharmaceuticals in kit form which can be used for a wide range of functional organ studies. The convenience of the production and availability of ^{99m}Tc, the suitability of its physical characteristics for γ camera imaging, and the large number of the different types of ^{99m}Tc-labelled radiopharmaceuticals have led to its wide use in diagnostic nuclear medicine: a ^{99m}Tc-labelled radiopharmaceutical was used in 82% of all imaging procedures carried out in the UK during 1989/1990 (1).

All attempts to identify the chemical species of ^{99m}Tc expressed in milk have indicated that it is largely in the form of free pertechnetate, and it was assumed for the dosimetry estimations that only this form passes into milk after administration of any ^{99m}Tc radiopharmaceutical. The value of effective dose per unit activity ingested is based on the ICRP data which assumes a fractional absorption of 80%, and on the distribution and retention of pertechnetate (2, 3).

REFERENCES

1. Elliott AT, Shields RA (1993) UK nuclear medicine survey, 1989/90. *Nucl. Med. Commun., 14,* 360–364.
2. International Commission on Radiological Protection (1980) *Limits for Intakes of Radionuclides by Workers* (ICRP Publication 30). Pergamon Press, Oxford.
3. International Commission on Radiological Protection (1991) *Annual Limits on Intake of Radionuclides by Workers Based on the 1990 Recommendations* (ICRP Publication 61). Pergamon Press, Oxford.

^{99m}Tc-DIISOPROPYLPHENYLCARBAMOYLMETHYL IMINODIACETIC ACID

GENERAL

There are several radiopharmaceuticals used for functional imaging of the hepatobiliary system based on derivatives of iminodiacetic acid. Breast milk data have been published for ^{99m}Tc-diisopropylphenylcarbamoylmethyl iminodiacetic acid (^{99m}Tc-DISIDA). Following intravenous administration, it is rapidly cleared from the circulation with the predominant uptake to the liver. Approximately 8% of the injected activity remains in the circulation at 30 min after injection, and about 9% of the injected activity is excreted in the urine during the first 2 h after injection. The remainder is cleared through the hepatobiliary system to the intestine with a peak gall bladder accumulation by about 30–40 min after injection. Pathological conditions of the liver and biliary tract should not affect the recommendation given below.

EVALUATION OF DATA

Analysis of the available data describing the passage of ^{99m}Tc into milk gives the following results.

No. of cases; route	Fractional ingested activity (%)			Effective half-life (h)			Administered activity (MBq)	Effective dose to infant (mSv)	Time to reach 1 mSv (h)	Ref
	Max.	Min.	Mean	Max.	Min.	Mean				
6; i.v.	0.28	0.10	0.16	9.1	3.8	5.5	150	0.2	–	1

RADIOACTIVITY IN MILK

The reference does not give details of the time course of the passage of radioactivity in the first few hours after administration, but the authors suggest that the low concentration in milk is probably because the ^{99m}Tc-IDA derivatives are not metabolised by the liver (1).

ASSESSMENT

After a single intravenous administration of 150 MBq of ^{99m}Tc-DISIDA, the maximum effective dose is estimated to be 0.2 mSv for uninterrupted breast-feeding with the first feed taken at 3 h after administration.

RECOMMENDATION

Category I. Interruption not essential

Breast-feeding need not be interrupted because the activity concentrations in milk and the estimated effective dose to the infant are small. In practice, a mother can be reassured by advising a short interruption (e.g. 4 h), at the end of which milk should be expressed and discarded.

REFERENCES

1. Rubow S, Klopper J, Wasserman H, Baard B, van Niekerk M (1994) The excretion of radio-pharmaceuticals in human breast milk: additional data and dosimetry. *Eur. J. Nucl. Med., 21,* 144–153.

^{99m}Tc-DIETHYLENETRIAMINEPENTAACETIC ACID

GENERAL

After intravenous administration, ^{99m}Tc-diethylenetriaminepentaacetic acid (^{99m}Tc-DTPA) is distributed initially throughout the extracellular space, and is then rapidly cleared from the body by glomerular filtration. The plasma clearance half-time is about 70 min and the biological half-life for clearance from the whole body is 1–2 h. Its plasma protein binding is negligible. The radiopharmaceutical is useful for the measurement of glomerular filtration rate, assessment of renal blood flow, renal function and morphology, and ureteric obstruction. It can also be used for the detection of vascular and neoplastic brain lesions.

EVALUATION OF DATA

Analysis of the available data describing the passage of ^{99m}Tc into milk gives the following results.

No. of cases; route	Fractional ingested activity (%)			Effective half-life (h)			Administered activity (MBq)	Effective dose to infant (mSv)	Time to reach 1 mSv (h)	Ref
	Max.	Min.	Mean	Max.	Min.	Mean				
7; i.v.	0.24	0.005	[a]	9.6	3.1	[a]	800	0.7	–	1–4
1; i.v.	7.9						800	22	46	4

[a] The combined mean value of all cases could not be estimated because separate data was not published for the 4 cases in reference (4). However, the above method of analysis was used in reference (4) which reported a mean fractional ingested activity for these 4 cases alone of 0.12%, and a mean effective half-life of 4.5 h. For the remaining 3 cases, the mean fractional ingested activity is 0.01% and the mean effective half-life is 5.9 h.

RADIOACTIVITY IN MILK

Individual data points were not published in 5 of the cases including the case producing the maximum fractional ingested activity (4). In 2 of the remaining 3 cases, the peak activity concentration was not in the first sample expressed, and occurred in samples expressed at 2 h and 4.5 h after administration (1,3). In each case, the activity concentration decayed monoexponentially after the peak value.

The fractional ingested activity derived from these 3 cases were 2–3 orders of magnitude less than the maximum value, varying from 0.005% to 0.015%. The peak fractional activity concentration recorded from these 3 cases varied from 0.8×10^{-5} % ml^{-1} at 4.5 h (3) to 4.4×10^{-5} % ml^{-1} at 2.8 h after administration (2). In 3 other cases with insufficient data for the above analysis, the fractional activity concentrations were similar to this range with values of 7.3×10^{-5} % ml^{-1} (5), 8.6 ×

10^{-5} % ml^{-1} (6) and 1.8×10^{-5} % ml^{-1} (7) at 3.6 h, 2.5 h and 5.5 h respectively after administration, indicating that their corresponding fractional ingested activities would also be at least 2 orders of magnitude less than the maximum above.

ASSESSMENT

Over all 8 cases, the fractional ingested activity varies by more than three orders of magnitude, and the maximum value was nearly the highest of all the ^{99m}Tc-labelled radiopharmaceuticals. This variation is by far the greatest out of all the ^{99m}Tc-labelled radiopharmaceuticals including those compounds whose administration will result in the presence of free ^{99m}Tc-pertechnetate in blood which is associated with varying and significant levels of ^{99m}Tc in milk. If the case producing the highest fractional ingested activity is ignored, then the variation reduces to less than two orders of magnitude, and the maximum fractional ingested activity reduces by a factor of ×0.03 to a value similar to other ^{99m}Tc-labelled radiopharmaceuticals where there should be negligible free ^{99m}Tc-pertechnetate in blood. The authors of this case have considered that its high value may have been due to a high percentage of free ^{99m}Tc-pertechnetate administered with the DTPA (3).

If the case producing the highest fractional ingested activity is ignored, then after a single intravenous administration of 800 MBq of ^{99m}Tc-DTPA, the maximum effective dose is estimated to be 0.7 mSv for uninterrupted breast-feeding with the first feed taken at 3 h after administration.

RECOMMENDATION

Category I. Interruption not essential

Breast-feeding need not be interrupted because the activity concentrations in milk and the estimated effective dose to the infant are small. In practice, a mother can be reassured by advising a short interruption (e.g. 4 h), at the end of which milk should be expressed and discarded.

REFERENCES

1. Ahlgren L, Ivarsson S, Johansson L, Mattson S, Nosslin B (1985) Excretion of radionuclides in human breast milk after the administration of radiopharmaceuticals. *J. Nucl. Med., 26,* 1085–1090.
2. Mountford PJ, Coakley AJ, Hall FM (1985) Excretion of radioactivity in breast milk following injection of ^{99m}Tc-DTPA. *Nucl. Med. Commun., 6,* 341–345.
3. Hawkins T (1989) Unpublished data.
4. Rubow S, Klopper J, Wasserman H, Baard B, van Niekerk M (1994) The excretion of radiopharmaceuticals in human breast milk: additional data and dosimetry. *Eur. J. Nucl. Med., 21,* 144–153.

5. Mountford PJ (1985) Unpublished data.
6. Merrick MV (1987) Unpublished data
7. Taylor W (1987) Unpublished data.

^{99m}Tc-DIMERCAPTOSUCCINIC ACID

GENERAL

^{99m}Tc-Dimercaptosuccinic acid (^{99m}Tc-DMSA) is used for the visualisation of the kidneys, particularly for the identification of renal scarring, and for quantifying divided renal function. After intravenous administration virtually all of the radioactivity is in the plasma. This plasma level falls from 55% of the injected activity at 5 min after administration to 7% at 6 h. Approximately 75% of the radioactivity is bound to plasma protein up to 6 h after administration. About 20–35% of the injected radioactivity is accumulated by each kidney 6 h after administration. A smaller component is taken up by the liver and spleen. It is excreted totally by the renal tract.

EVALUATION OF DATA

Analysis of the available data describing the passage of ^{99m}Tc into milk gives the following results.

No. of cases; route	Fractional ingested activity (%)			Effective half-life (h)			Administered activity (MBq)	Effective dose to infant (mSv)	Time to reach 1 mSv (h)	Ref
	Max.	Min.	Mean	Max.	Min.	Mean				
1; i.v.	0.03			5.9			80	0.008	–	1

RADIOACTIVITY IN MILK

The maximum fractional activity concentration of 7.2×10^{-5} % ml^{-1} occurred in the first sample expressed at 3 h after administration, thereafter the fractional activity concentration decreased monoexponentially with time after administration. In one other case with insufficient data for the above analysis, the fractional activity concentration at 4.9 h after administration was 4.8×10^{-5} % ml^{-1} (2).

ASSESSMENT

After a single intravenous administration of 80 MBq of ^{99m}Tc-DMSA, the maximum effective dose is estimated to be 8 μSv for uninterrupted breast-feeding with the first feed taken at 3 h after administration.

RECOMMENDATION

Category I. Interruption not essential

Breast-feeding need not be interrupted because the activity concentrations in milk and the estimated effective dose to the infant are small. In practice, a mother can be reassured by advising a short interruption (e.g. 4 h), at the end of which milk should be expressed and discarded.

REFERENCES

1. Taylor W (1987) Unpublished data.
2. Wells CP (1994) Unpublished data.

^{99m}Tc-DIPHOSPHONATES

GENERAL

Breast milk data has been obtained for ^{99m}Tc-methylene diphosphonate (^{99m}Tc-MDP), ^{99m}Tc-hydroxymethylene diphosphonate (^{99m}Tc-HMDP) and ^{99m}Tc-hydroxyethylidene diphosphonate (^{99m}Tc-HDP) which are all used for bone imaging. They have been grouped together because of their similar biokinetic behaviour which ICRP considers to justify the use of a common biokinetic model for their dosimetry. The main uptake is to the skeleton, with a further small uptake in kidneys, and the excretion is through the bladder. There may be higher bone uptake and longer retention in certain skeletal pathologies (e.g. osteomalacia, Paget's disease), and particularly in renal diseases (e.g. renal osteodystrophia).

Approximately 50% of intravenously administered activity remains in the blood at 3 min, falling to 3% at 3 h and less than 1% at 24 h. There is no significant binding to red blood cells and approximately 15% of the administered activity is loosely bound to plasma proteins at 1 h after injection, falling to 0.5% after 24 h. About 40% is excreted in the urine during the first hour rising to about 63% after 4 h.

EVALUATION OF DATA

Analysis of the available data describing the passage of ^{99m}Tc into milk gives the following results.

No. of cases; route	Fractional ingested activity (%)			Effective half-life (h)			Administered activity (MBq)	Effective dose to infant (mSv)	Time to reach 1 mSv (h)	Ref
	Max.	Min.	Mean	Max.	Min.	Mean				
8; i.v.	0.04	0.01	0.02	5.9	3.5	4.7	600	0.08	–	1–6

RADIOACTIVITY IN MILK

The peak activity concentration occurred in the first sample expressed at 2.0–5.1 h after administration in 5 cases (1, 3–5), but in the other 3 cases, it was delayed to the second sample expressed at 3.3, 4.2 and 5.5 h respectively (2, 5, 6), and thereafter it decayed monoexponentially in all cases. The maximum fractional activity concentration recorded was 1×10^{-4} % ml^{-1} in a sample expressed at 4.4 h after administration (5).

ASSESSMENT

After a single intravenous administration of 600 MBq of any of these ^{99m}Tc-diphosphonate compounds, the maximum effective dose is estimated to be 0.08 mSv for uninterrupted breast-feeding with the first feed taken at 3 h after administration.

RECOMMENDATION

Category I. Interruption not essential

Breast-feeding need not be interrupted because the activity concentrations in milk and the estimated effective dose to the infant are small. In practice, a mother can be reassured by advising a short interruption (e.g. 4 h), at the end of which milk should be expressed and discarded.

REFERENCES

1. Ahlgren L, Ivarsson S, Johansson L, Mattson S, Nosslin B (1985) Excretion of radionuclides in human breast milk after the administration of radiopharmaceuticals. *J. Nucl. Med., 26,* 1085–1090.
2. Cranage RW, Slade M (1987) Unpublished data.
3. Ormsby PL (1987) Unpublished data.
4. Ardley RG (1991) Unpublished data.
5. Mountford PJ (1993) Unpublished data.
6. Rose MR, Prescott MC, Prince JR (1996) Unpublished data.

^{99m}Tc-ERYTHROCYTES

GENERAL

Autologous ^{99m}Tc-erythrocytes are widely used for blood pool imaging, blood dynamic studies such as organ perfusion and ventricular function (ejection fraction), and spleen imaging with denatured radiolabelled red cells. Breast milk data have been obtained for cases where erythrocytes have been labelled in vivo with ^{99m}Tc for the purpose of assessing ventricular function and for cases where erythrocytes have been labelled in vitro with ^{99m}Tc for the same purpose. Slow leaching of activity from the labelled cells will result from both techniques. Excretion is by the renal tract.

EVALUATION OF DATA

Analysis of the available data describing the passage of ^{99m}Tc into milk gives the following results.

No. of cases; route	Fractional ingested activity (%)			Effective half-life (h)			Administered activity (MBq)	Effective dose to infant (mSv)	Time to reach 1 mSv (h)	Ref
	Max.	Min.	Mean	Max.	Min.	Mean				
7; i.v.	1.0	0.01	0.27	9.1	5.4	7.5	800	2.8	17	1–5

RADIOACTIVITY IN MILK

Compared to other ^{99m}Tc-labelled radiopharmaceuticals, the peak activity concentration occurred later (up to 9 h after administration (2)), and the mean effective half-life in milk was longer. This delayed passage of radioactivity into milk may be due to the slow leaching of radioactivity from the erythrocytes. The maximum fractional activity concentration recorded was $1.76 \times 10^{-3}\%\ ml^{-1}$ (2, 3), and in all cases the activity concentration decreased monoexponentially after the peak value. In vitro labelling should result in less free pertechnetate being present in plasma compared to in vivo labelling where a range of labelling efficiencies is to be expected, and in the two cases where in vitro labelling was used, the fractional ingested activity was estimated to be 0.02% and 0.03% (4). For in vivo labelling, even if only a few per cent of the administered activity (typically 500 MBq) is not cell-bound, the magnitude of this free activity circulating in plasma will lead to significant concentrations in milk.

ASSESSMENT

After a single intravenous administration of 800 MBq of ^{99m}Tc-erythrocytes, the maximum effective dose is estimated to be 2.8 mSv for uninterrupted breast-feeding with the first feed taken at 3 h after administration, requiring an interruption period of 17 h to reduce it to 1 mSv.

RECOMMENDATION

Category III. Interruption with measurement

Although the available data indicate that breast-feeding can be resumed after a period of interruption, they are too limited for a definite period to be recommended. Instead, the concentration of radioactivity in expressed milk should be measured, and feeding interrupted for a period (derived by the method described in the first part of this chapter) which will reduce the infant's effective dose to 1 mSv.

REFERENCES

1. Ahlgren L, Ivarsson S, Johansson L, Mattson S, Nosslin B (1985) Excretion of radionuclides in human breast milk after the administration of radiopharmaceuticals. *J. Nucl. Med., 26,* 1085–1090.
2. Rose MR, Prescott MC, Herman KJ (1990) Excretion of iodine-123-hippuran, technetium-99m-red blood cells, and technetium-99m-macroaggregated albumin into breast milk. *J. Nucl. Med., 31,* 978–984.
3. Rose MR, Prescott MC, Prince JR (1996) Unpublished data.
4. Rubow S, Klopper J, Wasserman H, Baard B, van Niekerk M (1994) The excretion of radiopharmaceuticals in human breast milk: additional data and dosimetry. *Eur. J. Nucl. Med., 21,* 144–153.
5. Mountford PJ (1990) Unpublished data.

^{99m}Tc-GLUCOHEPTONATE, GLUCONATE

GENERAL

These radiopharmaceuticals are used for the visualisation of kidneys, investigation of renal perfusion and morphology, and for brain studies. Following intravenous administration, they are rapidly cleared from the blood by glomerular filtration and tubular secretion. They rapidly equilibrate in extracellular space with little binding to plasma proteins. Some of the administered activity is retained for a long time in the renal cortex, and the rest is cleared by glomerular filtration.

EVALUATION OF DATA

Analysis of the available data describing the passage of ^{99m}Tc into milk gives the following results.

No. of cases; route	Fractional ingested activity (%)			Effective half-life (h)			Administered activity (MBq)	Effective dose to infant (mSv)	Time to reach 1 mSv (h)	Ref
	Max.	Min.	Mean	Max.	Min.	Mean				
3; i.v.	0.14	0.02	0.07	7.2	3.6	4.9	800	0.4	–	1–3

RADIOACTIVITY IN MILK

Individual data points were not published in the case producing the highest fractional ingested activity (1), but in the other two cases the maximum fractional activity concentration recorded was 1.8×10^{-4} % ml^{-1} (2) and 0.3×10^{-4} % ml^{-1} (3) at 3 h and 5.7 h respectively. In the latter case, the maximum fractional activity concentration was delayed to the second sample, but in all cases the activity concentration decayed monoexponentially after the peak value was reached.

ASSESSMENT

After a single intravenous administration of 800 MBq of ^{99m}Tc-glucoheptonate or ^{99m}Tc-gluconate, the maximum effective dose is estimated to be 0.4 mSv for uninterrupted breast-feeding with the first feed taken at 3 h after administration.

RECOMMENDATION

Category I. Interruption not essential

Breast-feeding need not be interrupted because the activity concentrations in milk and the estimated effective dose to the infant are small. In practice, a mother can be reassured by advising a short interruption (e.g. 4 h), at the end of which milk should be expressed and discarded.

REFERENCES

1. Rubow S, Klopper J, Wasserman H, Baard B, van Niekerk M (1994) The excretion of radiopharmaceuticals in human breast milk: additional data and dosimetry. *Eur. J. Nucl. Med., 21,* 144–153.
2. Mountford PJ, Coakley AJ (1987) Breast milk radioactivity following injection of $^{99}Tc^{m}$-pertechnetate and $^{99}Tc^{m}$-glucoheptonate. *Nucl. Med. Commun., 8,* 839–845.
3. Mountford PJ (1990) Unpublished data.

^{99m}Tc-HEXAKISMETHOXYISOBUTYLISONITRILE

GENERAL

^{99m}Tc-Hexakismethoxyisobutylisonitrile (^{99m}Tc-MIBI) is a cationic complex used primarily for ischaemic heart disease, localisation of myocardial infarction and assessment of global ventricular function. It has also been used in dual radiopharmaceutical studies with ^{99m}Tc-pertechnetate or sodium ^{123}I-iodide for localising parathyroid adenoma. After intravenous administration, 33% of the radioactivity clears from blood with a half-life of 4.3 min. It accumulates in muscle, liver and kidneys, and in the thyroid and salivary glands to a lesser degree. The major metabolic pathway is the hepatobiliary system with radioactivity appearing in the intestine via the gall bladder within 1 h after injection. Approximately 27% of the administered radioactivity is excreted in the urine within 24 h. Myocardial uptake is approximately 1.2% of the administered activity when the patient is at rest.

EVALUATION OF DATA

Analysis of the available data describing the passage of ^{99m}Tc into milk gives the following results.

No. of cases; route	Fractional ingested activity (%)			Effective half-life (h)			Administered activity (MBq)	Effective dose to infant (mSv)	Time to reach 1 mSv (h)	Ref
	Max.	Min.	Mean	Max.	Min.	Mean				
3; i.v.	0.03	0.01	0.02	6.7	4.5	5.6	1000	0.1	–	1,2
							400	0.04	–	

RADIOACTIVITY IN MILK

Individual data points have been published for two of the cases. The maximum fractional activity concentration of 1×10^{-4} % ml^{-1} (1) and 3×10^{-5} % ml^{-1} (2) occurred in both cases in the first sample expressed at about 3.3 h (1) and 1.9 h (2) after administration. Thereafter the activity concentration decreased monoexponentially.

ASSESSMENT

A myocardial perfusion study is carried out in two parts: an exercise scan followed by a resting scan. If these two scans are carried out as tomographic procedures on the same day, then the total maximum usual activity permitted in the UK is

1000 MBq. If the tomographic scans are carried out on separate days, then 400 MBq is the maximum usual activity for each scan.

After a single intravenous administration of 1000 MBq or 400 MBq of ^{99m}Tc-MIBI, the maximum effective dose is estimated to be 0.1 mSv and 0.04 mSv respectively for uninterrupted breast-feeding with the first feed taken at 3 h after administration. In practice for a same day protocol, the total activity would be administered as two injections separated by several hours, and therefore the total effective dose will be less than 0.1 mSv.

RECOMMENDATION

Category I. Interruption not essential

Breast-feeding need not be interrupted because the activity concentrations in milk and the estimated effective dose to the infant are small. In practice, a mother can be reassured by advising a short interruption (e.g. 4 h), at the end of which milk should be expressed and discarded.

REFERENCES

1. Rubow SM, Ellman A, Le Roux J, Klopper J (1991) Excretion of technetium 99m hexakis-methoxyisobutylisonitrile in milk. *Eur. J. Nucl. Med., 18,* 363–365.
2. Rubow S, Klopper J, Wasserman H, Baard B, van Niekerk M (1994) The excretion of radiopharmaceuticals in human breast milk: additional data and dosimetry. *Eur. J. Nucl. Med., 21,* 144–153.

^{99m}Tc-HEXAMETHYLPROPYLENEAMINE OXIME

GENERAL

^{99m}Tc-Hexamethylpropyleneamine oxime (^{99m}Tc-HMPAO) is a lipophilic complex used for regional cerebral blood flow scintigraphy. The complex is rapidly cleared from blood after intravenous injection, and reaches a maximum of 3.5–7.0% of the injected dose in the brain within one minute of injection. Up to 15% of the cerebral activity washes out of the brain after 2 min. Radioactivity not associated with the brain is distributed in muscle and soft tissue. About 30% of the dose is found in the liver and gastrointestinal tract immediately after injection, with about one-half being excreted through the gut by 48 h after administration. About 40% of the injected dose is excreted through the kidneys and urine by 48 h after administration.

EVALUATION OF DATA

Analysis of the available data describing the passage of ^{99m}Tc into milk gives the following results.

No. of cases; route	Fractional ingested activity (%)			Effective half-life (h)			Administered activity (MBq)	Effective dose to infant (mSv)	Time to reach 1 mSv (h)	Ref
	Max.	Min.	Mean	Max.	Min.	Mean				
1; i.v.	0.14			3.8			500	0.3	–	1

RADIOACTIVITY IN MILK

The maximum fractional activity concentration of 4.1×10^{-4} % ml^{-1} occurred in the second sample expressed at 6.5 h after administration. Thereafter the fractional activity concentration decreased monoexponentially with time after administration.

ASSESSMENT

After a single intravenous administration of 500 MBq of ^{99m}Tc-HMPAO, the maximum effective dose is estimated to be 0.3 mSv for uninterrupted breast-feeding with the first feed taken at 3 h after administration.

RECOMMENDATION

Category I. Interruption not essential

Breast-feeding need not be interrupted because the activity concentrations in milk and the estimated effective dose to the infant are small. In practice, a mother can be reassured by advising a short interruption (e.g. 4 h), at the end of which milk should be expressed and discarded.

REFERENCES

1. Marshall DSC, Newberry NR (1996) Measurement of the secretion of ^{99m}Tc-HMPAO into breast milk. *Eur. J. Nucl. Med.,* in press.

^{99m}Tc-MACROAGGREGATED HUMAN SERUM ALBUMIN

GENERAL

^{99m}Tc-Macroaggregated human serum albumin (^{99m}Tc-MAA) is a radiopharmaceutical used for diagnostic lung perfusion imaging. In combination with a lung ventilation scan, it is the technique of choice for the diagnosis of pulmonary embolism. This indication represents the most likely reason for a nuclear medicine procedure to be carried out on a breast-feeding mother, and therefore it is not surprising that ^{99m}Tc-MAA has the largest number of cases where the variation with time of the concentration of radioactivity in breast milk has been recorded. ^{99m}Tc-labelled agents in the form of either a ^{99m}Tc-DTPA aerosol or ^{99m}Tc-technegas can be used for the ventilation scan.

Approximately 100 000–400 000 particles of ^{99m}Tc-MAA, with a size range of 10–80 μm, are injected intravenously and trapped during the first-pass through the pulmonary capillary bed, lodging in the capillaries and precapillary arterioles. Their distribution reflects regional differences in pulmonary blood flow. The half-life of the particles in the lung is approximately 1.5 h. They are broken down in size by mechanical movement of the lungs and enzyme action, released into the circulation, and smaller particles are removed by phagocytosis in the reticuloendothelial system.

EVALUATION OF DATA

Analysis of the available data describing the passage of ^{99m}Tc into milk where the ventilation scan was not carried out with ^{99m}Tc-technegas, gives the following results.

No. of cases; route	Fractional ingested activity (%)			Effective half-life (h)			Administered activity (MBq)	Effective dose to infant (mSv)	Time to reach 1 mSv (h)	Ref
	Max.	Min.	Mean	Max.	Min.	Mean				
39; i.v.	7.1	0.2	[a]	7.9	2.5	[a]	100	2.5	13	1–15

[a] The combined mean value of all 39 cases could not be estimated because separate data was not published for the 6 cases in reference (7). However, the above method of analysis was used in reference (7) which reported a mean fractional ingested activity for these 6 cases alone of 3.1%, and a mean effective half-life of 3.7 h. For the remaining 33 cases, the mean fractional ingested activity is 2.9% and the mean effective half-life is 4.2 h.

Where the ventilation scan was carried out with ^{99m}Tc-technegas (15), analysis of the available data describing the passage of ^{99m}Tc into milk gives the following results.

No. of cases; route	Fractional ingested activity (%)			Effective half-life (h)			Administered activity (MBq)	Effective dose to infant (mSv)	Time to reach 1 mSv (h)	Ref
	Max.	Min.	Mean	Max.	Min.	Mean				
6; i.v.	9.1	2.2	5.4	5.8	2.7	4.7	20 + 100[a]	3.8	14[b]	15

[a] 20 MBq 99mTc-technegas + 100 MBq 99mTc-MAA.
[b] Based on the maximum value of effective half-life for this sub-group of data.

RADIOACTIVITY IN MILK

The rapid dissociation of the MAA particles in the pulmonary capillary bed produces circulating plasma levels of pertechnetate which result in significant levels of radioactivity in milk. Differences in the amount of free pertechnetate administered with the MAA particles and in the rate of breakdown in the capillary bed contribute to the variation in the quantity of ^{99m}Tc expressed in milk by different patients.

For the first group of cases where the ventilation scan was not carried out with ^{99m}Tc-technegas, the maximum recorded fractional activity concentration was 2.1×10^{-2} % ml^{-1} in a sample expressed at 2.5 h after administration (12). In two cases, a single milk sample was expressed between the ^{99m}Tc-DTPA aerosol and ^{99m}Tc-MAA administration and the fractional activity concentration due to the ^{99m}Tc-DTPA aerosol alone was found to be as low as 7.5×10^{-5} % ml^{-1} and 9.5×10^{-5} % ml^{-1} at 1.5 h and 0.75 h after administration (12). Therefore if ^{99m}Tc-DTPA aerosol had been administered, no allowance was made in the fractional activity estimations for the administered activity since its contribution to the total ^{99m}Tc concentration in milk was negligible compared to that from ^{99m}Tc-MAA. For several cases in this group, the peak activity concentration was delayed to the second sample expressed at times ranging from 2.5 to 7.0 h after administration (4, 10, 12–15). In all the other cases, the peak concentration occurred in the first sample, and in 6 of these other cases, this first sample was expressed earlier than 2.5 h after administration (6–8, 10, 12, 15). In all cases the activity concentration decayed monoexponentially after the peak value was reached.

For the second group of cases where the ventilation scan was carried out with ^{99m}Tc-technegas, a higher range of fractional activity concentrations and fractional ingested activities was probably due to the presence of pertechnegas contamination which will be quickly absorbed into blood as pertechnetate and produce significant levels of ^{99m}Tc in milk. The maximum recorded fractional activity concentration was 2.4×10^{-2} % ml^{-1} in a sample expressed at 4.8 h after administration (15). In all of these cases, the activity concentration was at a peak value in the first sample expressed at 2.3–5 h after administration of the ^{99m}Tc-MAA, and it decayed monoexponentially thereafter (15).

ASSESSMENT

After a single intravenous administration of 100 MBq of ^{99m}Tc-MAA, the maximum effective dose is estimated to be 2.5 mSv for uninterrupted breast-feeding with the first feed taken at 3 h after administration, requiring an interruption period of 13 h to reduce it to 1 mSv.

When 20 MBq of ^{99m}Tc-technegas is administered for a ventilation scan followed by 100 MBq of ^{99m}Tc-MAA, the combined maximum effective dose from the two radiopharmaceuticals is estimated to be 3.8 mSv for uninterrupted breast-feeding with the first feed taken at 3 h after administration, requiring an interruption period of 14 h to reduce it to 1 mSv.

RECOMMENDATION

Category II. Interruption for a definite period

There is sufficient published data to allow a definite period of interruption of 13 h after administration of 100 MBq of ^{99m}Tc-MAA alone to be recommended in order to reduce the estimated effective dose to 1 mSv.

However if ^{99m}Tc-technegas is administered for the ventilation scan, then the following recommendation should be made.

Category III. Interruption with measurement

Although the available data indicate that breast-feeding can be resumed after a period of interruption, they are too limited for a definite period to be recommended. Instead, the concentration of radioactivity in expressed milk should be measured, and feeding interrupted for a period (derived by the method described in the first part of this chapter) which will reduce the infant's effective dose to 1 mSv.

REFERENCES

1. Berke RA, Hoops EC, Kereiakes JC, Senger EL (1973) Radiation dose to breast-feeding child after mother has ^{99m}Tc-MAA lung scan. *J. Nucl. Med., 14,* 51–52.
2. Tribukait B, Swedjemark GA (1978) Secretion of ^{99}Tc^{m} in breast milk after intravenous injection of marked macroaggregated albumin. *Acta Radiol. Oncol., 17,* 379–382.
3. Mattson S, Johansson L, Nosslin B, Ahlgren L (1981) Excretion of radionuclides in human breast milk following administration of ^{125}I-fibrinogen, ^{99}Tc^{m}-MAA, and ^{51}Cr-EDTA. In Watson EE, Schlafke AT, Coffey JL, Cloutier RJ (Eds), *Proc. 3rd Int. Radiopharmaceut. Dosimetry Symp.,* HHS Publications FDA 81–8166, pp 102–110. US Department of Health and Human Services, Rockville, MD.
4. Pittard III WB, Merkatz R, Fletcher BD (1982) Radioactive excretion in human milk following administration of technetium Tc 99m macroaggregated albumin. *Pediatrics, 70,* 231–234.

5. Short MD, Todd JH, Mulvey PJ, Ramsey NW (1984) Radiation protection procedures in the use of $^{99}Tc^{m}$ *(Topic Group Report 39)*, pp 10–13. Hospital Physicists' Association, London.
6. Mountford PJ, Hall FM, Wells CP, Coakley AJ (1984) Breast milk radioactivity after a Tc-99m-DTPA aerosol/Tc-99m-MAA lung study. *J. Nucl. Med., 25,* 1108-1120.
7. Ahlgren L, Ivarsson S, Johansson L, Mattsson S, Nosslin B (1985) Excretion of radionuclides in human breast milk after the administration of radiopharmaceuticals. *J. Nucl. Med., 26,* 1085–1090.
8. Cranage R, Palmer M (1985) Breast milk radioactivity after ^{99m}Tc-MAA lung studies. *Eur. J. Nucl. Med., 11,* 257–259
9. Rose MR, Prescott MC, Herman KJ (1990) Excretion of iodine-123-hippuran, technetium-99m-red blood cells, and technetium-99m-macroaggregated albumin into breast milk. *J. Nucl. Med., 31,* 978–984.
10. Mountford PJ (1989) Unpublished data.
11. Marshall DSC (1989) Unpublished data.
12. Hesslewood SR (1990) Unpublished data.
13. Jansson LG (1990) Unpublished data.
14. Parker B (1990) Unpublished data.
15. Rose MR, Prescott MC, Prince JR (1996) Unpublished data.

^{99m}Tc-MERCAPTOACETYLTRIGLYCINE

GENERAL

^{99m}Tc-Mercaptoacetyltriglycine (^{99m}Tc-MAG3) has been developed for dynamic renal studies and for the investigation of urological disorders with improved imaging quality over ^{99m}Tc-DTPA. After intravenous administration it is distributed into the extracellular fluid, and then rapidly excreted by renal tubular secretion similar to hippuran. The renal transit time is assumed to be 4 min, but this is increased with bilateral impairment of renal function. Small amounts (1–2%) of ^{99m}Tc labelled impurities in the preparation may be localised in the liver and excreted via the gall bladder.

EVALUATION OF DATA

Analysis of the available data describing the passage of ^{99m}Tc into milk gives the following results.

No. of cases; route	Fractional ingested activity (%)			Effective half-life (h)			Administered activity (MBq)	Effective dose to infant (mSv)	Time to reach 1 mSv (h)	Ref
	Max.	Min.	Mean	Max.	Min.	Mean				
5; i.v.	0.86	0.10	0.39	6.0	3.2	4.2	400 100	1.2 0.3	5 –	1,2

RADIOACTIVITY IN MILK

In three cases, the peak concentration occurred in the first sample expressed at 2.6–5 h after administration (1, 2), and in the other two cases, it was delayed to the second sample expressed at 4.0 h (1) and 3.8 h (2) after administration. The former peak value was the maximum recorded fractional activity concentration of 3.3×10^{-3} % ml^{-1} (1). In all cases the activity concentration decayed monoexponentially after the peak value was reached.

ASSESSMENT

If ^{99m}Tc-MAG3 is to be administered for a renal perfusion study, then the maximum usual activity in the UK is 400 MBq, otherwise the maximum usual activity for a dynamic renal scan is 100 MBq.

After a single intravenous administration of 400 or 100 MBq of ^{99m}Tc-MAG3, the maximum effective dose is estimated to be 1.2 mSv and 0.3 mSv respectively for uninterrupted breast-feeding with the first feed taken at 3 h after administration, requiring an interruption period of 5 h in the former case to reduce it to 1 mSv.

RECOMMENDATION

Category I. Interruption not essential

For a dynamic renal scan, breast-feeding need not be interrupted because the activity concentrations in milk and the estimated effective dose to the infant are small. In practice, a mother can be reassured by advising a short interruption (e.g. 4 h), at the end of which milk should be expressed and discarded.

However, if a greater activity is to be administered for a perfusion study, then the following recommendation should be made.

Category III. Interruption with measurement

Although the available data indicate that breast-feeding can be resumed after a period of interruption, they are too limited for a definite period to be recommended. Instead, the concentration of radioactivity in expressed milk should be measured, and feeding interrupted for a period (derived by the method described in the first part of this chapter) which will reduce the infant's effective dose to 1 mSv.

REFERENCES

1. Evans JL, Herring AN, Richardson MA (1993) Secretion of radioactivity in breast milk following administration of ^{99}Tc^{m}-MAG3. *Nucl. Med. Commun., 14,* 108–111.
2. Rose MR, Prescott MC, Prince JR (1996) Unpublished data.

^{99m}Tc-MICROSPHERES

GENERAL

^{99m}Tc-Microspheres are made of human serum albumin, and can be used for lung perfusion imaging. After intravenous administration, the lung uptake is greater than 90% of the administered activity. The microspheres are biodegradeable in the lungs (by proteolysis) and the radioactivity is cleared from the lungs with an effective half-life of about 6 h. After lung clearance, the smaller particles are phagocytised by the reticuloendothelial system.

EVALUATION OF DATA

Analysis of the available data describing the passage of ^{99m}Tc into milk gives the following results.

No. of cases; route	Fractional ingested activity (%)			Effective half-life (h)			Administered activity (MBq)	Effective dose to infant (mSv)	Time to reach 1 mSv (h)	Ref
	Max.	Min.	Mean	Max.	Min.	Mean				
16; i.v.	11.3	0.88	[a]	7.0	2.9	[a]	100	4	17	1,2

[a] The combined mean value of all 16 cases could not be estimated because separate data was not published for the 14 cases in reference (2), but the above method of analysis was used in that reference which reported a mean fractional ingested activity for these 14 cases alone of 4.33%, and a mean effective half-life of 5.3 h.

RADIOACTIVITY IN MILK

Separation of free ^{99m}Tc from the microspheres both before and after lung clearance leads to significant levels of radioactivity in milk. Individual data points were only available for three of the cases. In two cases, the peak fractional activity concentration of 5.7×10^{-3} % ml^{-1} and 1.5×10^{-2} % ml^{-1} occurred in the first milk sample expressed at 7.5 h and 4 h after administration (1). In the third case, the peak fractional activity concentration was delayed until the third milk sample expressed at 9 h after administration. Thereafter, the activity concentration in each case decayed monoexponentially with time after administration.

ASSESSMENT

After a single intravenous administration of 100 MBq of ^{99m}Tc-microspheres, the maximum effective dose is estimated to be 4 mSv for uninterrupted breast-feeding with the first feed taken at 3 h after administration, requiring an interruption period of 17 h to reduce it to 1 mSv.

RECOMMENDATION

Category III. Interruption with measurement

Although the available data indicate that breast-feeding can be resumed after a period of interruption, they are too limited for a definite period to be recommended. Instead, the concentration of radioactivity in expressed milk should be measured, and feeding interrupted for a period (derived by the method described in the first part of this chapter) which will reduce the infant's effective dose to 1 mSv.

REFERENCES

1. Gadd R (1990) Unpublished data.
2. Rubow S, Klopper J, Wasserman H, Baard B, van Niekerk M (1994) The excretion of radiopharmaceuticals in human breast milk: additional data and dosimetry. *Eur. J. Nucl. Med., 21,* 144–153.

SODIUM ^{99m}Tc-PERTECHNETATE

GENERAL

^{99m}Tc in the form of the pertechnetate ion ($^{99m}TcO^{-}_4$) can be used for thyroid and brain imaging. Pertechnetate is water-soluble and partly bound to circulating serum proteins after intravenous injection. Equilibrium of the free ion between the vascular compartment and interstitial fluid is reached in 2–3 min. The ions are removed from the interstitial fluid compartment by the stomach, thyroid, salivary glands, bowel, choroid plexus of brain and kidney. The half-time clearance of pertechnetate from the blood is about 30 min, the normal route of elimination being the kidneys.

EVALUATION OF DATA

Analysis of the available data describing the passage of ^{99m}Tc into milk gives the following results.

No. of cases; route	Fractional ingested activity (%)			Effective half-life (h)			Administered activity (MBq)	Effective dose to infant (mSv)	Time to reach 1 mSv (h)	Ref
	Max.	Min.	Mean	Max.	Min.	Mean				
24; i.v.	32.7	0.1	[a]	6.8	2.2	[a]	800 80	92 9.2	47 25	1–11

[a] The combined mean value of all 24 cases could not be estimated because separate data was not published for the 11 cases in reference (10). However, the above method of analysis was used in reference (10) which reported a mean fractional ingested activity for these 11cases alone of 12.2%, and a mean effective half-life of 4.2 h. For the remaining 13 cases, the mean fractional ingested activity is 7.6% and the mean effective half-life is 4.1 h.

RADIOACTIVITY IN MILK

Animal studies have shown that free pertechnetate is concentrated by the mammary gland (12), and out of all the ^{99m}Tc-labelled radiopharmaceuticals, its administration produces the greatest value of, and a wide range in fractional ingested activity. The wide range may be due partly to the simultaneous administration of perchlorate in some cases to block thyroid pertechnetate uptake. Perchlorate has been shown by animal studies to suppress the secretion of ^{99m}Tc-pertechnetate in milk, and in human studies to be associated with a lower secretion of ^{99m}Tc-pertechnetate compared to the its absence (12).

In 4 of the 13 cases where individual data points were available, the peak fractional activity concentration did not occur in the first sample expressed, but appeared in samples expressed at about 3–5 h after administration (1, 7, 8). Thereafter, the activity concentration in each case decayed monoexponentially with time after administration. The maximum concentration recorded was 9.8×10^{-2} % ml^{-1} at 3.5 h after administration (7).

EFFECT ON INFANT

In only one report (with insufficient data for the above analysis) was an infant breast-fed after maternal administration of 555 MBq of ^{99m}Tc-pertechnetate (13). This occurred at 4 h after injection and was shown to have delivered 3 MBq to the infant through the milk. No adverse effects in the infant were reported.

ASSESSMENT

If the ^{99m}Tc-pertechnetate is administered for a first pass blood flow study or for a thyroid scan, then the maximum usual activity in the UK is 800 MBq and 80 MBq respectively. For uninterrupted breast-feeding with the first feed taken at 3 h after a single intravenous administration of 800 MBq and 80 MBq of ^{99m}Tc-pertechnetate, the maximum effective dose is estimated to be 92 mSv and 9.2 mSv respectively, requiring an interruption period of 47 h and 25 h respectively to reduce it to 1 mSv.

RECOMMENDATION

Category II. Interruption for a definite period

There is sufficient published data to allow a definite period of interruption of 47 h after administration of 800 MBq of ^{99m}Tc-pertechnetate and a period of 25 h after administration of 80 MBq of ^{99m}Tc-pertechnetate to be recommended in order to reduce the estimated effective dose to 1 mSv.

REFERENCES

1. Pittard III WB, Bill K, Fletcher BD (1979) Excretion of technetium in human milk. *J. Pediatr., 94,* 605–607.
2. Wyburn JR (1973) Human breast milk excretion of radionuclides following administration of radiopharmaceuticals. *J. Nucl. Med., 14,* 115–117.
3. Maisels JM, Gilcher RO (1983) Excretion of technetium in human milk. *Pediatrics, 71,* 841–842.
4. Ahlgren L, Ivarsson S, Johansson L, Mattsson S, Nosslin B (1985) Excretion of radionuclides in human breast milk after the administration of radiopharmaceuticals. *J. Nucl. Med., 26,* 1085–1090.
5. Mountford PJ, Coakley AJ (1987) Breast milk radioactivity following injection of $^{99}Tc^m$-pertechnetate and $^{99}Tc^m$-glucoheptonate. *Nucl. Med. Commun., 8,* 839–845.
6. Hedrick WR, Di Simone RN, Keen RL (1986) Radiation dosimetry from breast milk excretion of radioiodine and pertechnetate. *J. Nucl. Med., 27,* 1569–1571.
7. Hesslewood SR (1992) Unpublished data.
8. Hawkins T (1992) Unpublished data.

9. Mountford PJ (1988) Unpublished data.
10. Rubow S, Klopper J, Wasserman H, Baard B, van Niekerk M (1994) The excretion of radiopharmaceuticals in human breast milk: additional data and dosimetry. *Eur. J. Nucl. Med., 21,* 144–153.
11. Rose MR, Prescott MC, Prince JR (1996) Unpublished data.
12. Mountford PJ, Heap RB, Hamon M, Fleet IR, Coakley AJ (1987) Suppression of technetium-99m and iodine-123 secretion in milk of lactating goats. *J. Nucl. Med., 28,* 1187–1191.
13. Rumble WF, Aamodt RL, Jones AE, Henkin RI, Johnston GS (1978) Accidental ingestion of Tc-99m in breast milk by a 10-week-old child. *J. Nucl. Med., 19,* 913–915.

^{99m}Tc-PYROPHOSPHATE

GENERAL

^{99m}Tc-Pyrophosphate is used as a skeletal imaging agent and as an adjunct in the diagnosis of acute myocardial infarction. After intravenous administration, 40–50% of the radioactivity appears in the skeleton within 1–2 h. Approximately 10% remains in the vascular system and the remainder is excreted by the kidneys.

EVALUATION OF DATA

Analysis of the available data describing the passage of ^{99m}Tc into milk gives the following results.

No. of cases; route	Fractional ingested activity (%)			Effective half-life (h)			Administered activity (MBq)	Effective dose to infant (mSv)	Time to reach 1 mSv (h)	Ref
	Max.	Min.	Mean	Max.	Min.	Mean				
8; i.v.	0.44	0.15	0.28	6.8	3.5	4.9	600	0.9	–	1

RADIOACTIVITY IN MILK

Individual data points were not published for any of these cases but the authors had analysed each by the above method (1). One other case has been published but with insufficient data for analysis where the fractional activity concentration in a milk sample expressed at 5 h after administration was 2×10^{-3} % ml^{-1} (2).

ASSESSMENT

After a single intravenous administration of 600 MBq of ^{99m}Tc-pyrophosphate, the maximum effective dose is estimated to be 0.9 mSv for uninterrupted breast-feeding with the first feed taken at 3 h after administration.

RECOMMENDATION

Category III. Interruption with measurement

Although the maximum effective dose is less than 1 mSv, it is only just less than this critical value and only a limited amount of data is available. Therefore it is recommended that the concentration of radioactivity in expressed milk should be measured, and feeding interrupted for a period (derived by the method described in the first part of this chapter) which will ensure the infant's effective dose does not exceed 1 mSv.

REFERENCES

1. Rubow S, Klopper J, Wasserman H, Baard B, van Niekerk M (1994) The excretion of radiopharmaceuticals in human breast milk: additional data and dosimetry. *Eur. J. Nucl. Med., 21,* 144–153.
2. O'Connell MEA, Sutton H (1976) Excretion of radioactivity in breast milk following $^{99}Tc^{m}$-Sn polyphosphate. *Br. J. Radiol., 49,* 377–379.

^{99m}Tc-SULPHUR COLLOID

GENERAL

^{99m}Tc-Sulphur colloid particles (typically 100–1000 nm diameter) are used for the evaluation of the reticuloendothelial system. After intravenous administration, they are cleared from the blood with a half clearance time of approximately 3 min. Approximately 90% of the injected activity is taken up by the liver, 5% by the spleen and 5% by the bone marrow. Uptake to these latter two organs increases dramatically in diffuse parenchymal liver disease.

EVALUATION OF DATA

Analysis of the available data describing the passage of ^{99m}Tc into milk gives the following results.

No. of cases; route	Fractional ingested activity (%)			Effective half-life (h)			Administered activity (MBq)	Effective dose to infant (mSv)	Time to reach 1 mSv (h)	Ref
	Max.	Min.	Mean	Max.	Min.	Mean				
5; i.v.	1.5	0.16	0.67	8.3	5.1	6.2	80	0.4	–	1

RADIOACTIVITY IN MILK

Individual data points were not published for any of these cases but the authors had analysed each case by the above method (1).

ASSESSMENT

After a single intravenous administration of 80 MBq of ^{99m}Tc-sulphur colloid, the maximum effective dose is estimated to be 0.4 mSv for uninterrupted breast-feeding with the first feed taken at 3 h after administration.

RECOMMENDATION

Category I. Interruption not essential

Breast-feeding need not be interrupted because the activity concentrations in milk and the estimated effective dose to the infant are small. In practice, a mother can be reassured by advising a short interruption (e.g. 4 h), at the end of which milk should be expressed and discarded.

REFERENCES

1. Rubow S, Klopper J, Wasserman H, Baard B, van Niekerk M (1994) The excretion of radiopharmaceuticals in human breast milk: additional data and dosimetry. *Eur. J. Nucl. Med., 21,* 144–153.

RADIOACTIVE THALLIUM

The radionuclide ^{201}Tl is produced in a cyclotron and may contain up to 3% impurities as other radionuclides. It has a physical half-life of 73.1 h and decays by electron capture to stable mercury with the emission of 69–80 keV mercury X-rays, and 135 keV (3%) and 167 keV (10%) γ-rays.

The ICRP dosimetry data for ingested activity assumes a fractional absorption of 100% for thallium in its ionic form (1, 2).

REFERENCES

1. International Commission on Radiological Protection (1980) *Limits for Intakes of Radionuclides by Workers* (ICRP Publication 30). Pergamon Press, Oxford.
2. International Commission on Radiological Protection (1991) *Annual Limits on Intake of Radionuclides by Workers Based on the 1990 Recommendations* (ICRP Publication 61). Pergamon Press, Oxford.

^{201}Tl-CHLORIDE

GENERAL

^{201}Tl-thallous chloride is used for functional imaging of myocardial perfusion, and in dual radiopharmaceutical studies with ^{99m}Tc-pertechnetate or sodium ^{123}I-iodide for localising parathyroid adenoma. Approximately 88% of the intravenously administered activity is extracted in one pass through the coronary circulation and is taken up in the cells of all organs. The degree of uptake and the anatomical distribution depends largely on regional blood flow which in turn will depend on the state of physical exercise. After intravenous administration to a patient at rest, approximately 3.5% of the activity localises in the myocardium, increasing to 4.4% at exercise. Significant redistribution of the radionuclide occurs with time. Excretion is mostly by the gastrointestinal tract and partly by the renal tract.

EVALUATION OF DATA

Analysis of the available data describing the passage of ^{201}Tl into milk gives the following results.

No. of cases; route	Fractional ingested activity (%)			Effective half-life (h)			Administered activity (MBq)	Effective dose to infant (mSv)	Time to reach 1 mSv (h)	Ref
	Max.	Min.	Mean	Max.	Min.	Mean				
1; i.v.	0.7	–	–	27 (0.3%) 362 (0.4%)	–	–	80	0.7	–	1

RADIOACTIVITY IN MILK

Although two cases have been published with measurements of breast milk radioactivity up to 12 and 15 days after administration respectively (1, 2), the second case did not contain enough detail for the above analysis (2). Both cases showed a similar biexponential decrease in activity concentration in milk with a fractional activity concentration on the first day of about 2×10^{-4} % ml^{-1} (1) and about 1.4×10^{-4} % ml^{-1} (2). Using the method of least squares in the first case, the authors derived the following relation to describe the variation of the fractional activity concentration $A(t)$ (ml^{-1}) with time t (h) after administration (1):-

$$A(t) = 2.17 \times 10^{-6} \exp(-0.0255t) + 1.93 \times 10^{-7} \exp(-0.00191t)$$

ASSESSMENT

After a single intravenous administration of 80 MBq of ^{201}Tl-chloride, the effective dose is estimated to be 0.7 mSv for uninterrupted breast-feeding with the first feed taken at 3 h after radiopharmaceutical administration.

RECOMMENDATION

Category I. Interruption not essential

Breast-feeding need not be interrupted because the activity concentrations in milk and the estimated effective dose to the infant are so small. In practice, a mother can be reassured by advising a short interruption (e.g. 4 h), at the end of which milk should be expressed and discarded.

REFERENCES

1. Murphy PH, Beasley CW, Moore WH, Stabin MG (1989) Thallium-201 in human milk: observations and radiological consequences. *Health Phys., 56,* 539–541.
2. Toney MO, Landry A, Smith T (1992) Excretion of Tl in human breast milk. *Health Phys., 63,* 234.

OTHER RADIOPHARMACEUTICALS

Recommendations have also been derived for the following radiopharmaceuticals which are no longer in common use or where there is insufficient data for the above analysis:-

Category III. Interruption with measurement

^{99m}Tc-MACROAGGREGATED FERROUS HYDROXIDE
^{99m}Tc-PLASMIN
^{99m}Tc-ETHYLENEDIAMINETETRAACETIC ACID
^{99m}Tc-Sn-POLYPHOSPHATE
^{113m}In-CHELATE COMPLEX
^{125}I-ORTHOIODOHIPPURIC ACID

Although the available data indicate that breast-feeding can be resumed after a period of interruption, they are too limited for a definite period to be recommended. Instead, the concentration of radioactivity in expressed milk should be measured, and feeding interrupted for a period (derived by the method described in the first part of this chapter) which will reduce the infant's effective dose to 1 mSv.

Category IV. Cessation

^{125}I-FIBRINOGEN
^{131}I- MACROAGGREGATED HUMAN SERUM ALBUMIN
^{131}I-HUMAN SERUM ALBUMIN
CHROMIC ^{32}P-PHOSPHATE
SODIUM ^{32}P-PHOSPHATE
^{75}Se-METHIONINE

The period of interrruption is likely to be so long that the mother will have to be advised to discontinue feeding altogether.

Drugs and Human Lactation
P.N. Bennett, editor

9. Environmental and occupational chemicals

Allan Astrup Jensen

SUMMARY

Humans are exposed to innumerable chemicals from sources in the natural environment and the workplace. Some of these chemicals, especially the lipophilic and persistent organohalogens such as DDT, PCB and 'dioxins', accumulate in human fat tissues and are excreted mainly by breast milk. Toxic metals such as lead, cadmium and mercury may also be excreted in breast milk. Average concentrations of contaminants in breast milk from the general population differ between countries, states and districts and with time. Some of the recorded variation arises through differences in sampling techniques and chemical assay methods. Factors that influence the level of contamination include the fat content of milk, the sampling time in the lactation period, maternal age, parity, body weight, residence time in a locality, dietary habits, and certainly the occupation. Human milk contains more than ten times higher concentration of these contaminants than do cow's milk or milk substitutes. Even though the period of breast-feeding is short in relation to a lifetime, these chemicals persist in the body and enter it at a sensitive phase of its development. There should be a constant awareness of this source of potentially toxic substances for the breast-fed infant.

INTRODUCTION

Human milk is an ideal nutrient for infants. Unfortunately, it is also a major excretory pathway of lipophilic substances that are not effectively metabolised by the body. As early as the last century it was known that breast milk from a mother who was occupationally exposed to toxic chemicals, e.g. heavy metals, might contain amounts of the substance which could adversely effect her nursing infant (1). In the last 40 years a vast number of breast milk samples collected from the general population all over the world have been investigated and low concentrations of environmental chemicals, such as chlorinated pesticides, polychlorobiphenyls and 'dioxins' have been determined. Although, the concentrations are low, these contaminants may be potentially hazardous to the breast-fed infant (for reviews, see 2–5).

The concentrations of man-made organic chemicals in human milk are normally more than ten times higher than in cow's milk from the same area, and commercial infant milk formulas contain even lower levels (2, 6). Frequently, limit values established for contaminants in cow's milk are exceeded in human milk. Therefore, new-borns and infants, whose main foodstuff is breast milk, may have a much higher relative daily intake of these chemical pollutants than adults, and 'acceptable daily intakes' (ADIs), tolerable daily intakes (TDIs) or provisionally tolerable weekly intakes' (PTWIs) set by FAO/WHO for pesticides, contaminants and heavy metals, respectively, may be exceeded (2, 6).

GLOSSARY

Abbreviation	Chemical name
DDD	1,1-Dichloro-2,2-bis(*p*-chlorophenyl)ethane
DDE	1,1-Dichloro-2,2-bis(*p*-chlorophenyl)ethylene
DDT	1,1,1-Trichloro-2,2-bis(*p*-chlorophenyl)ethane
Dieldrin	1,2,3,4,10,10-Hexachloro-6,7-epoxy-1,4,4a,5,6,7,8,8a-octahydro-1,4-exo-5,8-*endo*-dimethanonaphthalene
HCB	Hexachlorobenzene
HCH/BHC	1,2,3,4,5,6-Hexachlorocyclohexane
Heptachlor epoxide	1,4,5,6,7,8,8a-Heptachloro-2,3-epoxy-2,3,3a,4,7,7a-hexahydro-4,7-methanoindene
Lindane	γ-HCH
PBB	Polybrominated biphenyls
PCB/Aroclor	Polychlorinated biphenyls
PCDD	Polychlorinated dibenzo-*p*-dioxins
PCDF	Polychlorinated dibenzofurans
TCDD	2,3,7,8-Tetrachlorodibenzo-*p*-dioxin
ppb	Parts per billion, 10^{-9}
ppm	Parts per million, 10^{-6}
ppt	Parts per trillion, 10^{-12}

ENVIRONMENTAL POLLUTANTS IN BREAST MILK

The first environmental chemical discovered in human milk in the general population was the insecticide DDT. The average concentration found by a colorimetric method in milk samples from 32 healthy black American women living in Washington, DC, was 130 ppb (7). During subsequent decades the development of gas-chromatographic methods made detection of organochlorine contaminants much easier and more reliable. Using this technique, Quinby et al. (8) determined DDT and its metabolites (DDE and DDD) in human milk from the United States, and Egan et al. (9) determined for the first time other organochlorine pesticides, including dieldrin, hexachlorocyclohexanes (HCH, BHC) and heptachlor epoxide in human milk from Great Britain.

Peters and co-workers, investigating a mass intoxication from bread contaminated with the fungicide hexachlorobenzene (HCB) in Turkey in the late 1950s, reported that several suckling infants were fatally poisoned by HCB received by breast-feeding (10). In a follow-up study, the same researchers found raised HCB concentrations in human milk from that same area 25 years after the incident (11).

Shortly after Søren Jensen (12) in 1966 discovered that the industrial chemical polychlorinated biphenyls (PCBs), e.g. Aroclors, were important environmental pollutants, PCBs were determined in human milk samples from Sweden by Westöö et al. (13) and from Germany by Acker and Schulte (14). Today, PCBs are probably the most widespread organochlorine contaminant of human milk in the general population of industrialised societies. While the early investigations quantified the mixture of PCB congeners, the most recent studies may quantify the single PCB congeners including the most toxic, so-called co-planar PCB congeners (15).

The first detection of organophosphorous pesticides in human milk was made in Taiwan by Yeh et al. (16), who found an average concentration of 1.9 ppm of malathion (used as a DDT substitute in Taiwan) in whole milk; this value was 50 times that of DDT in the same samples.

Brilliant et al. (17) detected polybrominated biphenyls (PBBs) in most human milk samples analysed from the State of Michigan (USA) after the 1973 pollution incident, in which animal feed was accidentally contaminated with PBBs, mainly hexabromobiphenyls.

Rappe et al. (18) were the first scientists who discovered 'dioxins' (chlorinated dibenzo-*p*-dioxins and chlorinated dibenzofurans) in human milk from European countries. 'Dioxins' included the extremely toxic compound 2,3,7,8-tetrachlorodibenzo-*p*-dioxin (TCDD) determined in concentrations of 1–2 ppt. TCDD is well-known from the 'Seveso' accident on 10 July 1976 in a chemical plant (ICMESA), located near the town of Seveso in northern Italy. Shortly after the explosion, up to 7.9 ppb of TCDD was detected in milk from cows grazing in contaminated zones (19). TCDD concentrations in human milk fat from the polluted area were 2–28 ppt with an average of 13 ppt (20).

Very recently the persistent and bioaccumulating 'nitro musks', which are widely used as fragrances in cosmetics and detergents, have been detected (up to 0.3 ppm) in human milk from the northern part of Germany (21).

Other potentially hazardous environmental chemicals have been detected in human milk, for instances, pentachlorophenol (22), traces of nitrosamines (23), and polycyclic aromatic hydrocarbons (PAHs) (24) and no doubt others will be discovered in the future. Pellizzari et al. (25) identified about 200 different volatile chemical compounds in 12 samples from four urban areas in the United States, indicating a much broader chemical contamination of human milk from the general population than had previously been expected (Table 1).

TABLE 1 *Volatile chemicals identified in at least 7 of 12 samples of human milk from 4 urban areas of the USA (25)*

Aliphatic hydrocarbons	Cyclic hydrocarbons	Halocarbons	Others
Pentanes	Benzene	Methylene chloride	Isopropylalcohol
Hexanes	Toluene	Methylchloroform	Acetone
Heptanes	Xylene	Chloroform	Acetophenone
Octanes	Ethylbenzene	Trichloroethylene	Pentanal
Nonanes	Styrene	Perchloroethylene	Hexanal
Decanes	Limonene	Dichlorobenzene	Carbon disulfide

ACCUMULATION OF POLLUTANTS IN BREAST MILK

Lipophilic, un-ionised organic chemicals readily penetrate the cellular barriers between blood plasma and breast milk and concentrate in the fat globules. In this way, chemicals can be transferred and attain significant concentrations in human breast milk, if exposures are either periodically high or life-long (26, 27).

Periodically high exposures to lipophilic chemicals, e.g. organic solvents, halocarbons and pesticides, may occur in some occupations, but are rare in the general population apart from a few incidences of mass intoxication. Of more relevance for the general population are life-long exposures to low levels of certain lipophilic and metabolically persistent environmental chemicals, such as the organohalogens DDT and PCBs, to which practically everyone is exposed, either directly or through food chain bioaccumulation (27).

In mammals these chemicals are efficiently absorbed through the skin, lungs and gastrointestinal tract, and they mainly bind to very low density lipoproteins (VLDL) in the blood. As they are only slowly or even negligibly metabolised by and eliminated from the body, most absorbed material is retained unchanged, and thus the body burden gradually increases. The main storage is in the adipose tissue (28).

In females, pregnancy and lactation change the accumulation and distribution of lipids in the body (26). Lipids and lipophilic contaminants are transferred into breast tissue from adipose tissues. A lactation period mobilises 10–20% of fat deposits in the body (29). In Germany it was estimated that a women during her pregnancy and delivery loses about 16 kg body weight (30). Lactation will in practice be the most important route of excretion for bioaccumulating, lipophilic chemicals (17). Experiments with lactating mice have indicated that essentially the entire body burden of persistent PCBs and HCB may be eliminated and transferred to nursing offspring by 20 days postpartum (31, 32, 26).

Under normal circumstances, the concentrations of organohalogens in human milk fat largely reflect the amounts in adipose tissue, and daily intakes of the chemicals during lactation are in general without great influence on the concentrations in breast milk (24, 33, 34).

CONCENTRATIONS AND TRENDS OF ENVIRONMENTAL CHEMICALS IN HUMAN MILK

During the past two decades, many scientists have reported contamination of human milk by environmental chemicals. Investigations differ greatly in purpose, scope, design, size, selection of milk donors, sampling methods and chemical analysis. Most studies involve too few samples and mothers to make any real conclusions about the origin of the contamination. Some studies ignore factors that are known to affect the concentrations of contaminants in human milk (see 'Factors that affect the level of contamination', p. 686), and other studies lack sufficient analytical quality control.

Differences in the method of assay may substantially affect the results, especially in the case of PCBs and dioxins. Therefore, it is not surprising that published data, even within the same country or district, may differ greatly, and comparisons of the findings of different research groups should be interpreted with great caution. With this reservation, some recent results of average DDT, PCB and 'dioxins' (PCDDs + PCDFs) concentrations in human milk fat obtained from individuals living in various countries are selected and shown in Figs. 1–4.

Typically, the concentrations of DDT are higher in samples from developing countries with current or recent usage of persistent pesticides. Levels are extremely high in areas of these countries where DDT is spayed The concentrations of PCBs and dioxins are higher in samples from industrialised countries, whereas these

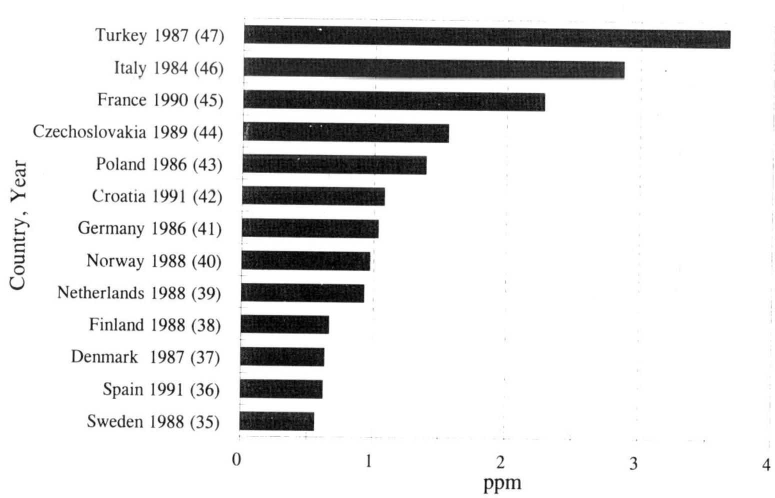

FIG. 1 *Average DDT + DDE in human milk fat from European countries. The number of individuals from whom samples were taken is shown in parentheses.*

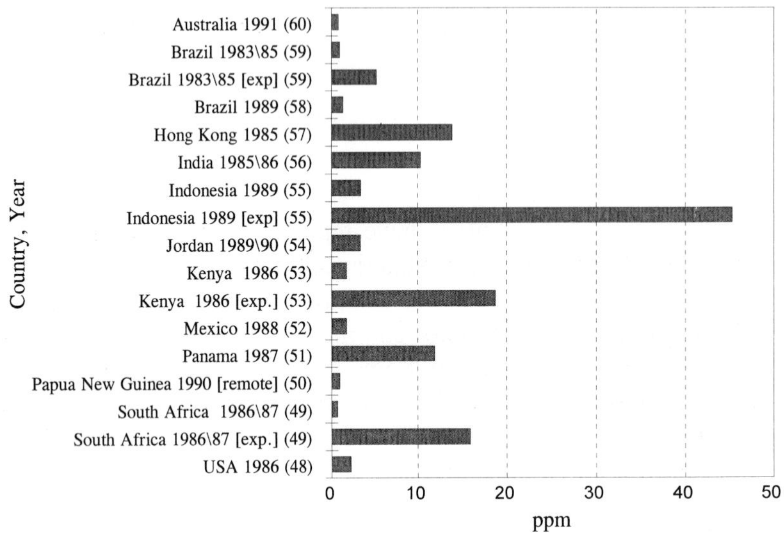

FIG. 2 *Average DDT + DDE in human mild fat from countries outside Europe. The number of individuals from whom samples were taken is shown in parentheses.*

chemicals often are not detectable in samples from developing countries. If only a few PCB peaks are used for the chromatographic quantitation, then PCB levels are approximately twice as high.

The trends in average DDT, DDE, and PCB concentrations in human milk dur-

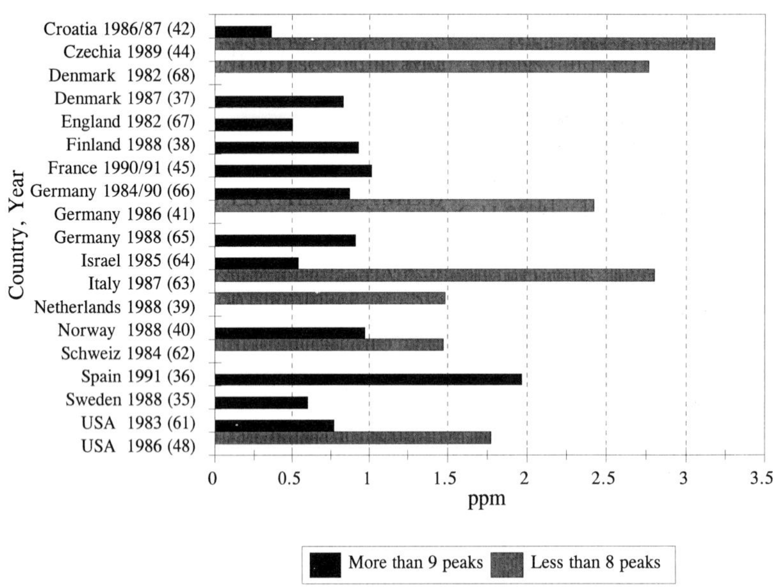

FIG. 3 *PCB in human milk fat: Average concentrations. The number of individuals from whom samples were taken is shown in parentheses.*

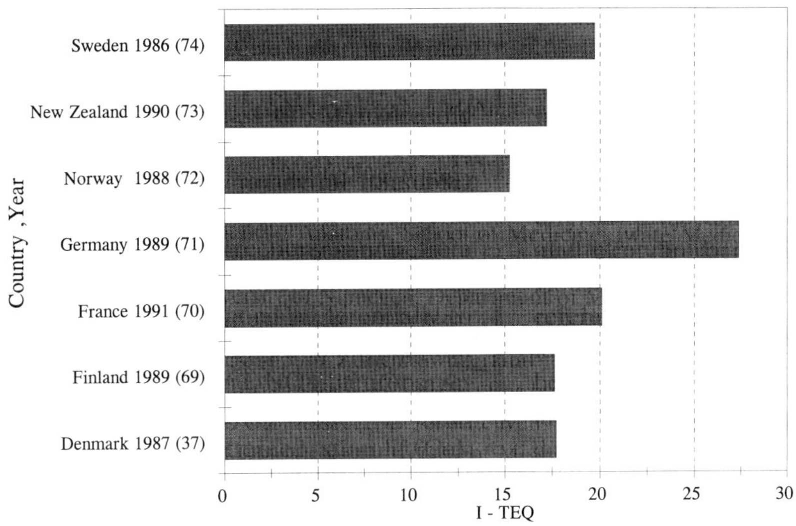

FIG. 4 *Average dioxin toxicity equivalents (I-TEQ) in human milk fat.*

ing more than a decade in Sweden are illustrated in Fig. 5. The samples are from a milkbank in Stockholm, and the contaminants were determined by the same laboratory and similar methods (35, 75).

Concentrations of DDT and its metabolite DDE decreased throughout the period

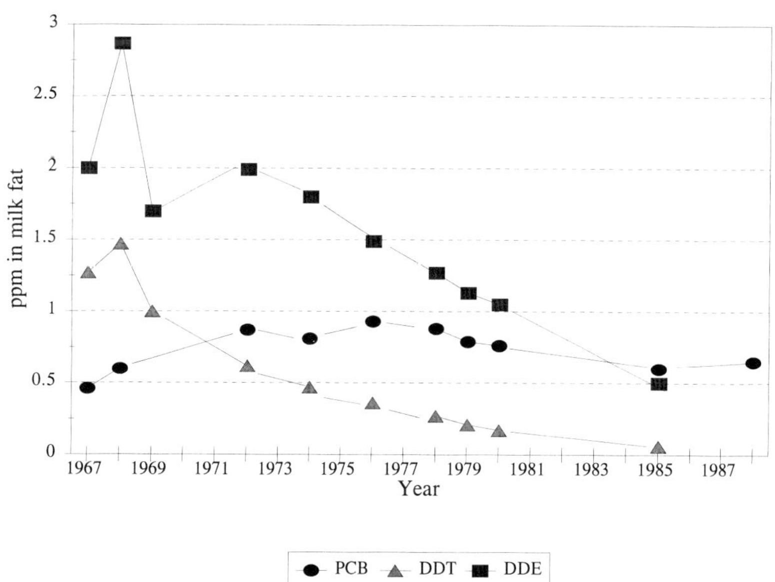

FIG. 5 *Trend of DDT, DDE and PCB levels in human milk from Stockholm.*

studied, DDT faster than the more persistent DDE. The levels of PCBs increased in the first years, followed by a weak downward trend. Investigations from other European countries have not indicated a clear decline of PCB concentrations in human milk (24, 29), if the same analytical method is used It is worth noting that the methods of chemical analysis that are most popular nowadays should give lower values than those that were used some years ago (76).

Heavy metals may also contaminate human milk. Concentrations direct toxic to the suckling infant (≤200 ppb mercury in whole milk) were, for instance, observed in connection with the tragic 1972 mercury poisoning episode in Iraq (77).

Some recent data on average concentrations of lead, cadmium and mercury from different countries are shown in Figs. 6–8, respectively. Again, some of the differences may be explained by the different analytical methods used

FACTORS THAT AFFECT THE LEVELS OF CONTAMINATION

Several factors may influence the actual amounts of environmental chemicals in individuals. These include: (a) fat content of breast milk, (b) sampling time in lactation, (c) maternal age, (d) maternal parity and history of delivery, (e) maternal weight, (f) maternal origin and residence, (g) maternal diet, (h) seasonal differences,, (i) maternal smoking, (j) maternal use of biocides, (k) maternal use of cosmetics, and (l) maternal occupation. Some of the published investigations include too few mothers/samples that the differences found were not statistical significant.

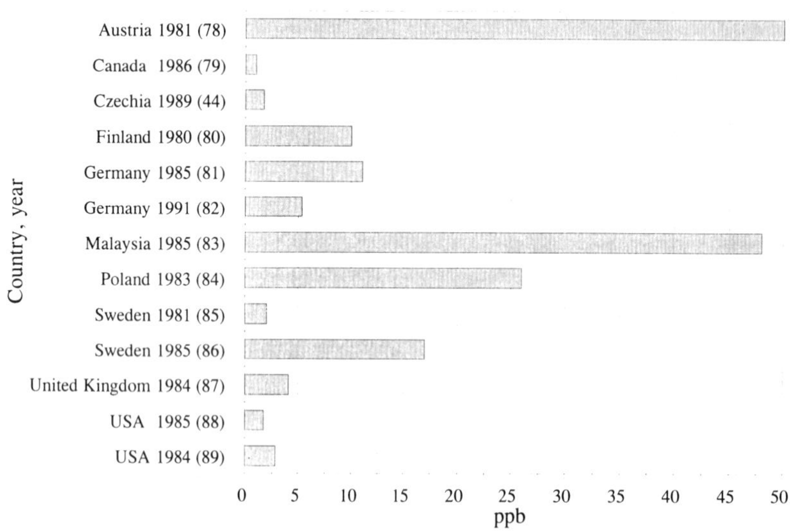

FIG. 6 *Lead in human milk average concentrations. The number of individuals from whom samples were taken is shown in parentheses.*

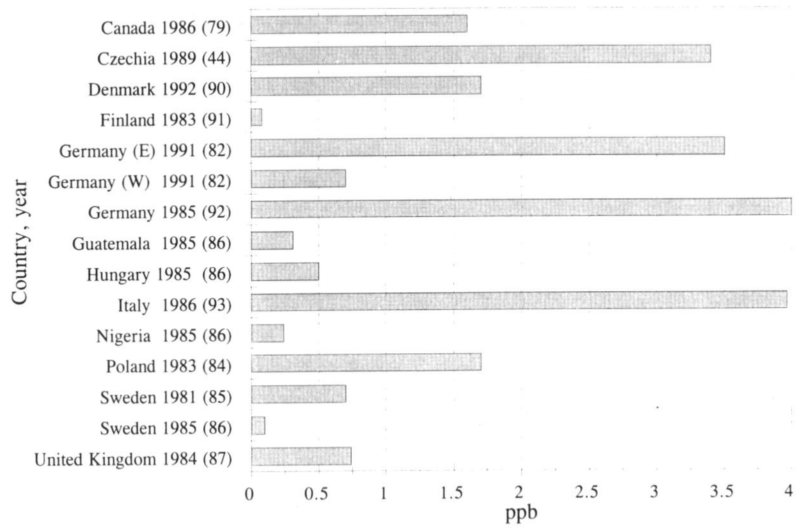

FIG. 7 *Cadmium in human milk average concentrations. The number of individuals from whom samples were taken is shown in parentheses.*

Fat content of breast milk and daily fluctuations

The average concentration of fat in breast milk is around 3–4% but varies between individuals and fluctuates within an individual during a feed, during a day, and from day to day (96). Since most residues are lipophilic and associated with the milk fat, the concentration of residues will also fluctuate.

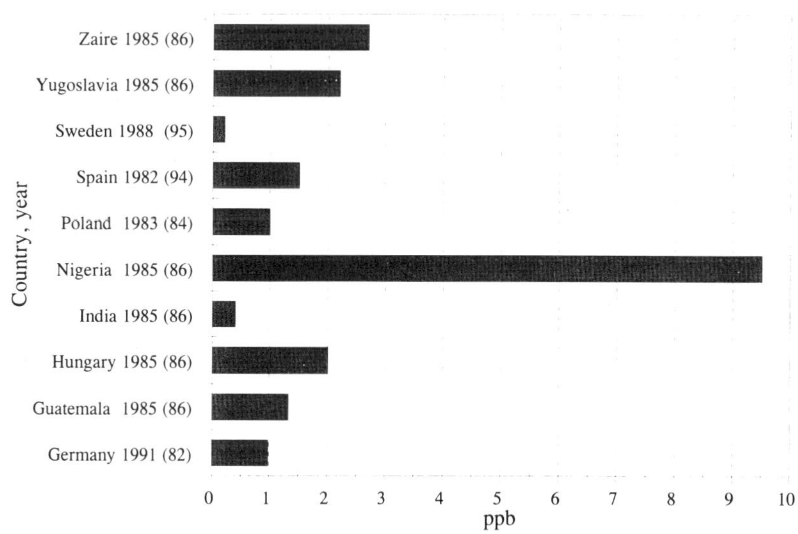

FIG. 8 *Mercury in human milk average concentrations. The number of individuals from whom samples were taken is shown in parentheses.*

Mes and Davies (97) reported 5-fold differences of PCB concentrations in whole milk during one feed, or during the day in single donors. There was a tendency to higher concentrations later in a feeding period. The same trend was reported by Wilson et al. (98) and Barnett et al. (99) with DDT. When the data were corrected for milk fat content, however, very small or no differences were observed Therefore, comparison of results of different investigations of lipophilic contaminants must take into account variation in milk fat.

Pluim et al. (100) have recently found significant higher dioxin concentrations in milk fat from mothers milk collected in the evening compared with collection in the morning.

Sampling time in lactation

During the lactation period the fat% in breast milk decreases (101). The concentrations of organohalogens are generally lower in whole colostrum (fat deficient) than in mature milk; but the quantities are higher in colostrum fat than in mature milk fat (102). The content of heavy metals are, however, higher in whole colostrum (81).

There appears to be a tendency towards a gradual decrease of organochlorine residues in both whole mature milk and milk fat during the first 6–12 months of lactation, especially if the concentration of the residues at the start of breast-feeding is relatively high. DDT and HCB in milk fat from 12 Austrian donors decreased to one-third of the initial level during about 10 weeks, and reached the current Austrian limits for cow's milk (1 and 0.5 ppm, respectively). The decrease continued to a lesser degree during the following weeks (103). Earlier, Acker and Schulte (104) reported a 30% decrease of DDT in human milk fat during the first 3 months of lactation. In an investigation of DDE and PCBs in milk fat from an occupationally exposed Japanese woman, concentrations of PCBs gradually decreased from about 15 ppm to less than 5 ppm after a year. In the same period, the DDE concentration decreased from 4 to 1 ppm in milk fat (105). In Canada, Mes et al. (106) reported a small but statistically significant decrease of β-HCH, HCB, DDE and DDT in milk fat during lactation. Rogan et al. (48) reported a 20% and 40% decrease in DDE and PCB in milk fat from the United States in 6 and 18 months, respectively. In Norway, PCB levels in milk fat decreased 30% in 4 months (107). Also dioxin levels may decrease up to 50% in 1 year (71, 108).

The heavy metals lead and cadmium, also show a decrease in human mature milk concentration with lactation time (81, 91, 109, 110).

Maternal age

The daily rate of elimination from the body of persistent organohalogens is generally less than the daily uptake rate. Increasing accumulation by age of these substances in adipose fat (111) and in blood serum (112, 113) is therefore not surprising. In studies involving a very large number of samples Rogan et al. (48) reported 20–30% lower levels of DDE and PCB in 16–24-year-old compared with 30–41-year-old mothers, and Ehrensdorfer et al. (29) found a gradually increase of 50% of DDT and PCB from the year 20 to 45. Dioxin concentrations in milk fat also increased significantly with age (114).

In many earlier human milk studies there was no clear relationship between maternal age and the concentration of residues in human milk, possibly because of low sample size, the relative youth of women giving birth and because of confounding factors such as parity (115).

Maternal parity and history of delivery

Since lactation is the most important route of excretion of persistent organohalogens, previous lactations are likely to deplete the deposits. Indeed most studies confirm that the concentrations of DDT/DDE (38, 48, 49, 66, 116–125, 127), PCBs (48, 66, 107, 121–125, 127), β-HCH (116, 128, 127), γ-HCH (129), HCB (128), dieldrin (130) and dioxins (71) in human milk or milk fat decrease with parity. Normally, significant differences first occur after the second birth.

Mothers giving birth to twins (or for other reasons having an increased milk production) excrete a relatively higher amount of DDT overall (131). Women undergoing premature delivery and stillbirth were found to excrete more DDT in their milk than those undergoing full-term, normal delivery (132).

Maternal weight

In general, slim persons have less fat deposits and higher concentrations of DDT and PCB in adipose fat tissues (57, 104, 133–135). In whole human milk, Polishuk et al. (133) observed higher concentrations of DDT, γ-HCH, dieldrin, heptachlor epoxide and PCBs in mothers who weighted less than 63 kg, compared to mothers who weighed more than 72 kg. A similar association with DDT in whole milk was found by Knoll and Jayaraman (117), and with dieldrin, heptachlor epoxide and γ-HCH in whole milk, and dieldrin and heptachlor epoxide in milk fat by Miller et al. (102). Other investigations have not observed the influence of maternal weight.

Maternal origin and residence

Investigations in the USA and Brazil have suggested a racial factor in human milk contamination. In both countries, mothers from black population groups had higher DDT concentrations in their milk than had white mothers (123, 136). It is more likely that these differences are attributable to socioeconomic factors as was observed by Davies et al. (137) who assessed the body burden of DDT.

In many industrial countries, female immigrants from less developed countries may have far more DDT and less PCBs in their breast milk than have native citizens (40, 138–142). These findings may be explained by higher exposure to DDT and lower exposure to PCB's in the less developed countries, and the persistence of these chemicals in body fat. A investigation of 33 mothers who emigrated from Turkey to Germany showed a significant positive correlation between PCB concentration in milk fat and residence time in their new country (143).

In general, mothers from urban areas have higher DDT concentrations in their milk than do mothers from rural areas, as long as DDT has not been used commercially in the area (58, 119, 144, 145). On the other hand, DDT may reach enormously high concentrations in rural and agricultural areas, where the pesticide is still in use (49, 53, 55, 99, 146).

PCB and dioxin concentrations are also higher in urban and industrial areas than in rural areas (129, 147, 148). The principal source may be air pollution. In a Canadian study, the highest concentration of PCBs was detected in milk from a woman who had lived close to a municipal waste incinerator for 5 years (129). In the Northern Canada, Dewailly et al. (149, 150) found that Inuit women had 2–10 times more PCB (including co-planar congeners) and dioxins in their milk than Caucasian women. The reason is the high intake of contaminated marine mammals (see later). In Germany and Brazil, the concentrations of β-HCH were highest in milk from mothers who lived in rural areas (58, 151).

Regional differences in both organochlorine pesticides and PCBs in human milk have been observed in Sweden (152). The concentrations of all residues were generally lower in the northern and less densely populated parts. DDT and β-HCH concentrations in milk from mothers living in the capital, Stockholm, were about the same as those from Lund, a southern, less-industrialised university city. The air fallout of PCBs is greater in southern Sweden, because of long-range carriage from central Europe. Concerning dioxins Fürst et al. (71) reported no difference between breast milk from urban and rural areas.

Area of residence also has an important influence on the heavy metal content of human milk. Breast milk from an area of Austria with high traffic density had a 50% higher lead content than that from rural areas (153). In Poland, both cadmium and lead in human milk were significantly higher in industrial compared to agricultural areas (84). In Mexico City close to a smelter, extremely high lead concentrations were found in blood and breast milk samples (154). Lead concentrations in milk from an industrial city in Romania were more than 10 times higher than those from a pollution-free town (155).

Maternal diet

Apart from direct exposure to chemicals, ingestion of contaminated foodstuffs is often recognized to be the main source of persistent environmental chemicals in the human body. Dietary habits will therefore to a great extent decide the level of residues in human milk.

High concentrations of organochlorine pesticides (DDT, HCH, dieldrin) in milk from, urban Japanese mothers have been explained by a high intake of animal proteins and animals fats by inhabitants of cities (144). These findings are in line with experience with organohalogens in Hawaii (156). In general, the greater the intake of calories by the individual, the higher is the DDE content of human milk (120).

In an earlier study from the USA higher concentrations of DDT were found in breast milk from women who consumed margarine than those who took butter (98). The finding may have been related to the use of contaminated cottonseed oil in the manufacture of margarine, because prior to 1973, spraying of cotton crops accounted for 70% of DDT consumption in the USA. A subsequent investigation in Brazil did not detect a difference between women who ate margarine or butter (123).

Recent studies have indicated that eating fish and marine products may often be the most important dietary factor that controls concentrations of DDT and PCBs in human milk (116, 119, 141, 157–160). The association with fish intake is also supported by findings that PCB concentrations in human milk in Japan were highest in fishing cities (161), and in Canada were highest in coastal provinces (162). A contrary conclusion was reached by a more recent Canadian study by Mes et al. (127).

In coastal areas with high intake of ocean fish (tuna, swordfish etc.) or marine mammals (whales, seals, etc.) increased levels of mercury have also been detected in human milk (163, 164).

Countries may differ in the origin of the residues in milk. In the former Federal Republic of Germany, relatively high PCB concentrations in human milk may be explained by dietary habits. Investigation showed that about 60% of the daily PCB intake in that country originated from meats and dairy products, 35% from vegetables, and only 5% from fish (165).

The origin of contamination of meat and dairy products may be cattle feed stored in silos previously coated with PCBs. From such indirect contamination, the wife of a Swiss farmer achieved 10 ppm PCBs in her milk fat by eating the farm's own dairy products when the average PCB concentration in the milk fat from their cows was 2.3 ppm (166).

The influence of intake of meat, dairy products and fish on the concentrations of organochlorine pesticide in human received support from Hergenrather et al. (167) in the USA, who reported lower concentrations, particularly of DDT, dieldrin, and β-HCH but also of DDE and heptachlor epoxide in vegetarians. On the other hand, PCB levels did not differ significantly between vegetarians and non-vegetarians, indicating sources of PCB contamination other than foodstuffs.

Cetinkaya et al. (151) observed lower concentrations of both HCB and PCBs in human milk from vegetarians in the former Federal Republic of Germany and significantly higher concentrations of HCB and β-HCH in meat eaters, but no association with intake of milk and milk products. From the Netherlands, Dagnelie et al. (168) reported that mothers on a macrobiotic diet (without meat and dairy products) had lower levels of HCB and PCB in their milk fat. Norén (124) found higher concentrations of PCBs, β-HCH and DDT in breast milk from women who regularly consumed fatty fish from the Baltic Sea, compared to non-fish eaters. Lacto-vegetarians had even lower concentrations of PCBs and DDT, while no differences were apparent with regard to dieldrin, α-HCH and HCB. Fürst et al. (71) recently observed higher dioxin levels in German lacto-vegetarians than in meat and fish eaters indicating that dairy products may be the main source in that country. A strong and very significant correlation between daily intake of animal protein and fat and dioxin concentration in breast milk indicated meat as a main source in the Netherlands (114).

It seems reasonable to add that where organochlorine pesticides are used on a large scale on crops, including vegetables, a vegetarian diet could be as bad as a non-vegatarian diet at contaminating breast milk.

Seasonal differences

Wilson et al. (98) observed that DDT concentrations in human milk were 60% higher during late summer than in late winter. Investigations in Norway, the former USSR and South Africa have shown a similar picture of seasonal variations of DDT in human milk (49, 141, 169). Wickizer et al. (170) in the USA also observed higher PCB concentrations in human milk in the summer as compared to the winter. These variations may, if real, be associated with use pattern of pesticides, meteorological factors or with variations in diet.

Maternal smoking

Some investigators have observed that cigarette smokers carry higher DDT concentration in their milk than do non-smokers (48, 58, 120, 129, 168, 171, 172). The explanation may be the use of DDT in tobacco fields or altered metabolism of the chemical in smokers. By contrast, Fürst et al. (71) observed lower levels of dioxins in breast milk from German smokers. Mothers living in houses with open fireplaces, however, had higher dioxin levels.

Maruna et al. (173) observed almost twice as high cadmium concentrations in breast milk from smokers as compared to non-smokers.

Maternal use of biocides

DDT preparations used to treat head lice in humans may be absorbed through the skin to a significant extent and elevated concentrations of DDT have been found in the milk after such therapy; the levels of DDE were lower (125, 159). Extensive use of some garden pesticides (including non-persistent pesticides) has, in some cases, been related to increased amounts of DDT in breast milk (98, 119, 174).

Maternal use of cosmetics

German investigations found that the use of cosmetic made from contaminated raw materials, for example lanolin, is associated with the appearance of residues in milk (175, 176).

Maternal occupation

Occupational exposure to toxic chemicals is potentially more extensive than is exposure by other means. In most human milk studies where the objective is to assess the degree of contamination of the general population, women with known occupational exposure are excluded Nevertheless, elevated concentrations of DDT in human milk from agricultural areas where DDT has been used, might be due partly to occupational exposure; indeed particularly high levels in individuals may subsequently be attributable to this source. This was the case in Brazil where agricultural workers had the highest DDT/DDE levels in their milk and more DDT than DDE indicating a recent source (59).

In a study from Portugal the highest DDT concentration was determined in a sample from an employee who for 6 years had cleaned glass equipment used for the analysis of pesticide formulations (177). Milk from Japanese mothers exposed to PCBs in a capacitor factory contained 10–100 times more PCBs than milk from non-occupationally exposed mothers (122). In the USA female farmers had lowest PCB and highest DDE levels in the milk. In highly skilled workers and students, opposing findings were made (48).

Increased lead concentrations have been detected in milk from women employed in the lead industry (178). Occupational exposure to various other substances has resulted in contamination of milk. Examples include perchloroethylene (179), methylene dichloride (180), ethylene dichloride (181), petroleum solvent (182) and carbon disulfide (183).

EXPOSURE OF SUCKLINGS AND RISE OF THE BODY BURDEN

At birth, the new-born may already be contaminated by toxic chemicals from transplacental exposure. Animal experiments and human experience indicate, however, that transfer of persistent organohalogens across the placental membranes is much smaller than the transfer through the milk (26, 27).

Takagi et al. (184), investigating PCBs in rats, observed a placental transfer of 0.03% of the administered doses, while sucklings received from 0.1 up to 2% by the milk, and their tissue concentrations were higher than those in the mother.

Similar results were obtained with mice by Masuda et al. (185), who found that 0.1–0.2% of the total PCB intake during pregnancy entered the foetus. By comparison, 5-week-old offspring contained 100 or more times as much PCBs, transferred by lactation. Some of the more toxic PCB congeners were transferred to a higher degree (186). In rats, Ando et al. (187) observed a relatively higher placental and milk transfer of DDT and 2,2′, 4,4′, 5,5′- hexachlorobiphenyl but there was still a difference; respectively 1.5 and 2.7% of the initial exposure passed through the placental barrier, while 21.5 and 39.2% were transferred in the milk.

Studies involving human beings have confirmed that PCB transfer via the milk is much more significant than is placental transfer (106, 188–192). In all studies, the concentrations of PCBs in maternal blood at delivery were significantly higher than in cord blood, and the individual concentrations were correlated

Kodama and Ota (191) observed that the PCB concentrations in the blood of breast-fed children after delivery increased rapidly and reached maternal levels after 3 months. The increase of blood-PCB concentrations in infants continued until breastfeeding was stopped, and values up to 4 times that of their mother's were recorded After termination of suckling, PCB concentrations declined again, mainly because of dilution in the growing fat deposits. In bottle-fed infants, blood-PCB concentrations declined after birth. Yakushiji et al. (192) found half-lives of 7.1 and 2.8 years for PCBs in the blood of mother and child respectively, the difference being ascribed to dilution, with a 14% gain in body weight per year in the child.

Niessen et al. (193) found significantly higher concentrations of organochlorine pesticide and PCBs in adipose tissue from children who had a high intake of human milk, compared to children with a low intake. The concentration in adipose fats were especially high (up to 5 ppm of PCBs) in infants less than 12 weeks of age. Teufel (194) detected a clearly increased PCB concentration in breast-fed children which was related to the duration of breastfeeding. Jacobson et al. (195) observed a dependence of blood PCB on breast-feeding duration in four-year-old children (see Table 2).

Both Wickizer et al. (170) and Mes et al. (106) calculated the rise in body burden of PCBs and other organohalogens in an hypothetical infant during breastfeeding and found that it took only a few month to a year before the infant reached adult levels of the chemicals in body fat. A steep rise in the PCB body burden during lactation has also been observed in a calf fed by a PCB-contaminated heifer (196). Heinsow (197) and Haschke et al. (198) modelled the development of body burden for dioxins in breast-fed and bottle-fed infants during the first 30 years. Haschke et al. (198) reported a steady decline in dioxin levels after lactation to reach levels similar to breast-fed and bottle-fed children at age 15 years. On the other hand Heinsow (197) reported higher contamination levels during the whole time-span in an individual who has been breast-fed The differences between the studies may be related to the input to the model calculations. Haschke et al. (198) used a rapid and probably unrealistic elimination rate of dioxins from the body.

TABLE 2 *Serum PCB levels in 4 years old children related to duration of their suckling (195)*

Breast-feeding duration	Mean serum PCB concentration (ng/ml, ppb)
0 to <3 months	0.6
0 to <6 months	2.3
0 to ≤6 months, ≤12 months	4.4
0 to ≥12 months	5.5

The same may apply to heavy metals; the mercury content in the hair of Spanish babies who were being nursed was about 1.5 times higher than that found in their mothers (199). In the Faroe Islands of the Atlantic Grandjean et al. (164) also reported increased mercury in infant hair depending on nursing length (Table 3).

For 15 children who were not breast-fed the geometric mean was 3.0 nmol Hg/g hair. At 1 year of age the mercury concentration in the child's hair was only 25% of that of the mother sampled at delivery, which indicated considerable mercury exposure of the adults from seafood intake. The average level of mercury in the milk was estimated to 10 ppb.

RISKS FOR THE DEVELOPING INFANT

Unfortunately, there are not many hard facts about the hazard of chemicals in human milk, especially any that may be associated with low, long-term exposure. Nevertheless there would appear to be a point of issue because most chemical contaminants in human milk are inherently toxic, especially the persistent organohalogens and heavy metals. Their adverse effect tend to be directed against the liver, skin, immune system and nervous system. In addition, some of the contaminants do have estrogen-like properties and are animal carcinogens and suspected human carcinogens.

The likelihood of overt toxic effect is presumed to relate to the quantity of contaminants consumed by the infant and to their duration in the body. There in no doubt that after exposure to high levels of pollutants, such as may occur after occupational exposure or accidental poisoning, breast-milk concentrations may be large enough to cause toxic effects. Under normal circumstances, however, the concen-

TABLE 3 *Mercury concentration in hair from 583 infants at approx. 12 months of age (164)*

Length of nursing (months)	No. of samples	Mercury concentration (geometric mean, nmol/g)
0–3	143	3.6
4–6	137	4.3
7–11	143	6.1
≤12	160	9.0

trations of the chemicals in breast milk are low, and direct intoxication is unlikely. The potential long-term effects are difficult to assess. The daily intake in many countries of dioxins and co-planar PCBs in an average breast-fed infant is at present 10–100 times higher than official recommended tolerable daily intake for adults (114, 200, 201). The Inuit population in Northern Canada display an unusually high body burden of organochlorine compounds; the birth heights of male Inuit newborns were reported negatively associated with the contamination levels of their mothers milk fat (202).

In 1984 a German expert group concluded (24) that the advantages of breast feeding compared with bottle feeding are pre-eminently important in the first few months of the infant's life and gradually decrease in importance after 4–6 months. They recommended exclusive breast feeding during the first 4 months and feeding increasing quantities of supplementary food thereafter, because of the steady risk from the contaminants in human milk.

A 1988 report (203) from WHO Regional Office for Europe recommended that breast-feeding should be encouraged and promoted, and that on the basis of the then-present knowledge neither limitation of breast-feeding nor the elimination of certain foods from the diet was justified. Further, Rogan et al. (204) have estimated that in the USA an average breast-fed infant would have a life-expectancy 67 days greater than that of a bottle-fed infant. Based on these calculations only unusually high levels of contamination in breast milk would represent a greater cancer hazard than the mortality hazard of refraining from breast feeding. On the other hand, in Sweden the authorities have recommended that women who are pregnant, lactating, or plan to be pregnant in the near future should not eat fish or fish liver which may be very contaminated by mercury and organochlorines (205).

The presence of potentially toxic chemical contaminants in the body should be a cause for concern: even though the period of breast-feeding is short in relation to a lifetime, the chemicals have a long half-life, enter the body at a sensitive phase in the development of the organism and persist in it (206). Any long-term hazards of exposure to chemical pollutants ingested in milk can be clarified only by continued surveillance.

REFERENCES

1. Reed CB (1908) A study of the conditions that require the removal of the child from the breast. *Surg. Gynecol. Obstet., 6,* 514–527.
2. Jensen AA (1983) Chemical contaminants in human milk. *Residue Rev., 89,* 1–128.
3. Broomhall J, Kovar IZ (1986) Environmental pollutants in breast milk. *Rev. Environ. Health, 6,* 311–337.
4. Jensen AA, Slorach SA (Eds) (1991) *Chemical Contaminants in Human Milk.* CRC Press, Boca Raton, FL.
5. Sim MR, McNeil JJ (1992) Monitoring chemical exposure using breast milk: a methodological review. *Am. J. Epidemiol., 136,* 1–11.

6. Jensen AA, Slorach SA (1991) Assessment of infant intake of chemicals via breast milk. In: Jensen AA, Slorach SA (Eds), *Chemical Contaminants in Human Milk,* Ch. 8. CRC Press, Boca Raton, FL.
7. Laug EP, Kunze FM, Prickett CS (1951) Occurrence of DDT in human fat and milk. *Arch. Industr. Hyg., 3,* 245–246.
8. Quinby GE, Armstrong JF, Durham WF (1965) DDT in human milk. *Nature, 207,* 726–728.
9. Egan H, Goulding R, Roburn J, Tatton JO'G (1965) Organochlorine pesticide residues in human fat and human milk. *Br. Med. J., 2,* 66–69.
10. Cripps DJ, Gocmen A, Peters HA (1980) Porphyria Turcica, twenty years after hexachlorobenzene intoxication. *Arch. Dermatol., 116,* 46–50.
11. Peters HA, Gocmen A, Cripps DJ, Bryan GT, Dogramaci I (1982) Epidemiology of hexachlorobenzene-induced porphyria in Turkey. *Arch. Neurol., 39,* 744–749.
12. Jensen S (1966) Report of a new chemical hazard. *New Sci., 32,* 612.
13. Westöö G, Norén K, Andersson M (1970) Klorpesticid- och polyklorbiphenylhalter i margarin, vegetabila matoljor och vissa animala livsmedel i svensk handel åren 1967–69. *Vår Föda, 22,* 10–31.
14. Acker L, Schulte E (1970) Über das Vorkommen von chlorierten Biphenylen und Hexachlorbenzol neben chlorierten Insektiziden in Humanmilch und menschlichem Fettgewebe. *Naturwissensch., 57,* 497.
15. Norén K, Lundén Å, Sjövall J, Bergman Å (1990). Coplanar polychlorinated biphenyls in Swedish human milk, *Chemosphere, 20,* 935–941.
16. Yeh C-Y, Kuo P-H, Tsai S-T, Wang G-Y, Wang Y-T (1976) A study on pesticide residues in umbilical cord blood and maternal milk. *J. Formosan Med. Assoc., 75,* 463–470.
17. Brilliant L, Amburg GV, Isbister J, Humphrey H, Wilcox K, Eyster J, Bloomer AW, Price H (1978) Breast-milk monitoring to measure Michigan's contamination with polybrominated biphenyls, *Lancet, ii,* 643–646.
18. Rappe C, Bergqvist P-A, Hansson M, Kjeller L-O, Lindström G, Marklund S, Nygren M (1984) Chemistry and analysis of polychlorinated dioxins and dibenzofurans in biological samples. In: Poland A, Kimbrough RD (Eds) *Biological Mechanisms of Dioxin Action (Banbury report 18),* pp 17–25. Cold Spring Harbor Laboratory, Cold Spring Harbor, NY.
19. Fanelli R, Bertoni MP, Bonfanti M, Castelli MG, Chiabrando C, Martelli GP, No, MA, Noseda A, Garrattini S, Binaghi C, Marazza V, Pezza F, Pozzoli D, Cicognetti G (1980) 2,3,7,8-Tetrachlorodibenzo-p-dioxin levels in cow's milk from the contaminated area of Seveso, Italy. *Bull. Environ. Contam. Toxicol., 24,* 534–539.
20. Reggiani G (1981) Medical survey techniques in the Seveso TCDD exposure. *J. Appl. Toxicol., 1,* 323–331.
21. Rimkus G, Rimkus B, Wolf M (1994) Nitro musks in human adipose tissue and breast milk. *Chemosphere, 28,* 421–432.
22. Butte W, Fooken C (1990) Simultaneous determination of pentachlorophenol and neutral organochlorine compounds in human milk. *Fresenius J. Anal. Chem., 336,* 511–514.
23. Lakritz L, Pensabene JW (1984) Survey of human milk for volatile N-nitrosoamines and the influence of diet on their formation. *Food Chem. Toxicol., 22,* 721–724.
24. Deutsche Forschungsgemeinschaft (1984) Rückstände und Verunreinigungen in Frauenmilch. Mitteilung XII der Kommission zur Prüfung von Rückstande in Lebensmitteln. Verlag Chemie, Weinheim.
25. Pellizzari ED, Hartwell TD, Harris BSH, Waddell RD, Whitaker DA, Erickson MD (1982) Purgeable organic compounds in mothers' milk. *Bull. Environ. Contam. Toxicol., 28,* 322–328.
26. Gallenberg LA, Vodicnik MJ (1989) Transfer of persistent chemicals in milk, *Drug Metab. Rev., 21,* 277–317.

27. Jensen AA (1991) Transfer of chemical contaminants into human milk. In: Jensen AA, Slorach SA (Eds), *Chemical Contaminants in Human Milk*, pp 9–19. CRC Press, Boca Raton, FL.
28. Bickel MH, Muehlebach S (1980) Pharmacokinetics and ecodisposition of polyhalogenated hydrocarbons: aspects and concepts. *Drug Metab. Rev., 11,* 149–190.
29. Ehrensdorfer S, Hiebl J, Lassek E, Rappi A (1991) Ergebnisse von frauenmilchuntersuchungen aus dem südbayerischen raum auf schadstoffgehalte. *Öff. Gesundh.-Wes., 53,* 784–791.
30. Winter R, Segerling M (1988) Organochlorverbindungen in der muttermilch. *Öff. Gesundh.-Wes., 50,* 72–76.
31. Vodicnik MJ, Lech JJ (1980) The transfer of 2,4,5,2′,4′,5′-hexachlorobiphenyl to fetuses and nursing offspring. *Toxicol. Appl. Pharmacol., 54,* 293–300.
32. Courtney KD, Andrews JE (1985) Neonatal and maternal body burdens of hexachlorobenzene (HCB) in mice: gestational exposure and lactational transfer. *Fund. Appl. Toxicol., 5,* 265–277.
33. Kanja LW, Skaare JU, Ojwang SBO, Maitai CK (1992) A comparison of organochlorine pesticide residues in maternal adipose tissue, maternal blood, cord blood, and human milk from mother/infant pairs. *Arch. Environ. Health, 22,* 21–14.
34. Pluim HJ, Boersman ER, Kramer I, Olie K, van der Slikke JW, Koppe JG (1994) Influence of short-term dietary measures on dioxin concentrations in human milk. *Environ. Health Perspect., 102,* 968–971.
35. Norén K (1988) Changes in the levels of organochlorine pesticides, polychlorinated biphenyls, dibenzo-p-dioxins and dibenzofurans in human milk from Stockholm, 1972–85. *Chemosphere, 17,* 39–49.
36. Conde C, Maluenda C, Arrabal C (1993) Organochlorine residues in human milk in Spain. Polychlorinated biphenyls (PCBs) from 1988 to 1991. *Bull. Environ. Contam. Toxicol., 51,* 832–837.
37. Sundhedsstyrelsen (1987): Dioxiner i modermælk, Sundhedsstyrelsens Hygiejnemeddelelser: 7, Copenhagen.
38. Mussalo-Rauhamaa H, Pyysalo H, Antervo K (1988) Relation between the content of organochlorine compounds in Finnish human milk and characteristics of the mothers, *J. Toxicol. Environ. Health, 25,* 1–19.
39. Drijver M, Duijkers TJ, Kromhout D, Visser TJ, Mulder P, Louw R (1988) Determinants of polychlorinated biphenyls (PCBs) in human milk. *Acta Paediatr. Scand., 77,* 30–36.
40. Skaare JU, Tuveng JM, Sande HA (1988) Organochlorine pesticides and polychlorinated biphenyls in maternal adipose tissue, blood, milk, and cord blood from mothers and their infants living in Norway. *Arch. Environ. Contam. Toxicol., 17,* 55–63.
41. Hahne K-H, Heeschen W, Blüthgen A (1986) Untersuchungen über Vorkommen und Eintragswege persistenter Chlorkohlenwasserstoffe in Frauenmilch. I. Chlorkohlenwasserstoff pestizide und polychloriete Biphenyle (PCB). *Milchwissenschaft, 41,* 269–272.
42. Krauthacker B (1991) Levels of organochlorine pesticides and polychlorinated biphenyls (PCBs) in human milk and serum collected from lactating mothers in the northern Adriatic area of Yugoslavia. *Bull. Environ. Contam. Toxicol., 46,* 797–802.
43. Lembrych S, Lorenz K, Kelm R (1986) Zawartosc insektycydow polichlorowych w mleka Poloznic z rejonu Opola. *Ginekol. Pol., 57,* 349–352.
44. Zahradnícek L, Jodl J, Sevcík, J, Lenek J, Cítková, M, Subrt P (1989) Cizorodé, látky v materském mléce. *Cs. Pediat., 44,* 80–83.
45. Bordet F, Mallet J, Maurice L, Borrel S, Venant A (1993) Organochlorine pesticide and PCB congener content of French human milk. *Bull. Environ. Contam. Toxicol., 50,* 425–432.
46. Focardi S, Fossi C, Fossi E (1984) Livelli di pesticidi clorurati e policlorobifenili nel latte umano. *Riv. Ital. Ped., 10,* 286–290.
47. Karakaya AE, Burgaz S, Kanzik I (1987) Organochlorine pesticide contaminants in human milk from different regions of Turkey. *Bull. Environ. Contam. Toxicol., 39,* 506–510.

48. Rogan WJ, Gladen BC, McKinney JD, Carreras N, Hardy P, Thullen J, Tingelstad J, Tully M (1986) Polychlorinated biphenyls (PCBs) and dichlorodiphenyl dichloroethene (DDE) in human milk: effects of maternal factors and previous lactation. *Am. J. Publ. Health, 76,* 172–177.
49. Bouwman H, Cooppan RM, Reinecke AJ, Becker PJ (1990) Levels of DDT and metabolites in breast milk from Kwa-Zulu mothers after DDT application for malaria control. *Bull. WHO, 68,* 761–768.
50. Spicer PE, Kereu RK (1993) Organochlorine insecticide residues in human breast milk: a survey of lactating mothers from a remote area in Papua New Guinea. *Bull. Environ. Contam. Toxicol., 50,* 540–546.
51. Gonzalez JE, Thiel R (1987) Restos de insecticidas en la leche materna de madres Panamenas. *Rev. Med. Panama, 12,* 139–143.
52. Viveros AD, Albert LA, Namihira D (1988) Contamination de leche humana por residuos de compuestos organoclorados. Paper presented at a Toxocology Congress in Cuba, November.
53. Kanja L, Skaare JU, Nafstad I, Maitai CK, Lökken P (1986) Organochlorine pestcides in human milk from different areas of Kenya 1983–85. *J. Toxicol. Environ. Health, 19,* 449–464.
54. Alawi MA, Ammari N, Al-Shuraiki Y (1992) Organochlorine pesticide contaminations in human milk samples from women living in Amman, Jordan. *Arch. Environ. Contam. Toxicol., 23,* 235–239.
55. Sardjoko SN, Untung K, Hammers WE (1992) Impact of DDT spraying on the residue levels in soil, chicken, fish-pond water, carp, and human milk samples from malaria infested villages in central Java. *Toxicol. Environ. Chem., 34,* 237–251.
56. Zaidi SSA, Bhatnagar VK, Banerjee BD, Balakrishnan G, Shah MP (1989) DDT residues in human milk samples from Delhi, India. *Bull. Environ. Contam. Toxicol., 42,* 427–430.
57. Ip HMH, Phillips DJH (1989) Organochlorine chemicals in human breast milk in Hong Kong. *Arch. Environ. Health, 18,* 490–494.
58. Sant'Ana, LS, Vassilieff I, Jokl L (1989) Levels of organochlorine insecticides in milk of mothers from urban and rural areas of Botucatu, SP, Brazil. *Bull. Environ. Contam. Toxicol., 42,* 911–918.
59. Matuo YK, Lopes JNC, Casanova IC, Matuo T, Lopes JLC (1992) Organochlorine pesticide residues in human milk in the Ribeirao Preto region, State of Sao Paulo, Brazil. *Arch. Environ. Health, 22,* 167–175.
60. Stevens MF, Ebell GF, Psaila-Savona P (1993) Organochlorine pesticides in Western Australian nursing mothers. *Med. J. Austr., 158,* 238–241.
61. Schwartz PM, Jacobson SW, Fein G, Jacobson JL, Price HA (1983) Lake Michigan fish consumption as a source of polychlorinated biphenyls in human cord serum, maternal serum, and milk. *Am. J. Publ. Health, 73,* 293–296.
62. Disler RL, Glatt V, Meier W (1984) Rückstände von chlorierten Insektiziden und polychlorierten Biphenylen in Humanmilch. *Mitt. Geb. Lenensmittelunters. Hyg., 75,* 205–213.
63. Dommarco R, Muccio AD, Camoni I, Gigli B (1987) Organochlorine pesticide and polychlorinated biphenyl residues from human milk from Rome (Italy) and surroundings. *Bull. Environ. Contam. Toxicol., 39,* 919–925.
64. Weisenberg E, Arad I, Grauer F, Sahm Z (1985) Polychlorinated biphenyls and organochlorine insecticides in human milk in Israel. *Arch. Environ. Contam. Toxicol., 14,* 517–521.
65. Kruse H, Benthe C, Heinzow B, Jessen H, Rimkus G (1988) Belastung der Muttermilch in Schleswig-Holstein mit Halogenkohlenwasserstoffen (OC) – Nachweis und toxikologische Bewertung. *Lebenmittelchem. Gerichtl. Chem., 42,* 64–66.
66. Gilsbach W (1991) Organochlorpestizide und Polychlorierte Biphenyle in Frauenmilch aus dem nordbayerischen Raum. *Dtsch. Lebensmittel-Rundsch., 87,* 144–150.

67. Collins CB, Holmes DC, Hoodless RA (1982) Organochlorine pesticide residues in human milk in Great Britain, 1979–80. *Hum. Toxicol., 1,* 425–431.
68. Unger M, Ipsen L, Clausen J (1982) Forekomsten af polyklorerede bifenyler i human ammemælk, komælksprodukter samt i kostprøver. *Ugeskr. Læger, 144,* 1849–1852.
69. Yrjänheikki EJ (Ed) (1989) Levels of PCBs, PCDDs and PCDFs in breast milk. Environmental Health Series No. 34, World Health Organisation, FADL, Copenhagen.
70. Gonnord MF, Gille P, Fraisse D, Bard D (1991) Total 2,3,7,8-TCDD toxic equivalent (TEQs) in breast milk from the Paris (France) area. Poster, Dioxin-91, Research Triangle Park.
71. Fürst P, Fürst C, Wilmers K (1992) PCDDs and PCDFs in human milk – statistical evaluation of a 6-years survey. *Chemosphere, 25,* 1029–1038.
72. Johansen HR, Becher G, Polder A, JU Skaare (1994) Congener-specific determination of polychlorinated biphenyls and organochlorine pesticides in human milk from Norwegian mothers living in Oslo. *J. Toxicol. Environ. Health, 42,* 157–171.
73. Bates MN, Buckland SJ, Hannah DJ, Taucher JA, van Maanen T (1990) Organo-chlorine residues in the breast milk of New Zealand women: a report to the Department of Health, May.
74. Rappe C, Nygren M, Lindström G, Hansson M (1986) Dioxins and dibenzofurans in biological samples of European origin. *Chemosphere, 15,* 1635–1639.
75. Norén K, Lundén Å (1991) Trend studies of polychlorinated biphenyls, dibenzo-p-dioxins and dibenzofurans in human milk. *Chemosphere, 23,* 1895–1901.
76. Jensen AA (1987) Polychlorobiphenyls (PCBs), polychlorodibenzo-p-dioxins (PCDDs), and polychlorodibenzofurans (PCDFs) in human milk, blood and adipose tissue, *Sci. Total Environ., 64,* 259–293.
77. Amin-Zaki L, El Hassani S, Majeed MA, Clarkson TW, Doherty RA, Greenwood MR, Giovanoli-Jakubczak T (1980) Methylmercury poisoning in mothers and their suckling infants. In: B. Holmstedt et al. (Eds), *Mechanisms of toxicity and hazard evaluation*, pp 75–78. Elsevier/North-Holland Biomedical Press, Amsterdam.
78. Haschke F, Steffan I (1981) Die Bleibelastung des jungen Sauglings mit der Nahrung in den Jahren 1980/81. *Wien. Klin. Wochenschr., 93,* 613–616.
79. Dabeka RW, Karpinski KF, McKenzie AD, Bajdik CD (1986) Survey of lead, cadmium and fluoride in human milk and correlation of levels with environmental and food factors. *Food Chem. Toxicol., 24,* 913–921.
80. Varo P, Nuurtamo M, Saari E, Koivistoinen P (1980) Mineral element composition of Finnish foods. VIII. Dairy products, eggs and margarine. *Acta Agric. Scand., 22 (Suppl),* 115–126.
81. Sternowsky HJ, Wessolowski R (1985) Lead and cadmium in breast milk. *Arch. Toxicol., 57,* 41–45.
82. Teufel M, Niessen K-H (1991) Rückstände in Muttermilch. *Ernährungs-Umschau, 38,* 142–147.
83. Ong CN, Phoon WO, Law HY, Tye CY, Lim HH (1985) Concentrations of lead in maternal blood, cord blood, and breast milk. *Arch. Dis. Child., 60,* 756–759.
84. Juszkiewicz T, Radomanski, T, Szprengier T, Szkoda J, Zmudzki J (1983) Pierwiastki toksyczne w mleku krowim i kobiecym. *Przegl. Lek., 40,* 525–526.
85. Larsson B, Slorach SA, Hagman U, Hofvander Y (1981) WHO collaborative breast feeding study. II. Levels of lead and cadmium in Swedish human milk, 1978–1979. *Acta Paediatr. Scand., 70,* 281–284.
86. Yengar GV, Parr RM (1985) Trace element concentrations in human milk from several global regions, *International Workshop about Composition and Physiological Properties of Human Milk*, Kiel.
87. Kovar IZ, Strehlow CD, Richmond J, Thompson MG (1984) Perinatal lead and cadmium burden in a British urban population. *Arch. Dis. Child., 59,* 36–39.

88. Rabinowitz M, Leviton A, Needleman H (1985) Lead in milk and infant blood: a dose-respons model. *Arch. Environ. Health, 40,* 283–286.
89. Rockway SW, Weber CW, Lei KY, Kemberling SR (1984) Lead concentrations of milk, blood and hair in lactating women. *Int. Arch. Occ. Environ. Health., 53,* 181–187.
90. Hansen JS, Beck D (1992) Forskellige faktorers indflydelse på Cd-indholdet i modermælk. *Dansk Kemi, 73,* 32–34.
91. Vuori E, Vetter M, Kuitunen P, Salmela S (1983) Cadmium in Finnish breast milk, a longitudinal study. *Arch. Toxicol., 53,* 207–211.
92. Narres H-D, Mohl C, Stöppler M (1981) Metal analysis in difficult materials with platform furnace Zeeman-atomic absorption spectroscopy. *Z. Lebensm. Unters. Forsch., 181,* 111–116.
93. Sartorelli E, Gori R, Sartorelli S, Buffi C (1986) Valori di piombo e cadmio nel sangue di partorienti non esposte professionalmente, nel sangue dei neonati e nel latte materno. *Med. Lav., 77,* 515–518.
94. Baluja G, Hernandez LM, Gonzalez J, Rico C (1982) Presence of organochlorine pesticides, polychlorinated biphenyls and mercury in Spanish human milk samples. *Bull. Environ. Contam. Toxicol., 28,* 573–577.
95. Skerfving S (1988) Mercury in women exposed to methylmercury through fish consumption, and in their newborn babies and breast milk. *Bull. Environ. Contam. Toxicol., 41,* 475–482.
96. Hall B (1979) Uniformity of human milk. *Am. J. Clin. Nutr., 32,* 304–312.
97. Mes J, Davies DJ (1978) Variation in the polychlorinated biphenyl and organochlorine pesticide residue during human breastfeeding and its diurnal pattern. *Chemosphere, 9,* 699–706.
98. Wilson JW, Locker DJ, Ritzen CA, Watson JT, Schaffner W (1973) DDT concentrations in human milk. *Am. J. Dis. Child., 125,* 814–817.
99. Barnett R, D'Ercole AJ, Cain JD, Arthur RD (1979) Organochlorine pesticide residues in human milk samples from women living in Northwest and Northeast Mississippi, 1973–75. *Pestic. Monit. J., 13,* 47–51.
100. Pluim HJ, Slot PC, Olie K, van der Slikke JW, Koppe JG (1992) Diurnal variations in concentrations of PCDDs and PCDFs in human milk. *Chemosphere, 25,* 307–311.
101. Prentice A, Prentice AM, Whitehead RG (1981) Breast-milk fat concentrations of most African women. 1. Short-term variation within individuals. *Br. J. Nutr., 45,* 483–494.
102. Miller HJ, Cucos S, Wassermann D, Wassermann M (1979) Organochlorine insecticides and polychlorinated biphenyls in human milk. In: Deichmann WB (Ed) *Toxicology and Occupational Medicine*, pp 379–386. Elsevier/North-Holland, New York.
103. Gyimothi J (1979) Über die Rückstandsbelastung von Frauenmilch an Organochlorpesticiden in Abhängigkeit zur Laktations Zeit (Forschungsberichte 4/79), pp 317–381. Bundesministerium für Gesundheit und Umweltschutz, Wien.
104. Acker L, Schulte E (1971) Zur Vorkommen von Hexachlorbenzol und polychlorierten Biphenylen neben chlorierten Insektiziden in menschlichem Fettgewebe und im Humanmilch. *Ernährungsforschung, 16,* 559–567.
105. Yoshida S, Nakamura A (1979) Residual status after parturition of methylsulfon metabolites of polychlorinated biphenyls in the breast milk of a former employee in a capacitor factory. *Bull. Environ,. Contam. Toxicol., 21,* 111–115.
106. Mes J, Doyle JA, Adams BR, Davies DJ, Turton D (1984) Polychlorinated biphenyls and organochlorine pesticides in milk and blood of Canadian women during lactation. *Arch. Environ. Contam. Toxicol., 13,* 217–223.
107. Skaare JU, Polder A (1990) Polychlorinated biphenyls and organochlorine pesticides in milk of Norwegian women during lactation. *Arch. Environ. Contam. Toxicol., 19,* 640–645.
108. Lindström G (1988) Polychlorinated dibenzo-p-dioxins and dibenzofurans: analysis of and occurrence in milk. Ph.D. Thesis, University of Umeå, Sweden.

109. Schulte-Löbbert FJ, Bohn G (1977) Determination of cadmium in human milk during lactation. *Arch. Toxicol., 37,* 155–157.
110. Sharda B, Bhandari B, Bhandari LM (1983) Copper, zinc, magnesium and cadmium levels of breast milk of indian women. *Trans. Royal Soc. Trop. Med Hyg., 77,* 201–203.
111. Luckas B, Predel W, Vietinghoff U (1981) Zur Kontamination von Humanfett Rostocker Bürger mit DDT und polychlorierten Biphenylen im Jahre 1979. *Nährung, 25,* 427–433.
112. Kreiss K, Zack MM, Kimbrough RD (1981) Cross-sectional study of a community with exceptional exposure to DDT. *J. Am. Med Assoc., 245,* 1926–1930.
113. Wolff MS, Anderson HA, Selikoff IJ (1982) Human tissue burdens of halogenated aromatic chemicals in Michigan. *J. Am. Med Assoc., 247,* 2112–2116.
114. Pluim HJ, Kramer I, van der Slikke JW, Koppe JG, Olie K (1993) Levels of PCDDs and PCDFs in human milk: dependence on several parameters and dietary habits. *Chemosphere, 26,* 1889–1895.
115. Jensen AA (1991) Levels and trends of environmental chemicals in human milk. In: Jensen AA, Slorach SA (Eds), *Chemical Contaminants in Human Milk,* pp 45–198. CRC Press, Boca Raton, FL.
116. Slorach SA, Vaz R (Eds) (1983) Global Environmental Monitoring System (GEMS). Assessment of Human Exposure to Selected Organochlorine Compounds Through Biological Monitoring, Swedish National Food Administration, Uppsala.
117. Wickström K, Pyysalo H, Siimes MA (1983) Levels of chlordane, hexachlorobenzene, PCB and DDT compounds in Finnish human milk in 1982. *Bull. Environ. Contam. Toxicol., 31,* 251–256.
118. Kroger M (1972) Insecticide residues in human milk. *J. Pediatr.*, 80, 401–405.
119. Knoll W, Jayaraman S (1973) Zur Kontamination von Humanmilch mit chlorierten Kohlenwasserstoffen. *Nährung, 17,* 599–615.
120. Bradt PT, Herrenkohl RC (1976) DDT in human milk. What determines the levels? *Sci. Total Environ., 6,* 161–163.
121. Yakushiji T, Watanabe I, Kuwabara K, Yoshida S, Koyama K, Hara I, Kunita N (1978) Long-term studies of the exretion of polychlorinated biphenyls (PCBs) through the mothers milk of an occupationally exposed worker. *Arch. Environ. Contam. Toxicol., 7,* 493–504.
122. Yakushiji T, Watanabe I, Kuwabara K, Yoshida S, Koyama K, Kunita N (1979) Levels of polychlorinated biphenyls (PCBs) and organochlorine pesticides in human milk and blood collected in Osaka Prefecture from 1972 to 1977. *Int. Arch. Occup. Environ. Health, 43,* 1–15.
123. Matuo YK, Lopez JNC, Lopez JLC (1980) DDT levels in human milk from Ribeirao Preto (Brazil). *Rev. Brasil. Biol., 40,* 293–296.
124. Norén K (1983) Levels of organochlorine contaminants in human milk in relation to dietary habits of the mother. *Acta Paediatr. Scand., 72,* 811–816.
125. Rasmussen HB, Ørskov G (1983) Forurening of Modermaelk med Chlorholdige Pesticider og PCB – en Undersøgelse og en Toksikologisk Vurdering. Thesis. Royal Veterinary and Agricultural University, Copenhagen.
126. Gilsbach W (1991) Organochlorpestizide und Polychlorierte Biphenyle in Frauenmilch aus dem Nordbayerischen Raum. *Dtsch. Lebensmittel-Rundsch., 87,* 144–150.
127. Mes J, Davies DJ, Doucet J, Weber D, McMullen E (1993) Levels of chlorinated hydrocarbon residues in Canadian human breast milk and their relationship to some characteristics of the donors. *Food Addit. Contam., 10,* 429–441.
128. Andersen JR, Orbæk K (1984) Organochlorine contaminants in human milk in Denmark, 1982. *Ambio, 13,* 266–268.
129. Dillon JC, Martin GB, O'Brien HT (1981) Pesticide residues in human milk. *Food Cosmet. Toxicol., 19,* 437–442.

130. Ackerman LB (1980) Overview of human exposure to dieldrin residues in the environment and current trends of residue levels in tissue. *Pestic. Monit.* J., *14,* 64–69.
131. Adamovic VM, Sokic BB, Milena Javanovic-Smiljanska (1978) Some observations concerning the ratio of the intake of organochlorine insecticides through food and amount excreted in the milk of breast-feeding mothers. *Bull. Environ. Contam. Toxicol., 20,* 280–285.
132. Siddiqui MKJ, Saxena MC (1985) Placenta and milk as excretory routes of lipophilic pesticides in women. *Hum. Toxicol., 4,* 249–254.
133. Polishuk ZW, Ron M, Wassermann M, Cucos S, Wassermann D, Lemesch C (1977) Organochlorine compounds in human blood plasma and milk. *Pestic. Monit. J., 10,* 121–129.
134. Acker L (1981) Zur Kontamination der Frauenmilch mit Chlororganischen Verbindungen. *Geburtshilfe Frauenheilkd., 41,* 882–886.
135. Hrubá D, Dubsk H, Totusek J, Koukalová H (1988) Residues of polychlorinated biphenyls in breast milk of women non-occupationally exposed to PCBs. *J. Hyg. Epidemiol. Microbiol. Immunol., 32,* 273–278.
136. Woodard BT, Fereguson BB, Wilson DJ (1976) DDT Levels in milk of rural indigent blacks. *Am. J. Dis. Child., 130,* 400–403.
137. Davies JE, Edmundson WF, Raffonelli A, Cassady JC, Morgade C (1972) The role of social class in human pesticide pollution. *Am. J. Epidemiol., 96,* 334–341.
138. Ritcey WR, Savary G, McCully KA (1972) Organochlorine insecticide residues in human milk, evaporated milk and some milk substitutes in Canada. *Can. J. Publ. Health, 63,* 125–132.
139. Luquet FM, Gorsaud J, Gaudier B (1972) Étude de la pollution des laits humains par les résidues de pesticides. *Pathol. Biol., 20,* 137–143.
140. Schüpbach MR, Egli H (1979) Organochlorpestizide und polychlorierte Biphenyl in Muttermilch. *Mitt. Geb. Lebensmittelunters. Hyg., 70,* 451–463.
141. Westöö G, Norén K (1978) Organochlorine contaminants in human milk, Stockholm 1967–1977. *Ambio, 7,* 62–64.
142. Miethke von H, Heffter A, Hörtig W (1988) Humanmilch-Untersuchungen 1980–1986. *Dtsch. Lebensmittel-Rundsch., 84,* 137–143.
143. Cetinkaya M, Duszeln JV, Thiemann W (1983) Organochlorrückstände in Muttermilch türkischer Frauen in der Bundesrepublik Deutschland und in der Türkei. *Akt. Ernähr., 8,* 213–217.
144. Hayashi M (1972) Pollution of mother's milk by organochlorine pesticides (in Japanese). *Jpn. J. Publ. Health, 19,* 437–441.
145. Newton KG, Greene NC (1972) Organochlorine pesticide residue levels in human milk. *Pestic. Monit. J., 6,* 4–8.
146. DeCampos M, Olszyna-Marzys AF (1979) Contamination of human milk with chlorinated pesticides in Guatemala and in El Salvador. *Arch. Environ. Contam. Toxicol., 8,* 43–58.
147. Juszkiewicz T, Niewiadowska A, Radomanski T (1977) Polychlorinated biphenyls in human milk from three different regions of the country (in Polish). *Bromatol. Chem. Toksykol., 10,* 263–266.
148. Ogaki J, Takayama K, Myiata H, Kashimoto T (1987) Levels of PCDDs and PCDFs in human tissues and various foodstuffs in Japan, *Chemosphere, 16,* 2047–2056.
149. Dewailly E, Nantel A, Weber J-P, Meyer F (1989) High levels of PCBs in breast milk of Inuit women from arctic Quebec. *Bull. Environ. Contam. Toxicol., 43,* 641–646.
150. Dewailly E, Tremblay-Rousseau H, Carrier G, Groulx S, Gingras S, Boggess S, Boggess K, Stanley J, Weber JP (1991) PCDDs, PCDFs and PCBs in human milk of women exposed to a PCB fire and of women from the general population of the province of Québec–Canada. *Chemosphere, 23,* 1831–1835.
151. Cetinkaya M, Gabel B, Podbielski A, Thiemann W (1984) Untersuchung über den Zusammen-

hang zwischen Ernährung und Lebensumständen stillender Mutter und der Kontamination der Muttermilch mit schwerflüchtigen Organochlorverbindunden. *Akt. Ernähr., 9,* 157–162.
152. Norén K (1983) Levels of organochlorine contaminants in human milk from different parts of Sweden. *Ambio, 12,* 44–46.
153. Lechner W, Battista HJ, Dienstl F (1980) Untersuchungen zum Bleigehalt in der Muttermilch in verkehrsreichen und verkehrsarmen Gegenden Tirols. *Gynäkol. Rundsch., Suppl. 20,* 268–270.
154. Namihira D, Saldivar L, Pustilnik N, Carreon GJ, Salinas ME (1993) Lead in human blood and milk from nursing women living near a smelter in Mexico City. *J. Toxicol. Environ. Health, 38,* 225–232.
155. Ghelberg NW, Ruckert I, Straus H (1972) The lead content of milk in an area with nonferrous metallurgical industry. *Igiena, 21,* 17–21.
156. Takahashi R, Saidin D, Takei G, Wong L (1981) Organochlorine pesticide residues in human milk in Hawaii, 1979–80. *Bull. Environ. Contam. Toxicol., 17,* 506–511.
157. Watanabe I, Yakushiji T, Kuwabara K, Yoshida S, Maeda K, Kashimoto T, Koyama K, Kunita N (1979) Surveillance of the daily PCB intake from the diet of Japanese women from 1972-76. *Arch. Environ. Contam. Toxicol., 8,* 67–75.
158. Wickizer TM, Brilliant LB (1981) Testing for polychlorinated biphenyls in human milk. *Pediatrics, 68,* 411–415.
159. Hofvander Y, Hagman U, Linder C-E, Vaz R, Slorach SA (1981) Organochlorine contaminants in individual samples of Swedish human milk, 1978–79. *Acta Paediatr. Scand., 70,* 3–8.
160. Schwartz PM, Jacobson SW, Fein G, Jacobson JL, Price HA (1983) Lake Michigan fish consumption as a source of polychlorinated biphenyls in human cord serum, maternal serum, and milk. *Am. J. Publ. Health, 73,* 293–296.
161. Fujiwara K (1975) Environmental and food contamination with PCB's in Japan. *Sci. Total Environ., 4,* 219–247.
162. Grant DL, Mes J, Frank R (1976) PCB residues in human adipose tissue and milk. In: *Proceedings, National Conference on Polychlorinated Biphenyls,* Chicago, November 1975, (EPA-560/6-75-004), pp 144–146. Environmental Protection Agency, Washington, DC.
163. Galster WA (1976) Mercury in Alaskian eskimo mothers and infants. *Environ. Health Perspect., 15,* 135–140.
164. Grandjean P, Jørgensen PJ, Weihe P (1994) Human milk as a source of methyl mercury exposure in infants. *Environ. Health Perspect., 102,* 74–77.
165. Klein H (1983) The PCB situation in the Federal Republic of Germany. In: Barros MC, Könemann H, Visser R (Eds) *Proceedings, PCB Seminar,* Scheveningen-The Hague, pp 66–79. Ministry of Housing, Physical Planning and Environment, The Hague.
166. Kantonaler Vollzug der Lebensmittelgesetzgebung (1983) *Mitt. Geb. Lebensmittelunters. Hyg., 74,* 256–257.
167. Hergenrather J, Hlady G, Wallace B, Savage E (1981) Pollutants in breast milk of vegetarians (letter). *N. Engl. J. Med, 304,* 792.
168. Dagnelie PC, van Staveren WA, Roos AH, Tuinstra LGMTh, Burema J (1992) Nutrients and contaminants in human milk from mothers on macrobiotic and omnivorous diets. *Eur. J. Clin. Nutr., 46,* 355–366.
169. Bakken AF, Seip M (1976) Insecticides in human breast milk. *Acta Paediatr. Scand., 65,* 535–539.
170. Wickizer TM, Brilliant LB, Copeland R, Tilden R (1981) Polychlorinated biphenyl contamination of nursing mothers milk in Michigan. *Am. J. Publ. Health, 71,* 132–137.
171. Vuori E, Tyllinen H, Kuitunen P, Paganus A (1977) The occurrence and origin of DDT in human milk. *Acta Paediatr. Scand., 66,* 761–765.

172. Miller GJ, Fox JA (1973) Chlorinated hydrocarbon pesticide residues in Queensland human milk. *Med. J. Austr., 2,* 261–264.
173. Maruna H, Maruna RFL, Eisner R (1976) Cadmium und Blei in Muttermilchproben. *Arztl. Prax., 28,* 6–7.
174. Weisenberg E, Ackerman E, Freier S, Reshef A, Sahm Z, Shoenberg J (1980) Pesticides in the milk of mothers in Jerusalem. In: Freier S, Eidelman AI (Eds) *Human Milk – Its Biological and Social Value*, pp 147–152. Excerpta Medica, Amsterdam.
175. Müller, B, Schröder H (1982) Biozide in menschlichen Organismus. *Ernähr. Umsch., 29,* 359–362.
176. Meemken H-A, Habersaat K, Groebel W (1982) Zur Belastung von Muttermilch mit Chlorkohlenwasserstoffen aus wollwachshaltigen Cremes. *Lebensm. Chem. Gerichtl. Chem., 36,* 51–53.
177. Graca I, Fernandes ANSS, Mourao HC (1974) Organochlorine insecticide residues in human milk in Portugal. *Pestic. Monit. J., 8,* 148–156.
178. Ryu JE, Ziegler EE, Fomon SJ (1978) Maternal lead exposure and blood lead concentration in infancy. *J. Pediatr., 93,* 476–478.
179. Bagnell PC, Ellenberger HA (1977) Obstructive jaundice due to a chlorinated hydrocarbon in breast milk. *Can. Med Assoc. J., 117,* 1047–1048.
180. Vozoveya MA, Malarova LK, Enikeeva PM (1974) Content of methylene dichloride in tissues during pregnancy and lactation in female workers in rubber industry (*in Russian*). *Gig. Tr., 18,* 42–43.
181. Davidson IWF, Sumner DD, Parker JC (1982) Ethylene dichloride: a review of its metabolism, mutagenic and carcinogenic potential. *Drug Chem. Toxicol., 5,* 319–388.
182. Novikov KI, Kolodina LN, Lipovskij SN, Badalova LV (1979) Lactation particulars in female workers of the chemical (rubber) industry (*in Russian*). *Gig. Tr., 23,* 45–48.
183. Cai SX, Bao YS (1981) Placental transfer, secretion into mother milk of carbon disulphide and its effect on maternal function of female viscose rayon workers. *Ind. Health, 19,* 15–29.
184. Takagi Y, Otake T, Kataoka M, Murata Y, Aburada S, Akasaka S, Hashimoto K, Uda H, Kitaura T (1976) Studies on the transfer and distribution of (C-14)polychlorinated biphenyls from maternal to fetal and suckling rats. *Toxicol. Appl. Pharmacol., 38,* 549–558.
185. Masuda Y, Kagawa R, Tokudome S, Kuratsune M (1978) Transfer of polychlorinated biphenyls to the foetuses and offspring of mice. *Food Cosmet. Toxicol., 16,* 33–37.
186. Masuda Y, Kagawa R, Kuroki H, Tokudome S, Kuratsune M (1979) Transfer of various polychlorinated biphenyls to the foetuses and offspring of mice. *Food Cosmet. Toxicol., 17,* 623–627.
187. Ando M, Hirano S, Itoh Y (1985) Transfer of hexachlorobenzene (HCB) from mother to newborn baby through placenta and milk. *Arch. Toxicol., 56,* 195–200.
188. Masuda Y, Kagawa R, Kuroki H, Kuratsune M, Yoshimure T, Taki I, Kusada M, Yamashita, F. Hayaski M (1978) Transfer of polychlorinated biphenyls from mothers to foetuses and infants. *Food Cosmet. Toxicol., 16,* 543–546.
189. Kuwabara K, Yakushiji T, Watanable I, Yoshida S, Koyama K (1978) Relationship between breast-feeding and PCB residues in blood of the children whose mothers were occupationally exposed to PCBs. *Int. Arch. Occup. Environ. Health, 41,* 189–197.
190. Kuwabara K, Yakushiji T, Watanabe I, Yoshida S, Koyama K, Kunita N, Hara I (1979) Levels of polychlorinated biphenyls in blood of breast-fed children whose mothers are non-occupationally exposed to PCBs. *Bull. Environ. Contam. Toxicol., 21,* 458–462.
191. Kodama H, Ota H (1980) Transfer of polychlorinated biphenyls to infants from their mothers. *Arch. Environ. Health, 35,* 95–100.
192. Yakushiji T, Watanabe I, Kuwabara K, Tanaka R, Kashimoto T, Kunita N, Hara I (1984) Rate of

decrease and half-life of polychlorinated biphenyls (PCBs) in the blood of mothers and their children occupationally exposed to PCBs. *Arch. Environ. Contam. Toxicol., 13,* 341–345.

193. Niessen KH, Ramolla J, Binder M, Brugmann G, Hofmann U (1984) Chlorinated hydrocarbons in adipose tissue of infants and toddlers: inventory and studies on their association with intake of mothers' milk. *Eur. Pediatr., 142,* 238–243.
194. Teufel M (1992) PCB-exposition von kindern in Ost- und Westdeutschland. *Klin. Pädiatr., 204,* 348–354.
195. Jacobson JL, Humphrey HEB, Jacobson SW, Schantz SL, Mullin MD, Welch R (1989) Determinants of polychlorinated biphenyls (PCBs), polybrominated biphenyls (PBBs), and dichlorodiphenyl trichlorethane (DDT) levels in the sera of young children. *Am. J. Publ. Health, 79,* 1401–1404.
196. Peterson LA, Ross PF, Osheim DL, Nelson HA (1983) PCB residues in a lactating beef cow and calf. *Bull. Environ. Contam. Toxicol., 31,* 263–266.
197. Heinzow B (1991) Dioxine in der Frauenmilch. *Internist.-Prax., 31,* 547–554.
198. Haschke F, Male C, Pietschnig, B, Yrjänheikki EJ (1992) Infant exposure to PCDDs and PCDFs through breast milk and an approach to calculate body burden. *Toxic Subst. J., 12,* 227–236.
199. Gonzalez MJ, Rico MC, Hernandez LM, Balaju G (1985) Mercury in human hair: a study of residents in Madrid, Spain. *Arch. Environ. Health, 40,* 225–228.
200. Matsueda T, Iida T, Hirakawa H, Fukamachi K, Tokiwa H, Nagayama J (1993) Toxic evaluation of PCDDs, PCDFs and coplanar PCBs in breast-fed babies of Yusho and healthy mothers. *Chemosphere, 27,* 187–194.
201. Körner W, Dawidowsky N, Hagenmaier H (1993) Fecal excretion rates of PCDDs and PCDFs in two breast-fed infants. *Chemosphere, 27,* 157–162.
202. Dewailly E, Bruneau S, Ayotte P, Lalibert, C, Gingras S, Belanger D, Ferron L (1993) Health status at birth of Inuit newborn prenatally exposed to organochlorines. *Chemosphere, 27,* 359–366.
203. World Health Organization (1988) PCBs, PCDDs and PCDFs in breast milk: Assessment of health risks. *WHO Environmental Health 29.* WHO Regional Office for Europe Copenhagen.
204. Rogan WJ, Blanton PJ, Portier CJ, Stallard E (1991) Should the presence of carcinogens in breast milk discourage breast feeding?. *Regul. Toxicol. Pharmacol., 13,* 228–2450.
205. Slorach S (1992) Kvicksilver och andra främmende ämnen i fisk–åtgärder för att begränsa hälsoriskerna. *Vår Föda, 44,* 163–170.
206. International Programme on Chemical Safety (1986) *Principles for Evaluation of Health Risks from Chemicals During Infacy and Early Childhood: the Need for a Special Approach (Environmental Health Criteria 59).* World Health Organization, Geneva.

Index